The Society for Healthcare Epidemiology of America

Practical Handbook for Healthcare Epidemiologists

SECOND EDITION

Edited by

Ebbing Lautenbach, MD, MPH, MSCE
Assistant Professor of Medicine and Epidemiology
Division of Infectious Diseases
Associate Hospital Epidemiologist
Hospital of the University of Pennsylvania
Center for Clinical Epidemiology and Biostatistics
University of Pennsylvania School of Medicine
Philadelphia, Pennsylvania

Keith Woeltje, MD, PhD
Associate Professor of Medicine
Washington University School of Medicine
Medical Director
Infection Control and Healthcare Epidemiology Consortium
BJC Health System
St. Louis, Missouri

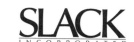

An innovative information, education, and management company
6900 Grove Road • Thorofare, NJ 08086

Practical handbook for healthcare epidemiologists / edited by Ebbing Lautenbach,
    Keith Woeltje ; The Society for Healthcare Epidemiology of America. -- 2nd ed.
        p. ; cm.
    Rev. ed. of: A practical handbook for hospital epidemiologists / The Society for
Healthcare Epidemiology of America. 1998.
    Includes bibliographical references and index.
    ISBN 1-55642-677-1 (hard cover : alk. paper)
    1. Nosocomial infections--Prevention. 2. Nosocomial infections--Epidemiology.
3. Cross infection--Prevention. 4. Health facilities--Sanitation.   I. Lautenbach,
Ebbing. II. Woeltje, Keith F. III. Society for Healthcare Epidemiology of America.
IV. Practical handbook for hospital epidemiologists.
    [DNLM: 1. Cross Infection--epidemiology. 2. Epidemiologic Methods. 3. Hospital
Administration. 4. Infection Control--methods. 5. Risk Management.   WX 167
P895 2004]
RA969.P728 2004
614.4'5--dc22

                                                        2004014489

Printed in the United States of America.

Published by: SLACK Incorporated
                 6900 Grove Road
                 Thorofare, NJ 08086 USA
                 Telephone: 856-848-1000
                 Fax: 856-853-5991
                 www.slackbooks.com

Contact SLACK Incorporated for more information about other books in this field or about the availability of our books from distributors outside the United States.

For permission to reprint material in another publication, contact SLACK Incorporated. Authorization to photocopy items for internal, personal, or academic use is granted by SLACK Incorporated provided that the appropriate fee is paid directly to Copyright Clearance Center. Prior to photocopying items, please contact the Copyright Clearance Center at 222 Rosewood Drive, Danvers, MA 01923 USA; phone: 978-750-8400; website: www.copyright.com; email: info@copyright.com.

For further information on CCC, check CCC Online at the following address: http://www.copyright.com.

Last digit is print number: 10   9   8   7   6   5   4   3   2   1

DEDICATION

To my wife, Gillian, and children, John, Kate, Thomas, and William.
Ebbing Lautenbach

For Maeve, John, Éile, and especially Gabrielle.
Keith Woeltje

CONTENTS

ACKNOWLEDGMENTS

We would like to first recognize Loreen Herwaldt and Michael Decker, editors of the first edition of this book, for recognizing the need for an entry-level text for aspiring healthcare epidemiologists. Lauren Biddle Plummer, Charlene Counsellor, and April Billick provided invaluable support at SLACK Incorporated. We'd like to thank our bosses—Harvey Friedman and Brian Strom at the University of Pennsylvania, Peter Rissing at the Medical College of Georgia, and Victoria Fraser at Washington University—for their encouragement and support. We would not be able to function in healthcare epidemiology without the tireless efforts of the many infection control practitioners with whom we work. We offer many thanks to all of our colleagues who contributed chapters to this book. We appreciate their adding even more hours to their already over-packed schedules to participate on this project.

Ebbing Lautenbach, MD, MPH, MSCE
Keith Woeltje, MD, PhD

ABOUT THE EDITORS

Ebbing Lautenbach, MD, MPH, MSCE is an Assistant Professor of Medicine in the Division of Infectious Diseases, Assistant Professor of Epidemiology in the Department of Biostatistics and Epidemiology, and Senior Scholar in the Center for Clinical Epidemiology and Biostatistics at the University of Pennsylvania School of Medicine. He is the Associate Hospital Epidemiologist and Codirector of Antimicrobial Management at the Hospital of the University of Pennsylvania. Dr. Lautenbach is a Fellow in the Institute on Aging and a Senior Fellow at the Leonard Davis Institute for Health Economics, both at the University of Pennsylvania. Dr. Lautenbach received his MD and MPH degrees from Columbia University in New York. He completed his Internal Medicine residency and Infectious Diseases fellowship at the University of Pennsylvania, where he also received a Master's Degree in Clinical Epidemiology. He is board certified in internal medicine, infectious diseases, and epidemiology. Dr. Lautenbach's clinical and research interests focus on the epidemiology and prevention of nosocomial infections, as well as the emergence of healthcare-acquired antimicrobial resistance.

Keith Woeltje, MD, PhD is an Associate Professor of Medicine in the Infectious Diseases Division, Department of Medicine, Washington University School of Medicine. He is the Medical Director of the BJC Health System Infection Control and Hospital Epidemiology Consortium. Dr. Woeltje earned his MD and PhD degrees at the University of Texas Southwestern Medical Center at Dallas. He did his Internal Medicine internship and residency at Barnes Hospital, St. Louis, then completed his Infectious Diseases fellowship at Washington University. He then served a year as Medicine Chief Resident at Barnes-Jewish Hospital. Dr. Woeltje was a hospital epidemiologist at the Medical College of Georgia prior to his current position. He is board certified in internal medicine and infectious diseases. Dr. Woeltje's interests are in epidemiology and prevention of nosocomial infections and in medical informatics.

Contributing Authors

ELIAS ABRUTYN, MD
Associate Provost and Associate Dean for Faculty Affairs
Interim Chief Infectious Diseases
Drexel University College of Medicine
Philadelphia, Pennsylvania

JUDENE BARTLEY, MS, MPH, CIC
Clinical/Safety Consultant, Safety Institute, Premier Inc
Vice President, Epidemiology Consulting Services Inc
Beverly Hills, Michigan

GONZALO M. L. BEARMAN, MD, MPH
Virginia Commonwealth University
Richmond, Virginia

CONSUELO BECK-SAGUE, MD
Division of Reproductive Health
Centers for Disease Control and Prevention
Atlanta, Georgia

WERNER ERNST BISCHOFF, MD, MSc
Wake Forest University School of Medicine
Department of Internal Medicine/Section on Infectious Diseases
Winston-Salem, North Carolina

HENRY M. BLUMBERG, MD
Professor of Medicine
Program Director, Division of Infectious Diseases
Emory University School of Medicine
Hospital Epidemiologist
Grady Memorial Hospital
Atlanta, Georgia

JOHN M. BOYCE, MD
Chief
Infectious Diseases Section and Hospital Epidemiologist
Hospital of Saint Raphael
New Haven, Connecticut
Clinical Professor of Medicine
Yale University School of Medicine
New Haven, Connecticut

PJ BRENNAN, MD
Professor of Medicine, Division of Infectious Diseases
University of Pennsylvania School of Medicine and the
Hospital of the University of Pennsylvania
Chief, Healthcare Quality and Patient Safety
University of Pennsylvania Health System
Philadelphia, Pennsylvania

CHERYL D. CARTER, RN, BSN
University of Iowa Hospital and Clinics
Iowa City, Iowa

HAROLD R. COLLARD, MD
Fellow
Division of Pulmonary Sciences and Critical Care Medicine
Department of Medicine
University of Colorado Health Sciences Center
Denver, Colorado

SHERRY A. DAVID, RN, BS, CIC
University of Iowa Hospital and Clinics
Iowa City, Iowa

H. GUNNER DEERY II, MD
Northern Michigan Infectious Diseases
Northern Michigan Hospital
Petoskey, Michigan

LOUISE M. DEMBRY, MD, MS
Hospital Epidemiologist
Yale-New Haven Hospital
Associate Professor of Medicine (Infectious Diseases) and
Epidemiology
Yale University School of Medicine
New Haven, Connecticut

ROBERT A. DUNCAN, MD, MPH
Harvard Medical School
Senior Staff and Hospital Epidemiologist
Center for Infectious Diseases & Division of Internal Medicine
Lahey Clinic
Burlington, Massachusetts

MICHAEL EDMOND, MD, MPH, MPA
Professor of Internal Medicine and Preventive Medicine
Virginia Commonwealth University
Richmond, Virginia

JOSE A. FERNANDEZ, RA
University of Iowa Hospital and Clinics
Iowa City, Iowa

LYNN SLONIM FINE, PhD, MPH, CIC
Infection Control Practitioner
University of Rochester Medical Center
Rochester, New York

SCOTT A. FLANDERS, MD
Clinical Associate Professor
Director, Hospitalist Program
Associate Director, Inpatient Programs
University of Michigan Health System
Ann Arbor, Michigan

MARY L. FORNEK, BSN, MBA, CIC
Director of Special Projects, Division of Epidemiology
New York City Department of Health & Mental Hygiene
New York, New York

RICHARD A. GARIBALDI, MD
University of Connecticut Health Center
Farmington, Connecticut

CAROLYN V. GOULD, MD
Fellow in Infectious Diseases
Division of Infectious Diseases
University of Pennsylvania
Philadelphia, Pennsylvania

DAVID K. HENDERSON, MD
Deputy Director for Clinical Care
Clinical Center
National Institutes of Health
Bethesda, Maryland

KELLY J. HENNING, MD
Director, Division of Epidemiology
New York City Department of Health & Mental Hygiene
New York, New York

LOREEN A. HERWALDT, MD
University of Iowa College of Medicine
University of Iowa Hospital and Clinics
Iowa City, Iowa

STEPHANIE HOLLEY, RN, BSN, CIC
Infection Control Professional
Program of Hospital Epidemiology
University of Iowa Hospitals and Clinics
Iowa City, Iowa

PATRICK A. HYMEL, MD
Section of Emergency Medicine, Department of Medicine
Louisiana State University Health Sciences Center
New Orleans, Louisiana
MedMined, Inc
Birmingham, Alabama

WILLIAM R. JARVIS, MD
Division of Healthcare Quality Research
Centers for Disease Control and Prevention
Atlanta, Georgia

LAURIS C. KALDJIAN, MD
University of Iowa
Carver College of Medicine
Iowa City, Iowa

YOUNG S. KIM, MD
Assistant Professor of Medicine
Drexel University College of Medicine
Division of Infectious Diseases
Hospital Epidemiologist and Chairman of Infection Control
Hahnemann University Hospital
Philadelphia, Pennsylvania

KENNETH R. LAWRENCE, BS, PHARMD
Clinical Pharmacy Specialist
Department of Pharmacy & Division of Geographic Medicine
and Infectious Diseases
Tufts New England Medical Center
Boston, Massachusetts

MARK LOEB, MD, MSC, FRCPC
Director, Infection Control
Hamilton Health Sciences
Hamilton, Ontario, Canada

DARREN R. LINKIN, MD
Instructor, Department of Medicine, Division of Infectious
Diseases
Faculty Fellow, Center for Education and Research on
Therapeutics, Center for Clinical Epidemiology and
Biostatistics
University of Pennsylvania
Hospital Epidemiologist
Philadelphia Veterans Administration Medical Center
Philadelphia, Pennsylvania

TAMMY LUNDSTROM, MD
Clinical Consultant, Safety Institute, Premier Inc
DMC Vice President, Chief Quality and Safety Officer and
DMC Medical Director of Epidemiology
WSU Assistant Professor of Medicine—Division of Infectious
Diseases
Detroit, Michigan

LISA L. MARAGAKIS, MD
Johns Hopkins University
Division of Infectious Diseases
Baltimore, Maryland

RICHARD A. MARTINELLO, MD
Clinical Instructor
Departments of Internal Medicine and Pediatrics, Infectious
Diseases
Yale University School of Medicine
New Haven, Connecticut
Hospital Epidemiologist
VA Connecticut Healthcare System
West Haven, Connecticut

JOEL MASLOW, MD, PHD
Chief of Infectious Diseases and ACOS for Research
Philadelphia Veterans Affairs Medical Center
Associate Dean for Research
University of Pennsylvania
Philadelphia, Pennsylvania

MARY D. NETTLEMAN, MD, MS
Chair, Department of Medicine
Michigan State University College of Human Medicine
East Lansing, Michigan

LINDSAY E. NICOLLE, MD
University of Manitoba
Winnipeg, Manitoba, Canada

DEBORAH M. NIHILL, RN, MS, CIC
Manager, Hospital Epidemiology and Infection Control
Barnes-Jewish Hospital
St. Louis, Missouri

TRISH M. PERL, MD, MSc
Division of Infectious Diseases, Department of Medicine
Department of Hospital Epidemiology and Infection Control
Johns Hopkins Medical Institutions and
Department of Epidemiology
Bloomberg School of Public Health
Johns Hopkins University
Baltimore, Maryland

DAVID L. PATERSON, MBBS, FRACP
Associate Professor
University of Pittsburgh School of Medicine
Director, Antibiotic Management Program
University of Pittsburgh Medical Center
Pittsburgh, Pennsylvania

LANCE R. PETERSON, MD
Division of Microbiology, Department of Pathology and
Laboratory Medicine
Evanston Northwestern Healthcare
Evanston, Illinois
Northwestern University's Feinberg School of Medicine
Chicago, Illinois

DIDIER PITTET, MD, MS
Professor of Medicine
Director, Infection Control Program
The University of Geneva Hospitals
Geneva, Switzerland
Honorary Professor
Division of Investigative Sciences
Hammersmith Hospital
Imperial College of Medicine, Science, and Technology
London, United Kingdom

JEAN M. POTTINGER, RN, MA, CIC
University of Iowa Healthcare
Iowa City, Iowa

GINA PUGLIESE, RN, MS
Vice President, Safety Institute, Premier Inc
Associate Faculty
University of Illinois School and Public Health and
Rush University College of Nursing
Chicago, Illinois

VIRGINIA R. ROTH, MD, FRCPC
Director, Infection Control
The Ottawa Hospital
Ottawa, Ontario, Canada

MARK E. RUPP, MD
Professor
Department of Internal Medicine
University of Nebraska Medical Center
Omaha, Nebraska
Medical Director
Department of Healthcare Epidemiology
Nebraska Medical Center
Omaha, Nebraska

SANJAY SAINT, MD, MPH
Research Investigator and Hospitalist,
Ann Arbor VA Medical Center
Director, VA/UM Patient Safety Enhancement Program
Associate Professor of Medicine
University of Michigan Medical School
University of Michigan
Ann Arbor, Michigan

DANIEL J. SEXTON, MD
Professor of Medicine
Division of Infectious Diseases
Duke University Medical Center
Durham, North Carolina

SHANON SMITH, MD
University of Iowa Hospital and Clinics
Iowa City, Iowa

VICTOR SOTO-CACERES, MD, MPH
Division of Reproductive Health
Centers for Disease Control and Prevention
Atlanta, Georgia

WILLIAM M. VALENTI, MD
Clinical Associate Professor of Medicine
University of Rochester School of Medicine and Dentistry
Founding Medical Director
Community Health Network/AIDS Community Health Center
Rochester, New York

MESUT YILMAZ, MD
University of Istanbul
Istanbul, Turkey

GETTING STARTED

CHAPTER ONE

PRACTICAL HOSPITAL EPIDEMIOLOGY: AN INTRODUCTION

Ebbing Lautenbach, MD, MPH, MSCE and Keith Woeltje, MD, PhD

It is with great pleasure that we introduce the second edition of the *Practical Handbook for Healthcare Epidemiologists*. As noted by Dr. Loreen Herwaldt in the introduction to the first edition of this textbook, "Hospital epidemiology and infection control have become increasingly complex fields."[1] While certainly true then, it may be even truer at present. The healthcare epidemiologist today faces an abundance of both challenges and opportunities. One needs to look no further than the recent emergence of severe acute respiratory syndrome (SARS) and monkeypox to appreciate the rapidly changing nature of this field. Recent emphasis on such issues as bioterrorism preparedness and patient safety, both closely related to infection control, highlights the need for the expertise of the healthcare epidemiologist in many arenas. The need for knowledgeable and well-trained healthcare epidemiologists has never been greater.

The reader may note that the title of this textbook has changed in a small but important way from the first edition. We have acknowledged substantial changes in the field by revising the title from focusing on the "hospital" epidemiologist to the "healthcare" epidemiologist. Indeed, this reflects an identical change made several years ago by the Society for *Healthcare* Epidemiology of America (SHEA). As more healthcare is delivered in the outpatient setting and a greater number of individuals are cared for in non-acute care health facilities (eg, skilled nursing facilities, long-term care facilities [LTCFs]), an understanding of infection control issues in these settings is vital. The focus of the contemporary infection control professional (ICP) is more accurately described as "healthcare" epidemiology. Indeed, issues facing the ICP (eg, healthcare acquired infections, adherence to hand hygiene guidelines, employee health) are not limited to the acute care hospital and do not respect geographic boundaries. Indeed, many examples of spread of infections across different healthcare settings exist in the literature. To recognize these changes in the field, we specifically focus on the "healthcare epidemiologist."

Healthcare infections exact a tremendous toll in morbidity, mortality, and costs.[2] Indeed, the number of nosocomial infections per 1000 patient days has actually gone up in the past 2 decades,[2] and there are reasons to suspect that healthcare infections will go up in the future. These include newer instruments and devices, more invasive procedures, sicker patient populations, stretched resources, and new patterns of antimicrobial resistance.

The primary focus of the healthcare epidemiologist remains the prevention of healthcare-associated infections. Effective infection control efforts have been shown to dramatically reduce nosocomial infections, with decreased morbidity, improvement in survival, and shorter duration of hospitalization.[3] Indeed, the healthcare epidemiologist must deal with all aspects of the healthcare setting to prevent patients or staff from acquiring infection. These include investigation of outbreaks, surveillance, development of policies, audits, teaching, advice, consultation, community links, and research. With the increasing acuity of the hospitalized patient population and the growing use of other healthcare facilities (HCFs) (eg, long-term care, outpatient, home care), the need for the healthcare epidemiologist will continue to increase dramatically in the coming years.[4]

The knowledge and skills of the healthcare epidemiologist also lend themselves extremely well to addressing many other issues at the forefront of patient care today. Knowledge of healthcare epidemiology is useful for drug use management, quality assessment, technology assessment, product evaluation, and risk management. In particular, application of healthcare epidemiology-based practices may offer much to the patient safety movement. These include establishing clear definitions of adverse events, standardizing methods for detecting and reporting events, creating appropriate rate adjustments for case-mix differences, and instituting evidence-based intervention programs.[5,6]

We recognize that several comprehensive textbooks of hospital epidemiology exist as excellent resources for ICPs.[7-9] This textbook is not meant to replicate these books but rather to complement them as a pragmatic, easy-to-use reference emphasizing the essentials of healthcare epidemiology. Our goal with this text is to provide a user-friendly and straightforward introduction to the field of healthcare epidemiology—one that fosters understanding the basics of this increasingly complex field. We anticipate that as the reader gains a greater knowledge of the essentials of healthcare epidemiology, he or she will desire, and should pursue, more in-depth knowledge of specific issues. Consultation with colleagues as well as a comprehensive infection control textbook would be an essential component of expanding one's expertise in the field. But as a starting point, this overview of the important aspects of healthcare epidemiology should provide a good foundation for those entering into the field of infection control. The practical nature of the textbook lends itself well to the very nature of healthcare epidemiology as a field that requires constant action (eg, surveillance, interventions). While daily decisions must be based on a thorough evaluation of the data, they must also be practical in the context of the healthcare setting and surroundings of the practitioner.

This textbook is also distinguished by its focus on experience. While based solidly on the existing medical literature, this resource also offers real-world advice and suggestions from professionals who have grappled with many of the longstanding and newer issues in infection control. As in the first edition of this textbook,[1] we asked the authors to write their chapters as if they were speaking to an individual who would be running an infection control program and who was just starting in this field. The authors' task was to prepare future hospital epidemiologists for their new career by summarizing basic data from the literature and by providing essential references and resources. In addition, we asked the authors to share their own experiences of what works and what does not work in particular situations.

To help you make the most of this textbook, we will briefly summarize the overall content of the chapters and how they are organized. Even in the 6 years since publication of the first edition, many changes have occurred in healthcare in general and in healthcare epidemiology in particular. Reflecting this, all chapters have been substantially revised. Furthermore, many new chapters have been added to address emerging issues in this rapidly changing field.

This textbook is divided into 6 sections. In the first section, "Getting Started," we include chapters on both the hospital epidemiologist and the infection control committee, recognizing that understanding their goals, responsibilities, and interaction with various other healthcare entities is a vital first step in organizing a successful infection control program.

In the second section, "Surveillance and Analysis," we include chapters on the basics of surveillance as well as essential epidemiological methods in infection control. Furthermore, specific sections addressing the most common and important healthcare-acquired infections are included.

The third section is entitled "Support Functions" and details the critical services, including microbiological support and molecular epidemiology, required to address the issues facing today's healthcare epidemiologist. Recognizing the increasingly important role of electronic surveillance and computer decision support, we have a chapter on the role of computers in hospital epidemiology.

The fourth section, "Antimicrobial Resistance," is new in this edition of the textbook, responding to the continually increasing threat to the hospitalized patient from resistant pathogens. Recognizing the close relationship between infection control and antimicrobial stewardship in preventing infections in the hospitalized patient, and the fact that the healthcare epidemiologist often has important input into antimicrobial formulary decision making, a chapter on antimicrobial stewardship is also included in this section.

The fifth section, "Special Topics," includes a variety of chapters that, while exceedingly important in healthcare epidemiology, do not fit neatly into one of the other sections. Many of these chapters are new and respond to issues that have emerged only in the past few years, issues to which the healthcare epidemiologist must respond. Acknowledging its critical role in infection prevention, a new chapter on hand hygiene has been added. Responding to issues for which awareness has grown dramatically in recent years, new chapters on patient safety and bioterrorism preparedness are also included. Finally, as noted previously, the scope of the "hospital" epidemiologist is ever expanding and often includes other healthcare settings. As such, chapters on infection control in long-term care and in the outpatient setting are included.

The final section, "Administrative Issues," highlights the many tasks that the hospital epidemiologist and infection control committee must tackle on an ongoing basis to ensure that their program remains responsive to current issues, mandates, and emerging problems. There are chapters describing development of policies and guidelines and preparing for surveys by the Joint Commission on Accreditation of Healthcare Organizations (JCAHO) and the Occupational Safety and Health Administration (OSHA).

We hope that this textbook will provide trainees and professionals in infection control, particularly the fledgling healthcare epidemiologist, the knowledge and tools to establish and maintain a successful and effective healthcare epidemiology program. Ours is a vibrant and exciting field that presents new challenges and opportunities daily. The prospects for the healthcare epidemiologist are virtually limitless, whether they are in infection control, antimicrobial stewardship, patient safety, or beyond. We hope that this textbook provides the foundation upon which many future years of further learning, innovation, and advancement are based.

REFERENCES

1. Herwaldt LA, Decker MD. An introduction to practical hospital epidemiology. In: Herwaldt LA, Decker M, eds. *A Practical Handbook for Hospital Epidemiologists*. Thorofare, NJ: SLACK Incorporated; 1998:3-5.

2. Weinstein RA. Nosocomial infection update. *Emerg Infect Dis*. 1998;4:416-420.

3. Scheckler WE, Brimhall D, Buck AS, et al. Requirements for infrastructure and essential activities of infection control and epidemiology in hospitals: a consensus panel report. Society for Healthcare Epidemiology of America. *Infect Control Hosp Epidemiol*. 1998;19:114-124.

4. Jarvis WR. Infection control and changing health-care delivery systems. *Emerg Infect Dis*. 2001;7:170-173.

5. Scheckler WE. Healthcare epidemiology is the paradigm for patient safety. *Infect Control Hosp Epidemiol*. 2002;23:47-51.

6. Gerberding JL. Hospital-onset infections: a patient safety issue. *Ann Intern Med*. 2002;137:665-670.

7. Bennett JV, Brachman PS, eds. *Hospital Infections*. 4th ed. Boston, Mass: Little, Brown and Company; 1998.

8. Mayhall CG, ed. *Hospital Epidemiology and Infection Control*. 3rd ed. Baltimore, Md: Lippincott Williams & Wilkins; 2004.

9. Wenzel RP, ed. *Prevention and Control of Nosocomial Infections*. 4th ed. Baltimore, Md: Lippincott Williams & Wilkins; 2003.

CHAPTER TWO

EDUCATIONAL NEEDS AND OPPORTUNITIES FOR THE HOSPITAL EPIDEMIOLOGIST

Richard A. Martinello, MD and Louise M. Dembry, MD, MS

INTRODUCTION

Hospital epidemiologists provide an essential service to healthcare institutions. In the past, their primary role was to oversee and manage the institution's infection control program in the traditional role of surveillance, prevention, and control of nosocomial infections. During the past decade, hospital epidemiologists have expanded their roles by increasing the spectrum of their activities. Hospital epidemiologists are now often involved in the institution's quality improvement, patient safety, and risk management programs. Some hospital epidemiologists have expanded their roles to become institutional healthcare epidemiologists who participate in or direct their institutions' comprehensive quality improvement and patient safety programs, evaluating a broad spectrum of healthcare outcomes.

Healthcare delivery is in transition. Today, greater numbers of sicker patients are being cared for in outpatient, long-term care, rehabilitation, and home settings, and increasing proportions of hospitalized patients are critically ill and/or immunocompromised. Multidrug-resistant bacteria such as methicillin-resistant *Staphylococcus aureus* (MRSA) and vancomycin-resistant enterococci (VRE) have become endemic in many institutions and are now beginning to spread in some communities. These changes present a challenge to programs aimed at preventing nosocomial transmission and subsequent infection with these pathogens. Individuals practicing hospital epidemiology must be capable of developing new approaches to prevent the spread of potential pathogens within the entire scope of healthcare settings. The prospect of bioterrorism has also become a reality, and hospital epidemiologists have been called upon to function as institutional experts in emergency preparedness with

regard to biological agents and to serve as the interface between the healthcare facility and public health.

The financial structure and stability of healthcare is also in flux. To survive the dramatic changes in healthcare delivery and financing, hospitals have had to optimize the process of care to balance costs. Numerous hospitals have compelled outcome measuring groups—quality improvement, risk management, and hospital epidemiology—to function together. Individuals who can apply the basic techniques of epidemiology, biostatistics, surveillance, and informatics to a broad range of infectious and non-infectious problems are in a position to help their hospitals and healthcare systems meet these challenges.

HOSPITAL EPIDEMIOLOGY TRAINING

Hospital epidemiologists come from diverse backgrounds. The majority of hospital epidemiologists have completed formal fellowship training in infectious diseases (ID). Some hospital epidemiologists are internists, surgeons, or other physicians with an interest in infection control. There is no formal accredited training process for hospital epidemiologists, though ample resources are available for formal and self-directed study. Several options are available to those interested in formal hospital epidemiology training. The path one chooses for hospital epidemiology training is dependent upon his or her current level of training and long-term goals. All people interested in a career in hospital epidemiology should gain experience and a working knowledge of the topics listed in Table 2-1. Subspecialty fellows training in ID should receive some formal exposure to hospital epidemiology. People who do not complete a fellowship in hospital epidemiology should pursue several training opportunities,

---

TABLE 2-1. TOPICS FOR THE HOSPITAL EPIDEMIOLOGIST

Biostatistics
Data collection and surveillance
Standard and transmission-based isolation precautions
Outbreak investigation
Prevention of nosocomial infections
      Medical devices
      Invasive procedures
      Special pathogens
            M. tuberculosis, VZV, Aspergillus, Legionella
      immunocompromised hosts
Antimicrobial resistance and antibiotic utilization
Sterilization and disinfection
Environment
      Construction and renovation
      Heating, ventilating, and air conditioning systems (HVAC)
      Water supplies
Techniques for influencing and impacting behavior (eg, hand hygiene)
Development of training and educational programs
Molecular typing
Emergency preparedness
Laboratory safety
Occupational hazards of healthcare workers (HCWs) (sharp injuries)
Risk management
Quality improvement
Regulatory, accreditation, and professional agencies
Administration, leadership, and personnel management

---

including short courses, summer programs, and national meetings.

People currently planning their formal ID training who are interested in hospital epidemiology should select an ID fellowship program that offers specific training in hospital epidemiology and infection control. A limited number of ID fellowship programs offer this training. ID fellow applicants should discuss their career goals in healthcare epidemiology with each institution's hospital epidemiologist to determine if the available training opportunities will meet their needs.

Some ID fellowship programs offer fellows the opportunity to train formally with the hospital epidemiologist for a 1- to 3-year period. The hospital epidemiologist, usually a member of the ID section, may serve as a mentor and supervise the fellow's research. The level to which fellows participate in the hospital epidemiology program varies. Programs that allow fellows to perform research and participate actively in the day-to-day activities of the hospital epidemiology program, including the administrative aspects, offer the most well-rounded experiences. Involvement in the daily functions of the hospital epi-

demiology service should provide adequate experience with topics and situations listed in Table 2-1 within a 6- to 24-month period. This period of training should include involvement in both short- and long-term hospital epidemiology projects such as annual influenza vaccination campaigns, hand hygiene improvement projects, and construction and renovation projects at the facility. Involvement with ongoing construction and renovation projects can provide an experience often only available once one's formal training has been completed. Specific experience with emergency preparedness planning would also be of benefit. Some people may gain from an organized curriculum to broaden the exposure to the hospital epidemiology literature and controversial topics.

Research in hospital epidemiology can take on multiple forms, and research careers in clinical and basic science aspects of hospital epidemiology are possible. Research training should include formal coursework in biostatistics, epidemiology, clinical study design, grant writing, and ethics. Interested people may choose to pursue fellowships such as the Robert Wood Johnson Foundation Clinical Scholars Fellowship or the Epidemiology

Intelligence Service fellowship coordinated through the Centers for Disease Control and Prevention (CDC) to provide a formal framework and experience with biostatistics, clinical research, and epidemiology. Many hospital epidemiologists have obtained formal epidemiology and biostatistics training as part of a master in public health (MPH) or master of science in clinical epidemiology (MSCE) program.

Funding specifically intended for training in hospital epidemiology research is available through the SHEA and the National Foundation for Infectious Diseases (NFID). The NFID sponsors grants for Postdoctoral Fellowships in Nosocomial Infection Research and Training (http://www.nfid.org/fellow/). SHEA offers grants to fund fellowship training for those interested in careers in healthcare epidemiology and related research. During the past several years, SHEA training grants have been awarded for research proposals ranging from the prevention of surgical site infections (SSIs) to the study and development of antimicrobial utilization programs. More information can be obtained online from the SHEA Web site (http://www.shea-online.org). Research training could also be potentially funded through the National Institutes of Health's National Research Service Award (NRSA) program (http://grants1.nih.gov/training/nrsa.htm#fellowships).

ADDITIONAL ASPECTS OF HOSPITAL EPIDEMIOLOGY

Perhaps one of the most intimidating aspects for the novice hospital epidemiologist is the alphabet soup of regulatory and accreditation agencies and their regulations and standards. In addition, numerous professional groups have published guidelines and voluntary standards for certain aspects of hospital epidemiology and the prevention of nosocomial infections. Many government agencies and professional organizations maintain Web sites and print publications outlining and describing many of their regulations, standards, and guidelines in-depth. The SHEA and the Association of Professionals in Infection Control (APIC) annual scientific meetings often have sessions or workshops specifically discussing these issues.

The hospital epidemiologist must be familiar with the OSHA Bloodborne Pathogens Standard, American Institute of Architecture's *Guidelines for Design and Construction of Hospital and Healthcare Facilities*,[1] the JCAHO *Prevention and Control of Infection* standards, the CDC *Guidelines for Preventing the Transmission of* Mycobacterium tuberculosis *in Health-Care Facilities*,[2] and Healthcare Infection Control Practices Advisory Committee (HICPAC) guidelines. The *APIC Text of Infection Control and Epidemiology*[3] and the *Infection Control Reference Service: The Experts' Guide to the*

Guidelines[4] are superb references providing in-depth information on hospital epidemiology and infection control standards and guidelines. (Further information is available in Chapter 29, discussing JCAHO, and Chapter 28, discussing OSHA, in this text.)

Molecular typing of pathogens is an important laboratory tool for investigating endemic and epidemic nosocomial infections. Strain typing techniques are used to determine genetic relatedness of organisms. The information gained from molecular typing can be used in conjunction with epidemiologic data to determine the extent of an outbreak, patterns of transmission, or the effectiveness of control measures. Organized training in this field is limited, although laboratories performing these techniques often are willing to train interested people on an individual basis. Perhaps the most important aspect of molecular typing is understanding when it is important to consider strain typing organisms and the inherent limitations in the interpretation of the results. Additional information can be found in Chapter 14 of this text. In addition, good reviews are available on the topic.[5,6]

TRAINING OPPORTUNITIES

In the following sections, a number of training opportunities that were available at the time this chapter was written are described briefly. Interested individuals may obtain detailed information regarding each program from the sponsoring institutions. Consultation with colleagues and Internet searches may reveal additional educational opportunities.

Short Training Courses

Individuals who have completed their formal training or who have limited time to devote toward further formal training in hospital epidemiology should consider taking the SHEA/CDC Training Course in Healthcare Epidemiology. This 4-day course is offered twice annually and provides an intensive overview of the principles of epidemiology, surveillance, outbreak investigation, transmission and control of nosocomial infection, disinfection and sterilization, occupational health, regulatory compliance, and quality improvement. Further course information can be obtained online at http://www.sheaonline.org/Courses.html.

The APIC offers a 3.5-day introductory course in infection control and epidemiology (ICE I). This course is offered twice each year and covers surveillance methodology, basic microbiology and an introduction to infectious processes, surveillance and data presentation, transmission-based infection control precautions, and an introduction to outbreak investigation. Further course information can be obtained online at http://www.apic.org/educ.

SHEA and APIC each offer continuing medical education during their annual scientific meetings. Courses in clinical epidemiology, biostatistics, and microbial pathogens are often available through medical schools and schools of public health. Some schools of public health offer specific courses in hospital epidemiology.

The University of Iowa Hospitals and Clinics, Program of Hospital Epidemiology organizes an annual "Extension Training Program" for infection control practitioners. This 5-day intensive course provides training in the fundamentals of surveillance, data management and analysis, outbreak investigation, and the prevention and control of nosocomial infections. Topics including antimicrobial resistance, regulatory agencies, and epidemic recognition are also covered. The course is directed toward infection control practitioners with at least 6 months of experience. Further information can be obtained from Dawn Folkmann, Extension Training Program, University of Iowa Hospitals and Clinics, 200 Hawkins Drive, C-52 GH, Iowa City, IA 52242; phone: (319) 356-1606 (http://www.uihc.uiowa.edu/corm/FolderHospitalEpiTraining.htm).

Summer Courses

Several schools of public health offer graduate summer programs in epidemiology and biostatistics. These courses, which vary in length from 1 to 4 weeks, are an alternative way for novice hospital epidemiologists to learn the principles of epidemiology. The courses also help more experienced individuals augment their knowledge and practical skills.

Generally, the summer epidemiology programs offer basic-, secondary-, and graduate-level courses in epidemiology, biostatistics, and study design. These programs often address specific topics including the epidemiology of acute and chronic diseases, occupational and environmental health, health policy, clinical epidemiology, and others. Some programs offer courses in hospital epidemiology, the epidemiology of ID, and methods in quality assessment. Some programs provide graduate-level credit through their respective universities.

The University of Michigan School of Public Health offers 1- and 3-week intensive courses covering a number of biostatistics and epidemiology topics. The Graduate Summer Session in Epidemiology is an independent course taught by faculty members from numerous institutions. This program offers several courses lasting from 1 to 3 weeks, including courses in the fundamentals of epidemiology and biostatistics, a course in computer applications for epidemiology (3 weeks), the epidemiology of ID (1 week), infection control (1 week), and methods in medical quality assessment (1 week). Further information can be obtained online at http://www.sph.umich.edu/epid/GSS/index.html.

The McGill University Department of Epidemiology and Biostatistics in Montreal, Quebec, Canada, offers a summer program intended for clinicians and other health professionals. The courses all last 4 weeks and include training in epidemiology, biostatistics, principles of epidemiology research, risk assessment and management, and the health services evaluation. Further information can be found at http://www.mcgill.ca/epi-biostat/summer.

The Graduate Summer Program in Epidemiology at The Johns Hopkins University School of Hygiene and Public Health, Baltimore, provides a number of courses in the principles and methods of epidemiology, study design, and biostatistics. The courses range between 1 weekend to 3 weeks in length. Further information can be obtained online at http://www.jhsph.edu/summerEpi.

Hospital Epidemiology and Infection Control at Johns Hopkins Hospital presents an annual Fellows Course. This 3-day course is focused on training fellows, physicians, and nurses in introductory hospital epidemiology and infection control. Further information can be found online at http://www.hopkins-heic.org/education/schedule.html#2.

The Summer Institute for Public Health Practice at the University of Washington, Seattle, conducts a 5-day course in introductory and advanced epidemiology. These courses cover the topics of surveillance, disease investigation, study design, and epidemiological principles. The extensive use of case scenarios and small group discussions create an interactive learning environment. Further information is available online at http://nwcphp.org/niphp.

Online Courses and Independent Education

The London School of Hygiene and Tropical Medicine offers a formal program in epidemiology that can lead to the awarding of an MSc degree. Students participate in the course via e-mail and online material. More information is available online at http://www.lshtm.ac.uk/cal/epp.

The University of Massachusetts Amherst School of Public Health and Health Sciences offers a web-based introduction course on the principles and methods of epidemiology and the application of these skills in the field of public health. More information is available online at http://www.umamherstonline.org.

An online course entitled "Health Care Statistics" is offered through the Pitt Community College. More information is available online at http://www.health.pitt.cc.nc.us/hit/.

Thomas Jefferson University offers a web-based course entitled "Epidemiology for Health Professionals." The course provides training in basic methods in epidemiology and their application to problems in health services. More information is available at http://jeffline.tju.edu.

The CDC offers a print-based education module entitled "Principles of Epidemiology" that presents the concepts, principles, and methods used in the surveillance and investigation of health-related events. More information is available online at http://bookstore.phf.org/prod12.htm. Completion of this coursework offers up to 42 hours of CME credit.

The CDC and the Public Health Training Network have developed a series of videotapes and a course workbook based upon a satellite course in epidemiology. This course is focused on statistics, data organization, public health surveillance, and outbreak investigation. More information is available by contacting the Alabama Department of Public Health/Video communications at (334) 206-5618.

The Global Health Network offers the "Supercourse," online, subtitled "Epidemiology, the Internet, and Public Health." More than 1400 lectures are available on a broad range of epidemiology topics, from faculty around the world. The main site is hosted by the University of Pittsburgh School of Public Health (http://www.pitt.edu/~super1), but international mirror sites are available.

Other courses may be found on the Public Health Foundation Web site http://www.TrainingFinder.org.

CONTINUING EDUCATION

Both APIC and SHEA hold annual scientific meetings that provide continuing education opportunities to attendees. APIC's meeting, held in late spring or early summer, provides scientific and practical information relevant to the practice of infection control. The SHEA meeting, held in early spring, includes workshops, symposia, and sessions for poster and oral presentations of original scientific work. The broad areas covered include nosocomial infections, occupational risks of HCWs, and quality assessment. Both meetings enable infection control personnel to learn about developments and research regarding the causes, modes of transmission, diagnosis, prevention, and control of nosocomial infections. In addition, division "L" of the American Society for Microbiology (ASM, http://www.asmusa.org/mbrsrc/ mbr41.htm), comprised of individuals who are interested in hospital epidemiology and nosocomial infections, sponsors sessions at the ASM national meetings that are relevant to hospital epidemiologists. Finally, the Infectious Diseases Society of America (IDSA) devotes a portion of its national meetings to important infection control topics (http://www.idsociety. org).

The Program of Hospital Epidemiology at the University of Iowa Hospitals and Clinics, in cooperation with the University of Iowa Colleges of Nursing and Medicine, offers a 2-day "Annual Infection Control Seminar" that is designed primarily for physician and nursing professionals in infection control. The course covers a variety of topics within infection control, including antimicrobial resistance, quality improvement, and bioterrorism. The seminar agenda varies each year to accommodate timely topics in hospital epidemiology.

Further information can be obtained online at http://www.uihc.uiowa.edu/corm/FolderHospitalEpiTraining.htm.

BOOKS AND JOURNALS

Several textbooks, including *Hospital Infections*,[7] *Prevention and Control of Nosocomial Infections*,[8] and *Hospital Epidemiology and Infection Control*[9] discuss the principles and practice of hospital epidemiology and provide excellent references. The textbooks are particularly useful for people who previously have learned basic epidemiologic concepts. The *APIC Text of Infection Control and Epidemiology*[3] and the *Infection Control Reference Service: The Experts' Guide to the Guidelines*[4] are excellent references providing in-depth information on hospital epidemiology and infection control standards and guidelines.

The official journal of SHEA is *Infection Control and Hospital Epidemiology*, which is published monthly. *Infection Control and Hospital Epidemiology* includes editorials on topical issues in hospital epidemiology, original articles, review articles, consensus papers, and special topics such as practical hospital epidemiology and molecular epidemiology, as well as information regarding the SHEA annual meeting and the SHEA/CDC/AHA Training Course. Further information can be obtained online at http://www.ichejournal.com.

APIC publishes the bimonthly journal *AJIC* (*The American Journal of Infection Control*). AJIC includes original research articles that focus on infection control practices, a commentary section, and APIC *Guidelines for Infection Control Practice*. AJIC also publishes information on upcoming meetings and courses in infection control. Further information can be obtained online at http://www.apic.org/ajic.

The Hospital Infection Society (HIS), based in the United Kingdom, publishes the *Journal of Hospital Infection*. The journal publishes original articles and review articles encompassing the scope of healthcare epidemiology. The HIS also supports educational programs as a part of its national and international meetings. Further information can be obtained online at http://www.elsevier-international.com/journals/jhin and http://www.his.org.uk.

Clinical Governance: An International Journal (formerly entitled *Clinical Performance and Quality Health Care* [CPQHC]) is published quarterly and contains articles addressing appropriateness of care, quality of care, outcome assessment, application of practice guidelines, and the economic aspects of quality improvement and assessment. Further information can be found online at http://www.emeraldinsight.com/vl=4012234/cl=12/nw=1/rpsv/cgij.htm.

REFERENCES

1. American Institute of Architects. *Guidelines for Design and Construction of Hospital and Healthcare Facilities*. Washington DC: American Institute of Architects; 2001.

2. Guidelines for Preventing the Transmission of *Mycobacterium tuberculosis* in Health-Care Facilities, 1994. *MMWR Morb Mortal Wkly Rep*. 1994;43(No. RR-13).

3. Pfeiffer JA, et al, eds. *APIC Text of Infection Control and Epidemiology*. Washington, DC: Association for Professionals in Infection Control and Epidemiology, Inc; 2002.

4. Abrutyn E, Goldmann DA, Scheckler WE, eds. *Infection Control Reference Service: The Experts Guide to the Guidelines*. Philadelphia, Pa: WB Saunders Company; 2001.

5. Sader HS, Hollis RJ, Pfaller MA. The use of molecular techniques in the epidemiology and control of infectious diseases. *Contemp Issues Clin Microbiol*. 1995;15:407-431.

6. Soll DR, Lockhart SR, Pujol C. Laboratory procedures for the epidemiological analysis of microorganisms. In: Murray PR, Baron JE, Jorgensen JH, Pfaller MA, Yolken RH, eds. *Manual of Clinical Microbiology*. Washington, DC: ASM Press; 2003:139-161.

7. Benett JV, Brachman PS, eds. *Hospital Infections*. 4th ed. Philadelphia, Pa: Lippincott-Raven Publishers; 1998.

8. Wenzel PR, ed. *Prevention and Control of Nosocomial Infections*. 4th ed. Philadelphia, Pa: Lippincott, Williams and Wilkins; 2003.

9. Maygall CG, ed. *Hospital Epidemiology and Infection Control*. 2nd ed. New York, NY: Lippincott, Williams and Wilkins; 1999.

CHAPTER THREE

HOW TO GET PAID FOR HEALTHCARE EPIDEMIOLOGY: A PRACTICAL GUIDE

H. Gunner Deery II, MD and Daniel J. Sexton, MD

INTRODUCTION

Every hospital in the United States is required to have an infection control program in order to be certified by the JCAHO. Recent publicity about widespread problems related to patient safety, which are literally an every day occurrence throughout the US healthcare system, has focused attention on preventable injuries related to the nosocomial acquisition of a wide array of serious infections. Despite these remarkable and important trends, many US hospitals do not have a paid hospital epidemiologist. Only 23% of members of the IDSA who responded to a survey in 1998 reported that they received payment for their role in their hospital's infection control program.[1] It is ironic that infectious diseases fellows are well trained in the science of infectious diseases, but most fellows receive minimal if any training or guidance in how to get paid for practicing healthcare epidemiology. In essence, learning how to get paid is left out of most training program's curriculums.

The professional and economic opportunities in infection control and healthcare epidemiology have never been greater. Mandates from the OSHA and JCAHO require that all hospitals develop and maintain programs to reduce the risk of transmission of infectious diseases to both patients and hospital employees. Furthermore, the risk of litigation alleging failure to provide for the safety of hospitalized patients has grown exponentially following the release of two landmark studies by the Institute of Medicine, each emphasizing the lack of patient safety programs in the US healthcare system. We believe these legal obligations will continue to increase as the public, press, and plaintiff bar incrementally increase their scrutiny on the causes and prevention of adverse patient outcomes. Real and theoretical threats of bioterrorism, pervasive problems with antimicrobial resistance, and a host of new and emerging infections add to the challenges facing US hospitals.

Indeed, each of the preceding challenges and problems represent an opportunity for infectious diseases physicians with an interest and training in hospital epidemiology.

Our hope is that this chapter will inspire you to think of yourself as valuable and useful to the mission of the infection control and patient safety program at your local institution. It is our thesis that these services and your expertise should receive appropriate compensation. Although in the past many infectious diseases specialists provided hundreds or even thousands of uncompensated hours of work and shouldered significant responsibility without monetary compensation, we believe that this model is as outdated as the technique of transtracheal aspiration. In the words of an experienced hospital epidemiologist: "If you still work for free [after reading this chapter] —shame on thee!"

HEALTHCARE EPIDEMIOLOGY "PRODUCT" (CREATE A VISION OF VALUE)

Nosocomial infections are one of the most serious patient safety issues in healthcare today.[2] Healthcare epidemiologists are in the primary business of infection prevention. Infection prevention is a critical part of continuous quality improvement and is fundamental to the goal and growing mandate to provide a safe environment for patients and employees. In order to explain the value of these services to hospital administrators, it is critical that a concept of "product" be carefully defined and explained. The concept of "product" may not be intuitive or immediately obvious. Thus, the services of a healthcare epidemiologist must be explicitly defined and the processes of care, infection rates, and compliance with standards of infection prevention need to be quantified, trended, and compared with objective benchmarks or goals. Hospital administrators are then more likely to grasp the value and rationale for providing compensation for healthcare epidemiology.

As individual expertise, interest, and time commitments to infection control vary widely among infectious diseases specialists, and as needs for infection control also vary between individual institutions, your product is highly dependent on how you define your job in infection control. This obvious but important matter should be examined carefully before you attempt to negotiate a contract for providing healthcare epidemiology services. In addition, as described in the section on negotiation skills (pp. 17-18), it is sometimes necessary to modify your product after you have discovered the interests, needs, and concerns of the other side involved in the negotiation process.

One of the best methods to define your "product" is to write a business plan. A typical business plan includes an introduction; a detailed description of the program (or product); a timeline containing short- and long-term goals; costs and required resources such as equipment, space, and personnel; a timetable; criteria for measuring success; and a summary statement. Writing a business plan requires that you set realistic goals, assess resources (including your compensation), outline strategies to achieve your goals, and most importantly, establish criteria to measure performance and success. Business plans are valuable to hospital administrators in several ways. First, they explain your "product" in terms they understand. Second, they provide a way to rationalize and explain the cost of a healthcare epidemiology contract. Finally, they provide an objective way to measure performance. Most business plans need to be updated, revised, and improved over time. For example, with time your "product" may change and grow to include a role in antibiotic management, staff education, or patient safety issues not directly related to infectious diseases (Table 3-1).

HEALTHCARE EPIDEMIOLOGY CUSTOMER (WHO IS THE PURCHASER OF YOUR PRODUCT?)

In most instances, the purchaser of your product is a hospital administrator. Thus, it is axiomatic that the crucial first step is to accurately identify the one administrator who will "purchase" your product. It is equally essential that this individual understand the scope of healthcare/hospital epidemiology, including the benefits and barriers to achieving specific goals. Until this individual understands your plan, your responsibilities, and the criteria used to assess performance, it is unlikely that he or she will be able to accurately value your product and justify the expenses needed to buy this product to his or her colleagues, superiors, or to the hospital governing board.

Before undertaking the above educational and promotional process, it is good to find convincing objective answers to these obvious questions: Why should the administration buy this product? What is the benefit to the institution? How do you explain the relationship between the costs of nosocomial infections and the costs of an infection control program? Hospital administrators can usually calculate the direct costs of an infection control program, but it is exceedingly difficult for most hospital administrators to quantify the benefit. Before negotiating the costs of an infection control program, it is wise to have extensive discussions and develop logical and simple explanations about the benefits of such a program.

The task of explaining the costs of nosocomial infections is difficult because the current total attributable cost of nosocomial infections to society is not known. However, in 1985, Haley estimated that the hospital related financial burden of nosocomial infections in the United States was approximately $3.9 billion per year.[3] This calculates to $6.8 billion per year in 2004 dollars.[4] Although the number of published studies that have rigorously assessed the costs and benefits of infection control programs are few, the existing literature clearly demonstrates that infection control interventions can produce enormous direct and indirect cost savings.[2,5] For example, Fraser and Olsen estimated that an infection control program similar to that advocated by current JCAHO standards was highly cost effective compared to standard health interventions such as cancer screening.[6] Fraser and Olsen estimated that the cost of infection control was $2000 to $8000 per year of life saved, a number considerably less than the estimated cost-effectiveness of *Papanicolaou* smears every 2 years ($650,000 per year of life saved) or even cholesterol reduction in high-risk persons >40 years of age ($32,500 per year of life saved).[6]

Deep sternal wound surgical site infections increase the direct cost of care by $20,000 to $30,000.[7] A follow-up study by the same group of authors demonstrated the economic impact of deep sternal surgical site infections was $14,211 after controlling for selection bias.[8] Even if the lower estimate of $14,211 per infection is used, the annual prevention of four deep surgical site infections at a single institution could save over $50,000/year.

Stone et al reviewed 55 studies published from 1990 to 2000 that contained original cost estimates of nosocomial infection.[2] The mean attributable cost of all nosocomial infections was $13,973. The mean cost of specific types of nosocomial infections was as follows: surgical site ($15,640), bloodstream ($38,703), pneumonia ($17,677), and MRSA ($35,367). A prospective controlled study of

TABLE 3-1. A Hospital Epidemiologist's Marketable Skills

➤ Supervises and collaborates with the infection control professionals
➤ Chairs infection control committee
➤ Supervises collection of surveillance data
➤ Analyzes surveillance data and implements control strategies
➤ Validates the surveillance system
➤ Supervises projects to decrease endemic "common-cause" nosocomial infections
➤ Investigates outbreaks
➤ Analyzes antibiotic resistance patterns and interprets their significance relative to antibiotic utilization
➤ Evaluates new products (eg, intravenous catheters)
➤ Evaluates the scientific validity of policies and procedures
➤ Interprets and implements, in a cost-effective manner, standards from regulatory agencies that are applicable to infection control, employee health, etc
➤ Consults with medical staff, hospital staff, and administration on epidemiological matters
➤ Analyzes trends in employee illness
➤ Supervises vaccination programs for medical staff and hospital employees
➤ Supervises pre-employment screening of new hospital employees
➤ Supervises the follow-up process for hospital employees who are exposed to infectious diseases (eg, blood-borne pathogens, tuberculosis, varicella, herpes zoster, meningococcus)
➤ Directs and supervises AIDS-related issues (eg, hospital employee education, case reporting)
➤ Consults with staff in the microbiology laboratory regarding the appropriate use of laboratory tests, antibiotic susceptibility reports, analysis of new rapid lab tests, etc
➤ Consults with architects, engineers, and contractors regarding infection risks associated with construction projects
➤ Consults with staff in risk management regarding actual or potential malpractice claims related to nosocomial infections
➤ Consults with the hospital's public relations personnel regarding release of information about outbreaks, endemic nosocomial infections, quality of care, epidemiological-based report cards, etc
➤ Serves as a liaison between hospital and medical staff in quality improvement initiatives
➤ Consults with other staff regarding epidemiological evaluations of noninfectious disease problems (eg, falls, decubitus ulcers)
➤ Supervises or consults with the hospital's pharmacokinetic dosing service
➤ Supervises the epidemiological initiatives in the hospital's long-term care facility, transitional care, and rehabilitation facility
➤ Directs the infection control and employee health initiatives in an expanded healthcare setting that includes the hospital or healthcare system, a home nursing program, and a home infusion therapy program
➤ Helps to develop an epidemiological-based quality management approach to noninfectious adverse outcomes of care
➤ Assists in outcome management initiatives
➤ Assists other staff as they develop clinical practice guidelines
➤ Serves as a liaison with staff from the local public health department
➤ Assists with epidemiology of medical error prevention and safety initiatives
➤ Assists with policy and program evaluation of reprocessing disposables/single-use items
➤ Assists with managing mask fit testing program
➤ Manages smallpox or other bioterrorism vaccination programs
➤ Assists with developing bioterrorism and emerging infection policies and procedures
➤ Assists with developing alcohol-based hand washing program
➤ Collects data on and assesses adequacy of processes related to infection control
➤ Designs, supervises, or oversees the scope, curriculum, and implementation of staff education related to infection control

ventilator-associated pneumonia found the attributable mean cost to be $11,897.[9] These data further affirm the point made above: annual prevention of only a small fraction of serious nosocomial infections can justify the costs of the entire infection control program in most community and tertiary care hospitals. Hospital administrators may logically point out that Medicare and many third-party payers actually reimburse hospitals for the cost of complications of care. Such reimbursement is nonexistent in patients without healthcare insurance and is limited in many patients covered exclusively by the Medicare program.

In a study done in 1999, Kirkland et al reported the total excess direct cost attributable to surgical-site infection as $5038.[10] In another study, from the same institution, Whitehouse et al reported the median direct excess cost of orthopedic surgical site infections was $17,708 and total (direct and indirect) median costs per patient were even higher ($27,969 per patient).[11] The 1-year study period reported by Whitehouse and colleagues involved a cohort of less than 100 orthopedic patients with surgical site infections, yet these patients' infections cumulatively resulted in total extra costs of $867,039.[11] These estimates undoubtedly underestimated the total cost of their patients nosocomial infection, as these authors were unable to measure the cost of outpatient services such as outpatient intravenous antibiotics, skilled nursing, and physical therapy.

Kaye et al recently reported that a structured and focused infection control program for small- and medium-sized community hospitals in North Carolina and South Carolina, which was administrated by a network employing trained physician epidemiologists and infection control nurse practitioners, resulted in dramatic reductions in the incidence of nosocomial infections over a 3-year span.[12] During the first 3 years of affiliation in the Duke Infection Control Outreach Network (DICON), annual rates of nosocomial bloodstream infections (BSI) decreased by 23% (p = 0.009) from year 1 to year 3 in study hospitals. Annual rates of nosocomial infection and colonization due to MRSA decreased by 22% (p = 0.002) and rates of ventilator-associated pneumonia decreased by 40% (p = 0.001). Rates of employee blood borne pathogen exposures decreased by 18% (p = 0.003).

These successes were attributed to feedback provided to the healthcare providers on nosocomial infection rates that were then linked to specific educational initiatives. This entire process in turn resulted in healthcare providers that were educated about the nature of the existing problems and as a consequence were secondarily motivated and stimulated to embrace effective strategies for preventing future infections.[12]

Other safety initiatives can also produce remarkable cost savings. The CDC estimates that 385,000 needle sticks and other sharps-related injuries are sustained in hospital-based healthcare personnel every year.[13] Treating a healthcare worker to prevent disease from a needle stick injury as reported in 1999 was estimated to cost between $500 and $3000 per event.[14] In 2004 dollars, this would calculate to $700 to $4300 dollars.[4]

The data cited above can be used to estimate the current cost of nosocomial infections to an individual hospital. It is possible to estimate the hypothetical cost of various infection control strategies using a simple spreadsheet. Various degrees of sophistication can be applied to such cost estimates depending upon the availability and reliability of existing data on the incidence of nosocomial infections, payer mix, rehospitalization rates, etc. Even if such data are not available, it is usually possible to develop a basic spreadsheet that provides meaningful data that can be used to define and explain your "product" to hospital administrators. Such spreadsheets are also useful to monitor subsequent cost savings (or increases) and to develop prevention strategies and set priorities.

It is important to realize that the process of assessing costs of nosocomial infections is substantially more complicated than simply assessing the aggregate costs of individual nosocomial infections. There are numerous other cost considerations when assessing the total costs of nosocomial infection. The institutional costs of a poor quality infection control program can be considerable. For example, the costs of poor or ineffective prevention measures (such as ineffective antibiotic prophylaxis); the existing appraisal costs of ineffective, meaningless, or improperly circulated surveillance data; internal failure costs (eg, repeat sterilization of loads that fail sterilization checks); and external failure costs (eg, reoperation for a wound infection) are cumulatively substantial.[15]

One often-neglected aspect of a well-designed infection control program is the economic benefit of a reduction in the costs of poor quality. For example, the waste of unnecessary or ineffective isolation gear and the waste incurred by unnecessary cultures (of staff or patients previously colonized with organisms such as vancomycin-resistant enterococci) can be considerable in many poorly managed infection control programs.

The elements comprising the intrinsic monetary value of an effective infection control program have been reviewed by Dunagan et al.[15] Monetary estimates that focus exclusively on measures to reduce direct operating costs caused by infections overlook savings to be gained by reducing malpractice claims, as well as lost opportunity costs resulting from failure of patients to return for further care. In addition, it is important to focus programs, policies, and practices that eliminate waste through wise product selection, avoid inappropriate use of expensive technology, and address employee safety. There is intrinsic monetary value in maintaining regulatory compliance, patient safety programs, and in programs that decrease the risk of resistant pathogens. Finally, it is important to link monetary arguments for effective infection control programs with an ethical rationale on the need to prevent morbidity and mortality involved with medical errors. In other words, an effective infection control program not only makes economic sense, it is also the right ethical decision for administrators.

FUNDAMENTAL SKILLS

Knowledge about the principles and practice of infectious diseases is the essential requirement of practicing hospital epidemiology, but in itself this is not sufficient to achieve success. Specific training in infection control/epidemiology during your fellowship greatly enhances your ability to take advantage of the opportunities in healthcare epidemiology in your subsequent career. We highly recommend taking the SHEA/CDC training course in healthcare epidemiology during your fellowship or prior to attempting to become a hospital epidemiologist. Such training is helpful, but the critical requirement is an interest in infection control and healthcare epidemiology. That interest must be accompanied by a willingness to learn the fundamental principles of hospital epidemiology. Additional reading, attendance at national meetings, and regular interaction with infection control nurse practitioners and other hospital epidemiologists is necessary and vital for the professional growth and development of all hospital epidemiologists—even those with advanced specific training and years of experience in epidemiology. As in all aspects of infectious diseases, life-long learning is fundamental to success, professional satisfaction, and excellence.

Although knowledge about the diagnosis, epidemiology, and prevention of nosocomial infection is a cornerstone of success in hospital epidemiology, there are many other skills that vie for equal importance as requirements for success in this endeavor. One of the most important of these skills is the ability to communicate. Arrogance, egotism, or "holier than thou" attitudes kill attempts to communicate. Learn to be humble, thoughtful, and appreciative in your interactions. Orderly rational problem-solving skills are also invaluable. Understanding the process of root cause analysis and quality improvement processes are important skills. All successful hospital epidemiologists learn to delegate responsibility and understand that the morale, professional education, growth, respect, and nurturing of their "infection control team" are priorities in virtually every management decision.

The skills required for success in healthcare epidemiology are similar in many ways to success in infectious diseases practice. The skill and respect a specialist earns in clinical infectious diseases often directly benefits one's effectiveness and reputation as a hospital epidemiologist and vice versa. In most cases, the two roles are complementary and mutually beneficial. However, it is important to clearly remember that the two roles are different. These different roles must sometimes be explicitly emphasized. The good of the entire institution and all patients is the paramount concern of a hospital epidemiologist, whereas the clinician is primarily concerned about the welfare of his or her individual patients.

It is vital for hospital epidemiologists to understand how hospitals or healthcare systems function. Hospital epidemiologists must understand and use the lines of authority. It is equally important to fully realize and comprehend who is making the decisions and how decision making occurs. Having an active imagination and ability to "think out of the box" provides new opportunities. Medical training programs seldom teach residents and fellows how to understand and solve the political and personal problems that beset all professionals in virtually any professional endeavor. Effective skills in these areas are vital in hospital epidemiology. It is beyond the scope of this chapter (and beyond our abilities) to effectively teach you these skills in a didactic manner. However, such skills are "learnable' (usually via a wise mentor), and self-learning is possible if there is true motivation, self-awareness, and openness to feedback.

THE PROCESS OF NEGOTIATING

The old axiom,"In business, you do not get what you deserve, you get what you negotiate," is widely quoted because it contains more than a modicum of truth. Actually, negotiation is a process of joint problem solving. When undertaken with careful forethought and a true understanding of basic negotiation skills, the process can be rewarding and useful to both parties in the negotiation. A successful negotiation educates others about one's individual concerns, interests, and needs. Just as important, the process of negotiation allows you to understand the concerns, interests, and needs of the other side. Thereafter, these considerations logically become the basis for a final agreement.

In practice, two basic models of negotiation exist: a confrontational (WIN-LOSE) approach and a collaborative (WIN-WIN) model. Although in practice, outcomes are often neither "wins" or "losses" but somewhere in between. The preceding terminology has utility in explaining two basic approaches to dispute resolution. The WIN-LOSE model is primarily based on taking an initial well-defined positional approach. Beginning a negotiation with a clear-cut position or a demand often seems the most efficient and desirable and thus it is the usual approach taken by many people in traditional disputes concerning money and other contentious issues. In fact, positional bargaining is the only form of negotiation many people know. However, such positional bargaining is often unsuccessful, highly contentious, and stressful. Paradoxically, a WIN-LOSS (positional) approach produces angry losers who will resist vigorously, resent the final agreement, and look for ways to undermine its implementation or success. A WIN-WIN negotiation approach is slower and more difficult; however, it is more likely to help you build long-term relationships, trust, and favorable outcomes. Such an approach is preferred in negotiating a contract for healthcare epidemiology services even though this approach, like any negotiation strategy, sometimes fails.

Negotiation techniques, pitfalls, and styles are extensively described in a practical manner in the excellent book, *Getting to Yes*.[16] This book is a defacto practical primer on the fundamentals of negotiation. The authors discuss a number of key principles. The most important one may be how to avoid "positional" bargaining; in other words, how to avoid talking only about what you are willing and unwilling to accept at the beginning of a negotiation. This approach is frequently a recipe for an unsuccessful negotiation (even if you happen to get what you request). Rather than bargaining over positions, the authors advocate a time-tested and widely used alternative approach called "principled negotiation" or "negotiation on the merits." This method includes four components:

1. Separate the people from the problem ("go to the balcony").
2. Focus on interests, not positions.
3. Generate a variety of possibilities before deciding what to do.
4. Insist that the results be based on some objective standard (to be the basis for the final agreement).

Another important and key concept outlined by the authors of *Getting to Yes* is understanding the concept of BATNA (ie, the "Best Alternative To a Negotiated Agreement"). Whether you should or should not agree on something in a negotiation depends entirely upon the attractiveness of your BATNA. It is also helpful to understand and know your opposition's BATNA. Sometimes it is helpful for the other side to understand your BATNA; yet other times, this information is best withheld during the early phases of negotiation. A clear understanding of one's BATNA greatly helps each side feel satisfied when a negotiation is over. A final result better than one's BATNA is often a success even if the final agreement was less than the original bargaining goal. For example, a hospital epidemiology contract for $20,000 per year may be better than one's BATNA (no income), even if the goal of the original contract negotiation was twice that amount. Similarly, the hospital administrator may leave the same negotiation realizing that his BATNA (no qualified hospi-

tal epidemiologist) was worse than his original position (no payment for hospital epidemiology oversight and management). If objective criteria were used as a basis for the final agreement, the hospital epidemiologist and the administrator have objective criteria to revisit the agreement and modify it at a later date.

Getting past "no" when a negotiation is going badly requires moving from "positions" to "merits" (ie, emphasizing and explaining interests, options, and standards). When negotiations are stalled or otherwise unsuccessful, it is generally best to concentrate on the merits of your and their proposal rather than the positions you or your opponent have expressed. In essence, it is often necessary to change the game by starting to play a new one when the original negotiation has stalled or failed.[16]

Successful negotiators must know their goals and link them to their interests as well as understand their strengths and those of the opposition. It is fundamental that a negotiator understands the needs, attitudes, interests, and positions of the person with whom he or she is negotiating and whom each negotiator represents. Generally, it is unwise to argue about "feelings." On the other hand, it is wise and good to choose your words carefully and listen carefully when the other side talks and then let them know you heard them. Successful negotiators always try to align interests and negotiate for objective criteria to decide contentious issues.

When initial negotiations fail, it is often a good idea to undertake "brainstorming sessions" to develop proposals attractive to the other side. These proposals should address common interests and they should be explicitly presented as proposals rather than final positions. In general, it is a bad idea to make threats or to close the door to future negotiations. It is always wise to be aware of and emphasize the importance of the relationship that precedes and will follow the negotiation.

Negotiating requires preparation and experience. However, it is not necessary to take advanced training to gain such experience. In fact, everyone uses negotiating skills in innumerable interactions with family, neighbors, employees, salesmen, lawyers, etc. When entering a negotiation for hospital epidemiology service or any professional contract, it is useful to remember these three maxims:

1. "You can't control the other side, you can't control the marketplace, but you can control your preparation."
2. "Much is lost for want of asking."
3. "Let us never negotiate out of fear, but let us never fear to negotiate."[17,18]

FUNCTIONAL MODELS OF HEALTHCARE EPIDEMIOLOGY INFECTION CONTROL MANAGEMENT

There are at least four ways that infectious diseases specialists have modeled their functional roles as healthcare epidemiologists. The *basic* model is limited individual institution oversight that may include functioning as chairing the hospital infection control committee, availability and willingness to answer questions of the infection control practitioner, and to "troubleshoot" ad hoc infection control-related problems while providing general support for existing infection control policies—all in the role as a local "opinion leader."

A second model is for an infectious disease specialist to take an expanded role in hospital epidemiology. This *expanded* model includes all of the "basic model" functions and a commitment to meet with the infection control practitioner(s) on a regular basis, directly participate in the education of staff related to infection control issues, and provide general "oversight" of the local infection control program. In most cases, the exact goals and expectations of the infectious diseases specialists are not clearly defined. Although in some cases, a time commitment is specified in the written or oral agreement for services. In many cases, reimbursement is linked directly to the preceding time commitment. If the goals and objectives of oversight and management of the infection control program can be clearly defined and objectively assessed, this model can have a definable value and can be considered a "product" using the criteria discussed previously; however, there can be problems with this model (such as hourly compensation) that will be discussed next.

A third model, the *advanced* model, includes all of the functions described above in the expanded model but also includes oversight of the infection control activities of the institution's entire healthcare system. Such systems may include one or more long-term care facilities or rehabilitation units as well as various outpatient facilities and/or affiliated hospitals. This model has significant potential to provide a valuable "product" to a healthcare system with commensurate compensation for the healthcare epidemiologist.

A fourth model is a *network* or *consortium* model, which is an advanced model that is duplicated at multiple unaffiliated hospitals by offering a menu of services to a potentially unlimited number of institutions. A prototype of this model is the DICON.[12] The DICON model provides a wide variety of resources to affiliated community hospitals, including training and support of local infection control practitioners, assistance with outbreak investigation, education, statistical expertise and analysis of local surveillance data, detailed programs to provide feedback of surveillance data on nosocomial infection, regional and national trends in nosocomial infections, and antimicrobial resistance to local practitioners. In addition, DICON utilizes all surveillance data collected in community hospitals with the explicit goal of providing time trended comparative data for individual hospitals. These data are also used for "benchmarking" of surveillance data on surgical site infections, blood stream infections, blood-borne pathogen exposures by hospital employees, and rates of device-specific infections for patients hospitalized in intensive care units so that individual DICON-affiliated hospitals can compare and contrast their data with hospitals of similar size and type in the region.

HOW TO GET PAID (WHAT IS THE "MARKET VALUE" OF A HOSPITAL EPIDEMIOLOGIST?)

Income potential from hospital epidemiology is related to your imagination, interests, expertise, and negotiating skills. Income also depends on the degree of your involvement and the amount of responsibility and accountability you agree to accept for the hospital epidemiology program.

It has been our experience and impression that too many infectious diseases physicians literally give away their time and expertise in infection control/hospital epidemiology activities. We believe that working as a healthcare epidemiologist and/or a chair of a hospital infection control committee without compensation is unwise. If you do not receive compensation for these positions of responsibility—resign! What have you lost? Your resignation will eliminate several meetings each year from a schedule that is already overloaded. In other words, your resignation from a job that requires substantial time and responsibility will allow you time for work that generates income or for leisure that makes your working hours more enjoyable. If you feel a "citizenship" obligation to your hospital, offer to be on the education committee or any other committee that does not represent the bread and butter of your specialty. If your colleagues or hospital administrators challenge the wisdom of your decision, you might ask them the following: "Do surgical colleagues operate au gratis for the hospital?" or "Do cardiologists donate a catheterization per day to the hospital?" Finally, it may be useful to point out that hospital and healthcare systems that rely on volunteerism for their infection control programs will at worst fail or at best lose important opportunities to be effective.

Determining appropriate compensation for supervision and management of a hospital infection control program is difficult but not impossible. For obvious reasons, there are no published data on the "market-rate" salary range for a hospital epidemiologist. As mentioned previously, the value of your work as hospital epidemiologist has to be defined in terms of your specific and unique job description, the goals of the program, your responsibility, the size of the local hospital, the type of infection control and/or patient safety problems at a specific institution, and objective criteria for performance. Networking with other epidemiologists or your SHEA liaison can give you general ideas of the range of regional or state ranges of compensation.

To our knowledge, no one has attempted to measure the economic value of infectious diseases specialists who function as healthcare or hospital epidemiologists. A SHEA membership survey in 1995 that involved 545 respondents reported that 44% of those responding to the survey received compensation for epidemiology services with an annual mean compensation of $52,000 and median of $40,000.[19] A second membership survey in 1998 involving 494 respondents reported that 60% of respondents received compensation for epidemiological services with an annual mean compensation of $45,700 and median of $40,000 (oral communication, SHEA). Our experience with colleagues involved in hospital epidemiology suggests that annual physician income for hospital epidemiology ranges from $2000 to greater than $250,000. Many healthcare epidemiologists work as employees in academic institutions. Their salaries include income for multiple activities such as research and teaching. Thus, it is frequently difficult or impossible to ascertain the percentage of annual income directly attributable to epidemiology services.

Many hospitals prefer to pay healthcare epidemiologists for each hour of service. Also, many hospital administrators contend that it is easier to defend compensation for hospital epidemiology service when logs of hours spent are provided to the administration who in turn can provide this data to the Center for Medicaid and Medicare Service auditors. We disagree with this approach. One does not "punch in and out" of hospital epidemiology activities like a shift or contract worker. Hospital epidemiological activities are integrated into the daily work of most infectious diseases specialists. Conversations related to infection control issues, controversies, and policies often occur in the context of patient care or in the daily routine of community hospitals. Billing by the hour, as is done by attorneys, is not feasible or practical. Also, the responsibility related to infection control issues is continuous and unpredictable. Decisions and guidance about isolation decisions are often made at night, weekends, or on holidays. Others in positions of leadership in the hospital, such as hospital administrators, are not paid by the hour and neither should a hospital epidemiologist. Indeed, the value of a hospital epidemiologist relates to his or her leadership, responsibility, and obligation to solve problems after hours or during emergencies.

We believe the issue of compensation must be directly related to the overall job description and the value of the total "product." We also believe establishing compensation linked to a "bounty," such as the percentage of money saved from appropriate antibiotic utilization or a specific reduction in the rate of any one infection or type of infection, has the potential to undermine credibility and distort motives. However, this concept is not the same as linking compensation to the overall goals and objectives of a sound business plan. Achieving the goals for such a program is a rationale basis for compensation and subsequent increases in compensation. The process of negotiation described above is the best way to resolve the fundamental question of the "market value" of a hospital epidemiologist.

COMMON DILEMMAS

If your hospital/healthcare system says they can't (or won't) pay for hospital epidemiology/infection control, what do you do? Obviously the answer to this question will vary depending upon the personalities and perceptions of the local administrators and infectious diseases specialist. We can provide the following general advice. First, it is often wise to solicit support for your proposals from key hospital staff (surgeons, pathologists, nursing personnel) to ask for their help and support for reopening negotiations and/or reviewing the respective positions of the involved parties. Second, it is also important to remember your BATNA. Finally, if an agreement that provides adequate compensation for time, effort, and responsibility cannot be successfully negotiated, it may sometimes be necessary to either simply refuse all further interaction with the infection control program, resign from the hospital staff and work at a neighboring hospital, or change your status from active staff to consulting staff. It is important to remember that the preceding are only a partial list of your options should the hospital refuse to negotiate a contract for infection control services. Indeed, you could consider some or all of the following options:

➤ Maintain a relationship with the infection control practitioner and look for opportunities to revisit the original negotiation.

➤ Offer to provide further assistance to the hospital if the need arises... for a price.

➤ Negotiate an agreement to revisit the pay issue in "x" months in exchange for continued participation in infection control/epidemiology activities.

➤ Barter your support for existing programs (such as formulary restrictions, antibiotic approval, or review of high-cost drugs) with the acceptance of an infection control contract.

➤ Negotiate an agreement to examine cost estimates of nosocomial infections at your institution (with or without compensation) in return for your continued participation.

➤ Negotiate an agreement to sponsor a position paper on the deficiencies and strengths of the current infection control program in return for your continued participation.

➤ Negotiate an agreement for the review of the current infection control program from local, regional, or outside experts in exchange for your continued participation in the current infection control program.

➤ Undertake a survey of infection control oversight processes and practices in local and regional peer institutions and provide these data to administration and to key members of the medical staff.

➤ Alternately, it may be best to devise new and innovative proposals such as the following:

➢ Offer to provide "x" presentations to medical and other professional staff about specific topics related to rational antibiotic use, antimicrobial resistance, and nosocomial infections.

➢ Offer to review antimicrobial therapy for each intensive care unit patient on Monday, Wednesday, and Friday mornings and make nonbinding recommendations in the patient's chart.

➢ Offer to supervise the establishment of a database on all patients with MRSA to develop a "scorecard" on nosocomial transmission of MRSA at your hospital.

Numerous other options and ideas undoubtedly exist, and some of these alternatives may be uniquely applicable to an individual hospital or healthcare system. If faced with a refusal to provide reasonable compensation for healthcare epidemiology services, use your imagination and energy to devise alternatives to the rejected plan.

HOSPITAL EPIDEMIOLOGY CONTRACTS

A contract is simply a written set of promises: "I promise to do something for you and, in return, you promise to something for me." The core components of any contract for healthcare epidemiology services should define the healthcare epidemiologist's roles and responsibilities, the lines of authority, and the compensation package. A typical contract for hospital epidemiology services often spec-

ifies access to data, computers, computer software, space, laboratory support, and secretarial support. It is also reasonable to contract for additional money for books, journals, and continuing medical education.

In general, contracts for hospital epidemiology should delineate roles and responsibilities either generically or specifically. Some of the many specific activities suitable for inclusion in a generic contract are outlined in Table 3-1. Although the language and style of most contracts is largely controlled by the attorneys who draft and review such agreements, we have a few specific caveats:

➤ You should never agree to do things that cannot be accomplished or for which you have responsibility but no authority.

➤ You should not spread yourself so thin that you cannot do anything well. It is better to commit to doing a few specific things well than an array of things that are not achievable.

➤ In general, it is best to have authority to supervise people actually involved in infection control activities rather than to rely on the good will of other administrators.

TIPS AND TRICKS OF THE TRADE (HOW TO KEEP YOUR JOB)

We believe the following practical tips and tricks are useful:

➤ Pick one or two major surveillance or intervention projects each year.

➤ Share the knowledge of and credit for your victories with administration, medical, and hospital staff.

➤ Communicate, communicate, communicate (especially with administration—they pay the bill).

➤ Provide feedback data to doctors, nurses, unit, and floor administrators at every opportunity. Repetition in this endeavor is rarely a tactical mistake.

➤ Only collect data that you intend to use.

➤ Use your data as often as possible.

➤ Pick your friends and adversaries carefully (rule of thumb—keep the ratio greater than 10 to 1).

➤ Listen to your adversaries and collect data to refute them.

➤ Bargain with your opponents.

➤ Little successes are important.

➤ Success begets success.

➤ Acknowledge and praise good behavior and good outcomes and use them as building blocks.

➤ Tell the truth politely and tactfully.

➤ Make all decisions based on the "60 Minute" rule (ie, whatever you say or do should play well with Mike Wallace interviewing you on "60 Minutes").

➤ Build slowly (eg, bloodstream infections and surgical site infection surveillance first).

➤ Set goals and develop an annual plan.

➤ Document everything: memos, meetings, and successes.

➤ Keep good records about what you did, when you did it, and why you did it.

➤ Create a monthly newsletter.

➤ Create an annual report to the hospital administration and other key people.

➤ Sponsor an annual symposium.

➤ Short memos are more effective than long memos.

➤ How you say something is as important, if not more important, than what you say.

➤ Avoid meetings when possible; when not possible, keep them short.

➤ Always set the meeting agenda and define the purpose at the beginning of each meeting.

➤ Make your decisions and get your votes before a meeting is held.

➤ Control the meeting agenda and watch the clock.

➤ Start meetings on time and finish early.

➤ Summarize at the end of the meeting.

➤ If there are tasks to be done after the meeting, do your task and follow up on those of others.

➤ Do not play the "They do not appreciate me" game.

➤ Do not fight with people when the outcome is not worth the fight (choose your enemies carefully).

➤ Learn to simplify your message (but have a message).

➤ Document your positions and big decisions with follow-up memos and letters.

➤ Do not ask for big things at big meetings unless you have notified your allies and solicited their support.

➤ Never say never and never say always.

➤ Note all cost savings.

➤ Establish local cost estimates using local infection control data.

➤ Assume that most people want to do the right thing. If they are not doing the right thing, assume the reason is lack of understanding rather than malice.

CONCLUSION

There is no limit to the opportunities available to healthcare epidemiologists with imagination and energy. Your skills as an infectious diseases specialist are extreme-

ly valuable. If you believe in your value as a healthcare epidemiologist and if you can explain this value to others and negotiate effectively, you can achieve appropriate monetary compensation and successfully fill an important and satisfying role. It is the right thing to do!

Finally, we advise you to remember these words: "A fair day's wages for a fair days work, it is as just a demand as governed men ever made of government. It is the everlasting right of man."[18]

REFERENCES

1. Slama TG, Sexton DJ, Ingram CW, Petrak RM, Joseph P. Findings of the 1998 Infectious Diseases Society of America membership survey. *Clin Infect Dis.* 2000;31: 1396-1402.

2. Stone WP, Larson E, Kawar LN. A systematic audit of economic evidence linking nosocomial infections and infectious control interventions: 1990-2000. *Am J Infect Control.* 2002;30(3):145-152.

3. Haley RW. Incidence and nature of endemic and epidemic nosocomial infections. In: Bennett JV, Brachman P, eds. *Hospital Infections.* Boston: Little, Brown; 1985:359-374.

4. Inflation Data. Inflation calculator. Available at: http://www.inflationdata.com/inflation/inflation_rate/infla tioncalculator.asp. Accessed July 22, 2004.

5. Graves N. Economics and preventing hospital-acquired infection. *Emerg Infect Dis.* 2004;10(4):561-566.

6. Fraser VJ, Olsen MA. The business of healthcare epidemiology: creating a vision for service excellence. *Am J Infect Control.* 2002;30(2):77-85.

7. Hollenbeak CS, Murphy DM, Koenig S, Woodward RS, Dunagan WC, Fraser VF. The clinical and economic impact of deep chest surgical-site infections following coronary artery bypass graft surgery. *Chest.* 2000;118: 397-402.

8. Hollenbeak CS, Murphy D, Dunagan WC, Fraser VS. Nonrandom selection and the attributable cost of surgical-site infections. *Infect Control Hosp Epidemiol.* 2002; 23(4):177-182.

9 Warren DK, Shukla SJ, Olsen MA, et al. Outcome and attributable cost of ventilator-associated pneumonia among intensive care unit patients in a suburban medical center. *Crit Care Med.* 2003;31(5):1312-1317.

10. Kirkland KB, Briggs JR, Trivette SL, Wilkinson WP, Sexton DJ. The impact of surgical-site infections in the 1990s: attributable mortality, excess length of hospitalizations, and extra costs. *Infect Control Hosp Epidemiol.* 1999; 20(11):725-730.

11. Whitehouse JD, Friedman ND, Kirkland KB, Richardson WI, Sexton DJ. The impact of surgical-site infections following orthopedic surgery at a community hospital and a university hospital: adverse quality of life, excess length of stay, and extra cost. *Infect Control Hosp Epidemiol.* 2002; 23(4):183-189.

12. Kaye KS, Engemann JE, Fulmer EM, Clark CC, Noga EM, Sexton DJ. Favorable impact of an infection control network on nosocomial infection rates in community hospital. *Infect Control Hosp Epidemiol*. 2004. In press.

13. Panlilo AL, Cardo DM, Campbell S, Srivastava PU, Jagger H, Orelien JG. Estimate of the annual number of percutaneous injuries in U.S. healthcare workers [Abstract S-T2-01]. *Program and Abstracts of the 4th International Conference on Nosocomial and Healthcare-associated Infections*. 2000:61.

14. United States General Accounting Office. Occupational safety: selected cost and benefit implications of needle stick prevention devices for hospitals. GAO-01-6OR; November 17, 2000.

15. Dunagan WC, Murphy DM, Hollenbeak CS, Miller SB. Making the business case for infection control: pitfalls and opportunities. *Am J Infect Control*. 2002;30(2):86-92.

16. Fisher R, Ury W, Patton B. *Getting to Yes*. New York, NY: Penguin Books; 1991.

17. Bunyan J. The pilgrim's progress, in the similitude of a dream: the second part. Paras. 112. In: Eliot CW, ed. *The Harvard Classics* vol. 15, part 1. New York, NY: PF Collier and Son; 1909-1914.

18. Kaplan J, ed. *Bartlett's Familiar Quotations*—17th Edition. Boston, New York, London: Little, Brown and Company; 2002: 434.24, 799.8.

19. Membership survey. *SHEA Newsletter*. 1997;6:4.

CHAPTER FOUR

ETHICAL ASPECTS OF INFECTION CONTROL

Loreen A. Herwaldt, MD and Lauris C. Kaldjian, MD

INTRODUCTION

Hospital epidemiologists and ICPs make countless decisions every day. In general, we do not make life and death decisions such as whether to withdraw life support or whether to withhold possibly life-sustaining therapies. Few of our decisions require court injunctions or provide the fodder for eager journalists. We simply decide whether to isolate patients, whether to let healthcare workers (HCWs) continue to work, or whether to investigate clusters of infections—all very routine decisions in the life of anyone who practices infection control. These decisions are so ordinary that they could not possibly have any ethical implications. Or could they?

In fact, many of the decisions we make everyday, even those we consider quite straightforward, are also ethical decisions—which is to say, they compel us to choose between competing moral values. Such choices are rarely easy, and their intrinsic difficulty is not eased by the fact that few of us have received more than cursory training in ethics. Moreover, if we attempt to train ourselves, we find that very little has been written about the ethics of our specialty, infection control. The following is brief introduction to the intricate intersection of ethics and infection control.

TAXONOMY

To date, no one has developed a taxonomy of ethical problems in infection control. On the basis of our experience in infection control and ethics, we have developed a taxonomy that we think will be helpful to infection control personnel as they think about their own work (Table 4-1).

This taxonomy not only describes the most important ethical problems in infection control, but it also helps us define the individuals, groups, and organizations to which infection control personnel have specific obligations. In particular, infection control personnel have obligations to inpatients and outpatients as groups, to individual patients, to visitors as a group, to individual visitors, to HCWs as a group, to individual HCWs, to the HCF for which they work, to public health entities both local and federal, to facilities to which their facility refers or transfers patients, to referring or transferring facilities, and to the public in general. The interests of these different groups are often in competition. We can use the taxonomy to help us identify the type of ethical problem that we are facing and the competing obligations that may surround that problem.

AN APPROACH TO ETHICAL PROBLEMS IN INFECTION CONTROL

Most discussions of medical ethics ignore the epidemiologist-population relationship and concentrate instead on the clinician-patient relationship.[1,2] Infection control personnel are frequently clinicians; however, we must differentiate their clinical and epidemiologic roles because their fiduciary duties do not always coincide. Medical ethics are "person-oriented," while epidemiologic ethics are "population-oriented" (Table 4-2).[3,4] Even so, the standard principles of medical ethics also apply to hospital epidemiology. These principles are:

➤ Autonomy (respecting the decisions of competent patients)

➤ Beneficence (doing good)

➤ Nonmaleficence (doing no harm)

➤ Justice (fairness and the equitable allocation of resources)[5,6]

TABLE 4-1. A TAXONOMY OF ETHICAL PROBLEMS IN INFECTION CONTROL

Control of Patient to Limit Spread of Pathogenic Organisms

Isolating patients who are colonized or infected with resistant organisms
Isolating patients who are infected with highly infectious/dangerous organisms

Control of Healthcare Workers to Limit Spread of Pathogenic Organisms

Restricting activities of HCWs who have been exposed to IDs
Restricting activities of HCWs who have IDs

Control of Medications to Limit Selection and Spread of Antimicrobial Resistance

Limit antimicrobial agents on hospital formulary
Develop guidelines regarding use of antimicrobial agents
Provide computer decision support to guide selection of antimicrobial agents

Mandating or Recommending Best Practice and Interventions to Reduce the Risk of Infection

Mandate or recommend treatment to eradicate carriage of resistant pathogens
Mandate implementation of isolation precautions
Mandate pre-employment vaccinations and/or immunity to certain pathogens
Organize and promote yearly influenza vaccine campaigns
Develop policies and procedures
Mandate postexposure testing of patients and HCWs
Mandate postexposure prophylactic treatment of patients and HCWs

Resource Allocation

Establish a threshold for investigating clusters of infections
Evaluate products to assess cost vs. safety and efficacy
Determine whether single-use items may be reused
Guide choices regarding materials, design, number of sinks, etc., for construction projects (cost vs. safety)
Limit hospital formularies to reduce costs and control antimicrobial resistance

Information Disclosure

Report exposure risks to staff and patients
Report outbreaks and reportable diseases to the public health department
Provide access to data on nosocomial infection rates
Identify patients colonized with resistant organisms before intra- or interinstitutional transfers
Protect confidentiality of patients' medical records and laboratory specimens
Protect identity of index cases of outbreaks
Protect confidentiality of patients who are HIV positive

Conflicting and Competing Interests

Manage Outbreaks

Staff, especially institutional leaders, may refuse to comply
The administration may balk at the cost of investigating outbreaks
Hospital epidemiologists who chose unpopular interventions may lose referrals and revenue

Manage Exposures

Staff members, especially institutional leaders, may refuse to comply

Select the Hospital Formulary

Relationships between staff on formulary committee and the pharmaceutical industry may compromise decisions
Staff physicians prefer specific agents not on the formulary

Individual Professionalism

Act altruistically (personal convenience vs. prompt intervention)
Mediate in-house disputes between administrators, clinicians, unions, hospital
Act when necessary despite inadequate or conflicting data
Keep up with new developments in field

Personal

Protect self from acquiring IDs
Protect family from acquiring secondary infections

TABLE 4-2. Differences in Emphasis Between Epidemiologic Ethics and Medical Ethics

	Epidemiologic Ethics	*Medical Ethics*
Scope of concern	Populations	Individuals
Goal	Prevent infection	Treat infection
Typical principles	Nonmaleficence	Beneficence
	Justice (fairness)	Respect for patient autonomy
Purpose of disclosure	Investigation	Diagnosis
Information handling	Confidential reporting	Confidential documentation

1. State the problem plainly
2. Gather and organize data
   a. Medical facts
   b. Goals and procedures of infection control
   c. Interests of patients, HCWs, hospital, and community
   d. Context
3. Ask: Is the problem ethical?
4. Ask: Is more information or discussion needed?
5. Determine the best course of action and support it with reference to one or more sources of ethical value:
   a. *Ethical Principles*: Beneficence, nonmaleficence, respect for autonomy, justice
   b. *Rights*: Protections that are independent of professional obligations
   c. *Consequences*: Estimating the goodness or desirability of likely outcomes
   d. *Comparable cases*: Reasoning by analogy from prior "clear" cases
   e. *Professional guidelines*: Example: APIC/CHICA-Canada professional practice standards
   f. *Conscientious practice*: Preserving epidemiologists' personal and professional integrity
6. Confirm the adequacy and coherence of the conclusion

Figure 4-1. An approach to ethical problems in infection control.

However, the principles are applied according to the public health model,[6] which requires commitment to improving the health of populations, not only individual patients.[7] Although both medical and epidemiologic ethics stress nonmaleficence and confidentiality, medical ethics emphasizes privacy and epidemiologic ethics emphasizes investigation and reporting to protect the population. Furthermore, medical ethics stresses patient autonomy, whereas epidemiologic ethics places special priority on justice. Put more practically, medical ethics demands that the clinician treat an infected patient while maintaining the patient's confidentiality, privacy, dignity, freedom, and contact with other human beings (see Table 4-2). In contrast, epidemiologic ethics might stress treating both infected and colonized patients to protect patients and HCWs. In particular cases, epidemiologic ethics might require HCWs to post labels on medical records and on the doors to the patients' rooms; insist that patients stay in their rooms except when going to essential tests, in which case they must wear gowns, gloves, and masks; or require HCWs to wear gowns, gloves, and masks to avoid direct contact with patients.

By now, it should be clear that ethically challenging situations are common in the practice of infection control and hospital epidemiology. To respond effectively to these challenges, infection control staff members must address each problem systematically. Kaldjian and colleagues developed an approach to ethics that is clinically oriented and helps the user state the problem clearly, collect data comprehensively, formulate an impression, and finally articulate a justified plan.[8] In outline form, we present a modified version of this approach tailored to the particular demands of infection control (Figure 4-1), and we employ this approach (in abbreviated form) as we discuss 4 core topics.

ETHICAL CORE TOPICS IN INFECTION CONTROL

Staff Vaccination Programs

Vaccines have been one of the public health movement's major triumphs during the 20th century, and in that very triumph are the seeds of a substantial controversy and an ethical problem. Because vaccines effectively decreased the incidence of many IDs, the public no longer remembers how dreadful these diseases were and how many complications and deaths these infections caused. The public is now more aware of the complications of vaccines than they are of the diseases the vaccines were developed to prevent. In addition, parents of "vaccine damaged children," the natural health movement, television, radio talk shows, and the Internet have all become important "players" or "instruments" in this debate.[9,10]

The controversy about the pertussis vaccine is illustrative. In the 1940s, pertussis was the leading cause of death in children younger than 14 years of age. Pertussis, in fact, killed more children than measles, scarlet fever, diphtheria, polio, and meningitis combined.[11] The incidence of pertussis was already decreasing before the killed whole cell vaccine was introduced, probably related to changes in social conditions, hygiene, and nutrition. However, the incidence declined significantly after the vaccine was introduced.[12]

The pertussis vaccine includes many toxic components because it is composed of dead gram-negative bacteria. Thus, it is quite reactogenic. Recipients often have significant pain, swelling, and erythema at the vaccine site, and they may develop fever, irritability, and any of a number of other systemic reactions, including even seizures.[13] The most severe complication of the pertussis vaccine is encephalopathy, which is very rare.[13] Opponents of the vaccine also allege that the vaccine not infrequently causes serious permanent neurological damage. In countries like Sweden, Japan, and the United Kingdom, the antivaccine movements gained such prominence that the countries either stopped vaccinating children or the rate of vaccination dropped significantly. All of these countries had subsequent outbreaks of pertussis that affected thousands of children and caused numerous deaths.[13]

The controversy over the pertussis vaccine suggests that the ethical debate over vaccines in both the public health arena and in the hospital revolves around providing the greatest good for the greatest number of people (ie, protecting them against harmful infections) and protecting the individual from harm that could be caused by a vaccination. The ethical dilemma occurs because, in highly vaccinated populations, a single person can elect to refuse a vaccine and may be able to avoid both the potential complications of the vaccination and the infection itself because he or she is protected by the vaccinated group.[14-18] However, the question arises as to whether this is fair to the people who took the risk and were vaccinated. Furthermore, if this scenario is repeated many times, the vaccination rate in the population will drop, and the non-immune people will be at risk.

The ethical dilemma described above also occurs in facilities that mandate that HCWs must be immune to certain infections. For example, most HCFs require that HCWs be immune to rubella, which means that employees

must present proof that they either had the infection or that they had at least 2 rubella vaccinations. The reasons HCFs have this requirement are that rubella is easily transmitted within HCFs and that this virus can cause severe congenital defects if a pregnant woman becomes infected.[19,20] However, the individual healthcare provider may not benefit from receiving this vaccine because rubella causes very mild disease in adults, and an adult vaccine recipient might develop complications. Thus, the hospital puts limits on the autonomy of its staff members and limits their freedom in order to be beneficent to their pregnant patients and employees.

The approach many facilities take to influenza vaccine illustrates another extreme. The influenza virus is quite contagious and can cause serious complications, hospitalization, and death among elderly people and those with significant underlying diseases. HCFs, particularly hospitals, care for many people who are at risk for complications of influenza. Thus, many hospitals offer the vaccine free of charge to employees each fall. But employees usually are not required to take the vaccine in order to work with high-risk patients.[21] Consequently, outbreaks of influenza have occurred in HCFs. These outbreaks are difficult to recognize and, therefore, are underreported.[22] In this case, hospitals have elected not to mandate a safe and effective vaccine that could prevent at least as many severe complications as does the rubella vaccine. Instead, they have elected to preserve their HCWs' autonomy and freedom rather than insist that vulnerable patients must be treated in an environment with the least risk of acquiring influenza.[21]

Why do hospitals choose to manage rubella one way and influenza another? To our knowledge, no one has studied this issue. However, we speculate about why this might be so. A single child who is born with congenital rubella is very dramatic, noticed, and considered a tragedy. The deaths of 100 elderly people who get influenza and then die of secondary bacterial pneumonia or congestive heart failure (CHF) are far less dramatic because we expect "old people" to get sick and die. Similarly, a damaged child represents many impaired life years, whereas, a frail elderly person who dies represents very few life years lost. In addition, because influenza outbreaks in HCFs are rarely recognized, most hospitals probably feel the risk to the patients is very low. On the other hand, the hospital would face a huge lawsuit if a woman could document that she acquired rubella while receiving prenatal care in that facility. The different approaches to rubella vaccine and influenza vaccine present major ethical issues. But these issues are rarely recognized and discussed even though employees' autonomy and freedom of choice do become prominent issues in HCFs.

We believe that HCWs have a moral obligation to restrict their own freedom when it comes to complying with interventions such as influenza vaccine if in so doing they might help preserve their patients' health. Rea and Upshur take this position in their commentary entitled *Semmelweis Revisited: The Ethics of Infection Prevention Among Health Care Workers*.[21]

"As Harris and Holm wrote of society in general, 'There seems to be a strong prima facie obligation not to harm others by making them ill where this is avoidable.'[23] But there is a special duty of care for us as physicians not simply to avoid transmission once infected, but to avoid infection in the first place whenever reasonable. Our patients come to us specifically for help in staying or getting well. We have not just the general obligation of any member of our community, but a particular trust: first do no harm."[20]

Isolating Patients Colonized or Infected With Resistant Organisms

The incidence of resistant microorganisms, particularly MRSA and VRE, has increased substantially over time. One of the primary roles for infection control personnel is to protect patients from acquiring pathogenic organisms, including these resistant organisms, from other patients, the environment, and HCWs. Infection control personnel have several means to accomplish this goal: educating staff, implementing isolation precautions (with or without active screening programs to identify carriers), implementing hand hygiene programs, controlling the use of antimicrobial agents, and developing cleaning protocols for patients' rooms and equipment. Of these methods for controlling spread of resistant organisms, implementing isolation precautions with or without active screening and controlling use of antimicrobial agents have been quite controversial and are associated with significant ethical issues. We will discuss ethical implications of isolation precautions in this section and ethical implications of formularies in the next. We will first address the arguments for and against controlling spread of MRSA and VRE and then the arguments for and against using isolation precautions to limit spread. Subsequently, we will discuss the ethical issues associated with isolating patients who are colonized or infected with MRSA or VRE.

There are numerous reasons to control spread of MRSA and VRE. Both organisms can cause serious infections.[24-27] Because MRSA and VRE are resistant to the first-line antimicrobial agents used to treat serious infections caused by *S. aureus* and enterococci, these infections may be difficult and expensive to treat. Moreover, if the genes for resistance are transferred from VRE to MRSA creating vancomycin-resistant *S. aureus* (VRSA), as has already occurred on at least 2 occasions,[28,29] such strains might be virtually untreatable with currently available antimicrobial agents. Data from numerous institutions document the effectiveness of aggressive control measures.[25] Infection control personnel who take this position would

also argue that as healthcare professionals we should first do no harm. MRSA and VRE harm many patients. Therefore, infection control programs are obliged to use reasonable means to prevent selection and spread of these organisms.[25]

Other infection control personnel argue to the contrary that there are numerous reasons not to invest substantial resources and time into efforts to control MRSA and VRE.[27,30] They insist that the incidence of these organisms is already so high that control measures are ineffective and waste precious resources. They would agree that aggressive measures have worked in some instances, primarily in outbreaks, but that the data on the overall incidence of MRSA and VRE indicate that infection control efforts have failed to stop transmission. They also argue that many colonized patients never become infected, colonization per se does not hurt these patients, and MRSA and VRE are not more virulent and do not cause greater morbidity and mortality than methicillin-susceptible *Staphylococcus aureus* (MSSA) and vancomycin-susceptible enterococci (VSE). Thus, these patients should not be subjected to treatment or to isolation. These infection control personnel also state that efforts to control MRSA and VRE impair patient care and, therefore, may actually cause worse patient outcomes than would have occurred if the patients were not isolated.[31-33] Finally, they would argue that eradication programs with agents such as mupirocin may actually increase antimicrobial resistance.[34]

Some infection control experts would argue that the real question is not whether to invest resources in attempts to control MRSA and VRE, but which means should be used to control spread. The major issue in this discussion is whether to use intensive active surveillance with contact isolation to control spread of these organisms[25,35-37] or to enhance compliance with standard precautions and hand hygiene.[30] The crux of this debate revolves around differing interpretations of the extant data. Those who support active surveillance and use of contact isolation believe that the data strongly support this approach,[25,36] while those who support enhancing general infection control precautions believe either that current data suggest these measures are not effective[30] or that more data are needed before hospitals spend large amounts of money and time doing active surveillance.[37]

As suggested in the preceding paragraphs, the major ethical dilemma with respect to using contact isolation to control spread of resistant organisms is that the health interests of patients who are not colonized or infected with a resistant organism conflict with those of the patients who are colonized or infected with one or more of these organisms. Both sides in this debate tell horror stories of what happened to patients when contact precautions were not used or when they were used. The authors of this chapter are aware of these arguments and stories and, in general, believe the arguments are stronger on the side of using contact isolation to protect patients from acquiring resistant organisms. We believe that the problems caused by contact precautions can be eliminated or ameliorated significantly if HCWs are educated properly and are taught to be flexible in the way they apply contact precautions and if there are an appropriate number of staff to care for patients in isolation. In addition, we believe that resistant organisms are often spread because contact precautions are breached. Thus, contact precautions have not failed; HCWs have failed to use contact precautions properly.

Inclusion and Restriction of Drugs by Formulary Committees

Infection control personnel routinely serve as members of hospital formulary committees that determine whether the pharmacy will stock particular antimicrobial agents and whether to restrict use of particular agents. Data from the literature suggest that up to 50% of antimicrobial usage in US hospitals is inappropriate. Thus, numerous investigators have attempted to identify mechanisms by which inappropriate use of antimicrobial agents can be reduced in order to curb costs and reduce the rate at which drug-resistant organisms are selected by antimicrobial pressure. Limiting which agents are on the healthcare organization's formulary appears to be the most direct method of accomplishing these goals.[38-40]

Ideally, formulary committees would make their decisions about antimicrobials based on explicit criteria and data from clinical, epidemiological, and pharmacoeconomic studies. However, some observers have suggested that additional factors, which are often not made explicit, such as clinicians' anecdotal clinical experience (positive or negative); personal or institutional financial interests; relationships with pharmaceutical industry representatives developed through interactions about clinical, educational, or research issues; or the demands of managed care organizations, may influence the decision-making process. The influence of the pharmaceutical industry is of special concern because studies have demonstrated that marketing strategies powerfully influence physicians' choices.[41]

Janknegt and Steenhoek have proposed that formulary committees use an evidence-based process to select drugs. These investigators created a "System of Objectified Judgment Analysis" (SOJA) that they believe helps formulary committees minimize the subjective biases that may hinder the committee's ability to make rational decisions.[42] Most importantly, Janknegt and Steenhoek insist that the committees *prospectively* define their selection criteria. These investigators recommend using 8 general criteria: clinical efficacy, incidence and severity of adverse effects, dosage frequency, drug interactions, acquisition cost, documentation (strength of evidence), pharmacoki-

netics, and pharmaceutical aspects.[42] In addition to these criteria, the investigators added group-specific criteria (eg, development of resistance when considering antimicrobial agents) for different classes of drugs. A panel of experts in a given field scores each drug in a class and gives each criterion a relative weight. Clinicians and pharmacists can apply this evidence-based expertise within the context of their local situations. Software has been developed to accommodate clinicians who want to modify the relative weights assigned to specific criteria by the experts because some decisions about relative weights may be controversial.[42] *Transparency* is a particular virtue of this selection process: Committees must make explicit the criteria (and their relative weights) upon which they base their decisions. This strategy also prevents committees from basing decisions on only a single criterion, such as cost.

Subjective interpretation cannot be entirely eliminated from the process that formulary committees use to make decisions; however, committees that implement procedures like SOJA can minimize the influence of personal or financial biases. Healthcare organizations can increase the transparency of this process by requiring committee members to disclose conflicts of interests, such as financial interests in pharmaceutical companies or products in a manner parallel to the disclosure statements required by journal editors and meeting planners. Healthcare organizations should hold to the highest standards of integrity and, thus, should require people who have conflicts of interest to remove themselves from voting on drugs or drug classes that pertain to those conflicts.[43] Similarly, healthcare organizations should consider whether criteria for membership on the formulary committee should include the absence of such conflicts of interest.

Postexposure Testing and Prophylaxis for Human Immunodeficiency Virus

HCWs knowingly accept the risks that they may be exposed to HIV through their work, and that if they are exposed, they may become infected with this virus. The risk of HIV infection is small but measurable. The average risk of HIV transmission is estimated to be 0.3% after percutaneous exposures to HIV-infected blood and 0.09% after mucous membrane exposures. Fortunately, exposure of intact skin to contaminated blood has not been found to be a risk for transmission. The CDC recommends postexposure prophylaxis (PEP) to diminish the risk of infection, as evidenced by seroconversion. This recommendation is based on direct and indirect evidence for the efficacy of prophylactic treatment and an overall positive risk-benefit ratio for treating exposed people prophylactically.[44] Although PEP decreases the risk of transmission, it is not 100% protective, and it is not without risks: at least 50% of treated people experience adverse drug reactions and about one third do not adhere to the treatment protocol. In addition, PEP may adversely affect the fetus if a pregnant woman is treated for an HIV exposure. Moreover, there is still much about PEP that we do not understand. For example, we do not know why 99.7% of exposed people do not become infected, we do not know how long after exposure PEP can be started and still be effective, and we have not identified the optimal duration of PEP or which regimens are most effective and safe. Gerberding recently reviewed the medical complexity surrounding PEP.[45]

After an exposure, PEP may be instituted based on an assessment of the risk of infection, the expected benefit of treatment, the risks of treatment, and the likelihood that the virus is susceptible to antiretroviral agents. The results of the source's HIV antibody testing are essential because, in the absence of symptoms of acute antiretroviral syndrome, negative test results mean that the risk of transmission can be assumed to be near zero. This would allow discontinuation of PEP that had been started empirically.

Conflict can arise if a potential source patient refuses to be tested. This situation presents a stressful ethical and legal dilemma that requires the HCW who is requesting permission to obtain the test to sensitively identify and address the causes of the patient's reluctance and still attempt to persuade the source patient to be tested. Such persuasion is justified because the source patient's serologic status determines whether the exposed HCW should take PEP, a fairly toxic combination of medications.

HCWs who evaluate the source patient must follow relevant local policies and regulations. These policies can vary substantially. Some states require consent from the source patient before blood is tested for HIV antibody and make stipulations about subsequent confidentiality surrounding a positive test result.[46] Other states presume consent, holding that "the individual to whom the HCW was exposed is deemed to consent to a test to determine the presence of HIV infection in that individual and is deemed to consent to notification of the care provider of the HIV test result."[47]

Situations in which source patients refuse to be tested are clearly ethical in that they pose problems related to ethical values, obligations, and rights. Infection control personnel who wish to use an organized ethical approach to these situations must carefully and sensitively assess the medical facts, the interests of all parties involved, and the particular context that surrounds the patient's refusal. To do this, infection control personnel may need to talk in-depth with the source patient about his or her concerns regarding testing, to explain the rationale behind testing, and to help enhance trust between the patient and the healthcare team. After this process is complete, not only may the risk of transmission be better defined, but also the interpersonal issues may be resolved to the point that the source patient and the healthcare team reach a consensus. In some cases, the source patient and the healthcare team may still disagree. At this point, infection control person-

nel may need to help identify a course of action that balances the interests of all involved people.

In such discussions, different ethical principles pertain to the exposed healthcare worker and to the source patient; beneficence, nonmaleficence, and justice (ie, fairness) are relevant for the exposed HCW, and autonomy is the primary principle that pertains to the source patient and his or her insistence on privacy and noninterference. Both the exposed HCW and the source patient have rights in these situations. The exposed worker has the positive right to assistance that does not impose significantly on others and the source patient has the negative right to be left alone. These situations are never easy but infection control personnel who prospectively think through the potential areas of conflict will be better able to resolve the situations when they occur.

ETHICAL CODES

Ethical codes emphasize a profession's core values and may help guide decisions and behavior. To our knowledge, neither the SHEA nor the APIC, the 2 societies concerned with infection control, have developed codes of ethics. Recently, APIC and the Community and Hospital Infection Control Association—Canada (CHICA-Canada) published a manuscript describing "professional and practice standards" for people practicing infection control.[48]

A well-developed and clearly stated ethical code is an essential guide, yet it is also insufficient. A code of ethics cannot identify all of the ethical dilemmas that individuals will face in the course of their practices. Alone, it cannot ensure ethical behavior. It must be taught, learned, affirmed, and lived if it is to affect our practice. An institution that acts not as it preaches encourages unethical behavior, at least implicitly. Institutions reward the conduct they prize.

As our financial and staff resources are stressed and as the pressures under which we work intensify, temptation amplifies. Barbara Ley Toffler of Resources for Responsible Management states:

> For many employees, being ethical is getting to be too risky—something they can't afford any more... The problem grows out of what I call the "move it" syndrome... That's when the boss tells a subordinate to "move it"—just get it done, meet the deadline, don't ask for more money, time, or people, just do it—and so it goes on down the line. For American companies, this peril from within is as serious as outside threats from competitors. As more employers are forced to "move it," companies are increasingly vulnerable—legally, financially, and morally—to the unethical actions of decent people trying to [move it just to keep their jobs].[49]

PRACTICAL ADVICE

What can you as an individual hospital epidemiologist or ICP do? We would recommend that you think about your job and identify the most common questions that you answer. Once you have identified the questions, you can try to identify the ethical dilemmas presented by those decisions. You can then develop a plan for dealing with the issues before you face them again, as one can usually think more clearly and dispassionately when not in the middle of a crisis. When designing such plans, you should obtain help, if necessary or prudent, from experts in medicine, law, ethics, or other appropriate disciplines.

We have described but a few of the manifold ethical challenges that confront us. Against our ambitions and our fears, we have only our values, commitments, and continual self-examination to rely on. Are we here to serve ourselves or to protect the health of patients and HCWs? Are we seeking to keep our jobs or are we pursuing beneficial knowledge?

As difficult as these questions may be, we must ask them or risk unethical conduct. In the quiet of our consciences, we must grade our answers candidly, guarding against our capacity to rationalize decisions that are expedient. We cannot afford to ignore the ethical aspects of infection control because in neglecting ethics we risk losing sight of our profession's goal—the health of individuals and populations.

ACKNOWLEDGEMENT

The authors thank Dr. Daniel Diekema for critiquing the chapter and suggesting helpful revisions.

REFERENCES

1. Jonsen AR. Do no harm. *Ann Intern Med*. 1978;88:827-832.
2. Last JM. Ethical issues in public health. In: *Public Health and Human Ecology*. East Norwalk, CT: Appleton & Lange; 1987:351-370.
3. IEA workshop on ethics, health policy and epidemiology. Proposed ethics guidelines for epidemiologists. *American Public Health Association Newsletter* (Epidemiology Section). 1990;Winter:4-6.
4. Beauchamp TL, Childress JF. *Principles of Biomedical Ethics*. 2nd ed. New York, NY: Oxford University Press; 1983.
5. Soskolne CL. Epidemiology: questions of science, ethics, morality, and law. *Am J Epidemiol*. 1989;129:1-18.
6. Herman AA, Soskolne CL, Malcoe L, Lilienfeld DE. Guidelines on ethics for epidemiologists. *Int J Epidemiol*. 1991;20:571-572.
7. Beauchamp TL, Cook RR, Fayerweather WE, et al. Appendix: ethical guidelines for epidemiologists. *J Clin Epidemiol*. 1991;44(1 suppl):151S-169S.
8. Kaldjian LC, Weir RF, Duffy TD. A clinician's approach to ethical reasoning. *J Gen Intern Med*. In press.
9. Clements CJ, Evans G, Dittman S, Reeler AV. Vaccine safety concerns everyone. *Vaccine*. 1999;17:S90-S94.
10. Freed GL, Katz SL, Clark SJ. Safety of vaccinations: Miss America, the media, and the public health. *JAMA*. 1996;276:1869-1872.
11. Gordon JE, Hood HI. Whooping cough and its epidemiological anomalies. *Am J Med Sci*. 1951;222:333-361.
12. Cherry JD. The epidemiology of pertussis and pertussis immunization in the United Kingdom and the United States: a comparative study. *Curr Probl Pediatr*. 1984;14:1-78.
13. Mortimer EA. Pertussis vaccine. In: Plotkin SA, Mortimer EA, eds. *Vaccine*. Philadelphia, Pa: WB Saunders Company; 1988.
14. Diekema DS. Public health issues in pediatrics. In: Post SG, ed. *The Encyclopedia of Bioethics*. 3rd ed. Farmington Hills, Mich: Thomson Gale; 2003.
15. Bazin H. The ethics of vaccine usage in society: lessons from the past. *Endeavour*. 2001;25:104-108.
16. Ulmer JB, Liu MA. Ethical issues for vaccines and immunization. *Natl Rev Immunol*. 2002;2:291-296.
17. Vermeersch E. Individual rights versus societal duties. *Vaccine*. 1999;17:S14-S17.
18. Hodges FM, Svoboda JS, Van Howe RS. Prophylactic interventions on children: balancing human rights with public health. *J Med Ethics*. 2002;28:10-16.
19. Poland GA, Nichol KL. Medical students as sources of rubella and measles outbreaks. *Arch Intern Med*. 1990;150:44-46.
20. Anonymous. Control and prevention of rubella: Evaluation and management of suspected outbreaks, rubella in pregnant women, and surveillance for congenital rubella syndrome. *MMWR Morb Mortal Wkly Rep*. 2001;50:1-23.
21. Rea E, Upshur R. Semmelweis revisited: the ethics of infection prevention among health care workers. *Can Med Assoc J*. 2001;164:1447-1448.
22. Evans ME, Hall KL, Berry SE. Influenza control in acute care hospitals. *Am J Infect Control*. 1997;25:357-362.
23. Harris J, Holm S. Is there a moral obligation not to infect others? *BMJ*. 1995;311:1215-1217.
24. Herwaldt LA. Control of methicillin-resistant *Staphylococcus aureus* in the hospital setting. *Am J Med*. 1999;106(5A):11S-18S.
25. Muto CA, Jernigan JA, Ostrowsky BE, et al. SHEA guideline for preventing nosocomial transmission of multidrug-resistant strains of *Staphylococcus aureus* and Enterococcus. *Infect Control Hosp Epidemiol*. 2003;24:362-386.

26. Farr BM. Protecting long-term care patients from antibiotic resistant infections: ethics, cost-effectiveness, and reimbursement issues. *J Am Geriatr Soc*. 2000;48:1340-1342.

27. Ostrowsky B, Steinberg JT, Farr B, Sohn AH, Sinkowitz-Cochran RL, Jarvis WR. Reality check: should we try to detect and isolate vancomycin-resistant enterococci patients. *Infect Control Hosp Epidemiol*. 2001;22:116-119.

28. CDC. *Staphylococcus aureus* resistant to vancomycin-United States, 2002. *MMWR Morbid Mortal Wkly Rep*. 2002;51:565-567.

29. CDC. Public Health Dispatch: vancomycin-resistant *Staphylococcus aureus*—Pennsylvania, 2002. *MMWR Morbid Mortal Wkly Rep*. 2002;51:902.

30. Teare EL, Barrett SP. Stop the ritual of tracing colonized people. *BMJ*. 1997;314:665-666.

31. Peel RK, Stolarek I, Elder AT. Is it time to stop searching for MRSA? Isolating patients with MRSA can have long term implications. *BMJ*. 1997;315:58.

32. Kirkland KB, Weinstein JM. Adverse effects of contact isolation. *Lancet*. 1999;354:1177-1178.

33. Pike JH, McLean D. Ethical concerns in isolating patients with methicillin-resistant *Staphylococcus aureus* on the rehabilitation ward: a case report. *Arch Phys Med Rehabil*. 2002;83:1028-1030.

34. Vasquez JE, Walker ES, Franzus BW, Overbay BK, Reagan DR, Sarubbi FA. The epidemiology of mupirocin resistance among methicillin-resistant *Staphylococcus aureus* at a Veterans' Affairs hospital. *Infect Control Hosp Epidemiol*. 2000;21:459-464.

35. Farr BM, Jarvis WR. Would active surveillance cultures help control healthcare-related methicillin-resistant *Staphylococcus aureus* infections? *Infect Control Hosp Epidemiol*. 2002;23:65-68.

36. Calfee DP, Giannetta ET, Durbin LJ, Germanson TP, Farr BM. Control of endemic vancomycin-resistant Enterococcus among inpatients at a university hospital. *Clin Infect Dis*. 2003;37:326-332.

37. Diekema DJ. Active surveillance cultures for control of vancomycin-resistant Enterococcus [letter]. *Clin Infect Dis*. 2003;37:1400-1402.

38. John JF, Fishman NO. Programmatic role of the infectious diseases physician in controlling antimicrobial costs in the hospital. *Clin Infect Dis*. 1997;24:471-485.

39. Shlaes DM, Gerding DN, John JF, et al. Society for Healthcare Epidemiology of America and Infectious Diseases Society of America Joint Committee on the prevention of antimicrobial resistance: guidelines for the prevention of antimicrobial resistance in hospitals. *Infect Control Hosp Epidemiol*. 1997;18:275-291 and *Clinical Infect Dis*. 1997;25:584-599.

40. Kollef MH, Fraser VJ. Antibiotic resistance in the intensive care unit. *Ann Intern Med*. 2001;134:298-314.

41. Wazana A. Physicians and the pharmaceutical industry: is a gift ever just a gift? *JAMA*. 2000;283:373-380.

42. Janknegt R, Steenhoek A. The system of objectified judgement analysis (SOJA): a tool in rational drug selection for formulary inclusion. *Drugs*. 1997;53:550-562.

43. Fijn R, van Epenhuysen LS, Peijnenburg AJM, Brouwers JRBJ, de Jong-van den Berg TW. Is there a need for critical ethical and philosophical evaluation of hospital drugs and therapeutics (D&T) committees? *Pharmacoepidemiol Drug Safety*. 2002;11:247-252.

44. Updated U.S. Public Health Service guidelines for the management of occupational exposures to HBV, HCV, and HIV and recommendations for postexposure prophylaxis. *MMWR Morbid Mortal Wkly Rep*. 2001;50(RR-11):1-52.

45. Gerberding JL. Occupational exposure to HIV in health care settings. *N Engl J Med*. 2003;348:826-833.

46. Catalano MT. Postexposure prophylaxis implementation issues: programmatic concerns in hospitals. *Am J Med*. 1997;102(5B):95-97.

47. Iowa Code 141A.8. Available at http://www.legis.state.ia.us/IACODE/2003/141A/8.html. Accessed August 16, 2004.

48. Horan-Murphy E, Barnard B, Chenoweth C, et al. APIC/CHICA-Canada infection control and epidemiology: professional and practice standards. *Am J Infect Control*. 1999;27:47-51.

49. Toffler BL. When the signal is 'move it or lose it.' *The New York Times*. November 17, 1991: F13.

SURVEILLANCE AND ANALYSIS

CHAPTER FIVE

EPIDEMIOLOGIC METHODS IN INFECTION CONTROL

Ebbing Lautenbach, MD, MPH, MSCE

INTRODUCTION

A good working knowledge of basic epidemiologic principles and approaches is essential for the healthcare epidemiologist. The ability to accurately quantify new patterns of IDs, design rigorous studies to characterize the factors associated with disease, and devise and evaluate interventions to address emerging issues are vital to effective job performance.

Epidemiology is commonly defined as the study of the distribution and determinants of disease frequency in human populations. This definition concisely encompasses the 3 main components of the discipline of epidemiology. The first, "disease frequency," involves identifying the existence of a disease and quantifying its occurrence. The second, "distribution of disease," characterizes in whom the disease is occurring, where it is occurring, and when it is occurring. Finally, the "determinants of disease" focuses on formulating and testing hypotheses with regard to the possible risk factors for disease.

MEASURES OF DISEASE FREQUENCY

Before setting about to identify the possible causes of a disease, one must first quantify the frequency with which the disease occurs. This is important both for measuring the scope of the problem (ie, how many people are affected by the disease), as well as for subsequently allowing comparison between different groups (ie, those with and without a particular risk factor of interest). The most commonly used measures of disease frequency in epidemiology are prevalence and incidence.

Prevalence

Prevalence is defined as the proportion of people with disease at a given point in time (eg, the proportion of hospitalized patients who have a nosocomial infection). This is also sometimes referred to as the "point prevalence."

$$\text{Prevalence} = \frac{\text{Number of diseased individuals}}{\text{Total population}}$$

A related, although infrequently used, measure is the "period prevalence," which is defined as the number of persons with disease in a given period of time divided by the number of persons observed during the period. Prevalence is a proportion and as such has no units. This measure of disease frequency is dependent on both the incidence (ie, the number of new cases that develop) as well as the duration of disease (ie, how long a disease lasts once it has developed). The greater the incidence and the greater the duration of disease, the higher the prevalence will be. Prevalence is useful for measuring the burden of disease in a population (ie, the overall proportion of persons affected by the disease), which may in turn inform decisions regarding such issues as allocation of resources and funding of research initiatives.

All populations are dynamic; individuals are constantly entering and leaving the population. Depending on the population, the prevalence may vary depending on when it is measured (Figure 5-1). If a dynamic population is at steady state (ie, cases leaving = cases entering), the prevalence will be constant over time.

Incidence

Incidence is defined as the number of new cases of diseases occurring in a specified period of time. Incidence may be described in several ways. Cumulative incidence is

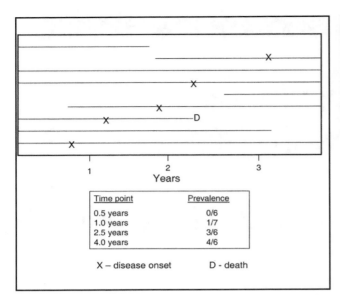

Figure 5-1. Measuring prevalence in a dynamic population.

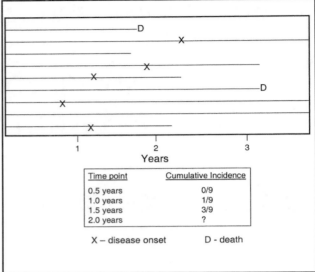

Figure 5-2. Cumulative incidence.

defined as the number of new cases of disease in a particular time period divided by the total number of disease-free individuals at risk of the disease at the beginning of the time period (eg, the proportion of patients who develop a nosocomial infection during hospitalization). In ID epidemiology, this traditionally has been termed the "attack rate."

$$\text{Cumulative Incidence} = \frac{\text{number of new cases of disease between } t_0 \text{ and } t_1}{\text{total disease-free individuals at risk of disease at } t_0}$$

The cumulative incidence, like the prevalence, is simply a proportion and thus has no units. In order to calculate the cumulative incidence, one must have complete follow-up on all observed individuals such that their final disposition with regard to having or not having the disease may be determined. Although this measure describes the total proportion of new cases occurring in a time period, it does not describe when in the time period the cases occurred (Figure 5-2).

For the cumulative incidence of nosocomial infections, the time period implied is the course of hospitalization until a first event or until discharge without a first event. However, patients do not all stay in the hospital and remain at risk for exactly the same period of time. Furthermore, most nosocomial infections are time related, and comparing the cumulative incidence of nosocomial infection among patient groups with differing lengths of stay may be very misleading. By contrast, if one is investigating events that come from a point source and are not

time related (eg, tuberculosis acquired from a contaminated bronchoscope), then the cumulative incidence is an excellent measure of incidence. Surgical site infections are also usually thought of as having a point source (ie, the operation).

Historically, nosocomial infection rates were often reported as a cumulative incidence (ie, the number of infections per 100 discharges). This definition had no unique quantitative meaning, as it did not separate first infections from multiple infections in the same patient, and allowed undefined multiple counting of individuals. The implications of 5 infections per 100 discharges would be entirely different, depending on whether it represented 5 sequential infections in a single moribund patient or 5 first infections in 5 different but healthy patients, such as women with normal deliveries.

The incidence rate (or incidence density) is defined as the number of new cases of disease in a specified quantity of person-time of observation among individuals at risk (eg, the number of nosocomial infections per 1000 hospital days).

$$\text{Incidence} = \frac{\text{number of new cases of disease during given time period}}{\text{total person-time of observation among individuals at risk}}$$

The primary value of this measure can be seen when comparing nosocomial infection rates in groups that differ in their time at risk (eg, short-stay patients vs. long-stay patients). When the time at risk in 1 group is much greater than the time at risk in another, the incidence rate, or risk per day, is the most convenient way to correct for time, and thus separate the effect of time (duration of

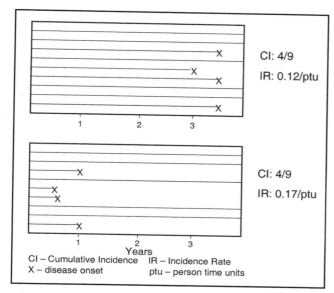

CI: 4/9
IR: 0.12/ptu

CI: 4/9
IR: 0.17/ptu

Years
CI – Cumulative Incidence   IR – Incidence Rate
X – disease onset   ptu – person time units

Figure 5-3. Cumulative incidence vs. incidence rate.

exposure) from the effect of daily risk. For convenience in hospital epidemiology, incidence rates for nosocomial infections are usually expressed as the number of first events in a certain number of days at risk (eg, nosocomial infections per 1000 hospital days) because this usually produces a small single- or double-digit number.

Incidence rate is usually restricted to first events (eg, the first episode of nosocomial infection). It is standard to consider only first events because second events are not statistically independent from first events in the same individuals (ie, patients with a first event are more likely to suffer a second event). For example, all hospitalized patients who have not yet developed a nosocomial infection would compose the population at risk. After a patient develops an infection, that patient would then be withdrawn and would not be a part of the population still at risk for a first event. Each hospitalized patient who never develops an infection would contribute all hospital days (ie, the sum of days the patient is in the hospital) to the pool of days at risk for a first event. However, a patient who develops an infection would contribute only those ventilator days before the onset of the infection.

Unlike cumulative incidence, the incidence rate does not assume complete follow-up of subjects and thus accounts for different entry and dropout rates. However, even when follow-up is complete (and thus cumulative incidence could be calculated), reporting the incidence rate may still be preferable. Cumulative incidence only reports the overall number of new cases occurring during the time period (regardless of whether they occur early or late in the time period). By comparison, the incidence rate, by incorporating the time at risk, accounts for poten-

tial difference in time to occurrence of the event. In considering the 2 examples in Figure 5-3, one will note that despite the fact that the cumulative incidence of disease at 4 years is the same for the 2 groups, subjects in the second group clearly acquire disease earlier. This is information is reflected in the different incidence rates.

Because the incidence rate counts time at risk in the denominator, the implicit assumption is that all time at risk is equal (eg, the likelihood developing a nosocomial infection in the first 5 days after hospital admission is the same as the likelihood of developing an infection during days 6 through 10 of hospitalization). If all time periods are not equivalent, the incidence rate may be misleading depending on when, in the course of their time at risk, patients are observed for the outcome.

STUDY DESIGN

One of the critical components of the field of epidemiology is identifying the "determinants of disease." This aspect of the field focuses on formulating and testing hypotheses with regard to the possible risk factors for disease. A number of study designs are available to the hospital epidemiologist when attempting to test a hypothesis as to the causes of a disease. These study designs, in order of increasing methodological rigor, include case report, case series, ecologic study, cross-sectional study, case-control study, cohort study, randomized controlled trial, and quasi-experimental study. Randomized controlled trials, case control studies, and cohort studies are considered analytic studies as opposed to the other study designs, which are considered descriptive studies. Analytic studies are most useful in identifying the "determinants of disease" (ie, risk factors for a particular outcome of interest). In determining the correct study design, the hospital epidemiologist must first carefully consider what the question is. Once this critical question has been clearly formulated, the optimal study design will likely also become evident. Other considerations (eg, available time, access to financial support, ethical considerations) may also influence the decision as to the type of study that should be undertaken.

Case Report/Case Series

A case report is the clinical description of a single patient (eg, a single case of a patient with a bloodstream infection [BSI] due to VRE). A case series is simply a report of more than one patient with the disease of interest. One advantage of a case report/series is its relative ease of preparation. In addition, a case report/series may serve as a clinical or therapeutic example for other health-care epidemiologists who may be faced with similar cases. Perhaps most importantly, a case report/series can serve to generate hypotheses that may then be tested in future analytic studies. For example, if a case report notes that a patient had been exposed to several courses of vancomycin in the month prior to the VRE infection, one hypothesis might be that vancomycin use is associated with VRE infection. The primary limitation of a case report/series is that it describes at most a few patients and may not be generalizable. In addition, because a case report/series does not include a comparison group, one cannot determine which characteristics in the description of the cases are unique to the illness. While case reports are thus usually of limited interest, there are exceptions, particularly when they identify a new disease or signify the index case of an important outbreak (eg, the first report of clinical VRE infection).

Ecologic Study

In an ecologic study, one compares geographic and/or time trends of an illness to trends in risk factors (ie, a comparison of annual hospital wide use of vancomycin with annual prevalence of VRE among nosocomial enterococcal isolates). Ecologic studies most often use aggregate data that are routinely collected for other purposes (eg, antimicrobial susceptibility patterns from a hospital's clinical microbiology laboratory, antimicrobial drug dispensing data from the inpatient pharmacy). This ready availability of data provides one advantage to the ecologic study in that such studies are often relatively quick and easy to do. Thus, such a study may provide early support for or against a hypothesis. However, one cannot distinguish between various hypotheses that might be consistent with the data. Perhaps most importantly, ecologic studies do not incorporate patient level data. For example, while both the use of annual hospital-wide use of vancomycin as well as the yearly prevalence of VRE in nosocomial clinical isolates might have increased significantly over a 5-year period, one cannot tell from these data whether the actual patients who were infected with VRE received vancomycin.

Cross-Sectional Study

A cross-sectional study is a survey of a sample of the population in which the status of subjects with regard to the risk factor and disease is assessed at the same point in time. For example, a cross-sectional study to assess VRE might involve identifying all patients currently hospitalized and assessing each patient with regard to whether they have a VRE infection as well as whether they are receiving vancomycin. One advantage of a cross-sectional study is it is relatively easy to carry out, given that all subjects are simply assessed at one point in time. As such, this type of study may provide early evidence for or against a hypothesis. A major disadvantage of a cross-sectional study is that this study design does not capture the concept of elapsed time (ie, it is not possible to determine

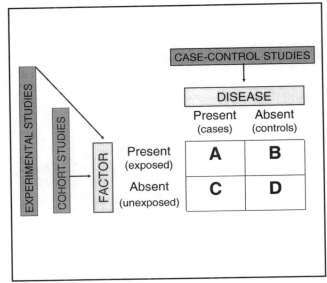

Figure 5-4. Study designs.

which came first, the proposed risk factor or the outcome). Furthermore, a cross-sectional study does not provide information about the transition between health states (eg, development of new VRE infection, resolution of VRE infection).

Case-Control Study

In distinguishing between the various types of analytic studies (eg, case-control, cohort, experimental), it is useful to consider the traditional 2-by-2 table (Figure 5-4). While all 3 study designs seek to investigate the potential association between a risk factor (or exposure) and an outcome of interest, they differ fundamentally in the way patients are enrolled into the study. In a case-control study, patients are entered into the study based on the presence or absence of the outcome (or disease) of interest. These 2 groups (ie, those with the disease and those without the disease) are then compared to determine if they differ with regard to their presence of risk factors of interest. Case-control studies are always retrospective.

A case-control study design is particularly attractive when the outcome being studied is rare because one may enroll into the study all patients with the outcome of interest. As such, this study design is much more efficient and economical than the comparable cohort study, in which a group of patients with and without an exposure of interest would need to be followed for a period of time to determine who develops the outcome of interest. Even if a large cohort is available, it may be more economical to conduct a small case-control study within the cohort. As such, a "nested" case-control study may produce the same information as the larger cohort study at a fraction of the cost. Another advantage of the case-control study is that one may study any number of risk factors for the outcome of interest. One disadvantage of a case-control study is that only one outcome may be studied. Another disadvantage of this approach is that one cannot directly calculate the incidence or relative risk from a case-control study because the investigator fixes the number of cases and controls to be studied.

Thoughtful consideration must be taken when selecting cases and controls in a case-control study. Cases may be restricted to any group of diseased individuals. However, they must arise from a theoretical source population such that a diseased person not selected is presumed to have arisen from a different source population. For example, in studying risk factors for nosocomial VRE infection, the theoretical source population could be considered to be the population of patients hospitalized at one institution. Thus, if any patient at that institution were to have a clinical isolate demonstrating VRE, they would be included as a case. However, a patient with VRE infection at a different hospital would not be included. Finally, cases must be chosen in a manner independent of their status with regard to an exposure of interest.

Careful attention is also required when selecting controls for a case-control study. Controls should be representative of the theoretical source population that gave rise to the cases. Thus, if a control were to have developed the disease of interest, they would have been selected as a case. In the example above, controls may be randomly selected from among all non-VRE infected patients in the hospital. In investigating the possible association between prior vancomycin use and VRE infection, these 2 groups (ie, patients with VRE infection and a random sample of all other hospitalized patients) could be compared to determine what proportion of patients in each group had experienced recent vancomycin exposure. In this case, the comparison being made answers the question, "Is prior vancomycin use a risk factor for VRE infection?" Another type of control group that is often selected, particularly in studies of risk factors for antimicrobial resistance, is the group of patients infected with the susceptible counterpart of the resistant infection of interest. In this example, patients with VRE infection would be compared to patients with VSE infections to determine what proportion of patients in each group had experienced recent vancomycin exposure. In this case, the comparison being made answers the question, "Among patients with enterococcal infections, is prior vancomycin use a risk factor for VRE?" A potential disadvantage of using this second type of control group is that it may result in an overestimate of the association between antimicrobial use and resistant infection. Finally, like cases, controls must be chosen in a manner independent of their status with regard to an exposure of interest and should not be selected because they have characteristics similar to cases.

Cohort Study

Unlike a case-control study in which study subjects are selected based on the presence or absence of an outcome or disease of interest, patients are entered into a cohort study based on the presence or absence of an exposure (or risk factor) of interest (see Figure 5-4). These 2 groups (ie, those with the exposure and those without the exposure) are then compared to determine if they differ with regard to whether they develop the outcome of interest. The investigator may select subjects randomly or according to exposure.

A cohort study may be either prospective or retrospective. Whether a cohort study is prospective or retrospective depends on when it is conducted with regard to when the outcome of interest occurs. If patients are identified as exposed or unexposed and then followed forward in time to determine whether they develop the disease, it is a prospective cohort study. If the study is conducted after the time the outcome has already occurred, it is a retrospective cohort study. In either case, subjects are selected into the study based on their exposure status with regard to a variable of interest, and these groups are then compared on the basis of the outcome of interest. For example, one might identify all patients who receive vancomycin in a hospital (ie, the exposed) and compare them to a randomly selected group of patients who do not receive vancomycin (ie, the unexposed). These groups could then be followed forward to determine what proportion of patients in each group develops the outcome of interest (ie, VRSA infection).

One advantage of a cohort study is that one may study multiple outcomes from a single risk factor or exposure. In addition, a cohort study allows the investigator to calculate an incidence as well as a relative risk in comparing the 2 groups. Potential disadvantages of a cohort study include heavy cost and time requirements because patients must be followed forward in time until a sufficient number develop the outcome of interest. Depending on the course of the disease, this may be a lengthy period of time. In addition, if the outcome is rare, a great many subjects will need to be followed until the necessary number develop the disease. Finally, the longer the study duration, the more likely that subjects will be lost to follow-up, potentially biasing the results of the study. Some of these limitations are lessened in a retrospective cohort study because outcomes have already occurred and patients do not need to be followed prospectively.

Randomized Controlled Trial

In clinical investigation, the closest approximation to a standard experiment in bench biology is the randomized controlled trial (RCT). In comparing the RCT to other analytic study designs (see Figure 5-4), it is very similar to the cohort study. However, in a cohort study, patients are enrolled already either having or not having the exposure of interest. In an RCT, the investigator assigns the exposure according to some scheme, such as randomization. This study design provides the most convincing demonstration of causality because patients in both groups should (provided randomization has worked appropriately) be equal on all important variables except the one variable (exposure) manipulated by the investigator. While RCTs may provide the strongest support for or against an association of interest, they are costly studies and there may be ethical issues that preclude their conduct. For example, in elucidating the association between vancomycin use and VRE infection, it would be unethical to randomly assign patients to receiving vancomycin if they did not require the drug.

Quasi-Experimental Study

A final study design often employed in investigations relating to infection control is the quasi-experimental study, also called the nonrandomized pre-post intervention design. The goal of a quasi-experimental study is typically to evaluate an intervention without using randomization. The most basic type of quasi-experimental study involves the collection of baseline data, the implementation of an intervention, and the collection of the same data following the intervention. For example, the baseline prevalence of VRE in a hospital could be calculated, an intervention to limit use of vancomycin would then be instituted, and, after some prespecified time period, the prevalence of VRE is again measured. Many different variations of quasi-experimental studies exist and include institution of multiple pretests (ie, collection of baseline data on more than one occasion), repeated interventions (ie, instituting and removing the intervention on sequentially), and inclusion of a control group (ie, a group on which baseline and subsequent data is collected but on which no intervention is implemented).

The quasi-experimental study design offers several advantages. This type of study design is frequently used when it is not ethical to conduct an RCT, such as for reasons noted above. In addition, when an intervention must be instituted rapidly in response to an emerging issue (eg, an outbreak), the first priority is to protect patients. In this case, it would be unethical to randomize the intervention across patient groups. Even in situations where an RCT would be ethical, it might not be logistically feasible to conduct one because broad interventions (eg, institution of new infection control guidelines, changes in the hospital antimicrobial formulary) are very difficult to randomize to individual patients or hospital floors/units.

There are several disadvantages to a quasi-experimental study design. In such studies it is often difficult to control for potential confounding variables. For example, other factors (eg, average patient severity of illness, quality of medical and nursing care) may also change over time

as the intervention is implemented. How much of the effect of any intervention that can be ascribed to these other changes often cannot be determined. Frequently, these other confounding variables are very difficult to measure and control. Another disadvantage of quasi-experimental studies is the principle of regression to the mean, which notes that trends in rates (eg, prevalence of antibiotic resistant bacteria) may fluctuate over time and while they may become elevated, often return to baseline levels even without intervention. Thus, without knowing the trends in disease that would have occurred in the absence of an intervention, it may be difficult to interpret the effects of an intervention. Use of a control group (ie, a group on which data are collected over time but on which no intervention is implemented) may help to address this limitation of quasi-experimental studies.

BIAS AND CONFOUNDING

Two common issues that arise when designing a study are the potentials for bias and confounding variables. A comprehensive discussion of bias and confounding variables is beyond the scope of this chapter and the reader is referred to several excellent texts (see Bibliography at the end of the chapter). Briefly, bias is the systematic error in the collection or interpretation of data. Types of bias include information bias (ie, distortion in the estimate of effect due to measurement error or misclassification of subjects on one or more variables) and selection bias (ie, distortion in the estimate of effect resulting from the manner in which subjects are selected for the study). The potential for bias must be addressed at the time the study is designed because it cannot be corrected during the analysis of the study.

Confounding occurs when the estimate of the effect of the exposure is distorted because it is mixed with the effect of an extraneous factor. To be a confounder, a variable must be associated with both the exposure and outcome of interest but cannot be a result of the exposure. Unlike bias, a confounding variable may be controlled for in the study analysis. However, in order to do this, data regarding the presence or absence of the confounder must be collected during the study. Thus, it is also important to consider the potential for confounding variables in the design of the study.

MEASURES OF EFFECT

Risk Versus Odds

Depending on which type of study one conducts, one will generally calculate either a relative risk (ie, in a cohort study or an RCT) or an odds ratio (ie, in a case-

		DISEASE	
		Present (cases)	Absent (controls)
FACTOR	Present (exposed)	A	B
	Absent (not exposed)	C	D

Relative Risk

Risk of disease among the exposed = A / (A+B)

Risk of disease among the unexposed = C / (C+D)

$$\text{Relative Risk} = \frac{A / (A+B)}{C / (C+D)}$$

Odds Ratio

Odds of exposure given disease = A / C

Odds of exposure given no disease = B / D

$$\text{Disease Odds Ratio} = \frac{A / C}{B / D} = \frac{AD}{BC}$$

Relationship Between Relative Risk and Odds Ratio

When disease is rare, B>>A, and D>>>C

$$\text{Relative Risk} = \frac{A / (A+B)}{C / (C+D)} \sim \frac{AD}{BC} = \text{Odds ratio}$$

Figure 5-5. Relative risk and odds ratio.

control study) to characterize the strength of an association between an exposure and outcome. Before describing these measures in greater detail, it is useful to briefly compare the concepts of risk and odds. In a risk (also referred to as a probability), the numerator contains the event of interest, while the denominator contains all possible events. For example, in throwing a die, the "risk" of throwing a "3" is 1 divided by 6 (because there are 6 possible events when throwing a die). Thus, the "risk of throwing a "3" equals 1/6 = 16.7%. In an odds, the numerator again contains the event of interest, while the denominator contains all possible events minus the event of interest. Using again the example of throwing a die, the "odds" of throwing a "3" is equal to 1 divided by 5 (ie, 6 minus 1). Thus, the "odds" of throwing a "3" equals 1/5 = 20.0%. Because the denominator in an odds is always smaller, the value for the odds is always somewhat greater than the comparable risk.

Relative Risk

The relative risk (also called the risk ratio) is the ratio of 2 probabilities: the probability of the outcome among the exposed divided by the probability of the outcome in the unexposed (Figure 5-5). A relative risk can be calculated from a cohort study or an RCT because from these study designs one can derive population based rates or proportions. A relative risk of 1.0 is called the value of no effect or the null value. A relative risk equal to 2.0 means the exposed subjects were twice as likely to have the outcome of interest as the unexposed subjects. On the other hand, a relative risk of 0.5 means that the exposed were half as likely to experience the outcome as the unexposed, indicating a protective effect of the exposure.

Odds Ratio

As noted previously, in a case-control study subjects are enrolled into the study based on the outcome of interest. One then compares these 2 groups (ie, those with the outcome and those without the outcome) to determine what proportion of subjects in each group demonstrate a risk factor of interest. In this setting, without additional information, one cannot determine how common the outcomes or the exposures are in the entire study population. Thus, unlike the cohort study, one cannot directly calculate a relative risk. What one can calculate in a case control study is the odds ratio. The odds ratio is defined as the odds of exposure in subjects with the outcome divided by the odds of exposure in subjects without the outcome (see Figure 5-5). An odds ratio of 1.0 is called the value of no effect or the null value.

As noted above, one cannot calculate a relative risk from a case-control study because the case-control study offers no insights into the absolute rates or proportions or disease among subjects. However, in situations in which the disease under study is rare (<10%), the odds ratio derived from a case-control study closely approximates the relative that would have been derived from the comparable cohort study. Figure 5-5 shows how the case control formula approaches the formula for relative risk when the rare outcome criterion is met.

Measures of Strength of Association

P Value

The most common method of measuring strength of association in a 2-by-2 table is the calculation of the chi-square test for the comparison of 2 binomial proportions. This calculation is identical for all 2-by-2 tables whether or not the data were derived from a cohort or case-control study. When one has calculated the value for the chi-square, one can then look up the associated probability that the observed difference between binomial proportions could have arisen by chance alone. The conventional interpretation of these probabilities is that a p value of <0.05 indicates that an effect at least as extreme as that observed in the study is unlikely to have occurred by chance alone, given that there is truly no relationship between the exposure and the disease. Although this is the conventional interpretation, there is nothing magical about the 0.05 cutoff for statistical significance. One limitation of the p value is that this value reflects both the magnitude of the difference between the groups being compared as well as the sample size. Consequently, even a small difference between groups (if the sample size is large enough) may be statistically significant, even if it is not clinically important. Conversely, a larger effect that would be clinically important may not achieve statistical significance if the sample size is insufficient.

95% Confidence Interval

Given the limitations of the p value noted above, it is generally preferable to report the 95% confidence interval (CI) for a given relative risk or odds ratio (depending on whether the study performed was a cohort or case control study, respectively). The 95% CI provides a range within which the true magnitude of the effect (ie, either the relative risk or the odds ratio) lies with a certain degree of assurance. Observing whether the 95%CI crosses 1.0 (ie, the value of null effect) provides the same information as the p value. If the 95%CI crosses 1.0, the p value will almost never be <0.05. In addition, the effect of the sample size can be ascertained from the width of the CI. The narrower the CI, the less variability was present in the estimate of the effect, reflecting a larger sample size. The wider the CI, the greater the variability in the estimate of the effect and the smaller the sample size. When interpreting results that are not significant, the width of the CI may be very helpful. A narrow CI implies that there is most likely no real effect or exposure, whereas a wide interval suggests that the data are also compatible with a true effect and that the sample size was simply not adequate.

CONCLUSION

A basic understanding of epidemiologic principles and approaches is essential for the healthcare epidemiologist. The ability to compute measures of disease occurrence, design and conduct appropriate studies to characterize the factors associated with disease, and rigorously evaluate the results of such studies are increasingly vital functions of someone in this position. To build on the foundation provided in this chapter, the healthcare epidemiologist is encouraged to refer to more comprehensive texts (noted at the end of the chapter) and to consult with other professionals (eg, epidemiologists, biostatisticians) as needed.

BIBLIOGRAPHY

Agresti A. *Categorical Data Analysis*. 2nd ed. New York: Wiley Interscience; 2002.

Hennekens CH, Buring JE, Mayrent SL. *Epidemiology in Medicine*. 1st ed. Philadelphia: Lippincott, Williams & Wilkins; 1987.

Hosmer DW, Lemeshow SL. *Applied Logistic Regression*. 2nd ed. New York: Wiley Interscience; 2000.

Kleinbaum DG, Kupper LL, Morgenstern H. *Epidemiologic Research: Principles and Quantitative Methods*. 1st ed. New York: Van Nostrand Reinhold; 1982.

Nelson KE, Williams CM, Graham NMH. *Infectious Disease Epidemiology: Theory and Practice*. 1st ed. New York: Aspen Publishers; 2000.

Rothman KJ, Greenland S. *Modern Epidemiology*. 2nd ed. Philadelphia: Lippincott, Williams & Wilkins; 1998.

Thomas JC, Weber DJ. *Epidemiologic Methods for the Study of Infectious Diseases*. 1st ed. Oxford: Oxford University Press; 2001.

CHAPTER SIX

BASICS OF SURVEILLANCE: AN OVERVIEW

Trish M. Perl, MD, MSc; Jean M. Pottinger, RN, MA, CIC; and Loreen A. Herwaldt, MD

INTRODUCTION

A good surveillance system does not guarantee that you make the right decisions but it reduces the chance of making the wrong ones.
Alexander Langmuir[1]

The cornerstone of any clinical outcomes program, including those responsible for healthcare epidemiology and infection control, is surveillance for complications of medical care. Specifically, this chapter reviews surveillance for healthcare-associated infection and epidemiologically important organisms. In the era of patient safety, this activity has been elevated from dark corners of hospitals into the public and legislative realms. This chapter describes the importance of these activities and includes components of a surveillance system, methods for surveillance, methods for finding events, and data sources. We describe methods used to stratify patients by their risk of developing infection or acquiring an epidemiologically significant organism. We also discuss the importance of calculating rates in a standardized fashion to ensure appropriate comparisons can be made. We review the importance of using computers and information technology that are becoming integral to efficient and effective surveillance. Although we focus on surveillance as it applies to healthcare acquired infections and epidemiologically significant organisms, the methods brought forth in this chapter are well established in healthcare settings and can also be applied to noninfectious complications of healthcare. We encourage the healthcare epidemiology and infection control team to use this information as they design surveillance systems that meet the goals of their individual institution's program. This reference should be supplemented with the training and resources needed to provide healthcare institutions with accurate and complex data.

In 1847, Ignaz Semmelweis reported an excessive mortality rate among mothers delivering babies at the Vienna Lying In Hospital. The process of identifying the complication rates and ultimately intervening describes a process called "surveillance." Surveillance is a dynamic process for collecting, concatenating, analyzing, and disseminating data concerning specific events that occur in a specific population.[2] Findings from surveillance are commonly linked to or should result in actions or decisions, often at the hospital policy level. As the cornerstone of hospital epidemiology and infection control programs, surveillance provides data that are used to determine baseline rates of nosocomial infections, epidemiologically important organisms, or other adverse events and to detect changes in previously established rates or in the distribution of these events. The changes that have been found may lead to investigations of each case, including the determination of time and space clustering of events or significantly increased rates, the generation of a hypothesis about risk factors, the institution of prevention and control measures, and ultimately, the determination of whether the interventions instituted were effective. Appropriately performed surveillance requires defined events and systematic case finding, and commonly uses stratification of risk to determine trends and evaluate the impact of interventions over time. Surveillance data should also be used to determine risk factors for the outcome of interest, to monitor compliance with established hospital policies and practices, to evaluate changes in practice, and to identify topics for further study. Importantly, such processes are critical to ensure appropriate rates are generated for inter-hospital comparisons.

Historically, the CDC, accrediting agencies, and hospital administrators accepted surveillance for nosocomial infections (now called "healthcare-associated infections")

as an important element of an infection control program. Despite increasing need for such programs, surveillance activities are commonly victims of cost saving efforts. In 1974, the CDC initiated the Study on the Efficacy of Nosocomial Infection Control (SENIC) to determine the magnitude of the problem associated with healthcare-associated infections, to evaluate the extent to which hospitals had adopted surveillance and control programs, and to examine whether infection control programs reduced rates of SSI, pneumonia, urinary tract infection (UTI), and BSI.[3] The SENIC investigators found that different combinations of infection control practices helped reduce infections at each site.[3] However, surveillance was the only component essential for reducing infections at all 4 sites. In addition, the SENIC project concluded that effective programs included surveillance for infections, adequate numbers of infection control practitioners (ICP), feedback of data to healthcare providers, and a trained hospital epidemiologist (ie, a physician trained in epidemiologic methods and infection control and prevention strategies).

Since this study was published, surveillance for healthcare-associated infections and epidemiologically important organisms, including those resistant to antimicrobial agents, is of an even greater import to facilitate the prevention of their transmission among an increasingly ill patient population. In addition, while much of the experience with surveillance for healthcare-associated events has taken place in North America, recently the Europeans and other international groups have developed large surveillance programs for healthcare-associated infections and resistant organisms that have enhanced our understanding of the expanding roles of surveillance. Several other new trends in surveillance should be mentioned. First, "syndromic" surveillance programs to track potential agents of bioterrorism and newly emerging diseases (eg, severe acute respiratory syndrome) have been integrated into healthcare epidemiology and infection control programs.[4] These data would be routinely transmitted to the public health authorities as an "early warning" system for a bioterrorism event. No data currently exist on how effective these efforts are or what components are required to make such surveillance efficient, valid, and effective. Secondly, several states in the United States have passed legislation requiring healthcare facilities to report healthcare-associated infections to public health authorities. The intended goal is to release these data to the public. With the public reporting of healthcare-associated infections looming, the importance of using standard definitions, systematically identifying cases, and choosing the appropriate population at risk (ie, denominator) is paramount.

WHAT DOES SURVEILLANCE ENTAIL?

Surveillance requires that relevant information be collected systematically. The purpose of and time frame for data collection should be specific. Data need to be analyzed and displayed to enhance interpretation and facilitate any necessary interventions. This chapter will focus on surveillance for healthcare-associated infections and epidemiologically important organisms. However, these principles can be applied for noninfectious adverse outcomes of medical care, such as falls and medication errors. The focus of this chapter is surveillance in the hospital, and although we recognize that an increasing number of patients have medical and surgical procedures in the outpatient settings, the principles set forth in this chapter can be used in any healthcare setting.

WHY CONDUCT SURVEILLANCE?

Surveillance is conducted for a myriad of reasons. Conducting or establishing surveillance allows an infection control program to do the following:

➤ Establish baseline rates.

➤ Detect time/space clustering (ie, outbreaks).

➤ Convince clinicians and administrators of a potential problem that may require additional resources.

➤ Generate hypotheses concerning risk factors.

➤ Identify a source of cases to test hypotheses concerning risk factors.

➤ Assess the impact of prevention and control measures.

➤ Guide treatment (eg, choice of antimicrobial agents) and/or prevention strategies (ie, vaccine or chemoprophylaxis).

➤ Reinforce practices and procedures.

➤ Satisfy patient care standards, guidelines, or regulatory requirements.

➤ Defend against lawsuits.

➤ Conduct research.

➤ Reduce healthcare-associated infections.

➤ Make inter/intra-hospital (or health system) comparisons.

TABLE 6-1. Needs and Resources for Surveillance Systems for Healthcare-Associated Infections and Epidemiologically Important Organisms

➤ Primary objective(s) and goal(s)
➤ Case definitions applied in a standard fashion
➤ Measure(s) of occurrence
➤ Numerators and denominators
➤ Access to data
➤ Resources (trained personnel, hardware, software)
➤ Data (information) to stratify by risk

WHAT IS NEEDED TO PLAN FOR AND CONDUCT SURVEILLANCE FOR HEALTHCARE-ASSOCIATED INFECTIONS?

Many infection control programs established surveillance systems (Table 6-1) because of CDC recommendations, regulatory agency requirements, or other external pressure such as competition from hospitals in the community with already established programs. Hospitals or healthcare settings that have established programs under such circumstances may not have established their own goals and priorities. Consequently, data collection became an end unto itself. Unfortunately, in these cases, the surveillance data often have had little influence on infection rates.

To be successful, a surveillance system needs clear and specific primary objectives. When developing a new surveillance system or revising an existing system, the staff must first define the priorities of the program. In this way, both the type of surveillance and the types of data to be collected are determined. After the hospital epidemiology and infection control staff have analyzed preliminary data from their own institution (ie, data obtained either through the previous surveillance system or through a hospital-wide prevalence survey), they can custom design a surveillance system specific for their own facility. Federal and state (provincial) regulatory issues, national guidelines, and local patient care standards that may dictate special surveillance needs must be considered. For example, some states require environmental surveillance for *Legionella*, while others require reporting of healthcare-associated infection rates.

When developing a surveillance program, hospital epidemiology and infection control personnel should consider characteristics of the institution, including the size, the hospital type (eg, private, university, federal, teaching, nonteaching), the patient populations served, the procedures and treatments offered, and the proportion of inpatient to outpatient care. Hospital epidemiology staff also should consider the resources available to the infection control program, including the budget, the number of personnel and their level of training and experience, and the computer hardware and software that is available. Hospital epidemiology staff should design a surveillance system that requires fewer resources than are available, so the staff can accomplish their other responsibilities (eg, education, developing interventions, monitoring efficacy).

An infection control program must consider which events to study and the data sources available when they choose the data sources and case-finding methods they will use. The staff should consider the advantages and disadvantages of different surveillance methods (Table 6-2) and the sensitivity of different case-finding methods (Table 6-3) as they design their surveillance system. Definitions must be standard and applied in the same fashion. Measures of occurrence should be determined and calculated using appropriate numerators and denominators. The ICP should collect basic information on all patients with healthcare-associated infections (Table 6-4). For some infections (eg, central venous catheter-associated bacteremia), one may want to collect additional data or collect information during certain time periods (eg, when conducting a study to evaluate the prevalence of certain infections and to identify risk factors for those infections).

Infection control programs that have bountiful resources may want to continue doing hospital-wide surveillance so they can detect healthcare-associated infections in all patient populations. However, programs that find themselves in this enviable position should develop innovative methods for conducting hospital-wide surveillance and not just use the traditional labor-intensive method-total chart review. Most infection control programs have severely limited budgets. Therefore, the staff must decide how to use these precious resources to their

TABLE 6-2. Advantages and Disadvantages of Surveillance Strategies for Surveillance of Healthcare-Associated Infections

Strategy	Advantages	Disadvantages
Hospital-Wide Surveillance		
Incidence	➤ Provides data on all organisms/infection sites and units ➤ Identifies clusters ➤ Establishes baseline rates ➤ Recognizes outbreaks early ➤ Identifies risk factors	➤ Expensive and labor intensive ➤ Large amounts of data collected and little time to analyze ➤ No defined prevention objectives; difficult to develop interventions ➤ Not all infections are preventable
Prevalence	➤ Inexpensive ➤ Time-efficient; can be done periodically	➤ Overestimates rates ➤ Can't compare with incidence rates/national benchmarks
Targeted Surveillance		
Site specific	➤ Flexible, can be mixed with other strategies ➤ No baseline rates at other sites ➤ Can include postdischarge component ➤ Simplifies surveillance effort	➤ No defined prevention strategies or objective ➤ May miss clusters at other sites ➤ Denominator data may be inadequate ➤ Easily adaptable to interventions
Unit specific	➤ Focuses on patients at greater risk ➤ Requires fewer personnel ➤ Simplifies surveillance effort	➤ May miss clusters in nonsurveyed units
Rotating	➤ Less expensive ➤ Less time-consuming and labor intensive	➤ May miss clusters during non-surveyed periods
Outbreak	➤ Valuable when used with all types of surveillance ➤ Thresholds are institution specific	➤ Can't compare data with national benchmarks ➤ No baseline rates provided
Limited periodic	➤ Liberates ICP to perform other activities, including interventions ➤ Increases efficiency of surveillance	➤ May miss clusters
Objective/Priority Based	➤ Adaptable to hospitals with special populations and resources ➤ Focus on specific problems at the institution ➤ Identifies risk factors ➤ Easily adaptable to interventions ➤ Can include postdischarge component	➤ No baseline infection rates ➤ May miss clusters or outbreaks

TABLE 6-3. Case Finding Methods for Healthcare-Associated Infection Surveillance

Method	Sensitivity	Estimated Time (hours)/500 beds/wk*
Physician self-report forms	0.14 to 0.34	3
Fever	0.47 to 0.56**	8
Antibiotic use	0.48 to 0.81**	13.8
Fever and antibiotic use	0.70**	13.4
Microbiology reports	0.33 to 0.84**	23.2
Gold standard	0.94 to 1.00	35.7 to 45
Selective chart review using "Kardex clues"	0.82 to 0.94**	35.7
Chart review		
Prospective	0.76 to 0.94	53.6
Retrospective (University of Virginia)	0.79	35.7
Retrospective (SENIC)	0.74 to 0.96	not specified
Infection Control Sentinel Sheet Survey (for ICU's or unit-based surveillance)	0.73 to 0.87	1 minute/chart
Ward liaison Surveillance	0.62	17.6
Laboratory-based ward liaison	0.76 to 0.89	32.0
Risk factor-based surveillance	0.50 to 0.89	32.4
Selective surveillance based on physician reports	0.74	not specified

* Time required for an infection control practitioner to perform surveillance in a 500 bed, acute care hospital
** The gold standard for healthcare-associated infection surveillance was determined by a trained physician who examined each patient, each medical record, and all "Kardexes" and who verified microbiologic data.

TABLE 6-4. Information to Collect About Patients With Healthcare-Associated Infections

General Information for All Infection Sites
- Patient name
- Patient identification number
- Age
- Gender
- Nursing unit
- Service
- Admission date
- Infection onset (date)/date of culture
- Site of infection
- Organism(s)
- Antimicrobial susceptibility pattern

Additional Information That an ICP May Want to Collect for Studies
- Presence of risk factor (eg, central intravenous line, urinary catheter, ventilator)
- Date of exposure or risk factor*
- Primary diagnosis*
- Comorbidities*

TABLE 6-4. Information to Collect About Patients With Healthcare-Associated Infections (Continued)

- Medications (antibiotics, steroids, chemotherapeutic agents)*
- Exposure or risk factor (immunosuppression, instrumentation, procedures)*
- Comments

Information for Surveillance of Resistant or Epidemiologically Important Organisms
General Information for All Infection Sites
- Site of culture
- Date of culture
- Current or prior roommates
- Previous rooms during this admission
- Previous hospitalizations in this hospital
- Intensive care unit stay

Additional Information That an ICP May Want to Collect for Studies
- Underlying disease(s)*
- History of antimicrobial use*
- Previous hospitalizations in another hospital*
- Previous stay in a long-term care facility*
- Previous vaccinations or history of infectious disease(s)*

Information for Selected Sites
Surgical Site Infection
- Surgical procedure
- Procedure date
- Surgeons (attending and resident)
- ASA score
- Wound classification
- Perioperative antibiotic(s)
- Timing perioperative antibiotic(s) administered*
- Time of incision
- Time procedure finished
- Other members of the surgical team*
- Operating room number*

Bloodstream Infection
- Intravascular catheters present (yes/no)
- Type of intravascular catheter (central placement vs. peripheral)
- Location of intravascular catheter insertion site
- Number of days catheter in place
- Person(s) who inserted catheter*

Lower Respiratory Infection/Pneumonia
- Endotracheal intubation (yes/no)
- Ventilator (yes/no)
- Number of ventilator days
- Date patient intubated

TABLE 6-4. Information to Collect About Patients With Healthcare-Associated Infections (Continued)

Urinary Tract Infection
- Urethral catheter present (yes/no)
- External catheter present (yes/no)
- Number of days catheter in place
- Persons who inserted catheter*
- Other urinary tract instrumentation*

ASA = American Society of Anesthesiologists

* Information to be collected under particular circumstances (eg, an outbreak).

greatest possible advantage. We believe that most infection control programs should not conduct hospital-wide surveillance. Instead, they should limit their surveillance to specific infections, pathogens, or patient populations.

Ideally, infection control staff should focus on infections that can be prevented, occur frequently, cause serious morbidity and mortality, are costly to treat, or are caused by organisms resistant to multiple antimicrobial agents. For example, because infections associated with medical devices are preventable, consider surveying those UTIs associated with indwelling catheters or those infections caused by resistant organisms. Another strategy is to limit surveillance to device-related infections in intensive care or step down units where such devices are commonly used. Healthcare-associated infections caused by *Legionella* spp or *Aspergillus* spp occur infrequently. However, these infections cause substantial mortality and environmental controls can prevent most cases. Therefore, the infection control staff may want to use microbiology laboratory data (and other sources of data if necessary) to identify all of these cases and set up an intervention designed to lower the rates. Vancomycin-resistant enterococci, methicillin-resistant *S. aureus,* and other bacteria resistant to multiple antimicrobials can spread rapidly within hospitals. Infections caused by these organisms can be very costly to treat or may not be treatable. Therefore, microbiology data may be used to do surveillance for patients who are infected or colonized with these organisms. Infection control personnel may choose to study infections that are relatively minor but occur frequently because these infections will increase the total cost to the healthcare system. For example, saphenous vein harvest site infections are less severe than sternal wound infections after coronary artery bypass graft (CABG) procedures. However, at least two-thirds of the surgical site infections after CABG are harvest site infections, with an attributable cost of nearly $7000 per infection.[5] Because harvest site infections occur much more frequently than do serious sternal infections, the total cost to a healthcare system for the former approximates that of the latter. Furthermore, harvest site infections may be caused by technique problems and thus could be prevented if the surgical technique was improved.

As medical care moves from the hospital to outpatient and alternative care settings, we should consider how healthcare-associated infections that develop in the ambulatory-care setting can be identified.[6,7] Unless infection control teams expand their boundaries, they will underestimate the frequency of infections associated with medical care. At present, many infection control programs monitor patients who develop surgical site infections after ambulatory operative procedures.[7] In addition, infection control staff might consider using surveillance to identify patients who acquire infections associated with outpatient treatments such as dialysis, chemotherapy, and intravenous therapy (eg, antimicrobials, antiviral agents, and parenteral nutrition) or in programs such as hospital-based home care.

ASSESSING A SURVEILLANCE SYSTEM

Infection control programs should annually evaluate their surveillance system to determine if it provides meaningful data. The staff should ask themselves a series of questions:
- Does the surveillance system measure meaningful outcomes? Are these outcomes relevant to the hospital population and infectious diseases that are prevalent or emerging in the community?
- Did the surveillance system detect clusters or outbreaks?

➤ How good is the system at identifying the events of interest (ie, the sensitivity and specificity)?

➤ How representative is the system, if it is not 100% sensitive? Can you generalize the findings?

➤ Were patient care practices changed based on surveillance data?

➤ How easy is it to collect data? What percentage of the ICP's time is spent collecting data? What is the burden to other groups within the institution?

➤ Were the data used to develop and implement interventions to decrease the endemic rate of infection?

➤ Are the data available in a timely fashion?

➤ How flexible is the system?

➤ Were the data used to assess the efficacy of interventions?

➤ Were the data used to ensure that infection rates did not increase when procedures were changed?

➤ Is the administrative and clinical staff aware of surveillance findings?

If no one, including the infection control staff, uses the data to alter practice, one must conclude that their current system is ineffective. At this point, it is more fruitful to abandon the surveillance and devise a new strategic plan with surveillance goals and objectives in mind. This strategic plan should include specific actions that use the collected data. If appropriate, one could develop interventions on the basis of currently available data. The staff could plan how they will use the revised surveillance system to monitor the efficacy of the proposed interventions.

Periodically, one must verify that the surveillance system is actually capturing the data the staff thinks they are getting. Hospital departments that provide data for the surveillance program may change their procedures and cause what appears to be a change in rates. Surveillance systems that use data from information systems are particularly vulnerable. If these departments notify infection control staff of procedural changes, the ICPs can modify surveillance appropriately. At such a time, the source of information will need to be revalidated. However, departments often change important procedures without informing staff in other departments. These changes could affect infection rates substantially; other changes do not affect the infection rates directly but alter the surveillance system's ability to obtain necessary data. Because changes in procedures instituted by other departments can be invisible and can affect infection rates substantially, ICPs would be wise to investigate dramatic changes in the rates or other important results before assuming the presence of an outbreak or a very successful intervention (Table 6-5).

For example, an ICP calculated that the proportion of *S. aureus* isolates resistant to methicillin had dropped precipitously from 34% to 0%. However, the ICP was suspi-cious that the decrease was not real. Much of the MRSA had been isolated from surgical wounds, so the ICP checked to see if the surgeons had changed their management of infected wounds. The ICP discovered that the surgeons were now treating SSI empirically without first obtaining wound cultures. Upon further investigation, the ICP discovered that the laboratory had changed the criteria for processing wound cultures. Laboratory personnel no longer plated specimens from wound cultures if the Gram stain did not show any white blood cells. The two unrelated changes factitiously reduced the proportion of MRSA isolates.

The overall infection rate in another hospital suddenly decreased (see Table 6-5). The infection control team discovered that the fiscal department had changed the bed-count procedure so that a patient was counted as an admission each time the patient transferred to another unit. Thus, the denominator was inflated and the resulting infection rate appeared low.

HOW SHOULD THE OUTCOMES OF INTEREST AND TARGETED POPULATIONS BE DETERMINED?

The infection control staff must first identify the event and the population they will study. Outcomes of interest should be determined based on the impact of the event on patients (ie, morbidity or mortality), its frequency, the impact on the institution (financial), and the regulatory requirements. Hospitals with only oncology, pediatric, ophthalmology, or trauma patients should prioritize outcomes of interest differently than general hospitals. Next, the staff should develop written definitions that are precise, concise, and nonambiguous. One of the greatest challenges is to use definitions to help differentiate patients who are colonized from those who have infections (Table 6-6). Definitions developed by the CDC are widely used and accepted for identifying healthcare-associated infections.[8,9] In some cases, such as SSIs among transplant recipients or bloodstream infections among hematopoietic transplant recipients, CDC definitions may need to be modified. In other cases, hospitals may need to develop their own definitions. Others can use the definitions as they are written or slightly modified. Importantly, CDC definitions should be used if infection control personnel wish to compare their institution's infection rates to those published by the National Nosocomial Infection Surveillance System (NNIS) of the CDC.[8,9] Such comparisons or "benchmarking" allow programs to determine

Table 6-5. Examples of Practices That Affect Observed Infection Rates

Change in Practice	*Apparent Effect on Infection Rate*
➤ Shift locus of treatment from the hospital to the outpatient setting	➤ Decrease overall infection rate because surveillance is rarely performed in the outpatient setting
➤ Length of hospital stay decreases as patients are discharged earlier	➤ Decrease overall infection rate
➤ Length of stay in hospital decreases after operative procedures	➤ Decrease surgical site infection rate because surveillance is rarely performed in the outpatient setting
➤ Low-risk operative procedures performed in separate ambulatory surgical facility	➤ Increase surgical site infection rates because patients who have a higher risk of infection have operative procedures performed in the hospital
➤ Patients residing on a boarding unit are not counted as hospital denominator	➤ Increased infection rate if surveillance is conducted on these admissions
➤ Patients counted as an admission each time they are transferred to a different unit	➤ Decreased overall infection rate because denominator is inflated artificially
➤ The accounting office changes from charging one general cost for a central-line insertion to charging for each catheter opened	➤ Decreased infection rate associated with central lines because the denominator (ie, the number of central lines inserted) appears to increase
➤ The business office assigns the surgical procedure to admitting physician, regardless of that physician's specialty, rather than to the surgeon doing the procedure	➤ Inaccurate surgeon-specific infection rates because some surgical site infections will be assigned to the wrong physician
➤ Physicians treat patients empirically for possible infections without obtaining cultures	➤ Decreased infection rates if case-finding method relies solely on microbiology report
➤ Microbiology laboratory changes screening criteria for processing specimens	➤ Decreased infection rates if case-finding method relies solely on microbiology reports
➤ Absence of written definitions or definitions used inconsistently	➤ Inaccurate infection rates
➤ ICD 9 codes used to identify patients with healthcare-associated infections	➤ Inaccurate infection rates

TABLE 6-6. Examples of Healthcare-Associated Infection/Colonization Definitions for Surveillance

Infection Sites	Criteria for Infection	Source	Comments	Issues	Reporting Refinements
Blood	Positive culture	Laboratory	Must rule out contaminant	Common skin contaminants such as *coagulase-negative staphylocci* may require different definition	State if primary or secondary to an infection at another site
Urine	10^5/colonies of bacteria per 1 mL WBC in urine	Laboratory	Lower counts may be accepted if associated with compatible symptoms and pyuria. Candida and mixed organisms frequently represent contamination	May miss many infections	Note if current or prior bladder catheterization
Postoperative wounds or surgical sites (SSI)	Pus at the incision site	Laboratory Clinical	Cellulitis is classified separately; depth of SSI classified as organ, space, deep, or incisional	May miss many infections	Stitch abscess should not be considered a SSI
Other wounds	Presence of pus	Laboratory Clinical	Includes decubitus ulcers, tracheotomy site	May require tissue biopsy to make diagnosis	
Burns	>10^6 organisms per 1 g of biopsied tissue; alternatively, new inflammation or new pus not present on admission	Laboratory Clinical	Success of skin grafts is reported to be greater if placed over burn sites with bacterial counts <10^5/g tissue	Commonly requires laboratories with specialized capacity	Note the antibiogram; organisms frequently resistant to multiple antibiotics

TABLE 6-6. Examples of Healthcare-Associated Infection/Colonization Definitions for Surveillance (Continued)

Infection Sites	Criteria for Infection	Source	Comments	Issues	Refinements Reports
Pulmonary	New or progressive infiltrate. Fever and sputum production with new inflammation or new pus not present on admission. New onset of purulent sputum	Clinical Radiographic	Clinical picture must be compatible; other entities (eg, atelectasis and pulmonary emboli or infarction) ruled out	No gold standard diagnosis for *Candida, enterococci,* and *coagulase-negative staphylococci,* which generally represent contaminants	Note if pneumonia associated with assisted ventilation; rule out colonization. Note antibiogram because the respiratory tract is a frequent source of resistant organisms
Gastrointestinal	Culture growing pathogen or unexplained diarrhea for >2 days	Laboratory Clinical	Pathogens are defined as salmonella, shigella, pathogenic, *E. coli,* viruses (rotavirus), or *C. difficile* toxin	Can have shorter incubation periods with some pathogens (generally food borne)	List any antibiotics patient is receiving
Skin/IV	Pus at site	Clinical	Includes permanent central venous catheters, artificial catheters. Catheter tip cultures may be helpful. Diagnosis of tunnel infections may be based on different clinical parameters	Neutropenic patients rarely have clinical signs of infection; criteria not well studied	Note site of IV, duration of placement. Note type of catheter; colony counts on catheter can be helpful
Miscellaneous (hepatitis, upper respiratory infections, peritonitis, etc)	Clinical picture	Clinical Laboratory	Need appropriate diagnostic tests	Viral infections can have longer incubation periods	Note if associated temporarily with any hospital procedure, blood products, drugs
Nasal/perirectal sites	Culture growing pathogen such as MRSA or VRE	Laboratory	Usually identifies by surveillance program(s). Need appropriate diagnostic tests	Patients rarely have signs of infection	Denotes colonization usually

Adapted from Wenzel RP, et al. Hospital acquired infections: I. Surveillance in a university hospital. *Am J Epidemiol.* 1976;103 (3):251–260; and based on Perl TM. Surveillance, reporting and the use of computers. In: Wenzel RP, ed. *Prevention and Control of Nosocomial Infections.* Baltimore, Md: Williams and Wilkens; 1997:127–162.

how their rates compare with data from other institutions and to evaluate the success of infection control interventions. Some larger institutions, or those with large volumes, can use control charts or 95% confidence intervals (95% CI) to compare rates.[10] The advantage of comparing one's self to internal rates is that the patient population(s) are likely consistent or similar in terms of underlying illness. The major disadvantage is that one cannot discern if the rates are higher or lower than they should be or than those reported by other institutions.

To collect data, ICP must apply the definitions consistently. Training of ICPs enhances their abilities to identify infections appropriately and consistently as shown by Cardo and colleagues.[11,12] These authors demonstrated that the sensitivity and specificity of SSI surveillance increased from approximately 84% to over 93% with training. This training is critical to ensure that appropriate definitions, sources of information, and case-finding strategies are used. Ehrenkranz et al described the severe consequences that may occur if collected data do not reflect objective, written definitions that are applied systematically.[13] The infection control team recorded SSI rates of 3% to 11% for a particular surgeon over a 3-year period. The infection control committee considered these rates excessive and repeatedly investigated this surgeon. After the surgeon decided to stop operating, the hospital administrator asked a consultant to review the findings. During the investigation, the consultant found that infection control staff did not use a specific definition of SSIs. The consultant concluded that a surveillance error, not poor operative technique, accounted for the surgeon's reported high infection rates.

The term "healthcare-associated infection" describes an infection that is not present or incubating at the time the patient is admitted to the institution. Thus, an infection is not considered healthcare associated if it represents a complication or extension of an infectious process present on admission. This allows ICPs to capture infections that are related to medical and surgical procedures performed in outpatient settings. Infections that occur more than 48 hours after admission and within 7 to 30 days after hospital discharge are defined as healthcare associated. The time frame is modified for infections that have incubation periods less than 48 to 72 hours (eg, gastroenteritis caused by *Norovirus*) or longer than 10 days (eg, hepatitis A or C). SSIs are considered healthcare associated if the infection occurs within 30 days after the operative procedure or within 1 year if a device or foreign material is implanted. Because of the changing paradigm of healthcare, infections that have been labeled nosocomial in the past are now called healthcare associated. Infections should be considered healthcare associated if they are related to procedures, treatments, or other events that occur immediately after the patient is admitted to the hospital or those performed in an alternative setting such as a surgical cen-

ter. For example, bloodstream infections associated with central venous catheters, pneumonia associated with mechanical ventilation, or urinary tract infections associated with urethral catheterization should be considered healthcare associated, even if the onset of infection occurs within the first 48 hours of hospitalization. An infection that occurs in a patient who has a surgical procedure in the outpatient surgical suite would be considered healthcare associated. Because bone marrow transplantation, chemotherapy, and other procedures are being performed in outpatient settings, high-risk patients treated in alternate settings will develop bloodstream infections. These infections are almost always related to indwelling intravenous catheters. Because of these situations, ICP will need to refine and validate definitions in order to capture infectious complications in new healthcare delivery settings.

COLLECTING DATA

One of the first mantras of surveillance is to remember that its purpose is to determine the burden of disease, identify trends and potential problems, and establish the epidemiologic features of the illness (person, place, and time). Hence, only the information needed to adequately analyze and interpret the data should be collected. If these data suggest a potential problem, the epidemiology team can design a more comprehensive study. Data can be collected either concurrently or retrospectively. In concurrent surveillance, data are collected at the time the event occurs or shortly thereafter. Concurrent (or prospective) surveillance requires the infection control staff to review the medical record, assess the patient, and discuss the event with caregivers at the time of the infection. Because the data are obtained close to the time the event occurs, additional information such as ward logbooks and nursing reports, which are not normally a part of the medical record, may be available. Clusters can be identified as they occur. Importantly, feedback of information about any adverse event, as it happens, helps healthcare workers appreciate the significance of the event as it becomes "real" and less theoretical and identify other potential prevention strategies. In retrospective surveillance, data are collected after the patient is discharged. The two methods have similar sensitivities, but retrospective surveillance depends on the completeness, accuracy, and quality of the medical records (see Table 6-3).[14] Because data are collected after the event, retrospective surveillance does not identify clusters or potential outbreaks as promptly as concurrent surveillance. In some cases, the "distance" of the event sometimes impedes interest and interventions.

To identify cases, highly sensitive methods for case-finding are preferred so that important cases are not missed. Commonly, ICPs employ several case-finding methods simultaneously. The practice of using information collected concurrently by from different sources has increased with early patient discharges and transfer of care to the outpatient setting. However, one must first identify strategies to increase the specificity of the surveillance process and thus reduce time wasted collecting irrelevant data. Using currently available computer systems that can identify patients who may have healthcare-associated infections or epidemiologically important organisms can reduce the time spent reviewing charts. Computer-based surveillance strategies are rapidly emerging as important adjuncts for surveillance.[6,7,15,16] As computers and software become more sophisticated and computer-based decision algorithms are developed and tested, these can be integrated into surveillance systems to identify healthcare-associated infections.[6,7,15,16] As an example, Yokoe and colleagues showed that the agreement rate between the microbiology data surveillance method and the CDC's NNIS review method was 91%.[15] The microbiology data method requires approximately 20 minutes less time per isolate than does routine surveillance.[15]

When an infection control program begins a new surveillance project, the staff should periodically look for flaws in the data, the collection tool, the data sources, and the surveillance process. In this manner, epidemiology personnel can identify problems or errors and correct them before reaching the end of the study. Infection control staff can determine the project's sensitivity and specificity by examining a random subset of medical records for a defined time period and comparing the number of events identified by this review with those identified by the usual surveillance system. In addition, changes in the surveillance system such as identifying a new data source or a new item, modifying definitions, or changing the personnel who collect the data can impact the integrity of the surveillance progress. This validation is necessary to ensure the quality of the data. Validation is also used to ensure that practitioners apply the definitions systematically and uniformly.[17]

MANAGING DATA

Managing the data or organizing it in a meaningful fashion is necessary to identify patterns and trends. One of the first processes is to catalogue "cases" identified systematically on a flow sheet or in a computerized "spread sheet." This process is called a line-listing and will include data pertinent to the problem. For example, a line list may include, in a single row, the patient name, hospital or medical record number, the admission data, infection site, date of infection onset, organism(s), and surgical procedure, if relevant. Pads of columnar accounting paper may suffice as a database in small hospitals, but relational databases on personal computers are generally used for larger

hospitals. Once the data are in a database, infection control personnel can easily plot numbers or rates over time to identify possible trends. Mini programs or "macros" using commonly available relational databases can be developed to present data to staff and facilitate work flow. Recently, several exciting computer software programs have been developed that can integrate information from various hospital computer systems (via HL7 messages) and provide data that are concatenated and presented in epidemiologic terms.

ANALYZING DATA

If the epidemiology team does not analyze their data, they have wasted the time, money, and effort they spent collecting and recording the data. The purpose of surveillance is not merely to count and record infections but to identify problems quickly and to intervene so that the risk of infection is reduced. The time factor inherent in this process requires data to be analyzed promptly. The frequency of data analysis is based on the nature of the healthcare-associated event, the frequency of the event, and the purpose of surveillance. The goal is to strike a balance between analyzing the data frequently enough to detect clusters promptly and collecting data for a long enough period of time to ensure that variations in rates are real. Computer programs are facilitating the latter as standard analyses can be generated automatically. In addition, the practitioner must also ensure that an adequate sample of cases has been reviewed so that the data are meaningful.

Infection control personnel commonly report only the number of events that occur in a specified time period (numerator). While there is merit to providing units with immediate feedback in the setting of an intervention or outbreak, to compare data over time one must calculate the incidence of the event being studied. This calculation requires both a numerator of events being studied in the defined population and a denominator—the population at risk during the same time period. The following example illustrates why the infection control team must select the appropriate denominator and why a denominator is important. Suppose 10 patients in a hospital developed MRSA bloodstream infections during 1 month. If the hospital discharged 1000 patients that month, the incidence rate of new MRSA bloodstream infections acquired in the hospital would have been 1%. However, if all 10 patients were on the medical service, which discharged 600 patients, the incidence rate of patients with MRSA bloodstream infections on the medical service would have been 1.7%. If 8 of the 10 patients developed MRSA bloodstream infections while in the medical intensive care unit (MICU), which discharged 90 patients, the incidence rate in the MICU would have been 9%. If, however, the number of admissions in the MICU drops to 45 patients for the month, the incidence of MRSA bloodstream infections would be 18%. Thus, one can assess the true incidence of an event in a defined population only if a denominator that accurately represents the patients who are at risk of experiencing the event is used.

Similarly, if one evaluates only summary reports of microbiology data, important trends in specific units may be missed. For example, the summary reports may obscure the fact that 90% of the *Pseudomonas aeruginosa* isolated from patients in the MICU are resistant to gentamicin, piperacillin, and cefotaxime. Stratton demonstrated that yearly summaries showed little variation in antimicrobial susceptibility patterns within the whole hospital.[18,19] Focused microbiologic surveillance on specific units, in contrast, showed that the predominant pathogens and their antimicrobial susceptibility patterns differed among specialty units and the entire hospital. Srinivasan and colleagues missed a doubling of the incidence of *P. aeruginosa* among patients undergoing bronchoalveolar lavage when they examined the overall hospital rates.[20] One can discern the endemic (baseline) rate after data have been collected for a sufficiently long period of time. Subsequently, it is easier to determine whether the current rates were substantially different from the baseline rate. In addition to calculating overall rates, the epidemiology staff can analyze the data further by calculating attack rates for specific nursing units, services, or procedures. The latter rates enable the staff to identify significant changes and important trends within subgroups of patients that might be missed if the entire population were analyzed as a whole. When comparing data, either within an institution or across institutions, one must use comparable surveillance methods, definitions, and time frames.

The infection control team must interpret the data. If the rate of a particular event increases substantially, the epidemiology staff should analyze the data thoroughly to determine if a problem really exists. Even if the increase is not statistically significant, it may be clinically significant and warrant control measures. Furthermore, the team should assess whether the incidence of an event is acceptable. For example, even if the rate of SSI is stable, the incidence may be higher than that reported by comparable institutions or may be higher than it would be if the process of care was improved. A study by Classen et al demonstrated that examining the process of care can decrease the rate of SSI significantly.[21] In their study, the SSI rate for patients who received prophylactic antibiotics 2 hours before surgery was significantly lower than for the patients who received their antibiotics either early (ie, 2 to 24 hours before surgery) or postoperatively (ie, more than 3 hours after the incision but less than 24 hours after surgery). Therefore, an infection control team that wants to decrease SSI rates in their hospital might want to review the time at which the prophylactic antimicrobial agents are given.

COMMUNICATING RESULTS

Finally, the infection control staff must communicate the data to the persons who need the information and who have the power to authorize changes. ICPs regularly report to the infection control committee or to the quality or performance improvement committee. Infection control staff should also communicate appropriate rates and numbers with key persons on individual nursing units, in each clinical service, in the nursing administration, and in the hospital administration. For example, as part of an intervention to reduce catheter related bloodstream infections, the first author's infection control team report bloodstream infections weekly to the ICU personnel. A banner is posted in the ICU that lists the number of weeks since the last infection. In addition, ICPs may need to report their data to the education service, the ICU committee, or the safety committee. When reporting data in any setting, epidemiology personnel must maintain confidentiality for patients and employees.

Simple reports that the target audience can understand in a few seconds (the amount of time usually given to a report at a busy committee meeting) are most effective. Graphical or tabular displays of the data can present important trends in pictures and help key clinicians and administrative personnel grasp key points quickly. The use of 95% CI can help staff understand the significance of change in rates. Comparing rates with the NNIS or other benchmark data can help staff determine if their rates are too high. Moreover, individuals who are unfamiliar with infection control issues may not understand the importance of a problem if they are presented only with the data. This is particularly true if the number of cases is small or the etiologic agent has not been discussed in the popular press. Thus, the ICP should include his or her assessment and conclusions in the report, so that he or she can persuade clinicians or hospital administrators that corrective action is necessary.

SURVEILLANCE FOR HEALTHCARE-ASSOCIATED INFECTIONS

Data Sources

Many different sources provide information about patients with infections (Table 6-7). In addition, ICPs can obtain data from databases maintained by other departments such as medical records, pharmacy, respiratory

> **TABLE 6-7.** General Sources of Data For Surveillance

Patient-Based

➤ Clinical ward rounds, including questioning nurses, review of temperature curves
➤ Electronic medical records, including review of notes, vital signs, antimicrobial use, surgical procedure data, radiology, and laboratory reports
➤ Hospital employees
➤ Laboratory, radiology, and pathology reports
➤ Pharmacy department
➤ Admissions department
➤ Emergency rooms and emergency transfer personnel
➤ Operating suite
➤ Outpatient clinics, including surgical centers
➤ Medical records department
➤ Employee or occupational health department
➤ Incident reports
➤ Postdischarge clinic visits
➤ Local/state/provincial public health officials
➤ National Public Health sources

Laboratory-Based

➤ Microbiology, virology, and serology reports
➤ Antimicrobial susceptibility patterns

Outside sources of Information

MMWR
NNIS or other national databases
WHO alerts
Promed
Alerts from state/provincial or local health departments

therapy, admissions, risk control, and financial management. However, it must be remembered that these databases are generally designed for billing or administrative purposes, not for collecting data on infections. Therefore, one must determine whether those databases include data needed for surveillance and whether the data are complete and accurate. For instance, an ICP who conducts surveillance and uses the daily surgery schedule to obtain the number and classification of operative procedures instead of using the list of completed operative procedures will not determine accurate rates. If surgeons add, cancel, and change operative procedures during the day, the denominator for calculating SSI rates will be inaccurate.

Surveillance Methods

Each infection control team must determine which of many surveillance methods is best suited to their hospital.

To help choose the most appropriate approach, we have described five basic surveillance methods and have summarized their advantages and disadvantages (see Table 6-2).

Hospital-Wide Traditional Surveillance

Hospital-wide surveillance, the most comprehensive method, requires the ICP to prospectively and continuously survey all care areas to identify patients who have acquired infections or epidemiologically significant organisms during hospitalization.[22,23] The ICP gathers information from daily microbiology reports and from the medical records of patients who have fever or cultures growing organisms and of patients who are receiving antibiotics or are on isolation precautions. The ICP also garners important information by frequently talking with nursing staff and by occasionally seeing patients. In addition, the ICP periodically reviews all autopsy reports and employee health records. Depending on the hospital size, the infection control team periodically calculates the overall hospital infection rates and the infection rates by site, nursing unit, physician service, pathogen, or operative procedure. This could be monthly, quarterly, or semi-annually.

Traditional hospital-wide surveillance is comprehensive. However, these systems are very costly, and they identify many infections that cannot be prevented. Consequently, many infection control programs have developed other surveillance methods that require fewer resources. With increasingly sophisticated electronic patient records, it is possible to capture many clinical details that facilitate and enhance surveillance for healthcare-associated infections. The information ICPs require can be displayed on one or two screens. With improved clinical informatics systems, the time commitment required for surveillance will need to be re-evaluated.

Periodic Surveillance

There are several ways to conduct periodic surveillance. In one method, the infection control program conducts hospital-wide surveillance only during specified time intervals, such as 1 month each quarter. Infection control programs that use this method frequently conduct targeted surveillance (see under "Targeted Surveillance") during the alternate periods. In another method, the infection control program conducts surveillance on one or a few units for a specified time period and then shifts to another unit or units. By rotating surveillance from unit to unit, the infection control team is able to survey the entire hospital during the year.

Prevalence Survey

In a prevalence survey, the ICP counts the number of active infections or epidemiologically significant organisms during a specified time period.[24] Active infections are defined as all infections present during the time of the survey, including those newly diagnosed and those being treated when the survey begins. The total number of active infections/organisms is divided by the number of patients present during the survey.

Because new *and* existing infections are counted, the rates obtained from prevalence surveys are usually higher than incidence rates. Prevalence surveys can focus on particular populations such as patients with central venous catheters or patients receiving antimicrobials.[25] Prevalence studies are also useful for monitoring the number of patients colonized or infected with important organisms such as VRE or MRSA.

Infection control programs also can use prevalence studies to assess risk factors for infection in a particular population. To determine why patients in this population are developing infections, the epidemiology staff could collect additional data about potential risk factors from all patients surveyed. Because prevalence studies assess all patients in the target population regardless of whether they have infections, infection control personnel can compare the rate of infection in patients who have the potential risk factor with the rate in those who do not have the potential risk factor.

Targeted Surveillance

There are several approaches to targeted surveillance. Many infection control programs focus their efforts on selected geographic areas such as critical care units or selected services such as cardiothoracic surgery. Other programs focus surveillance on specific populations such as patients at high risk of acquiring infections (eg, transplant or pediatric patients), patients undergoing specific medical interventions (eg, hemodialysis patients), or patients with infections at specific sites (eg, bloodstream or surgical site). Some infection control staff target surveillance to infections associated with specific devices such as ventilator-associated pneumonia (VAP). By limiting the scope of surveillance, ICPs can collect data on entire patient populations.

Some infection control programs use data from the microbiology laboratory to limit their surveillance. For example, the epidemiology team may focus either on specific microorganisms such as *Legionella* species or on organisms with particular antimicrobial susceptibility patterns such as VRE or MRSA.

Outbreak Thresholds

Some investigators have conducted surveillance to assess their baseline infection rates. On the basis of their data, they developed outbreak thresholds. Subsequently, they stopped conducting routine surveillance and only evaluated problems when the number of isolates of a particular species or the number of positive cultures exceeded outbreak thresholds.[26,27] For example, McGuckin used a threshold of an 80th percentile above the baseline for each bacterial species from a particular nursing ward for a specified time period.[27] Similarly, Schifman and Palmer established a threshold of double the baseline positive culture rate.[26] Wright and colleagues developed a computer based program set a threshold of 3-sigmas.[28]

Case-Finding Methods

ICPs should collect data only on infections that were acquired in their own facility or as a consequence of procedures or treatments done in their hospital or clinics. For example, a patient may become infected with *Clostridium difficile* while in Hospital A and then transfer to Hospital B while still infected. ICPs in Hospital B should not include this infection in their rates, even though it was acquired in a hospital. Inclusion of these infections will overestimate the extent of their problem and will underestimate the efficacy of their own programs. Although not included in the healthcare-associated infection rates, ICPs may want to identify all patients who on admission carry or are infected with particular organisms such as *C. diffi-*

cile, VRE, MRSA, and respiratory syncytial virus. Such data allow infection control staff to estimate the entire population of patients affected by these organisms. By determining the proportion of patients that acquires the organism in the hospital, infection control personnel can evaluate the efficacy of their infection control efforts.

Investigators have described various methods used to identify patients with healthcare-associated infections. We will review some of these methods in the following paragraphs and in Table 6-3.

Total Chart Review

When using the total chart review method, the ICP reviews nurses' and physicians' notes, medication and treatment records, and radiology and laboratory reports for each patient one to two times per week.[22,23] In addition, many ICPs review notes from respiratory therapy, physical and occupational therapy, dietetics, and any other specialty caring for the patient. Because the ICP requires between 10 and 30 minutes to review each medical record, this method is time-consuming and costly. As mentioned above, this review likely requires less time with improved electronic patient records that can display all the information needed for surveillance on several computer screens. Clinical information systems typically provide demographic and administrative information, microbiology, radiology and pharmacy data, and—in some cases—physician, physical therapy, respiratory therapy, and nursing notes and information about lines.

Laboratory Reports

Clinical laboratory reports often are the primary source for identifying infections, particularly if the ICP reviews virology and serology reports in addition to bacteriology results.[22,29,30] The ICP may find some healthcare-associated infections directly from reports of cultures growing organisms. For example, a patient whose cultured blood grows *S. aureus* likely has a healthcare-associated infection if the culture was obtained 10 days after admission. A laboratory report might prompt the ICP to review the patient's medical record. While reviewing the medical record, the ICP might identify a healthcare-associated infection for which a culture was not obtained. For example, a patient might have a blood culture from which *Klebsiella pneumoniae* was isolated. In the medical record, the ICP might learn that the chest radiographs revealed a new pulmonary infiltrate and the Gram stain of the sputum revealed many white blood cells and Gram-negative rods. This information might lead the ICP to conclude that the patient had pneumonia and a secondary bacteremia caused by *K. pneumoniae*. Alternatively, cultured urine might prompt the ICP to review a patient's medical record (Table 6-8). While reviewing the record, the ICP might discover a healthcare-associated pneumonia caused by another organism.

Most laboratories maintain log books or notebooks that ICPs can scan quickly to obtain preliminary results. In addition, the laboratory staff often will notify infection control of positive tests. Nonetheless, laboratory reports have some substantial limitations, and the infection control program should not use them as the sole source of data used for identifying patients with healthcare-associated infections. For example, clinicians may not obtain cultures from patients with clinical evidence of SSI or UTI, but instead may treat these patients empirically. In addition, cultures from some sites of infection may be negative. This is particularly true if the patient is on antimicrobial therapy, or if the organism is fastidious or does not grow on routine culture media. Consequently, the sensitivity of laboratory records is directly affected by the number of infections from which cultures are obtained and the culture methods used by the laboratory.[31]

Nursing Care Plans or Kardex Screening

Nursing care plans or nursing care plans such as Kardexes contain patient information and can provide the ICP "clues." The ICP surveys the nursing care plan one to two times each week to determine whether patients are receiving antibiotics, intravenous fluids, or parenteral nutrition and whether the patient has an indwelling urinary catheter, special orders for wound-dressing changes, or orders for isolation precautions.[22] If the ICP identifies one of these "clues" or other information that suggests the patient is at risk of healthcare-associated infection, the ICP reviews the patient's record. If the nursing care plan is complete and current, the method is highly sensitive and enables the ICP to spend less time reviewing charts.

Clinical Ward Rounds

ICPs who regularly visit clinical wards can gain insight into patients, infections, and other adverse events because much important information is not included in the patients' records.[32,33] This method allows the ICP to be highly visible in patient-care areas, to observe infection control practices directly, and to talk with the healthcare workers caring for patients. In this manner, the ICP not only can collect data but can also assess compliance with isolation precautions, answer questions on infection control issues, and conduct informal educational sessions.

Computer Alerts; Personal Device Assistants; and Computer Based, Automated Surveillance

Many organizations have "home grown" computer programs in place to facilitate surveillance or identification of patients colonized or infected with epidemiologically important organisms (flags). These tools are important to enhance the ICP's efficiency and to protect patients. Although, individual successes are reported in the literature, the ICP needs to determine the utility of the tool to them and their practice. Recently, several investigators have used small hand held computers to facilitate surveil-

TABLE 6-8. Clinical Clues to Help Identify High-Risk Patients With a Healthcare-Associated Infection

Unit	Infection Site	Are There Any Patients With the Following:
Medical	Urinary tract	1. Fevers? 2. Urinary tract catheters?
Surgical	Surgical site Lower respiratory Urinary tract	1. Fevers? 2. Productive coughs? 3. Draining or erythematous wounds? 4. Who returned to surgery? 5. Who had blood cultured? 6. Abnormal intravenous catheter sites? 7. Who received prolonged antibiotics? 8. Who had been readmitted?
Pediatric	Gastrointestinal Respiratory	1. Fevers? 2. Diarrhea? 3. Apnea/bradycardia spells? 4. Lethargy, irritability? 5. New respiratory symptoms?
Hematology/oncology	Bloodstream Permanent catheter	1. Fevers or new fevers? 2. New radiographic abnormalities or respiratory symptoms? 3. Placed on antibiotics? 4. Who had blood cultured? 5. Any erythematous intravenous catheter sites?
Intensive care	Pneumonia Intravenous catheters Urinary tract	1. Fevers? 2. Diarrhea? 3. Placed on antibiotics? 4. Who had cultured blood? 5. Any erythematous intravenous catheter sites or catheters that were changed?
Obstetrics and gynecology	Surgical site Lower respiratory	1. Fevers? 2. Foul-smelling drainage? 3. Erythematous wounds? 4. On new antibiotics? 5. Productive coughs?
Extended or chronic care	Urinary tract Lower respiratory	1. New fevers? 2. New mental status changes? 3. Recently placed on antibiotics? 4. Productive coughs or new respiratory symptoms? 5. Foul-smelling urine? 6. New diarrhea?

lance. Typically, these devices include administrative data about patients of interest. The ICP adds other details. These data are then downloaded into relational databases that allow the ICP to manipulate and analyze the data. Additionally, several companies have developed exciting computer software that merge microbiologic data with other clinically relevant data such as pharmacy, radiology, and device related data. These data, which are presented in a single screen, can be used to enhance and automate surveillance for healthcare-associated infections. Data can be easily viewed by the ICP and the data are collected in relational databases. These easy to use programs allow practitioners to "query" the system and to display data graphically. Some of these programs have data mining capabilities. The impact of one of these programs has been measured and it has been shown to be more efficient at identifying outbreaks than routine surveillance.[28] Eleven of the 18 alerts identified by the software were determined to be potential outbreaks, yielding a positive predictive value of 0.61.[28] Routine surveillance identified 5 of these 11 alerts during this time period. These systems have various degrees of sophistication and some can include data from electronic patient records. Such advances are likely to decrease time performing surveillance so the ICP can spend time on other activities.

Other investigators have mined large databases to look for novel ways of identifying healthcare-associated infections. As computerized medical records and administrative databases have become more common, there has been substantial interest in using such systems to conduct surveillance for healthcare-associated infections. The goals are to increase the sensitivity of surveillance, to decrease the need for chart reviews, and to reduce costs. Most of the work has been done with those systems that support large health systems that provide integrated healthcare. This facilitates identifying infections treated in outpatient or alternative settings. One common strategy is to use automated claims data to identify patients with infection related ICD-9 codes and with antibiotic use, readmissions, emergency room visits, or the use of other medical tests in a specified period of time. The overall sensitivity, specificity, and predictive values need to be tested as these systems are evaluated.[6,15,16,34] Of note, Sands et al examined the sensitivity of using the health plan administrative data base and found that the overall sensitivity was 72% as compared to 49% for the hospital-based surveillance.[6] Importantly, the sensitivity for detecting SSIs after discharge was 99%, far superior to routine surveillance.

Postdischarge Surveillance

As patients are discharged from hospitals earlier, the infection control team will have increasing difficulty detecting hospital-acquired infections. One way of obtaining these data is postdischarge surveillance. Infection control teams that do not conduct postdischarge surveillance will identify spuriously low healthcare-associated infec-

tion rates because traditional hospital-based surveillance methods only identify events that occur while the patient is in the hospital. In fact, studies have documented that postdischarge surveillance identifies 13% to 70% more SSIs than do methods that survey only inpatients.[35]

Most investigators who have studied methods for postdischarge surveillance have not evaluated all discharged patients but have focused on specific populations such as postoperative patients, postpartum women, or neonates. Investigators have assessed various methods for identifying infections after these patients are discharged, including directly assessing the patients, reviewing records from visits to clinics or emergency rooms, and contacting physicians or patients by mail or telephone. Although all of these methods identify patients who develop infections after discharge, the methods are time-consuming and can be insensitive. None of these methods have been accepted widely. Sands et al have used administrative billing data bases from an integrated health system to study the best methods to identify surgical site infections, 84% of which develop after discharge.[6,7] Unfortunately, most infection control programs do not have access to such resources.

WHICH CASE-FINDING METHOD IS BEST?

Each case-finding method has some merit, but each also has limitations. There is no agreement on which case-finding method is best. Some infection control personnel consider total chart review to be the gold standard for identifying healthcare-associated infections. However, in two studies that compared total chart review with combinations of two or more case-finding methods, the former method identified only 74% to 94% of the infections identified by the combined methods.[14,22] Investigators were unable to identify all infections by reviewing only the medical record because of the following:

➤ The records did not document all data required to determine whether the patients met criteria for specific infections.

➤ Laboratory or radiology reports were missing.

➤ Records were not available.

➤ The reviewer could not examine the patient.

Consequently, total chart review is no more sensitive than other case-finding methods or combination of methods.

Nettleman and Nelson conducted surveillance to identify adverse occurrences among patients hospitalized on general medical wards.[36] They used numerous data sources and found that no single source identified all adverse occurrences. In fact, the number of adverse occurrences the investigators identified in each category was dependent on which data source the investigators used. Certain data sources efficiently identified specific adverse occurrences. For example, the authors identified 77% of medication-related errors by reviewing the medication administration record, but detected only 10% of these events by reviewing the physicians' progress notes. Conversely, the authors identified 100% of procedure-related adverse occurrences by reviewing the physicians' progress notes but did not detect any of these events by reviewing the medication administration record.

Therefore, the infection control team must select case-finding methods that best identify the healthcare-associated infections they choose to study. For example, the ICP could identify most bloodstream infections by reviewing microbiology reports but would find very few bloodstream infections by observing the patient directly. On the other hand, the ICP might identify most SSIs by observing surgical wounds directly, but not by reviewing microbiology reports.

NATIONAL NOSOCOMIAL INFECTIONS SURVEILLANCE SYSTEM

In 1970, the CDC enrolled a sample of hospitals that voluntarily agreed to collect data on nosocomial infections, into the NNIS system. Currently, 202 hospitals participate in the program, and NNIS is the only source of national data on healthcare-associated infections in the United States.[37] The participating hospitals range in size from 80 to 1200 beds and include state, federal, profit, and nonprofit institutions. The NNIS program has several goals:

➤ To estimate the incidence of healthcare-associated infections.

➤ To identify changes in the pathogens causing healthcare-associated infections, the frequency of healthcare-associated infections at specific sites, the predominant risk factors, and the antimicrobial susceptibility patterns.

➤ To provide data on healthcare-associated infections with which hospitals can compare their data, including the distribution of healthcare-associated infections by major sites, device-associated infection rates by type of intensive care unit, and SSI rates by operative procedure.

➤ To develop strategies that infection control personnel can use for surveillance and assessment of healthcare-associated infections.

Initially, all hospitals participating in NNIS conducted prospective, traditional, hospital-wide surveillance. The CDC investigators subsequently identified methodological problems that made comparisons of data across hospitals unreliable. Thus, in 1986, the NNIS program created three

surveillance components in addition to hospital-wide surveillance: the adult intensive care unit or the pediatric intensive care unit, the high-risk nursery, and all surgical patients or patients undergoing specific procedures. The revised NNIS system has some advantages. First, the new components require ICPs to collect data on exposure to devices or to specific operative procedures. Thus, the CDC can adjust infection rates in the surveyed units for exposure to these devices and procedures. Hospitals that participate in NNIS regularly receive reports that compare their adjusted data with the aggregate adjusted data. ICPs in hospitals that do not participate in NNIS can compare their adjusted rates with the adjusted rates published by the CDC. Second, each hospital can choose the surveillance component in which it will participate. Thus, each infection control program can both design a surveillance program that meets the needs of their institution and participate in NNIS. Switzerland, Germany, Spain, the Netherlands, and France have developed remarkable surveillance systems for healthcare-associated infections that have elements of NNIS.[24,38-41]

HEALTHCARE-ASSOCIATED INFECTION RATES

Measures of frequency of healthcare-associated events have myriad names but can be categorized as incident and prevalent measures. The merits of these and some of the controversies are described below (see also Chapter 5). Prevalence measures the number of events (new or old) that are present during the period of interest. Prevalence is usually ascertained in surveys. This number is derived from a point in time (number of active current infections/number of patients at risk or studied). To measure incidence, the most common measures include the crude cumulative incidence (number of infections/100 admissions or discharges), the crude incidence density or the adjusted infection rate (number of infections/1,000 patient days), the specific cumulative or incidence density (by unit, procedure; or provider), and the adjusted cumulative or incidence density (adjusted for intrinsic host factors such as age). Finally, standardized infection ratios are used to compare surgical site infection frequency.[40] These are calculated by taking the ratio of the observed to the expected rate of infections with the expected rate derived using data from a reference facility or source and the distribution of operations by risk category.

Overall Hospital Infection Rates

Infection control programs that conduct hospital-wide surveillance sometimes track their overall infection rate. This rate is calculated by dividing the number of healthcare-associated infections identified in a given month by the number of patients admitted or discharged during the same month. However, the overall hospital infection rate has several inherent disadvantages:

➤ The overall rate treats all infections as though they are of equal importance. Furthermore, changes in uncommon but important infections (eg, bacteremia) might be hidden in the larger volume of common but less important infections (eg, urinary tract infections).

➤ The overall rate does not distinguish between patients who had one infection and those who had numerous infections.

➤ The overall infection rate may not be accurate and may underestimate the true rate because the ICP often cannot identify all healthcare-associated infections.

➤ The overall rate does not account for patients who are at increased risk for becoming infected because of their underlying diseases or exposure to procedures and medical devices; therefore, the overall infection rate tends to obscure important trends in intensive care units or among high-risk patients.

➤ The rate does not adjust for length of stay.

➤ The rate is not risk adjusted, therefore, it cannot be compared with rates from other hospitals.

In short, the accuracy and usefulness of the overall infection rate is limited. Therefore, we recommend that infection control personnel stop calculating their overall infection rate and begin calculating adjusted infection rates.

Site-Specific Infection Rates

Site-specific infection rates are a more appropriate measure of occurrence as they represent a more homogenous group of infections. Examples of site-specific infections include bloodstream infections, catheter related infections, UTIs, lower respiratory tract infections, or ventilator-associated pneumonia. These rates are calculated with a numerator divided by a denominator. The most common measure of frequency used is the specific cumulative or incidence density ratio.

Adjusting Rates

Comparison of infection rates within a single hospital over time may not be valid if the patient population or patient care changed substantially over the time period of interest. Further, comparisons among hospitals may not be valid because healthcare facilities are not standardized.[42] Patients in different hospitals have different underlying diseases and different severities of illness. In addition, patients who have the same disease and the same severity of illness but who are in different hospitals could undergo different diagnostic and therapeutic interventions and stay in the hospital for different periods of time.

Each hospital has its own unique environment, patient-care practices, and healthcare providers. Infection control programs vary substantially in the intensity of surveillance, the methods used for surveillance, the definitions of infections, and the methods used for calculating infection rates. Consequently, adjusted rates must be used to assess rates over time or to compare their rates with those in other hospitals. In the following paragraphs, we will discuss several methods for adjusting rates.

Adjusting Rates for Length of Stay

Infection rates more accurately reflect the risk of infection when they are adjusted for length of stay. Controlling for the length of stay has been achieved by calculating the number of healthcare-associated infections per patient day. This method uses the total number of healthcare-associated infections in a month as the numerator and the total number of patient days (ie, the sum of the number of days that each patient was on the unit) in that month as the denominator. For example, an obstetrics ward admits many patients who stay in the hospital for a very brief time and whose risk of infection is low, but a rehabilitation ward admits a few patients who stay for long periods of time and whose risk of infection is high. If the number of patients admitted to these units were used as the denominators, the rate for obstetrics probably would underestimate the risk of infection, whereas the rate on the rehabilitation ward most likely would overestimate the risk of infection. By using the number of patient-days as the denominator, infection control staff control for the effect of length of stay on the infection rate. However, this method does not control for the effect of other risk factors such as devices or for the severity of the patient's underlying illness.

Adjusting Rates for Exposure to Devices

Device-associated infection rates control for the duration of exposure to a device, which is one of the major risk factors for these infections. Therefore, device-associated rates can be compared more reliably over time and among institutions than can overall infection rates. To obtain this rate, the infection control team first chooses the device (eg, mechanical ventilators) and specifies the population (eg, patients in the medical intensive care unit) to be studied. Next, the team identifies the device-associated infections (eg, VAP) that occur in the selected population during a specified time period. The number of infections is the numerator. To obtain the denominator, the team sums the number of patients exposed to the device during each day of the specified period. For example, if the team surveyed the MICU for 7 days and the number of patients on ventilators each day was four, three, five, five, four, six, and four, respectively, the number of ventilator days would have been 31. If the team identified three cases of VAP during the week, the VAP rate would have been 0.097 (3/31) cases per ventilator-day or 97 per 1000 ventilator days.

Adjusting Rates for Severity of Illness

One would expect that a 28-year-old man who does not have underlying medical illnesses and who is undergoing an elective herniorrhaphy would have a lower risk of acquiring an SSI than would a 65-year-old man who has chronic lung disease treated with steroids, diabetes mellitus, and heart disease and who is undergoing an emergency exploratory laparotomy. Several investigators have developed scores to determine a patient's severity of illness. These scores range from simple, subjective scales based on clinical judgment to commercially available, computerized programs that use objective clinical data to assess the severity of a patient's underlying illnesses. Unfortunately, the currently available severity of illness scores cannot identify patients who are at high risk of developing a healthcare-associated infection. Thus, most infection control programs do not use these scores to risk-adjust healthcare-associated infection rates.

The risk index with which infection control personnel are most familiar is the surgical-wound classification. This classification system separates procedures into four categories: clean, clean-contaminated, contaminated, or dirty.[43] The incidence of infection increases as the wound classification changes from clean to dirty. However, this system does not account for each patient's intrinsic susceptibility to infection. Consequently, its ability to predict which patients are at highest risk of SSI is limited. Investigators in the SENIC and NNIS projects have developed risk indices that include variables assessing the patients' intrinsic risk of infection.[44,45] Culver et al used the NNIS risk index to stratify the risk of SSI and to standardize SSI rates.[45] However, other investigators tested the validity of the NNIS risk index and found that it did not predict which patients were at highest risk of developing an SSI after cardiothoracic surgery.[46] Hence, before risk indices can be used to identify high-risk patients or to adjust rates, they must be validated, and the population for which they are most predictive must be defined.

CONCLUSION

We believe that the surveillance systems of the 2000s must be extremely flexible so that they can be adapted to meet the needs of rapidly changing healthcare systems and to use the emerging information technology. We also think that effective infection control teams will not use a one-size-fits-all approach to surveillance, but will mix and match different case-finding methods and surveillance methods to create a surveillance system that meets the needs not only of their entire healthcare system but also of the individual components (eg, intensive care units and ambulatory-surgery center). That being said, as legislators pass laws asking hospitals to report infection rates, the importance of using standard definitions and standard approaches to identifying infections and calculating rates is paramount. In addition, we think infection control personnel must use computers and must develop surveillance systems that use the computerized databases already present in their hospital (eg, databases from the laboratory, surgical services, and financial management). They need to advocate to include newer information technology into their programs to enhance their efficiency with surveillance activities and increase interventions to prevent adverse events. Furthermore, the infection control team should collaborate with personnel from the information systems department to develop algorithms used to identify patients with possible healthcare-associated infections and thresholds used to identify likely outbreaks. As hospitals develop electronic patient records, computer-based surveillance should become easier. However, we would encourage infection control personnel not to wait until their hospital has electronic patient records, but to use whatever resources are available currently to streamline surveillance. Finally, computerized models that predict which patients are at highest risk of infection would allow infection control personnel to improve the efficiency of surveillance and stratify infection rates more appropriately. However, these models are not currently available. We would encourage the infection control community to make development of such models a priority for the future.

ACKNOWLEDGMENT

The author would like to thank Kathleen Speck for her critical review of this chapter.

REFERENCES

1. Langmuir AD. The surveillance of communicable diseases of national importance. *N Engl J Med*. 1963;268(Jan 24): 182-92.
2. Perl TM. Surveillance, reporting and the use of computers. In: Wenzel RP, ed. *Prevention and Control of Nosocomial Infections*. Baltimore, Md: Williams and Wilkens; 1997:127-162.
3. Haley RW, Quade D, Freeman HE, et al. The SENIC project: Study on the efficacy of nosocomial infection control (SENIC Project); summary of study design. *Am J Epidemiol*. 1980;111:472-485.
4. Bravata DM, McDonald KM, Smith WM, et al. Systematic review: surveillance systems for early detection of bioterrorism-related diseases. *Ann Intern Med*. 2004;140(11): 910-922.

5. Morales EM, Herwaldt LA, Nettleman M, et al. *S. aureus carriage and saphenous vein harvest site infection (HSI) following coronary artery bypass surgery.* Orlando, Fla: ICAAC; 1994.

6. Sands KE, Yokoe DS, Hooper DC, et al. Detection of postoperative surgical-site infections: comparison of health plan-based surveillance with hospital-based programs. *Infect Control Hosp Epidemiol.* 2003;24(10):741-743.

7. Sands K, Vineyard G, Livingston J, et al. Efficient identification of postdischarge surgical site infections: use of automated pharmacy dispensing information, administrative data, and medical record information. *J Infect Dis.* 1999;179(2):434-441.

8. Horan T, Gaynes R, Martone W, et al. CDC definitions of nosocomial surgical site infections, 1992: a modification of CDC definitions of surgical wound infections. *Am J Infect Control.* 1992;20:271-274.

9. Garner JS, Jarvis WS, Emori TG, et al. CDC definitions for nosocomial infections, 1988. *Am J Infect Control.* 1988;16:128-140.

10. Morrison AJJ, Kaiser DL, Wenzel RP. A measurement of the efficacy of nosocomial infection control using the 95 percent confidence interval for infection rates. *Am J Epidemiol.* 1987;126:292-297.

11. Cardo DM, Falk PS, Mayhall CG. Validation of surgical wound classification in the operating room. *Infect Control Hosp Epidemiol.* 1993;14(5):255-259.

12. Cardo DM, Falk PS, Mayhall CG. Validation of surgical wound surveillance. *Infect Control Hosp Epidemiol.* 1993; 14(4):211-215.

13. Ehrenkranz NJ, Richter EI, Phillips PM, et al. An apparent excess of operative site infections: analyses to evaluate false-positive diagnosis. *Infect Control Hosp Epidemiol.* 1995;16:712-716.

14. Haley RW, Schaberg DR, McClish DK, et al. The accuracy of retrospective chart review in measuring nosocomial infection rates. *Am J Epidemiol.* 1980;111:516-533.

15. Yokoe DS, Anderson J, Chambers R, et al. Simplified surveillance for nosocomial bloodstream infections. *Infect Control Hosp Epidemiol.* 1998;19(9):657-660.

16. Platt R, Yokoe DS, Sands KE. Automated methods for surveillance of surgical site infections. *Emerg Infect Dis.* 2001;7(2):212-216.

17. Broderick A, Mori M, Nettleman MD, et al. Nosocomial infections: validation of surveillance and computer modeling to identify patients at risk. *Am J Epidemiol.* 1990;131(4):734-742.

18. Stratton CW, Ratner H, Johnston PE, et al. Focused microbiologic surveillance by specific hospital unit as a sensitive means of defining antimicrobial resistance problems. *Diagn Microbiol Infect Dis.* 1992;15:11S-18S.

19. Stratton CW, Ratner H, Johnston PE, et al. Focused microbiologic surveillance by specific hospital unit: practical application and clinical utility. *Clin Ther.* 1993;15 Suppl A:12-20.

20. Srinivasan A, Wolfenden LL, Song X, et al. An outbreak of *Pseudomonas aeruginosa* infections associated with flexible bronchoscopes. *N Engl J Med.* 2003;348(3):221-227.

21. Classen DC, Evans RS, Pestotnik SL, et al. The timing of prophylactic administration of antibiotics and the risk of surgical-wound infection. *N Engl J Med.* 1992;326(5):281-286.

22. Wenzel RP, Osterman CA, Hunting KJ, et al. Hospital acquired infections: I. surveillance in a university hospital. *Am J Epidemiol.* 1976;103(3):251-260.

23. Haley RW, Culver DH, White JW, et al. The efficacy of infection surveillance and control programs in preventing nosocomial infections in US hospitals. *Am J Epidemiol.* 1985;121:182-205.

24. Pittet D, Harbarth S, Ruef C, et al. Prevalence and risk factors for nosocomial infections in four university hospitals in Switzerland. *Infect Control Hosp Epidemiol.* 1999;20(1):37-42.

25. Climo M, Diekema D, Warren DK, et al. Prevalence of the use of central venous access devices within and outside of the intensive care unit: results of a survey among hospitals in the prevention epicenter program of the Centers for Disease Control and Prevention. *Infect Control Hosp Epidemiol.* 2003;24(12): 942-945.

26. Schifman RB, Palmer RA. Surveillance of nosocomial infections by computer analysis of positive culture rates. *J Clin Microbiol.* 1985;21:493-495.

27. McGuckin MB, Abrutyn E. A surveillance method for early detection of nosocomial outbreaks. *Am J Infect Control.* 1979;19:18-28.

28. Wright MO, Perencevich EN, Novak C, et al. Preliminary assessment of an automated surveillance system for infection control. *Infect Control Hosp Epidemiol.* 2004;25(4):325-332.

29. Gross PA, Beaugard A, Van Antwerpen C. Surveillance for nosocomial infections: can the sources of data be reduced? *Infect Control Hosp Epidemiol.* 1980;1:233-236.

30. Glenister HM. How do we collect data for surveillance of wound infection? *J Hosp Infect.* 1993;24(4):283-289.

31. Manian F, Meyer L. Comprehensive surveillance of surgical wound infection in outpatient and inpatient surgery. *Infect Control Hosp Epidemiol.* 1990;10:515-520.

32. Glenister H, Taylor L, Bartlett C, et al. An assessment of selective surveillance methods for detecting hospital-acquired infection. *Am J Med.* 1991;91(suppl 3B):121S-124S.

33. Ford-Jones EL, Mindorff CM, Pollock E, et al. Evaluation of a new method of detection of nosocomial infection in the pediatric intensive care unit: the infection control sentinel sheet system. *Infect Control Hosp Epidemiol.* 1989;10:515-520.

34. Sands K, Vineyard G, Platt R. Surgical site infections occurring after hospital discharge. *J Infect Dis.* 1996; 173(4):963-970.

35. Holtz TH, Wenzel RP. Postdischarge surveillance for noso-comial wound infection: a brief review and commentary. *Am J Infect Control*. 1992;20(4):206-213.

36. Nettleman MD, Nelson AP. Adverse occurrences during hospitalization on a general medicine service. *Clin Perform Qual Health Care*. 1994;2(2):67-72.

37. Emori TG, Culver DH, Horan TC, et al. National nosoco-mial infections surveillance system (NNIS): description of surveillance methods. *Am J Infect Control*. 1991;19:19-35.

38. Gastmeier P, Gefers C, Sohr D, et al. Five years working with the German nosocomial infection surveillance sys-tem (Krankenhaus Infektions Surveillance System). *Am J Infect Control*. 2003;31(5):316-321.

39. Gastmeier P, Weigt O, Sohr D, et al. Comparison of hospi-tal-acquired infection rates in paediatric burn patients. *J Hosp Infect*. 2002;52(3):161-165.

40. Jodra VM, Rodela AR, Martinez EM, et al. Standardized infection ratios for three general surgery procedures: a comparison between Spanish hospitals and U.S. centers participating in the National Nosocomial Infections Surveillance System. *Infect Control Hosp Epidemiol*. 2003;24(10):744-748.

41. The French Prevalence Survey Study Group. Prevalence of nosocomial infections in France: results of the nationwide survey in 1996. *J Hosp Infect*. 2000;46(3):186-193.

42. Nosocomial infection rates for interhospital comparison: limitations and possible solutions. A report from the National Nosocomial Infections Surveillance (NNIS) System. *Infect Control Hosp Epidemiol*. 1991;12(10):609-621.

43. Garner J. CDC guidelines for the prevention and control of nosocomial infection. Guideline for prevention of surgical wound infection surveillance. *Am J Infect Control*. 1986; 14:71-82.

44. Haley RW, Culver DH, Morgan WM, et al. Identifying patients at high risk of surgical wound infection: a simple multivariate index of patient susceptibility and wound contamination. *Am J Epidemiol*. 1985;121(2):206-215.

45. Culver DH, Horan TC, Gaynes RP, et al. Surgical wound infection rates by wound class, operative procedure, and patient risk index. National Nosocomial Infections Surveillance System. *Am J Med*. 1991;91(3B):152S-157S.

46. Roy MC, Herwaldt LA, Embrey R, et al. Does the Centers for Disease Control's NNIS system risk index stratify patients undergoing cardiothoracic operations by their risk of surgical-site infection? *Infect Control Hosp Epidemiol*. 2000;21(3):186-190.

CHAPTER SEVEN

PREVENTING NOSOCOMIAL PNEUMONIA

Scott A. Flanders, MD; Harold R. Collard, MD; and Sanjay Saint, MD, MPH

INTRODUCTION

Nosocomial pneumonia (NP) is generally defined as pneumonia occurring 48 hours or more after hospital admission to exclude infections that may have been present but undetected at the time of admission. Ventilator-associated pneumonia (VAP) is a subgroup of NP and is defined as pneumonia developing more than 48 to 72 hours after initiation of mechanical ventilation (MV). The overwhelming majority of published work on NP involves patients in ICUs and, in particular, mechanically ventilated patients who develop VAP. Any evidence-based overview of NP, therefore, is largely based on experience in the ICU population. Thus, the hospital epidemiologist and infection control professional must extrapolate principles learned from the ICU population to the nonventilated patient residing on the general wards.

The incidence of NP varies depending on several factors, including patient characteristics such as illness severity and presence of comorbid disease; type of hospital (teaching vs. non-teaching); and method of diagnosis (clinical vs. bronchoscopic). Published estimates suggest rates of 5 to 10 cases per 1000 hospitalizations.[1] Patients with endotracheal tubes have rates that are up to 20-fold higher than patients without endotracheal tubes. A recent report from a large US database revealed that nearly 1 in 10 patients who required MV for more than 24 hours developed VAP.[2] The chance of infection increases with duration of MV, and thus rates presented per 1000 ventilator days more accurately reflect the risk of VAP. Overall, VAP rates of 15 per 1000 ventilator days are often reported, but again, rates will vary with patient population and setting.

Patients who develop NP often have significant underlying disease and thus have high overall (or crude) mortality rates. The attributable mortality, or deaths directly due to NP, is more difficult to discern. Some case-control and matched cohort studies have suggested attributable mortality rates for VAP as high as 30%, while others have been unable to demonstrate increased mortality. The fact that clinical outcomes improve with appropriate antibiotic therapy would argue that the attributable mortality is likely substantial. The economic burden of NP is sizable and actually easier to demonstrate. Multiple studies have shown that NP increases hospital length of stay by an average of 7 to 10 days. In patients with VAP, the duration of both MV and ICU stay is increased, and the attributable cost of VAP at one tertiary care medical center was nearly $12,000.[3] In another large epidemiologic study, patients who developed VAP had a mean increase of more than $40,000 in hospital charges when compared to matched control patients.[2]

Fortunately, the burden of this illness can be reduced via prevention. While our focus is on strategies for preventing NP, we initially consider pathogenesis, diagnosis, and treatment of NP. Importantly, the preventive strategies discussed in this chapter emphasize reducing rates of *bacterial* NP. The hospital epidemiologist and infection control professional, should be aware, however, that while uncommon, nosocomial viral and fungal pneumonia can occur, especially in highly immunocompromised patients or, in the case of viral infections, during community outbreaks.

PATHOGENESIS AND ETIOLOGY

NP is a result of microbial invasion of the normally sterile lung parenchyma. Given the rarity of hematological spread of infection to the lungs, most cases of NP are due to microaspiration of contaminated oropharyngeal or gas-

---

TABLE 7-1. RISK FACTORS FOR NOSOCOMIAL PNEUMONIA

Impaired Host Defenses/Increased Aspiration

Endotracheal tubes	Supine positioning
Nasogastric tubes	Impaired mental status
Enteral feeding tubes	Sedation

Large Inoculum of Organisms

Bacterial colonization	Sinusitis
Gastric alkalinization (enteral feeds/H_2 antagonists)	Malnutrition
Iatrogenic (forced hand ventilation)	Contaminated respiratory equipment

Overgrowth of Virulent Organisms

Prolonged antibiotic use	Comorbid illness
Iatrogenic (inadequate hand washing)	Frequent hospitalizations
Central venous lines	Prolonged hospital stays

---

tric secretions. A defect in normal host defenses (eg, endotracheal intubation), aspiration of a large inoculum of organisms, or aspiration of a particularly virulent organism may lead to infection. Table 7-1 highlights several key clinical factors associated with the development of NP. The use of endotracheal tubes is one of the most significant factors contributing to impaired host defenses, while bacterial overgrowth in both gastric and oropharyngeal secretions commonly results from the additive effect of multiple risk factors (see Table 7-1). Prolonged antibiotic exposure and iatrogenic spread of bacteria are key factors in the development of infection with a highly virulent organism. Modifiable risk factors serve as likely targets for preventive strategies and will be discussed in detail later in this chapter.

The clinician evaluating a patient with NP must consider a wide spectrum of causative organisms that range from relatively susceptible bacteria to highly resistant ones. As most initial antibiotic therapy is empiric, it is useful to identify whether a particular patient is at risk for a resistant organism.

Traditional thinking about bacterial etiologies of NP largely reflects the guidelines of the American Thoracic Society, which divide patients into those who develop pneumonia early in their hospital course (<5 days) and those who develop pneumonia later (>5 days).[1] In general, the spectrum of causative organisms in patients who develop early pneumonia reflects community isolates (*Streptococcus pneumoniae*, *Haemophilus influenzae*, *Escherichia coli*, non-resistant enteric gram-negative bacilli, methicillin-susceptible *Staphylococcus aureus*) and is unlikely to involve resistant organisms. Patients who develop late-onset NP are more likely to have resistant organisms (*Pseudomonas aeruginosa*, *Acinetobacter*

species, and MRSA). Importantly, many cases of NP, especially VAP, are polymicrobial.[4,5]

Clinical risk factors and comorbidities may be more important than time of onset in predicting the causative organism in NP. A recent prospective study of more than 3600 patients admitted to an intensive care unit compared patients with early (<5 days after ICU admission) vs. late-onset (>5 days after ICU admission) NP.[6] Of patients with early onset NP, *P. aeruginosa*, MRSA, and *Acinetobacter* spp. were isolated in 25%, 18%, and 6% of patients, respectively. In this sample, 78% of patients with early onset disease had received prior broad-spectrum antibiotics, and 49% had been in the hospital at least 24 hours prior to admission to the ICU. While some of the prevalence of resistant organisms may be due to sampling techniques (nonbronchoscopic sampling was allowed), the authors speculate that prior antibiotics and prior hospitalization may be more important than timing of onset when considering causative organisms. Other studies have demonstrated that in the absence of prior antibiotics or prolonged hospital stays, the risk of highly resistant organisms is much lower.[7,8]

Patients with coma, head trauma, diabetes, and renal failure are predisposed to infections with *S. aureus*,[1] while patients with prolonged ICU stays, prior antibiotics, corticosteroid use, and structural lung disease are at risk for *P. aeruginosa* infection. *Legionella* spp. infection in NP is usually seen in immunocompromised patients or in local hospital outbreaks due to contaminated water supplies. Anaerobic infection is historically associated with macroaspiration (aspiration of vomit), but at least one recent study questions this association. Marik and colleagues attempted to isolate anaerobic organisms from 143 patients with VAP and 25 patients with witnessed macroaspiration requiring intubation.[9] Only one nonpathogenic anaerobic organism was isolated. This study and others[10] argue that anaerobes do not appear to be a major cause of NP.

Most studies of the epidemiology of NP come from ICUs with a majority of patients receiving MV. Little is known about causative organisms in non-ICU-associated NP. Additionally, the incidence of resistant organisms varies widely between institutions and even on different wards within an institution. This underscores the importance of collecting institutional epidemiologic data regarding NP.

DIAGNOSIS

While most experts agree on the importance of diagnosing NP and identifying the etiologic agent, few can agree on *how* this should be done. Many conditions can present similarly to NP (eg, pulmonary embolism, atelectasis, congestive heart failure, acute respiratory distress syndrome), and an accurate diagnosis is critical to avoid both undertreatment (missed cases) and overtreatment (excess antibiotic use). In general, NP is diagnosed in 1 of 2 ways: clinically or invasively. A clinical diagnosis generally requires a new infiltrate on chest radiograph (CXR) not due to another process, along with signs consistent with infection such as fever, purulent sputum, and leukocytosis. Clinical diagnosis of NP is sensitive (ie, it is unlikely to miss true cases of NP) but not specific and can lead to antibiotic overuse. Invasive diagnostic strategies for NP generally use bronchoscopy to obtain quantitative cultures using a protected specimen brush (PSB) device to limit contamination. A patient is considered to have NP when culture results reveal more than 10^3 organisms/mL if bronchoscopy with PSB is performed or more than 10^4 organisms/mL with standard bronchoalveolar lavage (BAL). Invasive diagnosis is more specific but can lead to false-negative results, especially if antibiotics have been recently changed.[5,11]

A few diagnostic techniques fall between these extremes. Some have attempted to improve on clinical diagnosis by making it more quantitative. Pugin and colleagues evaluated patients with suspected VAP and assigned points for six clinical variables (temperature, white blood cell count, tracheal secretions, oxygenation, CXR abnormalities, and semiquantitative endotracheal aspirates) depending on their degree of abnormality and then assigned an overall score (the clinical pulmonary infection score [CPIS]) for each patient.[12] The score correlated well with quantitative BAL, and scores of more than 6 strongly suggested infection.[12] Endotracheal aspirates (ETA) with or without quantitative cultures have been shown to be highly sensitive (90% to 100%) when compared to anything other than a clinical diagnosis as the gold standard.[13] When compared to bronchoscopy, ETA usually identifies all organisms subsequently found on BAL or PSB.[13] The specificity, however, is much lower, and false positives are likely.

Few trials have prospectively compared clinical outcomes for NP patients undergoing different diagnostic strategies. The most notable was a multicenter trial of 413 patients with suspected VAP. Patients were randomized in an unblinded fashion to a diagnostic strategy of noninvasive ETA with qualitative cultures or an invasive diagnostic strategy that included either BAL or PSB with quantitative cultures. Patients managed with the invasive strategy had fewer positive cultures, which translated into more antibiotic-free days and reduced mortality at 14 days (16% vs. 26%, p = 0.02). At 28 days, a higher percentage of patients in the invasive group had received no antibiotics, and mortality was persistently lower, but this difference was no longer statistically significant (31% vs. 39%, p = 0.09).[14] The authors speculate that a negative invasive diagnostic workup led physicians to pursue mimickers of VAP more aggressively; patients in the invasive group were, in fact, more likely to be diagnosed and treated for an alternative infection. Other important observations in this study included the finding that a majority of the benefit was limited to patients with late-onset VAP (>5 days), and in patients who had negative cultures and no signs of severe sepsis, antibiotics could be safely withheld. Other studies, however, have found no difference in outcomes when comparing diagnostic strategies for NP.[15,16]

In summary, there are no convincing data that support one diagnostic strategy over another, but a few key principles are worth highlighting. First, a clinical diagnosis (new infiltrate, fever, purulent sputum, leukocytosis) is valuable in screening for patients with suspected NP. Some type of diagnostic test should be performed to evaluate for a causative organism. In non-ICU, nonventilated patients, although untested, an attempt should be made to obtain a sputum sample to help guide antibiotic therapy. In mechanically ventilated patients, an ETA should be obtained at a minimum. In patients with suspected VAP who have not had a recent change in their antibiotics (<72 hours) and do not have signs of sepsis, antibiotics can be safely stopped if respiratory cultures are negative. In these patients, an alternative diagnosis must be sought. An invasive workup with bronchoscopically obtained cultures may be the preferred strategy for patients with suspected late-onset VAP (after 5 to 7 days on the ventilator), patients who are failing empiric antibiotic therapy, patients who are at risk for an unusual pathogen (eg, immunocompromised patients), or patients suspected of having an alternative diagnosis.

TREATMENT

The most important treatment principle is that early appropriate antibiotic therapy of NP improves mortality. Several studies strongly suggest that patients treated with adequate initial empiric antibiotic therapy (ie, the antibiotics administered are shown to be active against all organisms isolated) have lower mortality rates than patients treated with inadequate initial antibiotic therapy.[17-19] In many of these studies, multivariable regression analysis showed inappropriate initial empiric therapy to be one of the strongest independent predictors of mortality.[20,21] The need to choose appropriate antibiotics correctly and expeditiously drives the use of broad-spectrum antibiotics. Recently, there has been significant effort to reduce the use of inappropriate broad-spectrum antibiotics in an attempt to prevent the development of highly resistant organisms.[22] Clinicians face the difficult task of balancing the need for appropriate empiric antibiotic coverage with the need to limit inappropriately broad antibiotic use.

There are 3 potential solutions to this dilemma. The first is to improve our diagnostic tests to help us identify causative organisms and allow for targeted antibiotic therapy. Unfortunately, as has been discussed, no diagnostic test performs well enough or provides results soon enough to allow this. The second is to identify patients who are at low risk for resistant organisms based on clinical factors. This would allow for more narrow, but reliably effective, antibiotic therapy. Such low-risk patients include those who are not critically ill, have not had multiple hospitalizations, have not received prior broad-spectrum antibiotics, and develop their infection within 4 to 5 days of hospitalization. In these patients, antibiotics should target common community-acquired organisms in addition to *S. aureus* and the Enterobacteriaceae. Appropriate initial selections would be a beta-lactam/beta-lactamase inhibitor or a non-pseudomonal third-generation cephalosporin.[1] Unfortunately, today's hospitalized population is becoming increasingly complex and, especially in ICUs, "low-risk" patients are uncommon. Higher risk patients need empiric antibiotic coverage active against gram-negatives such as *P. aeruginosa*, and in many centers *Acinetobacter*. This requires the use of drugs such as Imipenem (Merck & Co, Inc, Whitehouse Station, NJ) with or without an aminoglycoside or a beta-lactam/beta-lactamase inhibitor plus a fluoroquinolone, and in most situations the addition of a drug active against MRSA, such as vancomycin. In these cases, a third approach to limiting antibiotic overuse is "de-escalation therapy." This treatment principle acknowledges that broad therapy is warranted in many patients initially, but that treatment may be narrowed considerably as culture results identify the causative organism and its susceptibilities. De-escalation therapy focuses on limiting the duration of therapy and narrowing therapy as soon as possible.[23-26]

A potential approach to treatment of NP starts with the identification of low-risk patients who can receive narrower spectrum therapy. In higher risk or clinically unstable patients, initial empiric therapy should be broad, but quickly narrowed based on microbiological culture results. The data, while not conclusive, increasingly demonstrate that shorter treatment duration (1 week) is safe, effective, and less likely to promote the growth of resistant organisms in patients who are clinically improving.

PREVENTION

The high morbidity, mortality, and cost associated with NP mandates careful attention to strategies aimed at preventing its development. Preventive strategies are either directed at reducing the overall incidence of infectious complications in hospitalized patients, or they are specifically targeted at reducing the incidence of NP. In the case of the latter, preventive measures address the modifiable risk factors highlighted in Table 7-1. As is the case with most issues related to NP, a majority of the literature supporting preventive strategies is limited to patients in the ICU, and in particular, patients receiving MV.

GENERAL PREVENTIVE STRATEGIES

Most general preventive strategies are aimed at avoiding contamination of patients with antimicrobial resistant organisms that exist in hospitals or mitigating the emergence of antimicrobial resistant organisms in the first place.

Preventing Iatrogenic Spread

Careful handwashing both before and after patient contact has been shown to reduce the incidence of nosocomial infection,[27,28] but is often overlooked in the fast-paced hospital environment. Clusters of NP cases attributed to poor hand hygiene have been described, and careful handwashing remains an important defense against nosocomial spread. The use of plain soap and water are likely inferior to antibacterial soaps (chlorhexidine based) and alcohol-based hand rinses.[27] In addition, the use of alcohol-based hand wash in bedside dispensers has been shown to improve compliance with hand hygiene. The use of artificial fingernails among healthcare providers has come under recent attention as a significant risk factor for colonization and subsequent spread of resistant organisms.

Guidelines recommend against their use by personnel with direct patient contact, especially in ICU and surgical settings.[27] While not directly associated with reduced rates of NP, the use of protective gowns and gloves has been effective as part of multifaceted strategies to reduce transmission of resistant organisms.[29,30]

Reducing Emergence of Resistant Organisms

Indwelling devices such as central lines and urinary catheters increase the risk of colonization with resistant organisms and should be used only when absolutely necessary. When they are needed, efforts should focus on their timely removal. The use of sterile-barrier precautions (mask, cap, gown, gloves, and large sterile drapes) during insertion of central venous lines can reduce infectious complications including colonization and subsequent blood stream infections.[31]

The control of antibiotic use has been central to many preventive strategies. With regard to NP, use of antibiotics within the first week of ICU stay has been associated with reduced risk of developing VAP, but this effect is not significant after 1 week.[32] Prolonged use or unnecessary use of broad-spectrum antibiotics, however, is strongly associated with development and colonization of resistant organisms. Efforts focused on reducing use of broad-spectrum regimens and shortening treatment durations have reduced rates of colonization and recurrent episodes of NP. More recently, several investigators have combined antibiotic restriction with antibiotic rotation as a measure to control resistant organisms. Restriction of ceftazidime and ciprofloxacin and initiation of monthly rotation of empiric therapy for VAP were studied in the ICU of a large university hospital. In the period after implementation, there were marked decreases in rates of VAP, the number of resistant gram-negative bacilli isolated, and the percentage of MRSA isolates.[33] In a second study, a quarterly rotation in recommended empiric antibiotic therapy for a variety of infectious conditions was associated with marked decreases in resistant gram-negative rods and gram-positive cocci, as well as significant reductions in both VAP mortality and overall mortality in a before-after analysis.[34] Caution is required, however, in interpreting these studies. Both studies were unblinded and used before-after analysis, thus other factors could have led to the improvements seen. Also, it is unclear which antibiotics should be incorporated into rotational strategies, how frequently they should be rotated, and how long-lasting the results will be. One follow-up study suggested sustained reductions in the incidence of VAP at 5 years, but late increases in the incidence of potentially resistant gram-negative bacilli back to pre-intervention levels.[35]

TARGETED PREVENTIVE STRATEGIES

Preventive strategies to lower the incidence of NP focus on reducing or eliminating risk factors (see Table 7-1) for oropharyngeal or gastric colonization and subsequent aspiration of contaminated oropharyngeal or gastric secretions.

Noninvasive Ventilation

Endotracheal intubation is one of the most important risk factors contributing to pneumonia in patients requiring mechanical support for respiratory failure. Increasingly, the use of noninvasive (NIV) or positive pressure mask ventilation in selected groups of patients has been effective in preventing endotracheal intubation. In a randomized controlled trial of patients admitted with an acute exacerbation of chronic obstructive pulmonary disease (COPD), standard medical care combined with NIV was associated with significant reductions in endotracheal intubation, hospital length of stay (LOS), complications (including NP), and mortality when compared to standard medical care alone.[36] A subsequent case-control study of well-matched patients with acute exacerbations of COPD or CHF compared clinical outcomes between NIV and MV. The use of NIV was associated with lower rates of all nosocomial infections as well as NP (18% vs. 60%, p<0.001, and 8% vs. 22%, p = 0.04, respectively). Patients treated with NIV also had shorter ICU LOS and lower mortality and received fewer antibiotics.[37] While not appropriate for all patients, the use of NIV in selected populations with acute COPD[38,39] and CHF exacerbations appears safe and may reduce the likelihood of NP.

Semirecumbent Patient Positioning

Supine patient positioning may contribute to the development of VAP, likely due to an increased risk of gastric reflux and subsequent aspiration. Three trials have evaluated the efficacy of semirecumbent positioning (elevation of the head of the bed at least 45 degrees). Two small trials (each with 15 patients) used the surrogate outcomes of reflux and aspiration events, both of which were reduced with semirecumbent positioning.[40,41] The third was a randomized controlled trial in 86 mechanically ventilated patients that was stopped early after semirecumbent positioning was associated with a significant reduction in VAP (OR 0.16, 95% CI: 0.03 to 0.67).[42] In general, patients were excluded from these studies if they could not tolerate an upright position due to hemodynamic instability or recent abdominal or neurologic surgery. Unfortunately, scant data exist on patient positioning outside the ICU in nonventilated patients.

Subglottic Secretion Drainage

The pooling of contaminated secretions above the cuff of the endotracheal tube may predispose patients to aspiration and, subsequently, VAP. Removal of these secretions could theoretically reduce the risk of developing pneumonia. Subglottic secretion drainage requires specially designed endotracheal tubes with a separate lumen that opens into the subglottic region above the tracheal cuff. A recent systematic review summarizes the results of 3 randomized trials examining the effect of subglottic secretion drainage.[43] One trial showed a significant reduction in VAP for patients requiring more than 3 days of MV, one trial showed a trend toward reduced VAP, and one trial showed no difference. The third trial was in patients intubated for cardiac surgery who had a significantly shorter duration of MV. A fourth trial published after the systematic review showed a significant reduction in VAP with subglottic secretion drainage (relative risk = 0.22; 95% CI: 0.06 to 0.81), but in contrast to other studies, the investigators used a clinical diagnosis for VAP rather than an invasive strategy, so direct comparisons are difficult.[44] No study showed any difference in mortality. While these endotracheal tubes are more expensive, at least one cost effectiveness analysis showed cost savings of $1900 per case of VAP prevented.[45] In total, the data suggest that subglottic secretion drainage may safely reduce the incidence of VAP, but further study is warranted.

Oscillating Beds

Impaired clearance of secretions in immobile, critically ill patients predisposes to VAP. Efforts to improve clearance and prevent pneumonia with continuous rotational movement have been attempted with specially designed beds. A recent review of the use of oscillating beds found 6 randomized trials evaluating this practice.[43] A meta-analysis of these trials showed a 50% reduction in the risk for pneumonia with the use of oscillating beds.[46] Five of the trials, however, were limited to surgical patients. The sixth trial, as well as a subsequently published trial, did include medical patients, but results in both trials were not significant.[47,48] A recent prospective trial in 37 medical and surgical patients requiring long-term MV showed reduced odds for developing pneumonia with the use of oscillating beds (OR = 0.21, 95% CI: 0.05 to 0.98) as well as a delay in the onset of pneumonia when it occurred.[49] No trial has shown a mortality benefit. Oscillation has been associated with disconnected catheters, ventricular ectopy, pressure sores, and poor tolerance in conscious patients. Given the high cost of oscillating beds (approximately $200 per day), consideration of their use seems most justified in select populations (surgical patients and patients requiring long-term ventilatory care) where benefit potentially exists.

Stress Ulcer Prophylaxis

Medications that increase gastric pH, such as H_2 antagonists and antacids, allow for colonization of the upper gastrointestinal (GI) tract by potentially pathogenic organisms and may increase the risk for NP. Sucralfate, an agent often used for stress ulcer prophylaxis, has limited effect on gastric pH and therefore may not increase the risk for pneumonia. Seven meta-analyses of more than 20 randomized trials have evaluated the risk of NP in critically ill patients associated with the use of stress ulcer prophylaxis.[43] Four showed significant reductions in the incidence of pneumonia, and 3 showed similar but nonsignificant trends toward reduced pneumonia in patients treated with sucralfate when compared to H_2 antagonists. Three analyses found a mortality benefit with the use of sucralfate when compared to H_2 antagonists. A recent large randomized trial, however, compared sucralfate to H_2 antagonists and found no effect on pneumonia, but a significant increase in the risk of clinically important bleeding with the use of sucralfate.[50]

Healthcare practitioners must weigh the potential benefit in reduction of pneumonia with the use of sucralfate against the increased risk of GI bleeding when compared to H_2 antagonists. Of note, a majority of the patients included in these trials were mechanically ventilated, and no trial has assessed the risk of pneumonia associated with proton pump inhibitors, which are increasingly being used for GI bleeding prophylaxis in hospitalized patients. Importantly, the data currently do not support a mortality benefit in most patients who receive stress ulcer prophylaxis. Thus, given the risks and costs of stress ulcer prophylaxis, only patients with a high risk of GI bleeding should receive stress gastritis prophylaxis. This is especially important because all agents used as stress ulcer prophylaxis can increase the risk of NP. Therefore, identifying patients most likely to benefit from stress ulcer prophylaxis is imperative. Well-designed studies suggest this population is limited to patients with shock, respiratory failure, and coagulopathy.[51]

Selective Digestive Decontamination

Selective digestive decontamination (SDD) refers to sterilization of the oropharynx and GI tract in mechanically ventilated patients in hopes of preventing the aspiration of large numbers of organisms and subsequent VAP. Most evaluations of SDD have involved topical polymixin, aminoglycoside, and amphotericin. In many cases, investigators have added short-course IV therapy to topical therapy. There have been 7 meta-analyses of more than 40 randomized trials of SDD that have been recently summarized in a systematic review.[43] All 7 trials showed significant reduction in the risk of VAP with the use of SDD. Several meta-analyses also suggest that, in addition to reductions in VAP, the combination of topical and IV antibiotics may provide a mortality benefit.[43] A recent review of 32 trials of SDD, however, found an inverse relationship between reported benefit and methodologic quality.[52] In this context, the results of meta-analyses may overstate the benefit. In addition, it is unclear how routine use of SDD might affect antibiotic resistance patterns. Therefore, while promising as a preventive measure, further study with careful evaluation of delayed complications related to antibiotic resistance is warranted before SDD is widely implemented.

Ventilator Circuit Management Strategies

There has been substantial interest in the potential role of contaminated or colonized tubing, filters, and other components of the ventilator circuit in the pathogenesis of VAP. On the one hand, infrequent changes of ventilator circuitry may allow colonization with potentially pathologic organisms; on the other, frequent changes may increase the chance of iatrogenic introduction of bacteria into the circuit.

Several studies have looked at the frequency of ventilator circuitry changes and the impact on the development of VAP.[43] No difference in the occurrence of VAP has been found between frequent (usually 24 to 48 hours) and infrequent changes (usually 5 to 7 days). Frequent changes of ventilator heat and moisture exchangers or the use of alternative heating and humidification devices have also failed to show a significant effect on the occurrence of VAP. It remains unclear how ventilator circuits should be optimally managed to prevent VAP. As frequent changes of the ventilator circuitry are expensive, less frequent changes appear more cost effective.

Methods of Enteral Feedings

Enteral feeding of critically ill patients has been shown to increase the risk of NP.[53,54] This may occur by causing gastric distention and increasing the frequency of gastroesophageal reflux and aspiration of stomach contents contaminated with potentially pathogenic organisms. Unfortunately, the common practice of measuring gastric residual volume and suspending feeding should this volume increase appears to have little effect on the development of NP.[55]

Four approaches to limiting the risk of NP with enteral feedings have been investigated. Small intestinal (postpyloric) feeding appears to decrease gastroesophageal reflux and microaspiration.[56] Unfortunately, no difference in the incidence of NP with small intestinal feeding has been demonstrated.[57] A second approach evaluated was the use of the motility agent metoclopramide. Similarly, no effect on the incidence of NP was found.[58] The third approach compared intermittent with continuous enteral feeding and again found no difference in the incidence of NP.[59] Finally, enteral feedings have been acidified with the goal of decreasing gastric pH and thereby decreasing colonization with potentially pathogenic organisms.[60] Acidified feeding had no effect on the incidence of NP, but an alarming increase in acidemia and GI bleeding was observed. Based on the published literature to date, no method of enteral feeding can be recommended to prevent the occurrence of NP in critically ill patients.

CONCLUSION

NP is a common, costly, and morbid complication of hospitalization. While much is known about the epidemiology, pathogenesis, diagnosis, and treatment of this patient safety problem, additional studies are necessary. After carefully considering potential benefits and risks, we recommend the following for the prevention of NP: semirecumbent positioning in all eligible ventilated patients, the use of either sucralfate or no prophylaxis rather than H_2 antagonist in patients at low and moderate risk for GI tract bleeding, and subglottic secretion and oscillating beds in select patient populations. Selective digestive tract decontamination is not recommended because of the concern that routine use may increase antimicrobial resistance. Future studies should evaluate the cost effectiveness of various infection prevention methods because these types of analysis would help decision makers in choosing one strategy over another. Additionally, while data on mechanically ventilated patients are available, there is woefully little data derived from the nonventilated, noncritically ill patient residing on the general hospital ward. Finally, while some studies have focused on the impediments to and facilitators of successful translations of several of these proven preventive methods into practice,[61] additional research is required to better understand exactly how to translate research findings in this area into practice.

REFERENCES

1. Hospital-acquired pneumonia in adults: diagnosis, assessment of severity, initial antimicrobial therapy, and preventive strategies. A consensus statement. American Thoracic Society, November 1995. *Am J Respir Crit Care Med.* 1996;153(5):1711-1725.

2. Rello J, Ollendorf DA, Oster G, et al. Epidemiology and outcomes of ventilator-associated pneumonia in a large US database. *Chest.* 2002;122(6):2115-2121.

3. Warren DK, Shukla SJ, Olsen MA, et al. Outcome and attributable cost of ventilator-associated pneumonia among intensive care unit patients in a suburban medical center. *Crit Care Med.* 2003;31(5):1312-1317.

4. Combes A, Figliolini C, Trouillet JL, et al. Incidence and outcome of polymicrobial ventilator-associated pneumonia. *Chest.* 2002;121(5):1618-1623.

5. Chastre J, Fagon JY. Ventilator-associated pneumonia. *Am J Respir Crit Care Med*. 2002;165(7):867-903.

6. Ibrahim EH, Ward S, Sherman G, Kollef MH. A comparative analysis of patients with early-onset vs. late-onset nosocomial pneumonia in the ICU setting. *Chest*. 2000;117(5):1434-1442.

7. Rello J, Sa-Borges M, Correa H, Leal SR, Baraibar J. Variations in etiology of ventilator-associated pneumonia across four treatment sites: implications for antimicrobial prescribing practices. *Am J Respir Crit Care Med*. 1999;160(2):608-613.

8. Trouillet JL, Chastre J, Vuagnat A, et al. Ventilator-associated pneumonia caused by potentially drug-resistant bacteria. *Am J Respir Crit Care Med*. 1998;157(2):531-539.

9. Marik PE, Careau P. The role of anaerobes in patients with ventilator-associated pneumonia and aspiration pneumonia: a prospective study. *Chest*. 1999;115(1):178-183.

10. Morehead RS, Pinto SJ. Ventilator-associated pneumonia. *Arch Intern Med*. 2000;160(13):1926-1936.

11. Michaud S, Suzuki S, Harbarth S. Effect of design-related bias in studies of diagnostic tests for ventilator-associated pneumonia. *Am J Respir Crit Care Med*. 2002;166(10):1320-1325.

12. Pugin J, Auckenthaler R, Mili N, Janssens JP, Lew PD, Suter PM. Diagnosis of ventilator-associated pneumonia by bacteriologic analysis of bronchoscopic and nonbronchoscopic "blind" bronchoalveolar lavage fluid. *Am Rev Respir Dis*. 1991;143(5 Pt 1):1121-1129.

13. Cook D, Mandell L. Endotracheal aspiration in the diagnosis of ventilator-associated pneumonia. *Chest*. 2000;117(4 Suppl 2):195S-197S.

14. Fagon JY, Chastre J, Wolff M, et al. Invasive and noninvasive strategies for management of suspected ventilator-associated pneumonia. A randomized trial. *Ann Intern Med*. 2000;132(8):621-630.

15. Ruiz M, Torres A, Ewig S, et al. Noninvasive versus invasive microbial investigation in ventilator-associated pneumonia: evaluation of outcome. *Am J Respir Crit Care Med*. 2000;162(1):119-125.

16. Sole Violan J, Fernandez JA, Benitez AB, Cardenosa Cendrero JA, Rodriguez de Castro F. Impact of quantitative invasive diagnostic techniques in the management and outcome of mechanically ventilated patients with suspected pneumonia. *Crit Care Med*. 2000;28(8):2737-2741.

17. Luna CM, Vujacich P, Niederman MS, et al. Impact of BAL data on the therapy and outcome of ventilator-associated pneumonia. *Chest*. 1997;111(3):676-685.

18. Rello J, Rue M, Jubert P, et al. Survival in patients with nosocomial pneumonia: impact of the severity of illness and the etiologic agent. *Crit Care Med*. 1997;25(11):1862-1867.

19. Kollef MH, Bock KR, Richards RD, Hearns ML. The safety and diagnostic accuracy of minibronchoalveolar lavage in patients with suspected ventilator-associated pneumonia. *Ann Intern Med*. 1995;122(10):743-748.

20. Torres A, Aznar R, Gatell JM, et al. Incidence, risk, and prognosis factors of nosocomial pneumonia in mechanically ventilated patients. *Am Rev Respir Dis*. 1990;142(3):523-528.

21. Celis R, Torres A, Gatell JM, Almela M, Rodriguez-Roisin R, Agusti-Vidal A. Nosocomial pneumonia. A multivariate analysis of risk and prognosis. *Chest*. 1988;93(2):318-324.

22. Shlaes DM, Gerding DN, John JF Jr., et al. Society for Healthcare Epidemiology of America and Infectious Diseases Society of America Joint Committee on the Prevention of Antimicrobial Resistance: guidelines for the prevention of antimicrobial resistance in hospitals. *Clin Infect Dis*. 1997;25(3):584-599.

23. Hoffken G, Niederman MS. Nosocomial pneumonia: the importance of a de-escalating strategy for antibiotic treatment of pneumonia in the ICU. *Chest*. 2002;122(6):2183-2196.

24. Dennesen PJ, van der Ven AJ, Kessels AG, Ramsay G, Bonten MJ. Resolution of infectious parameters after antimicrobial therapy in patients with ventilator-associated pneumonia. *Am J Respir Crit Care Med*. 2001;163(6):1371-1375.

25. Ibrahim EH, Ward S, Sherman G, Schaiff R, Fraser VJ, Kollef MH. Experience with a clinical guideline for the treatment of ventilator-associated pneumonia. *Crit Care Med*. 2001;29(6):1109-1115.

26. Singh N, Rogers P, Atwood CW, Wagener MM, Yu VL. Short-course empiric antibiotic therapy for patients with pulmonary infiltrates in the intensive care unit. A proposed solution for indiscriminate antibiotic prescription. *Am J Respir Crit Care Med*. 2000;162(2 Pt 1):505-511.

27. Boyce JM, Pittet D. Guideline for Hand Hygiene in Health-Care Settings. Recommendations of the Healthcare Infection Control Practices Advisory Committee and the HICPAC/SHEA/APIC/IDSA Hand Hygiene Task Force. Society for Healthcare Epidemiology of America/ Association for Professionals in Infection Control/ Infectious Diseases Society of America. *MMWR Recomm Rep*. 2002;51(RR-16):1-45, quiz CE41-44.

28. Doebbeling BN, Stanley GL, Sheetz CT, et al. Comparative efficacy of alternative hand-washing agents in reducing nosocomial infections in intensive care units. *N Engl J Med*. 1992;327(2):88-93.

29. Montecalvo MA, Jarvis WR, Uman J, et al. Infection-control measures reduce transmission of vancomycin-resistant enterococci in an endemic setting. *Ann Intern Med*. 1999;131(4):269-272.

30. Ostrowsky BE, Trick WE, Sohn AH, et al. Control of vancomycin-resistant enterococcus in health care facilities in a region. *N Engl J Med*. 2001;344(19):1427-1433.

31. McGee DC, Gould MK. Preventing complications of central venous catheterization. *N Engl J Med*. 2003;348(12):1123-1133.

32. Cook DJ, Walter SD, Cook RJ, et al. Incidence of and risk factors for ventilator-associated pneumonia in critically ill patients. *Ann Intern Med*. 1998;129(6):433-440.

33. Gruson D, Hilbert G, Vargas F, et al. Rotation and restricted use of antibiotics in a medical intensive care unit. Impact on the incidence of ventilator-associated pneumonia caused by antibiotic-resistant gram-negative bacteria. *Am J Respir Crit Care Med.* 2000;162(3 Pt 1):837-843.

34. Raymond DP, Pelletier SJ, Crabtree TD, et al. Impact of a rotating empiric antibiotic schedule on infectious mortality in an intensive care unit. *Crit Care Med.* 2001;29(6): 1101-1108.

35. Gruson D, Hilbert G, Vargas F, et al. Strategy of antibiotic rotation: long-term effect on incidence and susceptibilities of gram-negative bacilli responsible for ventilator-associated pneumonia. *Crit Care Med.* 2003;31(7):1908-1914.

36. Brochard L, Mancebo J, Wysocki M, et al. Noninvasive ventilation for acute exacerbations of chronic obstructive pulmonary disease. *N Engl J Med.* 1995;333(13):817-822.

37. Girou E, Schortgen F, Delclaux C, et al. Association of noninvasive ventilation with nosocomial infections and survival in critically ill patients. *JAMA.* 2000;284(18): 2361-2367.

38. Keenan SP, Sinuff T, Cook DJ, Hill NS. Which patients with acute exacerbation of chronic obstructive pulmonary disease benefit from noninvasive positive-pressure ventilation? A systematic review of the literature. *Ann Intern Med.* 2003;138(11):861-870.

39. Ram F, Lightowler J, Wedzicha J. Non-invasive positive pressure ventilation for treatment of respiratory failure due to exacerbations of chronic obstructive pulmonary disease. Cochrane Review. In: The Cochrane Library, Issue 3, 2003. Oxford: Update Software. CD004104. 2003.

40. Torres A, Serra-Batlles J, Ros E, et al. Pulmonary aspiration of gastric contents in patients receiving mechanical ventilation: the effect of body position. *Ann Intern Med.* 1992;116(7):540-543.

41. Orozco-Levi M, Torres A, Ferrer M, et al. Semirecumbent position protects from pulmonary aspiration but not completely from gastroesophageal reflux in mechanically ventilated patients. *Am J Respir Crit Care Med.* 1995;152(4 Pt 1):1387-1390.

42. Drakulovic MB, Torres A, Bauer TT, Nicolas JM, Nogue S, Ferrer M. Supine body position as a risk factor for nosocomial pneumonia in mechanically ventilated patients: a randomised trial. *Lancet.* 1999;354(9193):1851-1858.

43. Collard HR, Saint S, Matthay MA. Prevention of ventilator-associated pneumonia: an evidence-based systematic review. *Ann Intern Med.* 2003;138(6):494-501.

44. Smulders K, van der Hoeven H, Weers-Pothoff I, Vandenbroucke-Grauls C. A randomized clinical trial of intermittent subglottic secretion drainage in patients receiving mechanical ventilation. *Chest.* 2002;121(3):858-862.

45. Shorr AF, O'Malley PG. Continuous subglottic suctioning for the prevention of ventilator-associated pneumonia: potential economic implications. *Chest.* 2001;119(1):228-235.

46. Choi SC, Nelson LD. Kinetic therapy in critically ill patients: combined results based on meta-analysis. *J Crit Care.* 1992;7:57-62.

47. Summer WR, Haponik EF, Nelson S, Elston R. Continuous mechanical turning of intensive care unit patients shortens length of stay in some diagnostic-related groups. *J Crit Care.* 1989;4:45-53.

48. Traver GA, Tyler ML, Hudson LD, Sherrill DL, Quan SF. Continuous oscillation: outcome in critically ill patients. *J Crit Care.* 1995;10(3):97-103.

49. Kirschenbaum L, Azzi E, Sfeir T, Tietjen P, Astiz M. Effect of continuous lateral rotational therapy on the prevalence of ventilator-associated pneumonia in patients requiring long-term ventilatory care. *Crit Care Med.* 2002;30(9): 1983-1986.

50. Cook D, Guyatt G, Marshall J, et al. A comparison of sucralfate and ranitidine for the prevention of upper gastrointestinal bleeding in patients requiring mechanical ventilation. Canadian Critical Care Trials Group. *N Engl J Med.* 1998;338(12):791-797.

51. Cook DJ, Fuller HD, Guyatt GH, et al. Risk factors for gastrointestinal bleeding in critically ill patients. Canadian Critical Care Trials Group. *N Engl J Med.* 1994;330(6):377-381.

52. van Nieuwenhoven CA, Buskens E, van Tiel FH, Bonten MJ. Relationship between methodological trial quality and the effects of selective digestive decontamination on pneumonia and mortality in critically ill patients. *JAMA.* 2001;286(3):335-340.

53. Byers JF, Sole ML. Analysis of factors related to the development of ventilator-associated pneumonia: use of existing databases. *Am J Crit Care.* 2000;9(5):344-349;quiz 351.

54. Rothan-Tondeur M, Meaume S, Girard L, et al. Risk factors for nosocomial pneumonia in a geriatric hospital: a control-case one-center study. *J Am Geriatr Soc.* 2003;51(7): 997-1001.

55. McClave SA, Snider HL. Clinical use of gastric residual volumes as a monitor for patients on enteral tube feeding. *JPEN J Parenter Enteral Nutr.* 2002;26(6 Suppl):S43-48; discussion S49-50.

56. Heyland DK, Drover JW, MacDonald S, Novak F, Lam M. Effect of postpyloric feeding on gastroesophageal regurgitation and pulmonary microaspiration: results of a randomized controlled trial. *Crit Care Med.* 2001;29(8):1495-1501.

57. Kearns PJ, Chin D, Mueller L, Wallace K, Jensen WA, Kirsch CM. The incidence of ventilator-associated pneumonia and success in nutrient delivery with gastric versus small intestinal feeding: a randomized clinical trial. *Crit Care Med.* 2000;28(6):1742-1746.

58. Yavagal DR, Karnad DR, Oak JL. Metoclopramide for preventing pneumonia in critically ill patients receiving enteral tube feeding: a randomized controlled trial. *Crit Care Med.* 2000;28(5):1408-1411.

59. Bonten MJ, Gaillard CA, van der Hulst R, et al. Intermittent enteral feeding: the influence on respiratory and digestive tract colonization in mechanically ventilated intensive-care-unit patients. *Am J Respir Crit Care Med*. 1996;154(2 Pt 1):394-399.

60. Heyland DK, Cook DJ, Schoenfeld PS, Frietag A, Varon J, Wood G. The effect of acidified enteral feeds on gastric colonization in critically ill patients: results of a multicenter randomized trial. Canadian Critical Care Trials Group. *Crit Care Med*. 1999;27(11):2399-2406.

61. Rello J, Lorente C, Bodi M, Diaz E, Ricart M, Kollef MH. Why do physicians not follow evidence-based guidelines for preventing ventilator-associated pneumonia?: a survey based on the opinions of an international panel of intensivists. *Chest*. 2002;122(2):656-661.

CHAPTER EIGHT

BASICS OF SURGICAL SITE INFECTION SURVEILLANCE

Lisa L. Maragakis, MD and Trish M. Perl, MD, MSc

INTRODUCTION

Our understanding of the pathogenesis and risk factors for SSIs has changed substantially over time. During the early years of modern surgery, many patients died from wound sepsis. Despite our increased knowledge, SSIs continue to cause substantial morbidity, mortality, and increased cost of healthcare. SSIs are the second most common healthcare-associated infection in the United States accounting for approximately 20% of all nosocomial infections.[1] Approximately 500,000 SSIs occur annually, accounting for 3.7 million excess hospital days and more than $1.6 billion in excess hospital costs.[2] In hospitals participating in the NNIS program of the CDC, 0.62% to 1.9% of patients with SSIs died from these infections.[3] These numbers likely underestimate the magnitude of the problem; yet, they highlight the tremendous human and financial costs that SSIs add to the healthcare system and, therefore, the importance of controlling them.

The CDC, motivated to document the cost-effectiveness of infection control activities, conducted the SENIC.[4] These investigators and many subsequent studies concluded that infection surveillance programs that report SSI rates to surgeons can decrease overall SSI rates by at least 32% to 50%.[4-6] However, several important questions about surveillance for SSIs remain:

➤ Which surveillance methods are best?

➤ Which surgical patients should we survey?

➤ How should we conduct postdischarge surveillance?

➤ How can we effectively use technology and automated systems for surveillance?

The purpose of this chapter is to explore these unanswered questions and to summarize the basic steps required to implement an in-hospital surveillance program for SSIs.

SURGICAL SITE INFECTION SURVEILLANCE

Objectives

When developing a surveillance system, the main objective is to reduce SSI rates, thereby reducing morbidity and improving patient care. To achieve this goal, infection control professionals (ICPs), including the hospital epidemiologist, must first perform surveillance to determine endemic or baseline rates of SSIs. As these rates are followed over time, epidemiology staff can identify both clusters of infections and time periods with SSI rates above baseline. The SSI surveillance program may be used to review the impact of interventions, including protocols for antimicrobial prophylaxis and aseptic precautions in the operating theater. ICPs should provide surveillance data to surgeons and other members of the surgical team to educate them and as an intervention to prevent SSIs.

Definition

Before implementing an SSI surveillance system, the ICP must agree on a precise definition for SSI. Ideally, in each hospital, the definition should remain unchanged so that infection control and surgical staff can compare data over time and evaluate interventions implemented to reduce these rates. The definition should be simple to use and accepted by nurses and surgeons. ICPs must apply the definition consistently.[7] A standard definition for SSI is available from the CDC (Figure 8-1).[8] Use of a standard definition allows for comparison of SSI rates across institutions and surgeons.

According to the CDC definition, SSIs are categorized as either incisional or organ space. Incisional SSIs are classified further as superficial (involving only the skin and subcutaneous tissue) or deep (involving deep soft tissues of the incision) (see Figure 8-1). The definition of superficial incisional SSI requires that at least one of the following occur within 30 days of the operative procedure:

➤ Purulent drainage from the superficial incision.

➤ Organisms isolated from an aseptically obtained culture of fluid or tissue from the superficial incision.

➤ At least one of the following signs or symptoms of infection: pain or tenderness, localized swelling, redness, or heat, and the surgeon deliberately opened the superficial incision, unless incision is culture negative.

➤ The surgeon or attending physician diagnosed a superficial incisional SSI.

Deep-incisional and organ-space SSIs are defined similarly.[7] When an implant is placed, infections that occur within 1 year of a procedure are considered to be nosocomial SSIs.

SURVEILLANCE METHODS

Hospitals use many different surveillance methods to identify healthcare-associated infections. The sensitivity and specificity of several surveillance methods have been assessed for nosocomial infections in general,[9,10] but not specifically for SSIs. Nevertheless, we will review several common surveillance methods and discuss whether each method can be used effectively to survey for SSIs (Table 8-1).

Daily Wound Examination and Chart Review

After conducting prospective SSI surveillance for 10 years, Olson and Lee concluded that daily hospital chart review and examination of postoperative wounds are probably the most sensitive and rigorous ways to perform SSI surveillance.[6] Although these methods are tedious and time consuming, some experts still consider them to be the gold standard and recommend that surveillance for SSI includes daily examination of operative wounds. To facilitate this method, ICPs or surgeons can train staff nurses who see the wounds during routine care to recognize signs of infection and report all clinically suspicious wounds to the ICP. The ICP then examines all such wounds and determines which ones meet the criteria for infection.[11]

Cardo and colleagues compared the following two approaches[12]:

1. Surveillance performed by an ICP who reviewed the patients' medical records and discussed each patient's progress with nurses and physicians.

2. Surveillance performed by a hospital epidemiologist who reviewed the patients' medical records and examined their wounds."

The ICP identified 84% of SSIs noted by the hospital epidemiologist. The authors concluded that accurate data

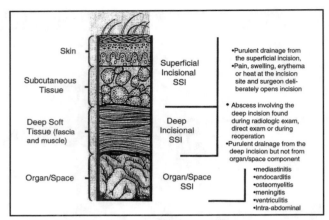

Figure 8-1. Schematic of SSI anatomy and appropriate classification. This figure depicts the cross-sectional anatomy of a surgical incision upon which is superimposed the most recent classification for SSI and the definition of an infection at each site.[7] (Reprinted with permission from Horan TC, Gaynes RP, Martone WJ, Jarvis WR, Emori TG. CDC definitions of nosocomial surgical site infections, 1992: a modification of CDC definitions of surgical wound infections. *Infect Control Hosp Epidemiol.* 1992;13(10): 606-608.)

on SSIs can be collected by people who do not examine the operative wounds directly.[12] Haley and colleagues corroborated this finding.[13] However, the quality of the information gleaned from medical records depends on their completeness and on the reviewer's experience. Furthermore, if the infection control team has limited resources for surveillance, review of the medical records of all surgical patients will not be possible. Such programs must either focus on specific surgical subpopulations or use other less time-consuming surveillance methods.

Selective Chart Review With Kardex Review

Wenzel and colleagues studied the sensitivity of reviewing selected medical records compared with reviewing all medical records.[10] In selective chart review, the ICP searched the Kardex (ie, a card-based system for ongoing documentation of patient care variables, including vital signs and medications) for clues, such as fever or antibiotic use. If one or more clues were noted, the ICP evaluated the patient's medical record more thoroughly. In Wenzel's study, the ICP, using Kardex review, correctly identified 82% to 94% of nosocomial infections identified when all medical records were reviewed. The Kardex method saved 15 to 19 hours of the ICP's time.[10] The Kardex may be a good source of information about patients at high risk of certain infections, but it is probably not a good source of

TABLE 8-1. SURVEILLANCE METHODS

Surveillance Methods	Type of Nosocomial Infections Surveyed	Sensitivity	References
Retrospective chart review	SSI	0.73 to 0.80	13
	All	0.90	10
Microbiology reports	All	0.33 to 0.71	10
Pharmacy records	All	0.81	17*
	All	0.48	10
Selective chart review using Kardex clues	All	0.85	10
Automated data collection	SSI	0.74 to 0.77	15
	All	0.91	18

SSI = surgical site infection
*Evaluated all nosocomial infections in patients after Cesarean section.

Adapted from Perl TM. Surveillance, reporting and the use of computers. In: Wenzel RP, ed. *Prevention and Control of Nosocomial Infections.* Baltimore: Williams & Wilkins; 1993:139-176.

information on patients with SSIs. Indeed, fever and antibiotic use are not necessarily good indicators of SSI. Unfortunately, more useful indicators, such as the frequency with which wound dressings are changed and descriptions of discharge from the wound, are not readily available from the Kardex. Moreover, the accuracy of the method is limited by the completeness and accuracy of the data in the Kardex.

Microbiology Reports

Surveillance for nosocomial infections that relies only on microbiology data has a sensitivity of only 33% to 65%.[9,10] Only two-thirds of inpatients' surgical wounds and even fewer outpatients' wounds are cultured, despite clinical evidence for SSI.[14] Therefore, surveillance for SSI that uses only microbiology data is even less sensitive than that for other healthcare-associated infections. Frequently, surgeons do not obtain cultures because they treat SSI with operative drainage and feel that they do not need to know the etiologic agent or its antibiotic susceptibility. It is important to note that a wound culture that grows does not prove that a patient has an SSI. Instead, the organisms may be colonizing the wound. The opposite is also true—a negative culture does not eliminate the diagnosis of SSI. For example, wound cellulitis often yields negative cultures, and organisms such as *M. tuberculosis*, other *Mycobacterium* spp., and *Legionella* spp. are not detected by routine culture methods. Although many programs use microbiology data to detect SSIs, these data should not be used as the sole source of case finding.

Pharmacy Files

Some investigators suggest that antimicrobial use is an indicator of healthcare-associated infection. Most studies that evaluate pharmacy data do not look at SSIs specifically. Healthcare-associated infection surveillance that relies on pharmacy data has low sensitivity.[9,10] There are several reasons why infection control programs should not use pharmacy data alone when conducting surveillance for SSIs. Some patients may continue to receive prophylactic antibiotics postoperatively, and some patients receive antimicrobial agents for infections that were present preoperatively (eg, peritonitis caused by a ruptured appendix). On the other hand, a patient whose infected wound is drained but who does not receive antimicrobials would not be identified by this surveillance method.

Automated Methods

Computerization of medical records and technological advances promise to improve the quality of data and make surveillance more automated. Infection control programs are trying to find new automated methods by which they can identify patients with SSIs, particularly those whose signs and symptoms occur after discharge. For example, Sands and colleagues found that individual components of an automated screening system could identify SSIs.[15] They determined that:

➤ Use of coded diagnoses, tests, and treatments in the medical record had a sensitivity of 74%.

➤ Specific codes and combinations of codes identified a subset of 2% of all procedures among which 74% of SSIs occurred.

➤ Use of hospital discharge diagnosis codes plus pharmacy dispensing data had sensitivity of 77% and specificity of 94%.

Platt and colleagues reported that automated claims and pharmacy data from several plans can be combined to allow routine monitoring for indicators of postoperative infection.[16,17] Bouam and colleagues demonstrated how

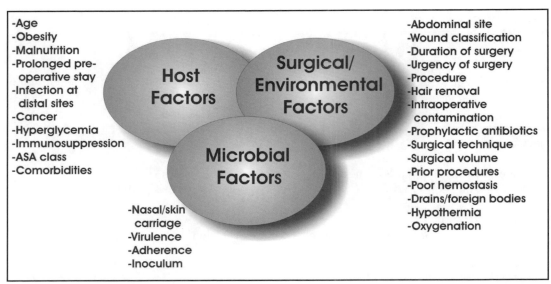

-Age
-Obesity
-Malnutrition
-Prolonged pre-
operative stay
-Infection at
distal sites
-Cancer
-Hyperglycemia
-Immunosuppression
-ASA class
-Comorbidities

Host Factors

Surgical/ Environmental Factors

Microbial Factors

-Nasal/skin
carriage
-Virulence
-Adherence
-Inoculum

-Abdominal site
-Wound classification
-Duration of surgery
-Urgency of surgery
-Procedure
-Hair removal
-Intraoperative
contamination
-Prophylactic antibiotics
-Surgical technique
-Surgical volume
-Prior procedures
-Poor hemostasis
-Drains/foreign bodies
-Hypothermia
-Oxygenation

Figure 8-2. Risk factors for surgical site infection. This figure indicates that the patient's risk of developing an SSI varies with numerous host factors, surgical and environmental factors, and microbial factors. A complex interaction of these factors determines whether the patient will acquire an SSI. ASA = American Society of Anesthesiologists.

cooperation between infection control and medical informatics can lead to an automated system of surveillance.[18] They compared computerized prospective surveillance of the electronic medical record with standard prospective review of lab data and charts by an ICP. The automated method required much less time and performed well with sensitivity and specificity of 91%.[18]

In a recent editorial, J. P. Burke suggested that computers can do more than simply automate traditional surveillance methods.[19] He cites studies that demonstrate how computerized event monitoring can be used to trigger epidemiologic investigations and how data mining can uncover small outbreaks and trends that might otherwise be missed. At the same time, he reminds us that time saved by automating surveillance will lead to more human work to interpret the new data, answer new questions, and design new interventions.[19] Unfortunately, many programs cannot currently take advantage of alternative data sources because their hospitals do not have integrated computer systems that enable ICPs to access the data.

Summary of Surveillance Methods

When selecting surveillance methods, ICPs must consider their objectives and the various sources from which the necessary data may be obtained. Sources available at one institution may not be available at others. Diagnostic procedures, such as computed tomography or magnetic resonance imaging, may help to identify deep or organ-space infections, and the operating room logbook may allow epidemiology staff to identify patients who return to the operating room for drainage and debridement. Computers and computerized databases can help ICPs perform surveillance efficiently. The availability of these resources will determine, in part, which surveillance methods are most useful in individual healthcare facilities.

ICPs should consider combining 2 or more surveillance methods to increase their sensitivity. For example, infection control staff can review both the medical records and the pharmacy files of selected patients. In-hospital surveillance for SSIs should include concurrent chart review, Kardex review, or direct examination of the wounds. Review of the pharmacy records or microbiology reports is not recommended as the sole method of identifying patients who have SSIs. No surveillance method is perfect, and any chosen strategy must be validated against the gold standard.

COLLECTING DATA

Data collected during surveillance can be classified into three categories: host factors, surgical and environmental factors, and microbial factors (Figure 8-2). Host factors are conditions that reflect the patient's intrinsic susceptibility to infection. These conditions usually are present when the patient is admitted to the hospital. Some of these factors increase the risk of SSI after many different operative procedures (eg, remote infection, age, preoperative length of stay),[20,21] while others increase the risk only after specific operative procedures (eg, obesity, poor glucose control, and cigarette smoking are associated with infections after cardiac surgery).[22] Surgical and environmental factors can increase the probability of bacterial contamination at the time of the surgical procedure and lead to SSI. For example, a contaminated wound, a long procedure, and poor surgical technique are risk factors for SSI.[20] Microbial factors, such as the virulence of the organism or the ability of the organism to adhere to sutures, may alter the risk of SSI, but few studies have addressed these issues systematically. To conduct routine surveillance for SSI, ICPs rarely need to know whether the patient carries specific organisms. However, during an outbreak, or when trying to answer specific research questions, they may need to obtain preoperative surveillance cultures from specific body sites.

The amount of data that the ICP should collect depends on the purpose of the surveillance program. In general, the basic data that should be collected include the following: the patient's identification, date of admission, date of surgery, type of procedure, wound category (ie, clean, clean-contaminated, contaminated, and dirty), surgeon's identification code, the date that the SSI was diagnosed, and the type of infection (ie, superficial, deep, or organ space). Other useful data are the American Society of Anesthesiologists' (ASA) score, the procedure's duration and urgency, the organism identified, and the type and timing of perioperative antibiotics.

Because surgical patients are readily identifiable, the denominator is easier to obtain than other healthcare-associated infections such as pneumonia, UTI, or bacteremia, for which the number of ventilator days, Foley catheter days, or intravenous catheter days must be determined retrospectively. All surgical patients can be included in a registry at the end of the operative procedure. Indeed, many hospitals maintain operating room logbooks or have computer databases for financial management that allow infection control staff to identify the appropriate denominators. Hospitals that have a separate database for surgical services may collect demographic data and patient, operative, and environmental data that are useful to the infection control program. In hospitals that do not collect these data, ICPs should seriously consider what information they need before they spend many hours collecting data. Several investigators have found that they collected data on variables that ultimately did not help them determine which patients were at highest risk of developing an infection.[23]

WHICH PATIENTS SHOULD BE SCREENED?

General Principles

Some infection control programs cling to the idea that they should survey all surgical patients, even healthy, young patients undergoing minor procedures. However, full-house surveillance consumes so much time that most programs must do some form of targeted surveillance.

In general hospitals, approximately 70% of operative procedures are categorized as clean operations. Some hospitals survey only clean operative procedures, assuming that SSIs in the other categories are rarely preventable. However, the SENIC project demonstrated that surveillance for SSIs after contaminated or dirty procedures reduced SSI rates as effectively as did surveillance for SSIs after clean or clean-contaminated cases.[24] Therefore, we advocate SSI surveillance that includes all categories of operative procedures.

Targeted surveillance may be more effective when focused on specific operative procedures. For example, SSIs after craniotomies or coronary artery bypass procedures cause higher morbidity and mortality than do SSIs after hernia repairs. Therefore, ICPs can focus surveillance on the former procedures, so that they can intervene immediately if SSI rates increase substantially. Alternatively, the infection control program can survey common operative procedures or operative procedures that have been identified to have high infection rates. Hospitals that limit SSI surveillance to the surgical intensive care unit (SICU) will miss many infections because the average SSI occurs 7 to 10 days postoperatively, and most patients leave the SICU within a few days of surgery. Rotating surveillance for SSIs on different surgical wards will also underestimate the SSI rates and may miss problems or epidemics that occur when a unit is not under surveillance.

Risk Indices to Direct Surgical Site Infection Surveillance

Another way to perform targeted surveillance is to stratify patients according to their risk of developing an SSI and then survey a select group of patients. The ideal risk index is a simple additive scale that can be calculated at the end of surgery and that predicts the patients who are at high risk of SSIs. In addition, the risk index should be validated prospectively on specific services or in individual hospitals to document that it predicts a patient's risk accurately.

TABLE 8-2. THE NATIONAL NOSOCOMIAL INFECTION SURVEILLANCE RISK INDEX[a]

Risk Factors	Score
ASA preoperative assessment score of 3, 4, or 5	1
Operative procedure lasting longer than "T" hours[b]	1
Operative procedure classified as either contaminated or dirty by the traditional wound classification system	1

[a] To calculate total score, sum factors present. Total score ranges from 0 to 3.
[b] "T" depends on the procedure being performed.

The idea of controlling for intrinsic risk is far from new. In 1964, the National Research Council's study of ultraviolet light in the operating room led to the development of the traditional wound-classification scheme, which stratifies wounds by level of intraoperative contamination.[25] Wound classification has limited ability to stratify patients because infection rates vary substantially within each group.[26] Therefore, investigators have developed risk indices that include other variables to better predict which patients are at highest risk of developing SSIs.

In 1985, Haley and colleagues published the SENIC risk index,[27] which includes 4 factors: abdominal operation, duration of surgery more than 2 hours, wound classification, and number of discharge diagnoses. The SENIC risk index predicts the risk of SSI twice as well as the traditional wound classification, but one of the index components—discharge diagnoses—must be obtained retrospectively. Therefore, Culver and colleagues adapted the SENIC risk index and assessed the underlying severity of illness with the ASA score rather than with discharge diagnoses.[28] This risk index, known as the NNIS risk index (Table 8-2), also includes a component that accounts for the expected variability in the duration of the operative procedure.[28] Instead of using a constant 2-hour cut point for length of surgery as used by the SENIC index, the NNIS index defines "T time" as the 75th percentile of the duration for each operative procedure. These 3 variables are easy to find because they are usually included in the anesthesia record.

The NNIS risk index is a simple additive scale; scores range from 0 to 3. In the CDC's study, the SSI rates increased from 1.5%, for a score of 1, to 13.0%, for a score of 3. The NNIS index has rarely been validated in populations other than in the NNIS participating hospitals or compared with other risk indices. As individual hospitals try to use the NNIS risk index, some report that the NNIS risk index does not stratify patients accurately by their risk of SSIs. We have shown that the NNIS risk index had a low sensitivity (24%) and poor predictive power (positive predictive value, 43%) for identifying SSIs after cardiotho-racic operative procedures.[23] Hence, we have chosen to use the NNIS risk index cautiously for SSI surveillance on our cardiothoracic surgery service.

A general risk index such as the NNIS risk index may predict poorly because the procedures and the patients are too diverse. Procedure-specific risk indices may solve the problems encountered with the NNIS risk index or its predecessors.[28-31] For example, Nichols and colleagues published a risk index that accurately predicted postoperative septic complications in a subset of patients who underwent operations after penetrating abdominal trauma.[29] In validating this risk index in a new population, they showed that the risk factors included in the index could identify high-risk patients who benefited from prolonged (5 days) antibiotic therapy and delayed wound closure and low-risk patients who did well with short-term (2 days) antibiotic therapy and primary wound closure.[29] Thus, this risk index not only stratifies patients by their risk of infection but also helps staff members predict which patients will benefit from costly preventive strategies.

POSTDISCHARGE SURVEILLANCE

The proportion of surgeries performed in the outpatient setting continues to increase. Postoperative length of stay following inpatient surgery is decreasing. Therefore, SSI frequently occurs in the outpatient setting. In recent studies, 45% to 84% of the SSIs were detected after discharge from the hospital.[32-34] Postdischarge SSI has been associated with a greater number of outpatient visits, readmissions, emergency room visits, home health services, and increased costs.[35]

The cost and time required to do postdischarge surveillance may discourage many infection control programs from instituting such systems. But infection control programs must acknowledge that inpatient surveillance alone will vastly underestimate the actual rates of SSI.[32,33,36,37] The CDC recommends that discharged patients be contacted 30 days after the procedure to determine whether an SSI has occurred.[38] Infection control programs therefore need to develop strategies that identify SSIs after discharge.

The census approach, surveying each patient or physician for a defined period, was used in several studies to measure nosocomial infection rates during the postdischarge recovery period.[33,39] Telephone surveys and questionnaires sent to patients or physicians also have been used.[34,40,41] Seaman and Lammers found that patients, despite using verbal or printed instructions, were unable to recognize infections.[40] They concluded that "reliance on printed instructions, telephone interviews, or any other means of patient self-evaluation may not allow early recognition of infection" and therefore should not be used for clinical investigations of wound healing."[40] Similarly, Sands and colleagues found that questionnaires sent to patients and to surgeons had sensitivities of 28% and 15%, respectively.[34]

In a later study of postdischarge surveillance, Sands and colleagues identified a method that appears more reliable.[34] They used automated pharmacy dispensing information, administrative data, and electronic records to identify postdischarge SSI.[15] In this method, specific codes for diagnoses, tests, and treatments were evaluated for their ability to predict postdischarge SSI. They found that an automated system of surveillance of hospital discharge diagnosis codes plus pharmacy dispensing data had a sensitivity of 77% and specificity of 94%.[15]

Delgado-Rodriguez and colleagues found that most of the postdischarge SSI occurred following clean surgery (ie, hernia, breast, or vascular surgery).[33] Clean-contaminated surgery of the biliary tract also had a significant number of SSIs in their study. This may give some guidance to ICPs when choosing procedures to target for postdischarge surveillance. Delgado and colleagues also found that risk factors for in-hospital SSI are not determinants of postdischarge SSI, with the exception of body mass index.[33]

We suggest that infection control programs link with home healthcare agencies or other agencies that provide care for patients at home to develop mechanisms by which SSIs can be identified. Furthermore, they must not conclude prematurely that same-day surgeries and endoscopic surgeries are not complicated by SSIs.

In the future, the severity of illness among surgical patients will increase, the operative procedures will become more sophisticated, the average length of stay after surgery will decrease, and more patients will have operative procedures in the outpatient setting. It is ironic that while these dramatic shifts in patient populations, operative techniques, and healthcare delivery will increase the need for outpatient surveillance, they will also increase the difficulty of performing accurate surveillance.

TABULATION, ANALYSIS, AND REPORTING OF DATA

Once data are collected, one can tabulate SSI rates. To calculate the rate of the outcome (ie, SSI) in a clearly delineated population for a given time (eg, 1 month, 1 quarter, or 1 year), divide the numerator (the number of patients with SSI) by the denominator (total number of patients in the population), and then multiply the result by 100 to obtain a percentage. Some examples follow.

1. Service-specific rates:

$$\frac{\text{Number of SSIs in patients on the neurosurgery service}}{\text{Number patients who had a neurosurgical procedure}} \times 100$$

2. Surgeon-specific rates:

$$\frac{\text{Number of SSIs in patients operated on by a particular surgeon}}{\text{Number of patients operated on by that surgeon}} \times 100$$

3. Procedure-specific rates:

$$\frac{\text{Number of SSIs occurring after a specific procedure (eg, appendectomy)}}{\text{Number of procedures (eg, appendectomy)}} \times 100$$

4. Risk-specific rates:

$$\frac{\text{Number of SSIs in patients with a NNIS risk index score of 2}}{\text{Number of patients with a NNIS risk index score of 2}} \times 100$$

Once the ICP identifies the population to be surveyed, the proper denominator is determined by searching the operating room logbook or the hospital's computerized database. All of the patients in the defined population are followed throughout the time frame designated by the definition of SSI (ie, 30 days postoperatively or one year postoperatively if an implant was inserted). Each patient who develops an SSI is included in the numerator. If the denominator is too broad (eg, all surgical patients in a large hospital), the group becomes very heterogeneous, and the calculated infection rate will be difficult to interpret. Consequently, ICPs may not identify clusters of SSIs or other problems. Surgeon-specific or procedure-specific rates more closely reflect true SSI rates. In general, data from at least 50 to 100 procedures should be included before calculating either overall or surgeon-specific rates.

The infection control program should stratify rates by type of procedures or by specific risk indices to allow comparisons among surgeons or among hospitals. The traditional wound classification system[25] has served this purpose for a quarter of a century, but it has some limitations, as mentioned earlier. The NNIS risk index, advocated by the CDC, is used widely today, but it does not perform well in certain circumstances.[23] Despite these limitations, it may be to a hospital's advantage to stratify the patients' risk by one of the available indices, particularly if the patients have numerous comorbidities or if the operative procedures performed in the hospital are quite complex.

The infection control program should report SSI rates to surgeons. SSI rates should be sent to the chief of surgery, and individual surgeons should receive their own rates. Confidentiality is of utmost importance in such a process. Therefore, codes should be used instead of names if surgeons are allowed to compare their rates with the rates of other surgeons or if surgeon-specific rates are reported to the infection control committee. Reporting SSI rates to practicing surgeons has been shown to reduce rates by the so-called Hawthorne effect (ie, the effect due to having one's performance observed).[4,6,8] However, one must interpret the conclusions with caution as most studies have included confounding factors.

Busy surgeons may ignore written reports. Therefore, ICPs should periodically present the data graphically and meet with the surgeons to discuss rates, clusters, and specific SSI cases. These discussions improve communication and cooperation between the infection control and the surgical teams. ICPs may learn ways to make the data more useful to the surgeons. The infection control staff can also use these feedback sessions as a means to introduce the surgical team to the state-of-the-art preventive measures to reduce the risk of SSIs.

The infection control program should report SSI rates, costs, lengths of stay associated with SSIs, and the effects of preventive measures to the hospital's administrators. Several investigators have demonstrated that SSIs are the primary independent determinant of hospital costs and length of stay after operative procedures.[42,43] Moreover, Olson and Lee demonstrated a $3 million cost savings in a 10-year wound surveillance program.[6] If an infection control program can show data that surveillance and interventions reduce SSI, length of stay, and cost, then hospital administrators will likely be more willing to provide the program with resources.

Finally, ICPs should periodically review their data to determine whether they should change their priorities or focus their energy on specific problems. For example, if a program analyzes its data and finds, after a few months, that the sensitivity of the case-finding method used for postdischarge surveillance is very low (eg, only 2% of SSIs are identified by this method), epidemiology staff may change their case-finding method instead of spending time and energy for a year or more before realizing that the method was not effective.

INTERVENTIONS TO REDUCE SURGICAL SITE INFECTIONS

Once data are collected, tabulated, and analyzed, the infection control program can develop and implement interventions to reduce SSI rates. These interventions will be dictated largely by the problems that have been identi-

fied through surveillance and data analysis. Epidemiology staff members examine factors in the preoperative, intraoperative, and postoperative periods for possible interventions to prevent SSI.[44]

Preoperative Intervention

Preoperative preparation of the patient is one area for intervention. Some variables cannot be modified (eg, age, gender), but others can be modified (eg, glucose control, steroid therapy). Several interventions, such as minimizing the duration of preoperative hospital stay and eradicating remote infections, have been shown to reduce SSI rates.[20] The preoperative stay should be as short as possible. Sometimes, it is prudent to send the patient home and readmit him or her for surgery.

ICPs need to ensure that best practices are followed for proper hair removal and antiseptic skin preparation. Patients who are colonized with *S. aureus* in the anterior nares are at increased risk of the development of SSI as well as other nosocomial infections.[45-48] A recent randomized double-blind clinical trial demonstrated that treatment with preoperative mupirocin decolonized the nares of patients and decreased *S. aureus* nosocomial infections in patients who were colonized.[48] Treated patients also had decreased *S. aureus* SSI, but the decrease was not statistically significant. Further study is needed to determine if this intervention can benefit a targeted subset of surgical patients.

The surgical team should perform appropriate antiseptic scrubs and avoid long or artificial nails. ICPs need to ensure that policies are in place (and followed) to restrict patient care of surgical staff with transmissible infectious diseases. If an epidemiologic investigation suggests that the source of the outbreak might be healthcare personnel who carry the organism, ICPs should obtain appropriate cultures from the implicated individuals (eg, cultures of nares and skin lesions for *S. aureus*, cultures of the throat, skin lesions, and, if necessary, the vagina and rectum for *Streptococcus* pyogenes). Finally, antimicrobial prophylaxis is crucial to preventing SSI and should be administered according to published guidelines for each given procedure. To be effective, prophylactic antibiotics must be given during the appropriate time interval. Recent studies have shown that there is much room for improvement in the administration of antimicrobial prophylaxis.[49-51]

Intraoperative Intervention

Interventions and institution of best practices during the intraoperative period can reduce SSI rates. Proper ventilation should be maintained in all operating rooms, including positive pressure and appropriate air filters. Traffic through the operating room should be kept to a minimum. ICPs need to monitor sterilization of surgical instruments to ensure that procedures conform to guidelines. Flash sterilization should be limited and never used solely for convenience. ICPs can work with the surgical staff to ensure that proper surgical attire and drapes are used. Observation in the operating room and collaboration with surgeons, surgical nurses, and surgical staff are important to maintain a high standard of asepsis and good surgical technique. Studies have demonstrated that intraoperative hypothermia approximately triples the risk of surgical site infection and leads to many other adverse events.[52-54] Therefore, normothermia should be maintained during surgery. The main methods of warming include passive insulation, fluid warming, and active warming of the patient with a forced-air system. Hyperglycemia increases mortality in critically ill patients and increases the risk of many adverse outcomes including SSI.[55-57] Interventions include screening for diabetes and hyperglycemia as well as intensive insulin therapy. The risk of surgical site infection is also directly related to tissue oxygenation.[58] Supplemental oxygen (80% vs. 30% inspired oxygen) during surgery and the immediate postoperative period has been shown to reduce rates of SSI by approximately half.[53,59]

Postoperative Intervention

Because most contamination happens during the operation through contact or airborne transmission, events that occur during the postoperative period (eg, improper dressing changes or isolation techniques) are less likely to contribute to SSIs. If epidemiological data indicate that postoperative care may be associated with increased SSI rates, the infection control staff may need to investigate practices during this period.

Implementation of Surgical Site Infection Surveillance

The ICP is a very important component of any surveillance program and should have personality traits that facilitate a good working relationship with surgeons. Particularly in programs that use direct wound examination to identify SSIs, a surgeon should train the ICPs so that they can evaluate subtle nuances of a wound's appearance.

Most importantly, the infection control program must involve the surgical staff so that they take the responsibility for controlling SSIs. To achieve this goal, infection control staff should do the following:

➤ Review the standard definitions of SSI with the surgeons, so they understand and accept the criteria.

➤ Ask the surgeons what data should be included in their infection control reports and whether they prefer a report with surgeon-specific or procedure-specific SSI rates.

➤ Confidentially report personal SSI rates to all staff surgeons and possibly to fellows and residents.

➤ Meet with surgeons and surgical nurses on a regular basis to build trust and to discuss issues such as surveillance methods.

➤ Visit the operating room routinely and during outbreaks to identify potential problems and to develop rapport and mutual respect.

➤ Encourage a surgeon or a surgical nurse to join the infection control committee.

➤ Join the Surgical Infection Society and attend its annual meeting to understand the surgeons' perspective on SSIs.

➤ Discuss protocols and goals for studies of SSIs with surgical staff and encourage them to participate.

➤ Develop creative strategies for identifying SSIs as the medical environment changes.

➤ Publish results of studies in surgical journals.

In addition, the infection control program requires adequate resources to conduct effective surveillance. Clerical support, computerized databases, and medical records personnel contribute significantly to the SSI surveillance program.

Conclusion

Surveillance for SSIs is a vital component of any infection control program, and it is a special form of continuous quality assurance in which the ultimate benefactors of control efforts are the patients. Therefore, the infection control program should define clear objectives, write precise definitions, and meticulously implement a surveillance system. Although methods of case-finding are hard to choose, the infection control team should focus on patients or procedures at high risk of infection if their resources are limited. Collecting data and calculating rates are useless if epidemiology and surgical staff do not use the data to reduce SSI rates. To succeed in such an effort, ICPs must collaborate with the surgical team.

As healthcare delivery shifts to the outpatient setting, numerous aspects of SSI surveillance must change because many factors that influence the risk of SSI also will change. Surveillance methods that worked well in the past and were supported by well-designed studies may no longer be efficacious. We desperately need creative research to determine how we should develop and apply risk indices and to identify which methods we should use for postdischarge surveillance. Indeed, exciting opportunities are open to those willing to accept the challenges.

REFERENCES

1. Burke JP. Patient safety: infection control—a problem for patient safety. *N Engl J Med*. 2003;348(7):651-656.

2. Martone WJ, Nichols RL. Recognition, prevention, surveillance, and management of surgical site infections: introduction to the problem and symposium overview. *Clin Infect Dis*. 2001;33 Suppl 2:S67-S68.

3. Emori TG, Gaynes RP. An overview of nosocomial infections, including the role of the microbiology laboratory. *Clin Microbiol Rev*. 1993;6(4):428-442.

4. Haley RW, Culver DH, White JW, et al. The efficacy of infection surveillance and control programs in preventing nosocomial infections in US hospitals. *Am J Epidemiol*. 1985;121(2):182-205.

5. Cruse PJ, Foord R. The epidemiology of wound infection. A 10-year prospective study of 62,939 wounds. *Surg Clin North Am*. 1980;60(1):27-40.

6. Olson MM, Lee JT Jr. Continuous, 10-year wound infection surveillance. Results, advantages, and unanswered questions. *Arch Surg*. 1990;125(6):794-803.

7. Ehrenkranz NJ, Richter EI, Phillips PM, Shultz JM. An apparent excess of operative site infections: analyses to evaluate false-positive diagnoses. *Infect Control Hosp Epidemiol*. 1995;16(12):712-716.

8. Horan TC, Gaynes RP, Martone WJ, Jarvis WR, Emori TG. CDC definitions of nosocomial surgical site infections, 1992: a modification of CDC definitions of surgical wound infections. *Infect Control Hosp Epidemiol*. 1992;13(10):606-608.

9. Perl TM. Surveillance, reporting and the use of computers. In: Wenzel RP, ed. *Prevention and Control of Nosocomial Infections*. Baltimore: Williams & Wilkins; 1993:139-176.

10. Wenzel RP, Osterman CA, Hunting KJ, Gwaltney JM Jr. Hospital-acquired infections. I. Surveillance in a university hospital. *Am J Epidemiol*. 1976;103(3):251-260.

11. Lee JT. Wound infection surveillance. *Infect Dis Clin North Am*. 1992;6(3):643-656.

12. Cardo DM, Falk PS, Mayhall CG. Validation of surgical wound surveillance. *Infect Control Hosp Epidemiol*. 1993;14(4):211-215.

13. Haley RW, Schaberg DR, McClish DK, et al. The accuracy of retrospective chart review in measuring nosocomial infection rates. Results of validation studies in pilot hospitals. *Am J Epidemiol*. 1980;111(5):516-533.

14. Manian FA, Meyer L. Comprehensive surveillance of surgical wound infections in outpatient and inpatient surgery. *Infect Control Hosp Epidemiol*. 1990;11(10):515-520.

15. Sands K, Vineyard G, Livingston J, Christiansen C, Platt R. Efficient identification of postdischarge surgical site infections: use of automated pharmacy dispensing information, administrative data, and medical record information. *J Infect Dis*. 1999;179(2):434-441.

16. Platt R, Kleinman K, Thompson K, et al. Using automated health plan data to assess infection risk from coronary artery bypass surgery. *Emerg Infect Dis*. 2002;8(12):1433-1441.

17. Hirschhorn LR, Currier JS, Platt R. Electronic surveillance of antibiotic exposure and coded discharge diagnoses as indicators of postoperative infection and other quality assurance measures. *Infect Control Hosp Epidemiol*. 1993;14(1):21-28.

18. Bouam S, Girou E, Brun-Buisson C, Karadimas H, Lepage E. An intranet-based automated system for the surveillance of nosocomial infections: prospective validation compared with physicians' self-reports. *Infect Control Hosp Epidemiol*. 2003;24(1):51-55.

19. Burke JP. Surveillance, reporting, automation, and interventional epidemiology. *Infect Control Hosp Epidemiol*. 2003;24(1):10-12.

20. Mayhall CG. Surgical infections including burns. In: Wenzel RP, ed. *Prevention and Control of Nosocomial Infections*. Baltimore: Williams & Wilkins; 1993:614-664.

21. Kernodle DS, Kaiser AB. Postoperative infections and antimicrobial prophylaxis. In: Mandell GL, Bennett JE, Dolin R, eds. *Principles and Practice of Infectious Diseases*. New York: Churchill Livingstone; 1995:2742-2756.

22. Nagachinta T, Stephens M, Reitz B, Polk BF. Risk factors for surgical-wound infection following cardiac surgery. *J Infect Dis*. 1987;156(6):967-973.

23. Roy MC, Herwaldt LA, Embrey R, Kuhns K, Wenzel RP, Perl TM. Does the Centers for Disease Control's NNIS system risk index stratify patients undergoing cardiothoracic operations by their risk of surgical-site infection? *Infect Control Hosp Epidemiol*. 2000;21(3):186-190.

24. Haley RW. Surveillance by objective: a new priority-directed approach to the control of nosocomial infections. The National Foundation for Infectious Diseases lecture. *Am J Infect Control*. 1985;13(2):78-89.

25. National Academy of Sciences-National Research Council. Postoperative wound infections: the influence of ultraviolet irradiation of the operating room and of various other factors. *Ann Surg*. 1964;160(suppl 2):1-132.

26. Ferraz EM, Bacelar TS, Aguiar JL, Ferraz AA, Pagnossin G, Batista JE. Wound infection rates in clean surgery: a potentially misleading risk classification. *Infect Control Hosp Epidemiol*. 1992;13(8):457-462.

27. Haley RW, Culver DH, Morgan WM, White JW, Emori TG, Hooton TM. Identifying patients at high risk of surgical wound infection. A simple multivariate index of patient susceptibility and wound contamination. *Am J Epidemiol*. 1985;121(2):206-215.

28. Culver DH, Horan TC, Gaynes RP, et al. Surgical wound infection rates by wound class, operative procedure, and patient risk index. National Nosocomial Infections Surveillance System. *Am J Med*. 1991;91(3B):152S-157S.

29. Nichols RL, Smith JW, Robertson GD, et al. Prospective alterations in therapy for penetrating abdominal trauma. *Arch Surg*. 1993;128(1):55-63.

30. Nichols RL, Smith JW, Klein DB, et al. Risk of infection after penetrating abdominal trauma. *N Engl J Med.* 1984;311(17):1065-1070.

31. Richet HM, Chidiac C, Prat A, et al. Analysis of risk factors for surgical wound infections following vascular surgery. *Am J Med.* 1991;91(3B):170S-172S.

32. Avato JL, Lai KK. Impact of postdischarge surveillance on surgical-site infection rates for coronary artery bypass procedures. *Infect Control Hosp Epidemiol.* 2002;23(7):364-367.

33. Delgado-Rodriguez M, Gomez-Ortega A, Sillero-Arenas M, Llorca J. Epidemiology of surgical-site infections diagnosed after hospital discharge: a prospective cohort study. *Infect Control Hosp Epidemiol.* 2001;22(1):24-30.

34. Sands K, Vineyard G, Platt R. Surgical site infections occurring after hospital discharge. *J Infect Dis.* 1996;173(4):963-970.

35. Perencevich EN, Sands KE, Cosgrove SE, Guadagnoli E, Meara E, Platt R. Health and economic impact of surgical site infections diagnosed after hospital discharge. *Emerg Infect Dis.* 2003;9(2):196-203.

36. Noy D, Creedy D. Postdischarge surveillance of surgical site infections: a multi-method approach to data collection. *Am J Infect Control.* 2002;30(7):417-424.

37. Kent P, McDonald M, Harris O, Mason T, Spelman D. Postdischarge surgical wound infection surveillance in a provincial hospital: follow-up rates, validity of data and review of the literature. *ANZ J Surg.* 2001;71(10):583-589.

38. Garner JS. CDC guideline for prevention of surgical wound infections, 1985. Supersedes guideline for prevention of surgical wound infections published in 1982. (Originally published in November 1985). Revised. *Infect Control.* 1986;7(3):193-200.

39. Burns SJ, Dippe SE. Postoperative wound infections detected during hospitalization and after discharge in a community hospital. *Am J Infect Control.* 1982;10(2):60-65.

40. Seaman M, Lammers R. Inability of patients to self-diagnose wound infections. *J Emerg Med.* 1991;9(4):215-219.

41. Rosendorf LL, Octavio J, Estes JP. Effect of methods of postdischarge wound infection surveillance on reported infection rates. *Am J Infect Control.* 1983;11(6):226-229.

42. Weintraub WS, Jones EL, Craver J, Guyton R, Cohen C. Determinants of prolonged length of hospital stay after coronary bypass surgery. *Circulation.* 1989;80(2):276-284.

43. Taylor GJ, Mikell FL, Moses HW, et al. Determinants of hospital charges for coronary artery bypass surgery: the economic consequences of postoperative complications. *Am J Cardiol.* 1990;65(5):309-313.

44. Mangram AJ, Horan TC, Pearson ML, Silver LC, Jarvis WR. Guideline for Prevention of Surgical Site Infection, 1999. Centers for Disease Control and Prevention (CDC) Hospital Infection Control Practices Advisory Committee. *Am J Infect Control.* 1999;27(2):97-132.

45. Perl TM, Golub JE. New approaches to reduce *Staphylococcus aureus* nosocomial infection rates: treating *S. aureus* nasal carriage. *Ann Pharmacother.* 1998;32(1):S7-S16.

46. Wenzel RP, Perl TM. The significance of nasal carriage of *Staphylococcus aureus* and the incidence of postoperative wound infection. *J Hosp Infect.* 1995;31(1):13-24.

47. Kluytmans J, van Belkum A, Verbrugh H. Nasal carriage of *Staphylococcus aureus*: epidemiology, underlying mechanisms, and associated risks. *Clin Microbiol Rev.* 1997;10(3):505-520.

48. Perl TM, Cullen JJ, Wenzel RP, et al. Intranasal mupirocin to prevent postoperative *Staphylococcus aureus* infections. *N Engl J Med.* 2002;346(24):1871-1877.

49. Silver A, Eichorn A, Kral J, et al. Timeliness and use of antibiotic prophylaxis in selected inpatient surgical procedures. The Antibiotic Prophylaxis Study Group. *Am J Surg.* 1996;171(6):548-552.

50. Classen DC, Evans RS, Pestotnik SL, Horn SD, Menlove RL, Burke JP. The timing of prophylactic administration of antibiotics and the risk of surgical-wound infection. *N Engl J Med.* 1992;326(5):281-286.

51. Zanetti G, Flanagan HL Jr., Cohn LH, Giardina R, Platt R. Improvement of intraoperative antibiotic prophylaxis in prolonged cardiac surgery by automated alerts in the operating room. *Infect Control Hosp Epidemiol.* 2003;24(1):13-16.

52. Kurz A, Sessler DI, Lenhardt R. Perioperative normothermia to reduce the incidence of surgical-wound infection and shorten hospitalization. Study of Wound Infection and Temperature Group. *N Engl J Med.* 1996;334(19):1209-1215.

53. Sessler DI, Akca O. Nonpharmacological prevention of surgical wound infections. *Clin Infect Dis.* 2002;35(11):1397-1404.

54. Melling AC, Ali B, Scott EM, Leaper DJ. Effects of preoperative warming on the incidence of wound infection after clean surgery: a randomised controlled trial. *Lancet.* 2001;358(9285):876-880.

55. Latham R, Lancaster AD, Covington JF, Pirolo JS, Thomas CS. The association of diabetes and glucose control with surgical-site infections among cardiothoracic surgery patients. *Infect Control Hosp Epidemiol.* 2001;22(10):607-612.

56. Van den BG, Wouters P, Weekers F, et al. Intensive insulin therapy in the critically ill patients. *N Engl J Med.* 2001;345(19):1359-1367.

57. Dellinger EP. Preventing surgical-site infections: the importance of timing and glucose control. *Infect Control Hosp Epidemiol.* 2001;22(10):604-606.

58. Hopf HW, Hunt TK, West JM, et al. Wound tissue oxygen tension predicts the risk of wound infection in surgical patients. *Arch Surg.* 1997;132(9):997-1004.

59. Greif R, Akca O, Horn EP, Kurz A, Sessler DI. Supplemental perioperative oxygen to reduce the incidence of surgical-wound infection. Outcomes Research Group. *N Engl J Med.* 2000;342(3):161-167.

CHAPTER NINE

SURVEILLANCE FOR INFECTIONS ASSOCIATED WITH VASCULAR CATHETERS

Werner Ernst Bischoff, MD, MSc

INTRODUCTION

Intravascular catheter-related infections (IV-CRIs) are one of the predominant causes of morbidity and mortality in the United States.[1] It is estimated that more than 150 million intravascular devices are purchased each year including more than 7 million central venous catheters (CVCs) alone.[2-4] These devices, and in particular CVCs, are the source of most primary bloodstream infections,[3,4] leading to approximately 250,000 to 500,000 hospital-acquired bloodstream infections in the United States annually.[2,5-9] These infections not only cause a significant economic burden with a marginal cost estimate of $25,000 per episode but are also related to a high mortality rate of 10% in hospitalized patients.[4,6,8,10-12]

Given these numbers, preventive measures are paramount for the control and reduction of IV-CRIs in the hospital setting. An accurate and practical surveillance system is essential for identifying the true scope of the problem and therefore allowing for implementation of effective strategies to reduce IV-CRI rates. Surveillance can provide the basis for an effective infection control program through the routine and orderly collection of data, subsequent analysis, and timely reporting. This chapter is intended to provide infection control personnel with the knowledge necessary to design and implement an effective surveillance program for IV-CRIs and to ensure the commitment of hospital personnel and administration in the continuing effort to reduce IV-CRI rates.

ARGUMENTS FOR SURVEILLANCE

Surveillance is an ongoing process, requiring a considerable amount of time and personnel resources. Therefore, convincing administration of the importance of surveillance is essential to guarantee adequate resources and a successful institution of such a program.

Evidence of the efficacy of surveillance programs in infection control has been best demonstrated in the SENIC.[13] Hospitals with a high-intensity control program, regardless of the level of surveillance activities, showed a moderate 15% reduction in nosocomial bacteremia rates. However, hospitals with a similar intensity control program but with at least a medium level of surveillance demonstrated a 35% reduction in nosocomial bacteremia rates. In a more recent study, Curran and colleagues showed a significant reduction in infections associated with peripheral vascular catheters from 8.5% to 5.3% using surveillance with feedback (p<0.001).[14] Similar results were also reported for CVCs.[15] The introduction of ongoing surveillance by an infection control professional in a 42-bed ICU achieved a significant reduction from 7.18 infections/1000 catheter-related exposure days to 4.29 infections/1000 catheter-related exposure days (p = 0.0045).[16] Lastly, the NNIS System of the CDC provides an indirect indication of the efficacy of a surveillance system by documenting a substantial decrease of BSI rates in different ICUs ranging from 31% (surgical ICUs) to 44% (medical ICUs) during 1990 to 1999.[17]

Another essential element is the cost effectiveness of a surveillance program. Estimates of the additional costs related to nosocomial BSI range from $4000 up to $56,000 per episode.[6,11,18-20] Slater calculated savings of $108,000 in the 9 months following introduction of a vascular catheter nurse in a surgical ICU by preventing an estimated 18 BSIs.[21] In a neonatal ICU setting, the cost estimates for one nosocomial BSI was approximately $22,980 with accommodation costs accounting for 70% of the total additional charges, while less than 30% accounted for physician fees, pharmaceuticals, and other ancillary services.[22] Critically ill patients with BSI are hospitalized for an average of 6.5 to 22 days longer than those without a BSI.[6,11,18,20] This suggests that the additional length of stay caused by IV-CRI contributes substantially to the overall costs and can also be used as an indicator for cost-benefit analyses.

GOALS AND ATTRIBUTES OF A SURVEILLANCE PROGRAM

There are 5 goals a successful IV-CRI surveillance program should meet[23]:

1. To define endemic ("background") rates of IV-CRI.
2. To identify increases in IV-CRI rates above the endemic level.
3. To identify specific risks for IV-CRI for patients undergoing routine hospital care or procedures.
4. To inform hospital personnel of the risks of the care or procedures they provide to patients.
5. To evaluate the utility and efficiency of control measures.

To accomplish these 5 goals, there are a number of attributes for public health surveillance systems published by the CDC that can be easily transferred to the surveillance of IV-CRI.[24]

Simplicity refers to understandable and easily manageable methods for data collection, analysis, and dissemination.

Flexibility describes the potential of a surveillance program to respond quickly and appropriately to changing information needs or operating conditions. Simpler systems can allow for fast reactions to these changes.

Data quality summarizes the completeness and validity of data recorded in the surveillance system. Counting the number of missing responses is an easy tool to assess the completeness of a database. Evaluation of the validity requires additional studies such as retrospective chart review of sampled data.

Acceptability refers to the willingness of people and organizations to participate in the surveillance program. This is affected by the user friendliness of the surveillance program and by the acceptance of the data from people inside and outside the sponsoring institution.

Sensitivity is another attribute that refers to the percentage of correct cases being reported by the surveillance program and also the ability to detect outbreaks as changes in the number of cases over time. Testing the validity of a program regarding sensitivity requires additional studies.

Predictive value positive is the proportion of reported cases actually having the health-related event under surveillance. The predictive value positive focuses on the sensitivity and specificity of the case definition by confirma-

tion of cases reported through the surveillance system. Low values mean that noncases are investigated, leading to unnecessary interventions and use of resources.

Representativeness describes the accuracy of the data reflecting the actual occurrence of events in a population over time. To achieve generalizability or high external validity, the population should be well defined, and results should be comparable to other surveillance systems.

Timeliness of the individual steps in a surveillance system is paramount to ensure effective responses to changing conditions. Transparency and simplicity of the program structure support the success of the surveillance program.

Stability refers to the ability of the program to collect, analyze, and report data without gaps.

These universal attributes should be kept in mind when planning and implementing a surveillance program.

SURVEILLANCE OPTIONS

Three major surveillance strategies can be distinguished, including hospital-wide, objective-directed, and targeted surveillance. The most extensive effort is the hospital-wide surveillance covering the entire institution for an extended period of time.[25-27] Objective-directed surveillance is based on an identified problem such as high rates of IV-CRI in a specific ICU and the allocation of surveillance and intervention resources to address this problem.[28] Unfortunately, no long-term data are collected because surveillance efforts are redirected once the specific objective is met. Targeted surveillance combines elements of the 2 previous approaches by focusing long-term surveillance efforts on an infection site such as BSI or on a location such as ICUs without having a specific problem objective.[29-31] This allows collecting data in areas of high risk with a longitudinal surveillance component. Because financial resources are limited in most institutions, the focus has shifted toward targeted surveillance. Published data demonstrate that IV-CRI occur most often in the intensive care and oncology settings.[30,31] Therefore, it is recommended that targeted surveillance efforts be directed to these high-risk areas.

OUTPATIENT SURVEILLANCE

The classic approach limits surveillance to the hospital stay of patients. Admission and discharge dates mark the time points of observation activities. However, the length of hospital stay has decreased in recent years, and in some cases, admission is completely replaced by outpatient care.[32-35] The first reduces the probability of detecting an event, whereas the second requires an entirely different approach to access data. The extension of surveillance efforts after discharge of patients appears to be very difficult, showing a wide range of outcomes depending on the methods used and the institution involved.[36,37] However, targeted postdischarge surveillance for catheter-related BSI has recently been suggested as a rational alternative.[38]

Outpatients are also a difficult population to monitor because contact with a healthcare provider is time limited and variable. The first controlled attempt to study these patients was initiated by the CDC in 1999 with the Dialysis Surveillance Network.[39] Focusing primarily on vascular access infections, this study should help to better define the surveillance tools necessary to monitor outpatients. Forms and guidelines can be downloaded from the CDC Web site (http://www.cdc.gov/ncidod/hip/Dialysis/procedure.htm).

Feasibility and cost effectiveness should be taken into account for individual facilities when considering whether outpatient surveillance should be initiated and what components would provide the most valuable and accurate data.

CASE DEFINITION

A surveillance program is based on a clear definition of an event, in this case an IV-CRI. Unfortunately, there is still no universal agreement as to which findings constitute this particular outcome. The clinical signs of catheter-related bloodstream infections are unreliable with low sensitivities and specificities.[2,40-45] Fever, erythema, or purulence around the catheter insertion site can be indicators for an infection but are not conclusive. In comparison, the microbiologic diagnosis of catheter-related infections is overall more precise. However, there are numerous definitions based on processing and culturing suspected catheters and other materials that make selection of one method versus another quite difficult. One can make up his or her own definition of an IV-CRI, but to ensure comparability with other studies, it is best to rely on existing standards. The following clinical definitions for IV-CRI are listed in the *Guidelines for the Prevention of Intravascular Catheter-Related Infections* by the CDC and have been used in numerous local and national studies[45]:

➤ *Catheter colonization* is defined as growth from a culture of the catheter tip, subcutaneous segment, or hub of more than 15 colony-forming units (CFUs) by semiquantitative roll-plate technique[42] or more than 10^3 *cfus* by the quantitative sonication method.[44]

➤ *Exit site infections* are defined as erythema or induration within 2 cm of the catheter exit site, in the absence of concomitant BSI and without concomitant purulence.

➤ *Clinical exit site infections or "tunnel" infections* require tenderness, erythema, and site induration more than 2 cm from the catheter site along the subcutaneous tract of a tunneled (eg, Hickman or Broviac) catheter, in the absence of concomitant BSI.

➤ *Pocket infections* in totally implanted intravascular devices show purulent fluid that might or might not be associated with spontaneous rupture and drainage or necrosis of the overlaying skin, in the absence of concomitant BSIs.

➤ *Infusate-related BSIs* require the concordant growth of the same organism from the infusate and blood cultures (preferably percutaneously drawn) with no other identifiable source of infection.

➤ *Catheter-related BSIs* require one of the following in addition to clinical manifestation of infections (ie, fever, chills, and/or hypotension) and no apparent source for the BSI except the catheter: the isolation of the same isolate (species and antibiogram) from the catheter (semiquantitative or quantitative colonization) and peripheral blood; simultaneous quantitative blood cultures with a > 5:1 ratio CVC versus peripheral, and differential period of CVC culture versus peripheral blood culture positivity of more than 2 hours.

In addition to the clinical definitions for catheter-related infections, CDC has published surveillance definitions for primary BSIs used for the NNIS System.[45] After fulfilling the CDC criteria for a laboratory confirmed BSI, these definitions include the following:

➤ A BSI is considered to be associated with a central line if the line was in use during the 48-hour period before development of the BSI.

➤ A vascular access device is one that terminates at or close to the heart or one of the great vessels including an umbilical artery or vein catheter.

➤ If the time interval between onset of infection and device use is more than 48 hours, there should be compelling evidence that the infection is related to the central line.

Using these guidelines in a surveillance program promotes the acceptability of the results internally and externally and the generalizability of the outcomes. Deviations from these widely accepted standards should be carefully considered given the potential problems in future interpretation.

COLLECTION OF DATA

Information is generally derived from at least 2 sources. Clinical data are collected routinely by infection control personnel, and microbiology data are provided by the hospital laboratory. It is paramount to coordinate the surveillance efforts of both parties to ensure a timely and efficient collection process.

The microbiology laboratory determines the occurrence of an IV-CRI by culturing patient samples such as catheter tips or blood cultures and identifying pathogens and their resistance patterns. As clinical signs are mostly inconclusive, the lab results play a crucial role in the diagnosis of catheter-related BSI. Therefore, a strong collaboration between the hospital epidemiologist and the microbiology lab should be established before initiating surveillance. It is recommended that well-established guidelines be adopted such as those laid out by the CDC and NNIS for BSI.[45] Standardized lab techniques are found in the National Committee for Clinical Laboratory Standards (NCCLS).[46] This allows comparison among one's own lab results and that of other investigators. One important caveat regarding the microbiology laboratory is the time delay between sampling and result reporting. The surveillance program should allow for at least a 48-hour period before conclusively determining the presence or absence of an IV-CRI in a patient.

Trained infection control professionals are preferred for collection of clinical data. Active surveillance provides the most reliable estimate of the "real" infection rate as compared to passive surveillance performed by individuals other than infection control personnel.[47] This applies in particular to IV-CRI because the complexity of event definitions and the combination of laboratory and clinical signs demand a high standard of knowledge and experience.

The means to collect data range from simple spreadsheets to hand held computer devices. Selection criterion should be the feasibility and acceptability of the method by the users. Minimal data collected should include demographic information (name, hospital identification number, age or date of birth, gender), admission information (date of hospital admission/unit admission, dates of catheter-related procedures), and clinical and laboratory information (criteria of infection, pathogens isolated). In addition, a multitude of other information such as underlying diseases, severity of symptoms, or antibiotic use data can be gathered. Accessibility of electronic medical records can streamline the collection process.

DATA VALIDATION

A central part of the management process is validation of the collected data. Validity or the lack of systematic error is separated in an internal and external component.[48] Applied to the surveillance of IV-CRI, the internal component focuses on the accurate measurement of these infections. Missing or misidentifications of such events

can jeopardize the entire surveillance effort. Data completeness and accuracy are crucial because all further evaluation of potential associations is based on the information obtained by surveillance. Therefore, routine testing of the internal validity should be implemented from the beginning.

The completeness of the data collection can be easily addressed by listing missing data from the surveillance forms. Clusters of blank spots can pinpoint problems in the ascertainment of information and provide clues as to how to improve the overall collection process. The accuracy of the data can be determined by a concurrent surveillance activity. During these spot checks, a dedicated person such as the hospital epidemiologist or an experienced infection control practitioner repeats the data collection and compares the outcomes of both efforts. The individual routinely assigned for the surveillance should be unaware of the time and location of these spot checks to avoid any bias. Deviations in the 2 outcomes can identify problems in the case definitions or misconceptions of the observer.

External validity addresses the generalizability of the inferences derived from the surveillance efforts to people or patient populations outside that particular surveillance group. This does not imply that the scientific value of surveillance is greater to more diverse patient groups. Because it is often not feasible and also unnecessary to include everyone in the surveillance, one has to make choices as to which subgroup of the population is most likely to represent a valid sample for the specific scientific problem in question. For IV-CRI, this sample selection can be based on risk assessments leading, for example, to patients in critical care, oncology, or hemodialysis. External validity requires the sound definition of the sample group and its environment. This includes demographic data of the patients but also hospital demographics, including number of beds, variety of services, ratio of HCWs to patients, and infection control measures in place. The collection of this information allows for the comparison of the characteristics of the patient group studied with other populations.

ANALYSIS, PRESENTATION, AND FEEDBACK OF DATA

The initial analysis of IV-CRI surveillance data is mostly descriptive in nature. Trends in infection rates, outbreak detection, or comparisons with other datasets are best visualized in graphic form accompanied by more detailed tables. The following is intended to provide a template for the initial analysis and presentation of IV-CRI rates.

The most commonly used formula to calculate IV-CRI rates reads as follows[1]:

$$\frac{\text{Number of IV-CRI (for a specific site)}}{\text{Number of intravascular catheter device days}} \times 1000 = \text{IV-CRI by 1000 device days}$$

Placing the number of device days in the denominator reflects the actual exposure to the devices. It is also useful to specify the unit in which the surveillance took place (eg, number of IV-CRIs in surgical ICUs). Both measures help to stratify one's own data for comparison to other units or hospitals.

There are multiple time periods for reporting, such as weekly, monthly, quarterly, or yearly intervals. However, one has to be aware that the shorter the interval, the less precise the results may become, particularly in small datasets. On the other hand, long intervals tend to cover more minute changes, making the detection of unusual clusters difficult. It is recommended that different intervals be applied when analyzing a dataset to observe overall trends and detect self-limiting outbreaks in IV-CRI.

Once the rates of IV-CRI have been determined, the data from the microbiology lab should be more closely inspected. Species identification and resistance patterns can indicate particular trends or clusters as well as the endemic occurrence of specific pathogens. Additional methods such as molecular typing can be used to identify clonal similarities among pathogen strains but are costly and time consuming.

One's own IV-CRI rates can also be compared internally (eg, to other units) or externally to other facilities. The majority of reported and accepted comparison data have been generated by the NNIS Program.[1] As mentioned previously, it is crucial to match the underlying surveillance techniques and adjust for potentially confounding factors to achieve a meaningful comparison.

The last step is the feedback and dissemination of the findings to the appropriate personnel. To effect change, in this case reduce IV-CRI rates, individuals directly and indirectly involved in patient care must be aware of the data generated by the surveillance effort. Without the understanding of the data and accountability of these individuals, surveillance efforts, regardless of how good, may be in vain. Therefore, the report of surveillance results, even if seemingly unimpressive, should be firmly implemented into the program.

CONCLUSION

For most institutions, the primary goal for the implementation of an IV-CRI surveillance program is to determine the IV-CRI rates, monitor the trends over time, and compare these rates to findings from other surveillance systems such as NNIS. A surveillance program should start with a small well-defined patient group such as those found in an ICU. Once the techniques and methods are mastered, the surveillance efforts can be extended to include all patient groups identified "at risk."

The directions a surveillance program can take are numerous and include detection of trends or outbreaks in infection rates and pathogen distribution, comparison of new techniques or devices such as catheters with antimicrobial coatings, or testing the impact of behavioral changes among healthcare professionals.[1,17,49-51]

Surveillance of IV-CRI is a time-consuming, personnel-intensive undertaking. However, without the information gathered by dedicated infection control practitioners, there would be no scientific evidence of the endemic rates of IV-CRI, the occurrence of outbreaks, or the usefulness of new methods or techniques to reduce IV-CRI.

REFERENCES

1. National Nosocomial Infections Surveillance (NNIS) System. Report, data summary from January 1992 to June 2002, issued August 2002. Am J Infect Control. 2002;30:458-475.
2. Maki DG, Mermel LA. Infections due to infusion therapy. In: Bennett JV, Brachman PS, eds. Hospital Infections. Philadelphia: Lippincott-Raven; 1998:689-724.
3. Jarvis WR, Edwards JE, Culver DH, et al. Nosocomial infection rates in adult and pediatric intensive care units in the United States. Am J Med. 1991;91(suppl 3B):185S-191S.
4. Maki DG. Pathogenesis, prevention and management of infections due to intravascular devices used for infusion therapy. In: Bison AL, Waldvogel F, eds. Infections Associated With Indwelling Medical Devices. Washington, DC: American Society for Microbiology; 1989:161-177.
5. Banerjee SN, Emori TG, Culver DH, et al. Secular trends in nosocomial bloodstream infections in the United States, 1980-1989. National Nosocomial Surveillance System. Am J Med. 1991;91(3B):86S-89S.
6. Heiselman D. Nosocomial bloodstream infection in the critically ill. JAMA. 1994;272:1819-1820.
7. Maki DG. Nosocomial bacteremia. Am J Med. 1981;70:183-196.
8. Mermel LA. Prevention of intravascular catheter-related infections. Ann Intern Med. 2000;132:391-401.
9. Raad I. Intravascular catheter-related infections. Lancet. 1998;351:893-898.
10. Arnow PM, Quimosing EM, Beach M. Consequences of intravascular catheter sepsis. Clin Infect Dis. 1993;16:778-784.

11. Pittet D, Tarara D, Wenzel RP. Nosocomial bloodstream infection in critically ill patients: excess length of stay, extra costs and attributable mortality. *JAMA*. 1994;271:1598-1601.

12. Smith RL, Meixler SM, Simberkoff MS. Excess mortality in critically ill patients with nosocomial bloodstream infections. *Chest*. 1991;100:164-167.

13. Haley RW, Culver DH, White JW, et al. The efficacy of infection surveillance and control programs in preventing nosocomial infections in US hospitals. *Am J Epidemiol*. 1985;121:182-205.

14. Curran ET, Coia JE, Gilmour H, et al. Multi-centre research surveillance project to reduce infections/phlebitis associated with peripheral vascular catheters. *J Hosp Infect*. 2000;46:194-202.

15. Curran ET, Booth MG, Dickson L, et al. Catheter-related sepsis in an ICU. In: *Eighth annual meeting of the Society of Healthcare Epidemiology of America (SHEA)*. Orlando: SHEA; 1998:S7.

16. Vandenberghe A, Laterre PF, Goenen M, et al. Surveillance of hospital-acquired infections in an intensive care department—the benefit of the full time presence of an infection control nurse. *J Hosp Infect*. 2002;52:56-59.

17. CDC. Monitoring hospital-acquired infections to promote patient safety-United States, 1990-1999. *MMWR*. 2000;49:149-153.

18. Pittet D, Wenzel RP. Nosocomial bloodstream infections in the critically ill [letter]. *JAMA*. 1994;272:1820.

19. Di Giovine B, Chenoweth C, Watts C, et al. The attributable mortality and costs of primary nosocomial bloodstream infection in the intensive care unit. *Am J Resp Crit Care Med*. 1999;160:976-981.

20. Dimick JB, Pelz RK, Consunji R, et al. Increased resource use associated with catheter-related bloodstream infection in the surgical intensive care unit. *Arch Surg*. 2001;136:229-234.

21. Slater F. Cost-effective infection control success story: a case presentation. *Emerg Infect Dis*. 2001;7:293-294.

22. Mahieu LM, Buitenweg N, Beutels PH, De Dooy JJ. Additional hospital stay and charges due to hospital-acquired infections in a neonatal intensive care unit. *J Hosp Infect*. 2001;47:223-229.

23. Perl TM. Surveillance, reporting, and the use of computers. In: Wenzel RP, ed. *Prevention and Control of Nosocomial Infections*. 3rd ed. Baltimore, Md: Williams & Wilkins; 1997:127-161.

24. CDC. Updated guidelines for evaluating public health surveillance systems. Recommendations from the guidelines working group. *MMWR*. 2001;50:1-36.

25. Freeman J, McGowan JE Jr. Methodologic issues in hospital epidemiology: I. Rates, case-finding, and interpretation. *Rev Infect Dis*. 1981;3:658-667.

26. Wenzel RP, Osterman CA, Hunting KJ, Gwaltney JM. Hospital-acquired infections: I. Surveillance in a university hospital. *Am J Epidemiol*. 1976;103:251-260.

27. Emori TG, Culver DH, Horan TC, et al. National nosocomial infections surveillance methods. *Am J Infect Control*. 1991;19:19-35.

28. Haley RW, Aber RC, Bennett JV. Surveillance of nosocomial infections. In: Bennett JV, Brachman PS, eds. *Hospital Infections*. Boston: Little, Brown & Co.; 1986:51-71.

29. Hambraeus A, Malmborg A. Surveillance of hospital infections: at the bedside or at the bacteriology laboratory? *Scand J Infect Dis*. 1977;9:289-292.

30. Wenzel RP, Thompson RL, Landry SM, et al. Hospital-acquired infections in intensive care unit patients: an overview with special emphasis on epidemics. *Infect Control Hosp Epidemiol*. 1983;4:371-375.

31. Pittet D, Wenzel RP. Nosocomial bloodstream infections. *Arch Intern Med*. 1995;155:1177-1184.

32. Owings MF, Kozak LJ. *Ambulatory and inpatient procedures in the United States, 1996*. National Center for Health Statistics. *Vital Health Stat*. 1998;13:19.

33. Pokras R, Kozak LJ, McCarthy E, et al. *Trends in hospital utilization: United States, 1965-86*. National Center for Health Statistics. *Vital Health Stat*. 1998;13:28.

34. Haupt BJ, Jones A. *National Home and Hospice Care Survey: annual summary, 1996*. National Center for Health Statistics. *Vital Health Stat*. 1999;13:8.

35. Popovic JR, Hall MJ. *National Hospital Discharge Survey*. National Center for Health Statistics. *Advance Data*. 2001;319:10.

36. Sands K, Vineyard G, Platt R. Surgical site infections occurring after hospital discharge. *J Infect Dis*. 1996;173:963-970.

37. Gaynes RP, Culver DH, Horan TC, et al. Surgical site infection (SSI) rates in the United States, 1992-1998: the National Nosocomial Surveillance System, basic SSI risk index. *Clin Infect Dis*. 2001;33 (suppl 2):69-77.

38. Hugonnet S, Eggimann P, Touveneau S, et al. ICU-acquired nosocomial infections: is post-discharge surveillance worth it? In: *41st Intersciences Conference on Antimicrobial Agents and Chemotherapy (ICAAC)*. Chicago, IL 2001;K1128.

39. Tokars JI, Miller ER, Stein G. New national surveillance system for hemodialysis-associated infections: initial results. *Am J Infect Control*. 2002;30:288-295.

40. Mayhall CG. Diagnosis and management of infections of implantable devices used for prolonged venous access. *Curr Clin Top Infect Dis*. 1992;12:83-110.

41. Kiehn TE, Armstrong D. Changes in the spectrum of organisms causing bacteremia and fungemia in immunocompromised patients due to venous access devices. *Eur J Clin Microbiol Infect Dis*. 1990;9:896-872.

42. Maki DG, Weise CE, Sarafin HW. A semi-quantitative culture method for identifying intravenous-catheter-related infection. *N Engl J Med*. 1977;296:1305-1309.

43. Maki DG, Cobb L, Garman JK, et al. An attachable silver-impregnated cuff for prevention of infection with central venous catheters: a prospective randomized multicenter trial. *Am J Med*. 1988;85:307-314.

44. Sherertz RJ, Raad II, Belani A, et al. Three-year experience with sonicated vascular catheter cultures in a clinical microbiology laboratory. *J Clin Microbiol*. 1990;28:76-82.

45. CDC. Guidelines for the prevention of intravascular catheter-related infections. *MMWR*. 2002;51:1-31.

46. National Committee for Clinical Laboratory Standards Web site at http://www.nccls.org.

47. Brachman PS. Nosocomial infections surveillance. *Infect Control Hosp Epidemiol*. 1993;14:194-196.

48. Rothman KJ, Greenland S. Precision and validity in epidemiologic studies. In: Rothman KJ, Greenland S, eds. *Modern Epidemiology*. 2nd ed. Philadelphia: Lippincott-Raven; 1998:115-134.

49. Wenzel RP, Edmond MB. The evolving technology of venous access. *N Engl J Med*. 1999;340:48-50.

50. Eggiman P, Pittet D. Overview of catheter-related infections with special emphasis on prevention based on educational programs. *Clin Microbiol Infect*. 2002;8:295-309.

51. Sherertz RJ, Wesley E, Westbrokk DM, et al. Education of physicians-in-training can decrease the risk for vascular catheter infection. *Ann Intern Med*. 2000;132:641-648.

CHAPTER TEN

OUTBREAK INVESTIGATIONS

Consuelo Beck-Sague, MD; Victor Soto-Caceres, MD, MPH; and William R. Jarvis, MD

INTRODUCTION

Epidemics or outbreaks of nosocomial infections are defined as hospital- or healthcare facility (HCF)-acquired infections among patients or staff members that represent an increase in incidence over expected rates. Epidemic-associated infections are often clustered temporally or geographically, suggesting that the infections are from a common source or are secondary to person-to-person transmission and are associated with specific procedures or devices. Although epidemic HCF-acquired infections occur infrequently, in some settings, such as ICUs, they account for a substantial percentage of hospital-acquired infections.[1] It has been estimated in the NNIS System that approximately 5% of nosocomial infections occurred as part of epidemics.[2]

Many factors have contributed in the past decade to increasing the proportion of nosocomial epidemics that may be recognized as outbreaks. Among them is the increasing availability of laboratory assays that can establish relatedness of patient isolates, as documented in Chapter 14 and elsewhere.[3-5] Even pathogens frequently causing endemic infections may be identified as likely to be transmitted as part of an outbreak if their relatedness is established based on currently available molecular typing methods. However, other factors, particularly increasing regulation related to privacy of patient information and vulnerability of HCFs to scrutiny or legal liability, may have resulted in a decline in recognition or reporting of nosocomial epidemics.[6] Moreover, declining hospitalization rates and shorter durations of hospitalizations may reduce the likelihood of nosocomial epidemic transmission and/or recognition of epidemics.[7] The declining numbers of hospitalizations among people with human immunodeficiency virus (HIV) may also play a role because such patients are particularly vulnerable to nosocomial infection and were over-represented among case-patients in *M. tuberculosis* epidemics in the early 1990s.[8-11] The widespread adoption of effective strategies to reduce the risk of nosocomial *M. tuberculosis* transmission,[11-13] and of other effective nosocomial infection prevention practices,[14] may have played a role as well. In addition, more healthcare is being provided in nonhospital settings (eg, ambulatory outpatient day surgery) where little or no nosocomial infection surveillance is conducted.

The investigation of epidemics of HCF-acquired infections continues to play a critical role in the identification of new agents, reservoirs, and modes of transmission. It is worth noting that the understanding of modes of transmission of emerging infectious diseases, particularly multidrug-resistant (MDR) tuberculosis, SARS, HIV, and hepatitis C infections during the 1990s and early years of the new millennium, was greatly advanced by investigation of HCF-acquired epidemic transmission.[11,15-17] As such, the recognition and effective investigation of epidemic transmission in the healthcare settings is among the most important activities of infection control.

RECOGNIZING OUTBREAKS

Hospitals need reliable, sensitive, surveillance systems that allow infection control personnel to detect increased infection rates in a defined time period and geographic area, suggestive of epidemic transmission. Although recognition of outbreaks often is believed to be among the major functions of surveillance, many outbreaks are recognized not as a part of routine surveillance, but because of the occurrence of sentinel events. In most of those incidents, even one episode of an uncommon or newly recognized pathogen, such as HCF-acquired SARS or SSIs caused by group A streptococcus or *Rhodococcus*

TABLE 10-1. IDENTIFIED CAUSES OF VARIOUS TYPES OF NOSOCOMIAL OUTBREAKS, CDC, 1990 TO 2003

Outbreak	Cause
Group A streptococcal surgical site infection	Colonized HCW disseminator
Tuberculosis, including multidrug-resistant	Exposure of immunosuppressed patients to infectious tuberculosis patients in absence of adequate source or engineering controls
SARS	Hospitalization of people with symptoms, workers SARS before enhanced respiratory precautions for patients and contacts were known to be necessary and implemented
Bloodstream infection with gram-negative organisms in patients with prescribed narcotics	Use of injected narcotics by substance-dependent HCWs, with contamination
Bloodstream infections in patients receiving medications from single- or multiple solutions; sharing of	Multiple use of single-use containers with preservative-free solutions; sharing of multiple dose containers among patients
Pyrogenic reactions in newborns prescribed single-dose gentamicin	High pyrogen levels in injectable gentamicin
Multi-state outbreaks of one organism	Intrinsic contamination
Outbreaks of postoperative infections, different	Extrinsic contamination of lipid-based medications microorganisms after introduction of medications such as propofol, which support rapid bacterial growth
Bacteremia, pyrogenic reactions, in hemo-dialysis patients	Dialysis machine waste handling options; poor water quality; reprocessing of dialyzers without prior hand antisepsis, glove change
Blood borne pathogen nosocomial epidemics	Multiple dose vials, syringes, used for more than 1 patient

Adapted from references 16 to 36.

bronchialis, can indicate epidemic nosocomial transmission.[15,18,19] In other instances, an increased incidence of HCF-acquired infections caused by unusual organisms, such as *Mycobacterium chelonae,* unusual strains of more common organisms, or in hosts where they are seldom diagnosed, may indicate epidemic transmission (Table 10-1).[16-36] During the late 1990s, several vehicles, organisms, and common sources that had been very problematic declined (eg, MDR-tuberculosis in people with HIV infection), and other hitherto unrecognized pathogens emerged. Some, such as *Candida* spp. bloodstream infections, continue to contribute to HCF-acquired epidemic infection.[32] Finally, after a long period of declining importance, some pathogens may be re-emerging, notably gram-negative bloodstream infection in newborns.[34,35]

Even if pathogens or anatomic sites are not unusual, an increased proportion of patients with infections in specific hospital units may indicate epidemic transmission. This is true particularly of units caring for highly vulnerable patients such as ICUs, units for HIV-infected patients, and organ transplant or hemodialysis units. Similarly, temporal increases in infection rates over well-established baseline rates often result from epidemic spread.

Some procedures, vehicles, and technical errors repeatedly are associated with HCF outbreaks (see Table 10-1). Infection control personnel will be able to investigate outbreaks more efficiently if they are aware of these associations. For example, substance-dependent personnel have been implicated in several bloodstream infection epidemics in which the use of a narcotic is identified as a risk factor. In these outbreaks, the dilution of the narcotic with water to replace the volume taken by the substance-dependent staff member appears to have been the route of introduction of gram-negative "water" organisms to the patients. When investigating outbreaks of gram-negative bloodstream infections in patients who are being prescribed narcotics, the investigation should include attempts to determine whether receipt of narcotics and

---

TABLE 10-2. STEPS IN OUTBREAK INVESTIGATIONS

Preliminary Investigation and Descriptive Study

➤ Review existing information
➤ Determine the nature, location, and severity of the disease problem
➤ Verify the diagnoses
➤ Create a case definition
➤ Find and ascertain case patients
➤ Request that the laboratory save isolates from affected patients and any suspected sources or vehicles
➤ Graph an epidemic curve
➤ Summarize case-patient data in a line listing
➤ Establish the existence of an outbreak
➤ Institute or assess adequacy of emergency control measures

Comparative Study and Definitive Investigations

➤ Review records of existing case patients
➤ Develop hypotheses
➤ Conduct comparative studies (case-control or cohort) to test hypotheses
➤ Conduct microbiologic or other laboratory studies and surveys
➤ Conduct observational studies, including interviews and questionnaire surveys
➤ Conduct experiments to confirm the mode of transmission

Acting on results

➤ Communicate results of investigation to administration and involved departments (as well as any necessary regulatory bodies), along with a plan for definitive control measures
➤ Implement definitive control measures
➤ Maintain surveillance for a sufficient time period to ensure that control measures are effective

---

specific personnel are associated with bloodstream infection. Likewise, improperly reprocessed hemodialyzers, inadequately processed water used to admix dialysate, or inadequacy of waste handling options have caused epidemics in hemodialysis units. Thus, infection control personnel should review procedures for reprocessing hemodialyzers and water treatment, as appropriate, early in the management of dialysis-related outbreaks.

INVESTIGATING OUTBREAKS

The First Steps

Once the infection control team suspects an outbreak, it should take steps to confirm whether it is actually occurring (Table 10-2). Both the possibility of an outbreak of true infections or of pseudo-infections should be evaluated. Obviously, an increase in the incidence of a serious or rare type of infection should be investigated even if it only approaches, but does not achieve, statistical significance. Infection control personnel should review some or all medical records from putative "case patients" to pro-

vide the basis for a preliminary case definition. A case definition states who (person) had the symptoms or findings, delineates a finite time period (time) during which the symptoms began or were recognized, and specifies the location (place) in which transmission occurred. A case definition may be based on clinical, laboratory, radiologic, pathologic, or other data, and the definition may change, becoming broader or more specific, as additional information becomes available. The following statement is an example of a case definition: "A case of *R. bronchialis* SSI is defined as a Hospital A patient with a surgical site culture positive for *R. bronchialis* who had undergone open heart surgery between May 1 and December 31, 1993."[19]

A variety of computer programs can provide invaluable assistance in investigating outbreaks (see Chapter 15). Epi Info (Centers for Disease Control and Prevention, Atlanta, Ga) is one such software package that allows public health and other staff to collect and analyze data generated in their epidemiologic investigation.[37] It is available for Microsoft Windows (an older version is available for MS-DOS). The program, which can be downloaded at no cost from the CDC Web site (http://www.cdc.gov/epiinfo/), enables the investigator to:

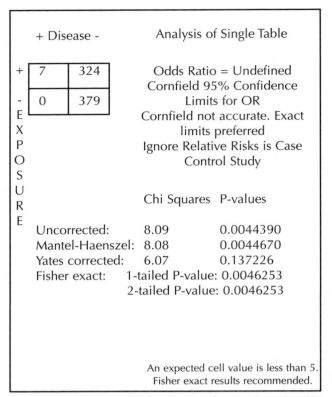

+ Disease -		Analysis of Single Table
+	7	324
-	0	379

Odds Ratio = Undefined
Cornfield 95% Confidence
Limits for OR
Cornfield not accurate. Exact
limits preferred
Ignore Relative Risks is Case
Control Study

Chi Squares	P-values
Uncorrected:	8.09	0.0044390
Mantel-Haenszel:	8.08	0.0044670
Yates corrected:	6.07	0.137226
Fisher exact:	1-tailed P-value: 0.0046253
	2-tailed P-value: 0.0046253

An expected cell value is less than 5.
Fisher exact results recommended.

Figure 10-1. Using the "Statcalc" option in Epi Info Utilities, the numbers of *R. bronchialis* infections[7] after open heart surgery procedures performed during the epidemic period (N = 331) were compared to the number of *R. bronchialis* infections during the 12 months preceding the epidemic period (0/379) to determine whether the increase in the number of *R. bronchialis* infections was statistically significant. The difference between the pre- and epidemic periods' rates was significant (Fisher's exact 2-tailed p = 0.0046).[19,37]

➤ Quickly determine, using summary data, whether an increase in a HCF-acquired infection rate, or a difference in risk between 2 groups, is statistically significant (Figure 10-1).

➤ Develop questionnaires.

➤ Enter data for descriptive and comparative investigations easily.

➤ Calculate odds ratios or relative risks, 95% confidence intervals, χ^2 (chi square), and p-values (for a more detailed discussion of choosing statistical tests, see Chapter 5).

It contains modules for training public health staff, including infection control personnel, on how to use Epi

Info to investigate epidemics. A training module for the *R. bronchialis* SSI epidemic investigation used as an example in this chapter is found in Epi Info's main screen Help file, titled "Rhodococcus."

Once an outbreak is suspected, potential sources or vehicles should be promptly removed from clinical areas to prevent HCWs from using (and possibly causing additional cases) or discarding these items (and preventing their confirmation as a source). Because impressions and recollections change rapidly during times of stress, infection control personnel should interview staff and review procedures immediately after they recognize a potential epidemic. Interviews should be conducted in a neutral and supportive manner, respecting staff members' and patients' rights to privacy. It is natural for staff to be defensive and wary of investigations that may be seen as attempts to "blame" them for an outbreak. Techniques that are seen clearly as fact-finding and guarantee confidentiality obviously are far more effective than interviews that appear to target specific tasks or staff members. Particularly effective strategies at this stage include questionnaire surveys that include all staff members using open-ended questions administered face-to-face by a neutral party.

Infection control personnel should request that the clinical laboratories save all isolates and/or other relevant specimens from patients possibly related to the outbreak. Infection control personnel can identify additional case-patients by searching in a variety of sources for people who meet the case definition, including records from infection control, microbiology, pathology, radiology, surgery, and pharmacy departments. After identifying all suspected case-patients, infection control personnel can chart an epidemic curve and calculate rates of infection during the pre-outbreak and outbreak periods. The shape of the epidemic curve may suggest the possible source and mode of transmission of the etiologic agent(s) (Figure 10-2). Comparison of rates during the outbreak and pre-outbreak periods will determine whether the observed rate increase is unlikely to be due to chance (see Figure 10-1).

If the observed infections suggest an epidemic, infection control personnel should review the medical records of patients identified as case-patients to produce a line-listing. The line-listing enumerates all affected patients and displays characteristics of the patients that may be important to the investigation (Table 10-3). The line-listing is used to characterize the outbreak, assess its extent, and generate hypotheses. In the *R. bronchialis* outbreak, the line-listing was helpful in generating hypotheses that could be tested quickly in a comparative epidemiologic study.[19] All patients who met the case-definition were men; surgeon A (MD-A) and circulating nurse A (CN-A) were involved in all of their surgical procedures, which were all CABGs. Among the hypotheses tested were that perhaps procedures to clip or shave chest hair (a procedure performed preferentially on men) could be implicat-

TABLE 10-3. LINE LISTING OF CHARACTERISTICS OF CASE PATIENTS IN THE *R. BRONCHIALIS* SURGICAL SITE INFECTIONS INVESTIGATION, USING THE EPI INFO 2002 COMMAND "LIST"[a]

Line	Age	Sex	Smoking	CABG	DrA	DrB	CN-A	CNB
1	66	M	Yes	Yes	Yes	Yes	Yes	No
2	60	M	Yes	Yes	Yes	No	Yes	No
3	53	M	Yes	Yes	Yes	Yes	Yes	Yes
4	56	M	Yes	Yes	Yes	Yes	Yes	Yes
5	65	M	No	Yes	Yes	Yes	Yes	Yes
6	57	M	No	Yes	Yes	No	Yes	No
7	55	M	No	Yes	Yes	No	Yes	No

[a] This line-listing shows that all case-patients were men between the ages of 53 and 66 years, all had CABGs, and in all cases, Dr. A and circulating nurse A (CN-A) participated in the procedure.[19,37]

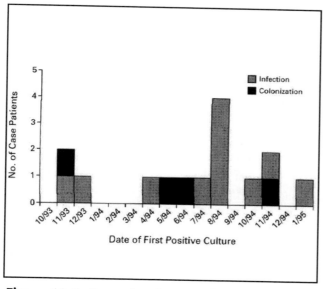

Figure 10-2. Example of an epidemic curve of a nosocomial outbreak: distribution of case-patients according to the date of the first positive culture for *Mycobacterium pachydermatis,* during the period from October 1993 through January 1995.[36]

ed. Of course, the possibilities that MD-A or CN-A were involved were also selected to be tested. The infection control staff also should review relevant policies and procedures and verify compliance or noncompliance. In addition, the infection control staff should review the literature to identify the source(s) and mode(s) of transmission in similar outbreaks. On the basis of all available data, infection control personnel should develop hypotheses to explain how the epidemic developed. Then, they can plan how to design a study to confirm or discard hypotheses, and they can use these data to plan rational control measures.

These steps should be taken in an atmosphere of rational, calm, systematic, and deliberate action. Systematic and transparent action can avert an atmosphere of fear and can result in effective outbreak investigations. If staff members panic, they may discard vital materials inadvertently, introduce various procedural changes, or disinfect possible reservoirs before appropriate samples are obtained. Interventions that are not chosen on a rational basis may impair or impede the investigation.

Emergency Measures

If infection control personnel confirm that an epidemic is occurring, they must decide immediately whether to:
➤ Conduct a full epidemiologic study.
➤ Obtain cultures from equipment or suspected vehicles, ideally, after epidemiologic data suggest them as a source.
➤ Call local, state, and federal agencies or a private consultant for assistance.
➤ Institute emergency control measures.

When making these decisions, infection control personnel should consider the following factors:
➤ The severity of illness, including mortality, associated with the epidemic.
➤ The public health importance of the outbreak and implications of restricting access to essential clinical services.
➤ The frequency of infection versus colonization.

➤ The possibility of a common source.

➤ The size of the outbreak.

➤ The characteristics of the pathogen.

➤ Local and state regulations that may require HCF personnel to report epidemics.

HCF personnel should identify a spokesperson who will update appropriate internal (eg, staff or patients) and external (eg, regulatory and advisory governmental agencies) constituencies regularly. The spokesperson(s) should present enough data to ensure these parties that HCF personnel are investigating the problem thoroughly and carefully. However, the spokesperson should not prematurely divulge the potential hypotheses being tested or offer premature reassurances or predictions that may under- or over-estimate the threat of the suspected epidemic. The credibility and effectiveness of spokespeople are ensured by frank explanations of the process that is being undertaken to explore the event and admission that the source of the epidemic is, at the time, unclear. Conversely, confidence and credibility are likely to be irretrievably lost by premature assertions that the cause of the epidemic has been identified or that it is under control.

Closing the Ward

The infection control staff must weigh carefully the benefit of closing a ward or unit against the risk of decreased access to care. There are no laws or regulations dictating when a ward should be closed. In general, a HCF should close wards only for conditions that cause high mortality or permanent disability, that had a clear onset, and that continue despite implementation of infection control precautions. Before deciding to close the ward or to discontinue surgery or specific procedures, the infection control staff should determine what criteria must be met before the suspended activities may be resumed.

Reporting Outbreaks

State and federal laws require that HCF personnel notify public health authorities of certain conditions. Infection control personnel should consult their state's laws. However, at a minimum, infection control programs should report to the county and state health departments all outbreaks that have potential public health implications at the state or national level. These, of course, include epidemic transmission of emerging diseases, such as SARS, *S. aureus* with intermediate or high resistance to vancomycin, etc. Outbreaks that may be the result of criminal, including terrorist, activity such as those related to illicit narcotic tampering also should be reported. In addition, infection control personnel should report suspected intrinsic contamination of sterile products, fatal blood transfusion reactions, infections caused by contaminated blood products, and infections associated with defective devices to the Division of Healthcare Quality,

CDC at (404) 498-1250 or (800) 893-0485, and the FDA's MED WATCH Program at (800) FDA-1088.

In many HCFs, infection control staff struggle with concerns regarding the protection of the privacy of living case-patients, their families, and healthcare staff. Occasionally, personnel may be contributing to epidemic transmission. As described in Chapter 25, a HCF culture that focuses on systemic changes to protect patients and HCF staff is clearly preferable to one that appears to focus primarily on blame. HCF personnel may also be concerned about the medico-legal implications of admitting that an epidemic may be occurring in their hospital. Hospitals that report outbreaks to state and national agencies often find that they benefit by receiving help as they evaluate and control the problem. Moreover, federal agencies, such as CDC, are bound by regulations to protect the privacy of patients. The CDC receives numerous calls each day from infection control personnel who request either advice on managing outbreaks or on-site assistance.

Conducting an Epidemiologic Study

Reviewing the Line-Listing

Before conducting a comprehensive epidemiologic study, infection control personnel should review the line-listing (see Table 10-3) and the epidemic curve (see Figure 10-2) because these tools may suggest the cause of the outbreak. This is true particularly if the problem is an acute, self-limited, one-time incident, such as those associated with a recognized or suspected contamination.

Comparative Studies

Infection control personnel usually must review the patients' medical records to determine which exposures might be important. Hospitalized patients usually do not know or recall details essential to the investigation. Moreover, patients may be too ill to answer questions. Infection control personnel may learn important information from short, open-ended interviews with patients. In general, the medical and laboratory records and other documents provide the most information (Table 10-4). Infection control personnel should design a standardized form on which to collect demographic data, information about exposures, and other data regarding the study subjects. The form ensures that personnel will collect data uniformly and that they will not need to review records repeatedly to find missed items.

A putative risk factor can be confirmed only if it meets certain criteria. First, the risk factor must have been present before the onset of the disease. Second, the risk factor will generally be associated with the condition statistically (ie, case patients will be significantly more likely to have the risk factor than other patients). To confirm the latter point, infection control staff must perform a comparative study, usually either a case-control study or a cohort study. The relative advantages and disadvantages of these study

TABLE 10-4. SOURCES OF INFORMATION

Log books
  Operating or delivery room
  Emergency department
  Nursing unit
  Intensive care unit (census, or admission, discharge
    log books)
  Procedure room
Microbiology record
Employee health records
Infection control surveillance data
Patient medical records
Operative notes
Pathology reports
Microbiology, other laboratory reports
Radiology procedure notes and records
Pharmacy records
Hospital billing records
Central-service records
Purchasing records

designs are described in detail in Chapter 5. Case-control studies are typically faster to conduct than cohort studies.[38,39] They may more rapidly and easily produce the important information (ie, what factors were statistically associated with becoming a case) than cohort studies.

Infection control staff should consider several factors, including what resources are available, before they decide to conduct a comparative study. Ongoing outbreaks generally deserve to be evaluated by a comparative study. This is true particularly of outbreaks associated with high mortality or severe disease that might be caused by a new or unusual agent, those potentially caused by a new or unusual agent, or outbreaks in which reservoirs or modes of transmission may be detected. Because epidemics of pseudo-infections or other nonfatal conditions may also affect patient care negatively, infection control personnel may also need to evaluate such clusters with comparative studies.

Each variable that is evaluated as a possible risk factor will increase the time and expense required for the outbreak investigation. Furthermore, each additional variable increases the likelihood that a characteristic entirely unrelated to the outbreak will appear to be a risk factor (ie, statistically significant by chance alone). To avoid these pitfalls, infection control personnel should include few, if any, characteristics that are not plausible risk factors. Obviously, a narrow interpretation of biologic plausibility may inappropriately restrict investigation to only previously suspected or confirmed risk factors. Such inappropriate restriction may be avoided by ensuring during the early phase of the studies (particularly the design of the line-listing) that a careful review of cases casts a very wide "net" for hypothesis generation, but that the data collection and analysis for the comparative study be more limited.

For example, in the *R. bronchialis* epidemic, it was noted during the line-listing that smoking was only reported by four case-patients (see Table 10-3.) The likelihood that smoking was associated with a statistically significant increased risk of being a case was thus low. The biological plausibility of a protective role for cigarette smoking also was extremely doubtful. As such, it was appropriate to not pursue this variable. Similarly, infection control staff would be wise to avoid investigating characteristics that would be "interesting" but are unlikely, according to the literature, the line listing, and expert advice, to be related to the outbreak.

Infection control personnel should consider carefully whether or not to perform a matched study. It should be remembered that variables on which case patients and controls are matched cannot be evaluated as potential risk factors.[38] Furthermore, matching may make controls and case patients so similar that the investigators would miss all but the most obvious risk factors. Matching is very useful when numerous characteristics are associated with the epidemic condition but are not the real cause(s) ("confounders"). These confounders can obscure the real causative factors.

Many investigators choose not to match, but to control for confounding variables by either stratifying the analysis by possible confounders or by using multivariate analysis. Matching may be useful in selected investigations where a considerable amount of risk is experienced by a specific subpopulation. Another alternative to matching is to restrict analysis to the subpopulation at highest risk, if only patients in this risk category appeared to be among the cases (for example, infants with birth weights less than 1300 grams).[36] The analysis of a study that is designed as a matched study has to be conducted in a matched fashion.[38]

In small outbreaks or clusters, the causative factor may not achieve statistical significance. If the power of the study is low, infection control personnel should explore any factor with an odds ratio or relative risk that suggests an association, even if the difference between cases and controls only approaches, but does not achieve, statistical significance. Aside from identifying an implicated procedure, product, or staff member, analysis of epidemiologic data can help determine which of a variety of modes of transmission is most likely. For example, the finding that the length of time that a surgical wound is open does not differ significantly between cases and controls suggests that the organism is not being disseminated by being suspended in the air; conversely, a strong, statistically significant association with a staff member in an analysis of a small outbreak is extremely compelling (Table 10-5).[19] This may be of great importance in not abandoning pre-

TABLE 10-5. EXAMPLE ANALYSIS FROM THE CASE CONTROL STUDY DATA FOR THE *R. BRONCHIALIS* SURGICAL SITE INFECTIONS EPIDEMIC[19,37] a

1)

		Obs	Total	Mean	Variance	Std Dev	p-value
	Cases	7	1785.00	255.00	4214.67	64.92	0.84
	Controls	28	7381.00	263.61	9886.10	99.43	

2)

		Case		Total
CN-A		Yes	No	
Yes		7	6	13
No		0	22	22
Total		7	28	35

Fisher Exact Test <0.001

a (1) shows that the median duration of the procedures in cases did not differ significantly from that of controls, suggesting that airborne transmission of suspended microorganisms did not play a major role. However, two cases were significantly more likely to have had circulating nurse A (CN-A) in the procedure.

maturely the search for other modes of transmission once an epidemiologically implicated staff member is shown to be colonized with the epidemic strain of an organism and to be able to aerosolize it.

Clinical Observations

Infection control personnel should observe HCWs perform procedures, particularly patient care techniques that might be related to the outbreak. Observational studies help infection control staff generate hypotheses regarding the origin of the outbreak and confirm comparative study findings. For example, if an epidemiologic study suggests that a vehicle is associated with the epidemic, an observational study allows infection control personnel to determine how the etiologic agent was transmitted from the contaminated source. Infection control staff should also review written protocols, interview supervisory staff, and identify procedural changes implemented before, during, or after the epidemic. Infection control personnel should observe procedures that are implicated and question personnel who perform these techniques directly. Infection control staff may obtain valuable information by observing different personnel on the same and different shifts as they perform procedures. In the *Rhodococcus* epidemic, a particularly striking finding was that CN-A's hands would become wet during the clotting time procedure.[19] Semi-structured interviews with similar questions posed to all staff members may be effective in identifying procedures that are being undertaken in different ways by specific staff members.

Culture Surveys

Experts disagree about the value of obtaining cultures from staff and the environment as a means of identifying the source of an outbreak. Organisms that cause nosocomial outbreaks (eg, gram-negative water organisms; fungi, including *Aspergillus* species; and gram-positive cocci, including *S. aureus*) can be isolated frequently from nonsterile environmental sources or from the staff. However, in our experience, culture survey results are only rarely helpful in the absence of epidemiologic data linking these sources to the outbreak. In fact, random culture surveys may increase the cost of an investigation substantially and may fail to identify the source, or may implicate the wrong source.

For example, some staff may become transiently colonized with the epidemic strain after working with infected or colonized patients but may not transmit the organism to other patients. Thus, infection control personnel generally should obtain cultures from staff members who are linked epidemiologically to the epidemic and should compare results to those staff who are not implicated instead of using the culture results to determine who is linked to the epidemic. CN-As' hands were only culture-positive for the outbreak strain of *R. bronchialis* when they were wet; a culture survey of HCWs' hands without the epidemiologic and observational study data would probably have missed her link to the epidemic.[19] Likewise, we recommend that infection control personnel obtain cultures only from environmental sources implicated by epidemiologic data and observational studies. Culture surveys of nonsterile areas (eg, floors, sinks, walls) that do not have plausible connections to the outbreak waste valuable resources and frequently yield uninterpretable data because there are no standard limits or acceptable levels of contamination of HCF floors, walls, or nonsterile equipment.

Conversely, infection control personnel should not abandon their hypothesis if cultures do not recover the organism from a source or reservoir that was implicated strongly in the epidemiologic study. For example, only a small proportion of the individual units of an intrinsically contaminated commercially prepared medication may be contaminated. Similarly, individuals who disseminate the epidemic strain may shed the organism only intermittently (for example, when their hands are wet),[19] may be colonized intermittently (ie, when they have a viral respiratory infection), or may be colonized in an unusual site (eg, the rectum or scalp,[18] but not the hands). Thus, infection control personnel should never use negative cultures alone to vindicate a source that was identified by a well-designed epidemiologic study.

In contrast, the isolation of the outbreak organism in a potential vehicle or disseminator implicated in the epidemiologic study and not in other sources or staff members is a very compelling finding, suggesting that an implicated source is, in fact, causing the outbreak. In the *R. bronchialis* sternal wound infection epidemic investigation, the isolation of the epidemic strain from CN-A's hands only when they were wet, in conjunction with the finding during observational studies using bile esculin that her technique for warming blood specimens in the water bath was associated with contamination of sterile surgical instruments with water micro-droplets, strongly supported the hypothesis that she was implicated in the *R. bronchialis* sternal wound infection outbreak.[19] Techniques for obtaining cultures vary considerably by organism and source. Infection control personnel can save time and resources if they consult with a microbiologist before they collect specimens or consume a limited supply of the suspected vehicle. For example, settle plates or devices, such as the Anderson or Reyneirs air sampler, can help identify the source of some airborne infections.[18] In some outbreaks (eg, outbreaks associated with hemodialysis fluid), the laboratory may need to use special techniques for cultures of large volumes of fluid and review standards of water quality for hemodialysis.[40-42]

Demonstrating Biological Plausibility

Because many epidemics in hospitals are caused by hitherto unappreciated events, infection control personnel must prove conclusively that the event can happen. Thus, the investigators should design and conduct additional experimental studies based on the observational studies to confirm that the reservoir and the mode of transmission are biologically possible. The infection con-

trol staff should use data gathered from procedure reviews, staff interviews or questionnaires, and observational studies to generate a possible scenario for how the organism was transmitted. Then, the staff should simulate the implicated procedure to establish that the organism could be transmitted in the postulated manner. In the investigation of the *R. bronchialis* epidemic, the ingenious use of bile esculin in the water-bath showed how water micro-droplets from CN-A's wet hands contaminated the sterile equipment; these droplets, invisible to the naked eye, fluoresced brightly in the presence of ultraviolet light.[19] Infection control personnel can, and often should, simulate some procedures on-site, but may use in vitro laboratory studies to simulate others. Settle plates may confirm that a staff member's activities in an area can disseminate the organism.[18] In outbreaks of infections due to airborne pathogens, such as *M. tuberculosis* or *Aspergillus niger*, infection control personnel may need chemical smoke tubes to evaluate the direction of air flow.[11-13]

In many instances, infection control personnel will want to confirm that outbreak-associated isolates are identical to each other and to those recovered from the implicated source. Molecular typing is available and is widely used for evaluating relatedness of strains for a wide variety of organisms, including fungi, viruses, and bacteria (Figure 10-3, see also Chapter 14).[3-5,11,16-23,26,32]

ACTING ON RESULTS

Infection control personnel should focus their interventions on the immediate cause of an outbreak and should institute the simplest measures that will correct the problem. The more focused the control measures, the more feasible their implementation and the more likely HCWs will be to adhere to the measures. Infection control personnel should emphasize the specific measures required to stop the outbreak and also encourage staff to comply with routine procedures. Sometimes, during an investigation, infection control personnel will identify deficiencies other than those directly associated with the epidemic strain and may be tempted to use the epidemic as an opportunity to revamp the entire infection control program. This is often counterproductive, distracting staff from the implementation of essential programs and diluting their efforts and potential impact.

Infection control personnel should develop a plan and timeline for implementing the control measures. After implementing the control measures, the staff should continue to work closely with the staff in the affected area to ensure that they understand and efficiently implement the recommendations and that they continue to comply with the recommendations over time. Obviously, infection control personnel must determine whether the measures are effective and, ideally, assess whether the decline in num-

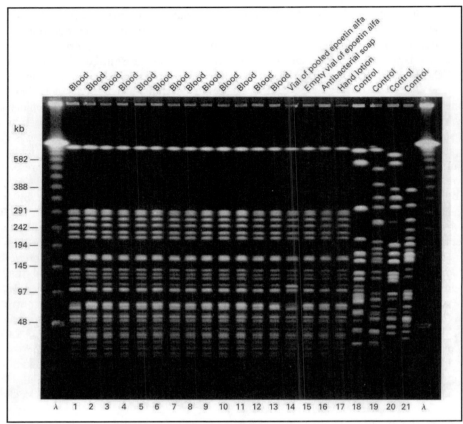

Figure 10-3. Pulsed-field gel electrophoresis of *Serratia liquefaciens* isolates in a bloodstream infection outbreak in which *S. liquefaciens* infection was epidemiologically linked with receipt of epoetin alfa in a hemodialysis center shows that isolates from case-patients, from full and empty vials of pooled epoetin alfa, antibacterial soap, and hand lotion in the center were identical, but that isolates from other centers in the state that were not associated with the outbreak were different from each other and from the outbreak strain.[23]

ber of cases of the epidemic condition was associated with implementation of one or more measures. Often, infection control personnel can prove that the interventions were effective by demonstrating that no new cases occurred after the control measures were implemented, even though patients continued to be at risk. If the pathogen causes endemic infections (eg, MRSA), the staff may need to conduct prospective surveillance cultures to ensure that the outbreak has ended.

CONCLUSION

Most nosocomial infections are endemic, and epidemics are relatively infrequent. However, in some settings, such as ICUs, outbreaks account for a substantial percentage of hospital-acquired infections. Outbreaks can cause substantial morbidity and mortality and can increase the cost of medical care significantly. Infection control personnel who identify outbreaks quickly and investigate them thoroughly and systematically using optimal epidemiologic and laboratory methods can improve medical care, advance medical knowledge, and ensure patient safety.

ACKNOWLEDGMENTS

This work was performed by Dr. Beck-Sague while she was an employee of the US government. Epi Info epidemiologic software and the tutorials in its help file are in the public domain. The graphics and photographs used in

Figures 10-1 through 10-3 and Tables 10-3 and 10-5 were based on work performed by Drs. C. Beck-Sague, H. Chang, A. Dean, L. Grohskopf, W. Jarvis, and H. Richet while they were US government employees. As such, there is no copyright on these graphics and photographs.

REFERENCES

1. Wenzel RP, Thompson RL, Landry SM, et al. Hospital-acquired infections in intensive care unit patients: an overview with emphasis on epidemics. *Infect Control.* 1983;1:371-375.

2. Doebbeling BN. Epidemics: identification and management. In: Wenzel RP, ed. *Prevention and Control of Nosocomial Infections.* 2nd ed. Baltimore, Md: Williams & Wilkins; 1992:177-206.

3. Jarvis WR. Usefulness of molecular epidemiology for outbreak investigation. *Infect Control Hosp Epidemiol.* 1995;16:63.

4. Grundmann H, Schneider C, Daschner FD. Fluorescence-based DNA fingerprinting elucidates nosocomial transmission of phenotypically variable *Pseudomonas aeruginosa* in intensive care units. *European J Clin Microbiol Infect Dis.* 1995;14:1057-1062.

5. Iovo J, Mateo E, Munoz A, Urquijo M, On SL, Fernandez-Astorga A. Molecular typing of *Campylobacter jejuni* isolates involved in a neonatal outbreak indicates nosocomial transmission. *J Clin Microbio.* 200;41:3926-3928.

6. Vermund SH, Fawal H. Emerging infectious diseases and professional integrity: thoughts for the new millennium. *AJIC.* 1999;27:497-499.

7. Popovic JR, Hall MJ. 1999 National Hospital Discharge Survey. Advance Data No. 319. 18 pp. (PHS) 2001-1250.

8. Fleishman JA, Hellinger FH. Recent trends in HIV-related inpatient admissions 1996-2000: a 7-state study. *JAIDS.* 2003;34(1):102-110.

9. Floris-Moore M, Lo Y, Klein RS, et al. Gender and hospitalization patterns among HIV-infected drug users before and after the availability of highly active antiretroviral therapy. *JAIDS.* 2003;34:331-337.

10. Pulvirenti JJ, Gerding DN, Nathan C, et al. Difference in the incidence of *Clostridium difficile* among patients infected with human immunodeficiency virus admitted to a public hospital and a private hospital. *Infect Control Hosp Epidemiol.* 2002;23:641-647.

11. Jarvis WR. Nosocomial transmission of multidrug-resistant *Mycobacterium tuberculosis.* *AJIC.* 1995;23:146-151.

12. Maloney SA, Pearson ML, Gordon MT, Del Castillo R, Boyle JF, Jarvis WR. Efficacy of control measures in preventing nosocomial transmission of multidrug-resistant tuberculosis to patients and health care workers. *Ann Intern Med.* 1995;122:90-95.

13. Manangan LP, Bennett CL, Tablan N, et al. Nosocomial tuberculosis prevention measures among two groups of US hospitals, 1992 to 1996. *Chest.* 2000;117:380-384.

14. Manangan LP, Banerjee SN, Jarvis WR. Association between implementation of CDC recommendations and ventilator-associated pneumonia at selected US hospitals. *AJIC.* 2000;28:222-227.

15. Booth CM, Matukas LM, Tomlinson GA, et al. Clinical features and short-term outcomes of 144 patients with SARS in the greater Toronto area. *JAMA.* 2003;289:2801-2809.

16. El Sayed NM, Gomatos PJ, Beck-Sague CM, et al. Epidemic transmission of human immunodeficiency virus in renal dialysis centers in Egypt. *J Infect Dis.* 2000;181:91-97.

17. Krause G, Trepka MJ, Whisenhunt RS, et al. Nosocomial transmission of hepatitis C virus associated with the use of multidose saline vials. *Infect Control Hosp Epidemiol.* 2003;24:122-127.

18. Mastro TD, Farley TA, Elliott JA, et al. An outbreak of surgical-wound infections due to group A streptococcus carried on the scalp. *New Engl J Med.* 1990;323:968-972.

19. Richet HM, Craven PC, Brown JM, et al. A cluster of *Rhodococcus (Gordona) bronchialis* sternal-wound infections after coronary-artery bypass surgery. *New Engl J Med.* 1991;324:104-109.

20. Freitas D, Alvarenga L, Sampaio J, et al. An outbreak of *Mycobacterium chelonae* infection after LASIK. *Ophthalmology.* 2003;110(2):276-285.

21. Ostrowsky BE, Whitener C, Bredenberg HK, et al. *Serratia marcescens* bacteremia traced to an infused narcotic. *N Engl J Med.* 2002;346(20):1529-1537.

22. Maki DG, Klein BS, McCormick RD, et al. Nosocomial *Pseudomonas pickettii* bacteremias traced to narcotic tampering: a case for selective drug screening of health care personnel. *JAMA.* 1991;265:981-986.

23. Grohskopf LA, Roth VR, Feikin DR, et al. *Serratia liquefaciens* bloodstream infections from contamination of epoetin alfa at a hemodialysis center. *N Engl J Med.* 2001;344:1491-1497.

24. Buchholz U, Richards C, Murthy R, et al. Pyrogenic reactions associated with single daily dosing of intravenous gentamicin. *Infect Control Hospital Epidemiol.* 2000;2:771-774.

25. Duffy R, Tomashek K, Spangenberg M, et al. Multistate outbreak of hemolysis in hemodialysis patients traced to faulty blood tubing sets. *Kidney International.* 2000;57:1668-1674.

26. Wang SA, Tokars JI, Bianchine PJ, et al. Enterobacter cloacae bloodstream infections traced to contaminated human albumin. *Clin Infect Dis.* 2000;30:35-40.

27. Labarca JA, Trick WE, Peterson CL. A multistate nosocomial outbreak of *Ralstonia pickettii* colonization associated with an intrinsically contaminated respiratory care solution. *Clin Infect Dis.* 1999;29(5):1281-1286.

28. Wang SA, Levine RB, Carson LA, et al. An outbreak of gram-negative bacteremia in hemodialysis patients traced to hemodialysis machine waste drain ports. *Infect Control Hosp Epidemiol.* 1999;20:746-751.

29. Jochimsen EM, Frenette C, Delorme M, et al. A cluster of bloodstream infections and pyrogenic reactions among hemodialysis patients traced to dialysis machine waste-handling option units. *Am J Nephrol.* 1998;18:485-489.

30. Wenger PN, Brown JM, McNeil MM, Jarvis WR. *Nocardia farcinica* sternotomy site infections in patients following open heart surgery. *J Infect Dis.* 1998;178:1539-1543.

31. Mangram AJ, Archibald LK, Hupert M, et al. Outbreak of sterile peritonitis among continuous cycling peritoneal dialysis patients. *Kidney International.* 1998;54:1367-1371.

32. Welbel SF, McNeil MM, Kuykendall RJ, et al. *Candida parapsilosis* bloodstream infections in neonatal intensive care unit patients: epidemiologic and laboratory confirmation of a common source outbreak. *Ped Infect Dis J.* 1996;15:998-1002.

33. Saiman L, Ludington E, Dawson JD, et al. The National Epidemiology of Mycoses Study Group Risk factors for Candida species colonization of neonatal intensive care unit patients. *Ped Infect Dis J.* 2001;20:1119-1124.

34. Dent A, Toltzis P. Descriptive and molecular epidemiology of gram-negative bacilli infections in the neonatal intensive care unit. *Curr Opinion Infect Dis.* 2003;16:279-283.

35. Schuchat A, Zywicki SS, Dinsmoor MJ, et al. Risk factors and opportunities for prevention of early-onset neonatal sepsis: a multicenter case-control study. *Pediatrics.* 2000;105(1 Pt 1):21-26.

36. Chang HJ, Miller HL, Watkins N, et al. An epidemic of *Malassezia pachydermatis* in an intensive care nursery associated with colonization of health care workers' pet dogs. *New Engl J Med.* 1998;338:706-711.

37. Dean AG, Arner TG, Sangam S, et al. *Epi Info 2000, a database and statistics program for public health professionals for use on Windows 95,98, NT, and 2000 computers.* Atlanta, Ga: Centers for Disease Control and Prevention; 2000.

38. Rotham KJ. Types of epidemiologic study. In: Rotham KJ, ed. *Modern Epidemiology.* Boston, Mass: Little, Brown and Co; 1986:51-76.

39. Schlesselman JJ. *Case Control Studies.* New York, NY: Oxford University Press; 1982.

40. *American National Standard for Hemodialysis Systems.* Arlington, Va: Association for the Advancement of Medical Instrumentation; 1992. (ANSI/AAMI no. RD5-1992.).

41. Luehman DA, Keshaviah PR, Ward RA, Klein E. *A Manual on Water Treatment for Hemodialysis.* Rockville, MD: US Department of Health and Human Services; 1989:109-115.

42. Keshaviah PR. Pretreatment and preparation of city water for hemodialysis. In: Maher JF, ed. *Replacement of Renal Function by Dialysis: A Textbook of Dialysis.* 3rd ed. Dordrecht: Kluwer Academic Publishers; 1989:189-198.

CHAPTER ELEVEN

EXPOSURE WORKUPS

Loreen A. Herwaldt, MD; Jean M. Pottinger, RN, MA, CIC; and Stephanie Holley, RN, BSN, CIC

INTRODUCTION

It is 5:25 on Friday afternoon. Everyone else in the infection control program has gone home already, but you stayed late to organize your desk. You have just finished filing the last paper when the telephone rings. Thinking that the caller is your husband, you pick up the telephone and greet the caller eagerly. But the voice is not your husband's. It takes you a minute to realize that the caller is John Smith, the head nurse on the pediatric hematology and oncology inpatient unit. He is talking very rapidly about a child on his unit. When you get him to slow down, you learn that a 6-year-old patient, who has been in the hospital for 5 days, broke out with chicken pox this afternoon. This child has been in the playroom with numerous immunocompromised children. He also was in the waiting rooms of the pediatric clinic and the radiology department. To make matters worse, a nurse on the unit is 2-months' pregnant, and she is not sure whether she has had chicken pox.

You ask Mr. Smith to start making a list of all unit staff who worked during the time this patient has been hospitalized and to ask the HCWs whether they have had chicken pox. You tell him that you will come out to the unit in about 20 minutes, after you have had a chance to call radiology and several other departments whose staff might have been exposed. After hanging up the telephone, you sink back into your chair, groan, and berate yourself for not insisting that the hospital develop a computer database of the employees' immune status. You then pick up the telephone to call your husband and ask him to cancel your long-planned dinner reservations.

This fictional scenario actually comes close to the experience of many infection control staff who have practiced for any length of time. The scenario illustrates several axioms about exposures in the hospital. First, they always come at inconvenient times. There is no good time for an exposure even if it's not Friday. The corollary to this axiom is that exposure workups always interrupt other important infection control activities. The second axiom is that exposures usually involve more than one department and that at least one of the affected areas will be a large, open room in which many persons congregate who may be very difficult to identify. The third axiom is that exposures almost always involve the most vulnerable patients or HCWs. The corollary to this axiom is that exposures are guaranteed to cause great anxiety among patients and staff.

Infection control personnel define exposures as events in which persons were exposed to infectious microorganisms or ectoparasites. The goals of an exposure workup are to prevent disease, if possible, in the persons who were exposed to the agent, and to prevent further transmission if exposed persons become ill. To achieve this goal, infection control personnel must identify all patients, visitors, and staff members who might have been exposed and then determine whether these persons are susceptible or immune. If the exposed persons are immune to the etiologic agent, they do not require further investigations or interventions. If exposed persons are not immune to the etiologic agent or do not know their immune status, infection control personnel may need to obtain further data, prescribe prophylactic treatment, and institute work restrictions. In this chapter, we will describe exposure workups for a number of important pathogens.

Many nosocomial exposures do not cause secondary cases of infection, or, if secondary cases occur, they are often mild. However, on occasion, patients, visitors, or HCWs acquire infections that cause serious short- or long-term consequences, including prolonged absence from work, exposure to toxic treatments, incurable chronic illness, irreversible disability, or death.[1] Regardless of the ultimate consequences, exposure workups consume considerable time, money, and other resources.[2-4] Therefore, the infection control staff should strive to prevent exposures with the following measures:

➤ Implementing policies that reduce the number of susceptible persons exposed (eg, requiring all HCWs to be immune to measles, mumps, and rubella or requiring all clinics to screen patients for symptoms consistent with communicable diseases)

➤ Teaching HCWs to recognize when they should stay home to prevent the spread of infectious agents

➤ Teaching HCWs to apply standard and expanded precautions properly

Given the serious consequences that can result from exposures, HCFs must manage exposures in a systematic and consistent manner. Many HCFs assign this responsibility to infection control personnel. In this chapter, we have described the steps in exposure investigations.

We have summarized our recommendations in a generic algorithm for working up exposures (Figure 11-1) and in a table (Table 11-1, p. 127). When developing the recommendations in this chapter we used the *2000 Red Book*,[5] *Control of Communicable Diseases Manual*,[6] the guidelines published by the HICPAC[7] and the APIC,[8] the Web sites created by the CDC and the World Health Organization (WHO), other published studies, and our own experience. We also consulted *Principles and Practice of Infectious Diseases*.[9] Infection control personnel who prefer the recommendations published in other references will need to modify our recommendations to suit their needs. We excluded bloodborne pathogens from this discussion and we included only the agents that cause most exposures in hospitals. Hospitals vary; thus, some facilities may have numerous exposures to agents that we have not discussed. In addition, new agents, such as the coronavirus that caused SARS and monkeypox virus, can and will continue to afflict hospitals. Therefore, infection control personnel need to know what is happening in their communities and around the world. One way infection control personnel can keep abreast of what is happening is to join list serves such as the Emerging Infections Network sponsored by the Infectious Diseases Society of America. In addition, some state or local health departments inform infection control personnel of important developments through emails or faxes.

GENERAL RECOMMENDATIONS REGARDING EXPOSURE WORKUPS

Obtain Mandate From the Administration

If the hospital administration assigns the responsibility for doing exposure workups to the infection control program, the administrators also must define the scope of that responsibility and delegate the authority for the associated activities to staff in the infection control program. The hospital administration must prospectively define what tests and prophylactic treatments the hospital will provide. In addition, the hospital administration must specify if exposed HCWs will be granted administrative leave, leave with pay, leave without pay, or if they will be allowed to work in nonpatient-care areas during the period in which they might be infectious.[10,11]

Develop Policies and Procedures

Once the infection control program has been given the authority to do exposure workups, the staff must develop specific policies that define exposures to various bacterial and viral pathogens and to ectoparasites and describe the investigative and preventive measures that should be undertaken for exposures caused by each agent. The staff also should develop general policies and procedures that define what tasks should be undertaken and who will do them.

Collaborate With Employee Health

In many institutions, the infection control staff members initiate the exposure workup and recommend the prophylaxis and work restrictions for exposed HCWs. However, staff members in the employee health service actually evaluate whether the employee was exposed and susceptible, examine the HCW, enforce work restrictions, and give permission for HCWs to return to work. Thus, as they develop policies and procedures, infection control personnel must collaborate extensively with the employee health staff.

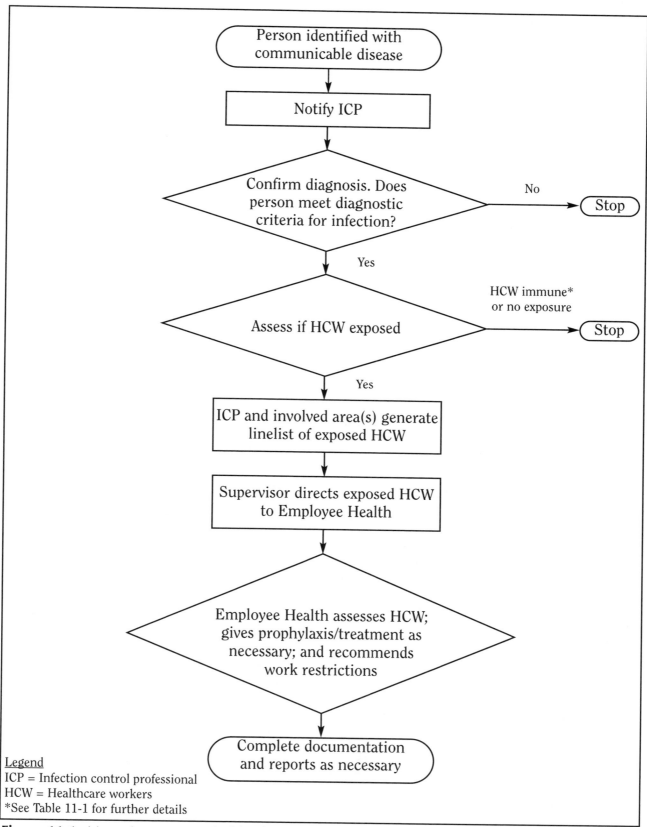

Figure 11-1. Managing communicable disease exposures at the University of Iowa Hospitals and Clinics.

Develop a Database on the Immune Status of Healthcare Workers

Infection control personnel will save countless hours if they have a database in which they store information on the immune status of all HCWs. The most important data are the employee's immune status to chicken pox, measles, mumps, rubella, and hepatitis B. However, some hospitals might find it useful to test employees for antibody to parvovirus B19 if they work in antipartum clinics or with patients who are immunocompromised or have hemolytic anemias. The employee's tuberculosis skin-test results and the results of respirator fit testing should be recorded in the database. The database also could store information on the employee's immunity to diphtheria, tetanus, and hepatitis A. Baseline data should be obtained from all new HCWs before they start working in the institution. If the hospital is establishing a new database, the same information should be obtained from all current employees.

In small hospitals, the database could be a paper line-list or a card file. The infection control staff or the staff in various departments or units could maintain the file or list. In large hospitals, the database should be computerized. The persons who develop and maintain the database could be in the hospital's information management group, in the infection control program, or in the employee health service. Regardless of who manages the database, the persons investigating exposures must have unobstructed access to the database so that they can use the data regardless of when the exposure occurs.

Develop a Data Collection Form

Infection control staff members must investigate exposures in a consistent fashion. Therefore, in addition to developing policies and procedures, infection control staff members should design a form (either paper or electronic) with which they can collect the necessary data for each exposure. For most exposures, we currently use the hospital's mainframe computer to generate a list of HCWs who were in the affected areas and, when appropriate, either the immune status of these employees or the date of their last tuberculin skin test. In the past we used a paper form that has 4 carbonless copies. Once the forms were completed, we distributed copies to the departments that needed to be informed of the exposure. We recently developed a computerized form that staff in the infection control program and in Employee Health can access on a common computer drive. Infection control personnel enter the names of exposed persons into the database and staff members in Employee Health have immediate access to that information so they are prepared when exposed employees come to them for follow-up.

Educate Staff

As noted in the introduction, infection control staff members can prevent exposures by educating HCWs. For example, HCWs should know the modes of transmission for common communicable pathogens and basic infection control practices that limit the spread of microorganisms. In addition, exposure workups will go more smoothly if infection control personnel prospectively educate HCWs about exposure workups in general and about the specific steps taken during common exposure workups. Infection control staff members also will need to educate and calm the staff while doing many exposure workups because staff who think they have been exposed to meningococcus or to lice frequently panic and act irrationally.

Collect and Evaluate Data on Exposures

Infection control personnel should collect data on the exposure workups that they conduct. They can tabulate the data on paper, or they can develop a computer database in which to store the information. At least once per year the infection control staff should assess the following:
➤   Number of exposures
➤   Etiologic agents
➤   Affected locations
➤   Number of susceptible HCWs, patients, and visitors exposed
➤   Number of secondary cases
➤   Number of HCWs who were placed on leave
➤   Number of leave days
➤   Breaks in infection control technique that led to the exposures
➤   Prophylactic treatments given
➤   Cost in time and dollars

Infection control personnel should report these data to the infection control committee and should use these data to do the following:
➤   Document their effort to the administration
➤   Identify topics for in-service educational programs
➤   Identify interventions (eg, offer influenza vaccine free of charge to all employees)
➤   Identify areas for collaboration with other departments (eg, work with staff in other departments to develop methods for screening and triage of potentially infectious patients)
➤   Identify areas for improvement
➤   Document quality improvement efforts required for accreditation

Disease-Specific Exposure Workups

Viral Diseases

Varicella-Zoster Virus

Varicella-Zoster virus (VZV) causes a primary infection, chicken pox, and a recrudescent infection, herpes zoster, or shingles. VZV can be transmitted through the air by persons with chicken pox or through direct contact with fresh chicken pox or herpes zoster lesions. Thus, patients with chicken pox or disseminated zoster should be placed on airborne and contact precautions until all lesions are crusted to prevent exposures within hospitals.[12] Nonimmune patients who have been exposed to chicken pox should be placed on airborne precautions between days 8 and 21 after their exposure (day 28 if the person is immunocompromised or received varicella-zoster immune globulin [VZIG]). Because VZV rarely is spread through the air from persons with localized herpes zoster, patients, visitors, and HCWs with this entity do not need to be restricted if their lesions can be covered.

Approximately 4% to 15% of susceptible HCWs will develop chicken pox each year.[13] Currently, 2% to 5% of all HCWs are not immune to VZV,[13,14] and 28% of those with no known history of chicken pox are susceptible to this virus.[13] A recent study of US Coast Guard recruits found similar results; only 4.1% of the recruits were seronegative for VZV.[15] Ninety-nine percent of recruits with a history of chicken pox had positive serology as did 73% of those who thought they had not had chicken pox or who were not sure.

Nonimmune HCWs who have been exposed to a person with chicken pox could be incubating the infection. To prevent the spread of VZV, infection control personnel must identify those HCWs and restrict their work during the incubation period. A few HCFs allow exposed nonimmune HCWs to wear masks and continue working.[16] Most HCFs do not allow susceptible, exposed HCWs to continue their patient-care duties during the incubation period. Some HCFs place such staff on leave,[10,11] and other facilities reassign exposed susceptible staff to nonpatient-care areas if all the employees in that area are immune.[17] Exposed staff members who are permitted to work must take care not to expose persons as they enter and exit the building. At the University of Iowa Hospitals and Clinics, we have used the latter approach since 1977 without difficulty. We require those HCWs to use the most direct route to the area in which they work (ie, excluding the main entrances), and we do not allow them to be in areas in which many people congregate (eg, waiting areas, lobbies, lounges, gift shop, cafeteria). Staff members who develop active disease must not work until all lesions are crusted.

Exposed visitors who are not immune should not be allowed to enter the hospital during the incubation period. Exposed visitors who do not know their immune status should not enter the hospital during the incubation period until they have antibody levels obtained and are documented to be immune.

Infection control personnel should work with employee health staff, expert clinicians, pharmacists, and hospital administrators to determine whether exposed persons will be offered the chicken pox vaccine (Varivax, Merck & Co, West Point, Pa) or VZIG. If the HCF provides one or both of these agents, this group should decide prospectively which persons will be offered either agent. In addition, this group should decide whether their HCF will offer the chicken pox vaccine to all nonimmune HCWs. This decision may not be a simple one for the following reasons:

➤ Five percent of HCWs who receive the vaccine will develop a varicella-like rash that will require them to miss work because transmission of the vaccine virus has been documented.

➤ For approximately 6 weeks after receiving the vaccination, HCWs should not care for susceptible, high-risk persons, including immunocompromised persons, pregnant women who do not have a history of chicken pox or detectable antibody to VZV, and newborns of such women.

➤ A substantial portion of vaccinated persons will have subclinical or breakthrough varicella infection after close exposure to a person with chicken pox.[18-21]

VZV used to be one of the most common communicable agents causing exposures at the University of Iowa Hospitals and Clinics, but since 1999 we have had 0 to 1 exposures per year. In these rare instances, a HCW or patient with community-acquired chickenpox exposed other HCWs or patients. We have been fortunate because very few of the exposures have caused secondary cases. Some HCFs have not been as fortunate and have experienced substantial transmission of VZV.[2,3,22] Several investigators found that varicella vaccine would be cost effective.[23-25] In nonhealthcare settings, the cost per case prevented may be prohibitive.[26]

Table 11-1 outlines an approach to managing HCWs who have been exposed to VZV.[5,11,21] Infection control personnel who want additional information about VZV exposures should consult the appropriate references.[6,9,13,14,17,27]

Measles Virus

Measles is a febrile illness that is characterized by Koplik's spots on the buccal mucosa and by an erythematous rash. The measles rash starts on the face and spreads to the trunk and extremities and also progresses from maculopapular to confluent. Measles virus, which is highly communicable, is spread by airborne transmission. Despite sensitivity to acid, strong light, and drying, the measles virus can remain viable in airborne droplets for hours, especially if the relative humidity is low. Consequently, outbreaks have occurred in HCFs when the index patient was no longer present.[28,29] To prevent the spread of measles virus within HCFs, patients with measles should be placed on airborne precautions.[12]

Before the measles vaccine was licensed in 1963, 500,000 cases of measles occurred in the United States each year. Subsequently, the number of measles cases in the United States declined dramatically, reaching a nadir in 1983. Thereafter, the incidence of measles increased for several years. More recently, increased immunization rates and routine use of 2 doses of the vaccine have helped decrease the number of measles cases. Measles now occurs most frequently in preschool children, many of whom are too young to be vaccinated. Seo et al recently reported that measles seropositivity rates among HCWs in their 20s was lower for those hired between 1998 and 1999 than for those hired between 1983 and 1988.[30] These authors reminded infection control staff members that HCWs who were born after 1989 should have their antibody levels checked when they are hired.

Despite the declining incidence of measles and recommendations that all persons receive 2 doses of measles vaccine and that all HCWs should be immune to measles, outbreaks and nosocomial transmission continue to occur.[28,29,31-48] Steingart et al reported that 8 of 31 persons in Clark County, Washington who acquired measles in 1996 were HCWs and 5 were patients or visitors in HCFs.[47] HCWs who acquired measles worked in facilities that did not require proof of measles immunity. Compared with adults in Clark County, the relative risk of measles in HCWs was 18.6 (95% confidence interval, 7.4 to 45.8; $p < 0.001$). Only 47% of facilities surveyed by these authors had measles immunization policies and only 21% met the APIC recommendations and enforced their policies. Kelly et al described several outbreaks of measles in Australian HCFs.[49] They concluded that the outbreaks occurred because published guidelines for preventing nosocomial measles were not followed.[49] They stated that transmission of measles in a HCF could be considered "a sentinel sign of system failure."[49]

At present, 5% to 10% of HCWs are susceptible to measles,[13] including 4.7% of those born before 1957, 16% of those born in the 1960s, and 34% of those born in the 1970s.[44] In fact, HCWs are the source of 5% to 10% of all measles cases and account for 28% of measles cases acquired in medical settings in the United States.[13] A case in South Dakota demonstrates that HCWs still acquire measles while caring for patients.

Measles exposures are relatively uncommon in many hospitals. At the University of Iowa Hospitals and Clinics, we have not had a patient with the diagnosis of measles admitted in the last 2 years. However, a representative from a specialty bed company became ill with measles 1 day after delivering beds to 5 patient-care areas. Fifteen HCWs were possibly exposed, 13 of these employees were born before 1957 (and thus presumably immune), and 2 were vaccinated 3 to 4 years before the exposure. Three patients were possibly exposed, 2 were born before 1957, and the third had detectable antibody. No secondary cases were identified.

Although measles exposures are infrequent, infection control personnel still must develop policies that will limit the spread of measles if it is introduced into the hospital. A study conducted by Enguidanos et al suggests that infection control programs may be ignoring measles because the incidence is low.[44] These investigators noted that 74 adults employed in acute-care hospitals acquired measles during a community-wide outbreak in 1987 through 1989. The investigators surveyed all 102 infection control professionals in the acute-care hospitals in Los Angeles County to determine whether infection control policies were adequate. Only 17% of the hospitals required HCWs to document immunity to measles, and only 4% had policies that covered students or volunteers. The investigators also surveyed the HCWs who became ill. Of these 74 persons, 46% worked in hospitals that did not have measles infection control policies, 43% were born before 1957, and 31% were working in jobs that have not been considered to increase the risk of measles exposure.[44]

As discussed previously, infection control personnel should work with the employee health department to develop a database that has each HCW's history of measles vaccination. If such a database is not available and a person with measles comes to the hospital, the infection control staff must identify exposed personnel and then determine whether these persons are immune. Nonimmune patients who have been exposed to measles should be placed on airborne precautions between day 5 and day 21 after their exposure.[12] Nonimmune family members and friends who have been exposed to a person with measles should not come to the hospital during the incubation period. Table 11-1 provides information necessary for managing a measles exposure.[5]

Rubella Virus

Rubella (German measles) is an acute exanthematous viral infection that affects children and adults. Postnatal rubella, which resembles a mild case of measles, is characterized by rash, fever, and lymphadenopathy. In contrast, rubella acquired in pregnancy can cause fetal death, premature labor, and severe congenital defects. Consequently, it is very important to prevent spread of rubella in HCFs. However, the mild clinical symptoms associated with rubella have, at times, facilitated nosocomial spread of rubella virus because HCWs have continued to work while they were ill. The literature documents numerous outbreaks of rubella in medical settings, some of which affected many susceptible pregnant women.[50-58]

Furthermore, these institutions had to invest large amounts of time and money to control the outbreaks.[54,56,58]

The epidemiology of rubella has been changing. Data from the CDC indicate that the incidence of rubella has been decreasing among children less than 15 years old but increasing in adults, primarily those born outside the United States.[59,60] In fact, 21 of 23 infants with congenital rubella syndrome reported to the CDC between 1997 and 1999 were born to foreign-born women, most of whom were Hispanic. Sheridan et al in the United Kingdom reported a case of nosocomial transmission of rubella from one neonate to another whose bed was nearby.[61] The mother of the index case was from Bangladesh and apparently had a mild flu-like illness without a rash when she was 10 weeks pregnant. The infant was not recognized as having congenital rubella.

Rubella virus is spread in droplets that are shed from the respiratory secretions of infected persons. Persons with rubella are most contagious when the rash is erupting. In addition, persons with subclinical illness also may transmit the virus. To prevent nosocomial spread, patients with rubella should be placed on droplet precautions until 7 days after the onset of the rash. Infants with congenital rubella shed large quantities of virus for many months, despite having high titers of neutralizing antibody. Such patients should be placed in droplet precautions each time they are admitted during the first year of life unless nasopharyngeal and urine cultures after 3 months of age are negative.

Nonimmune patients who have been exposed to rubella should be placed on droplet precautions between days 7 and 21 after their exposure.[12] Nonimmune family members and friends who have been exposed to a person with rubella should not come to the hospital during the incubation period.

Despite vaccination campaigns, 10% to 20% of hospital personnel are susceptible to rubella.[13] Given the adverse effects of rubella virus on the fetus, many HCFs require employees, especially those working in obstetrics, to be immune to rubella.[33,50]

Table 11-1 provides information infection control personnel need for evaluating exposures to persons with rubella.[5] Infection control personnel will be able to investigate such exposures more readily if the HCF maintains a computer database that includes information about the employees' immune status.

Mumps Virus

Mumps is characterized by fever and parotitis. In postpubertal men, mumps virus also can cause orchitis, which can be the primary manifestation of the infection. The mumps virus is transmitted through direct contact with contaminated respiratory secretions, inhalation of droplet nuclei, or through contact with fomites contaminated by respiratory secretions. Transmission of mumps virus requires more intimate contact with the infected person than does transmission of either measles virus or VZV. To prevent exposures in HCFs, persons with mumps should be placed on droplet precautions until 9 days after parotid (or other glandular) swelling began.[12]

The incidence of mumps decreased substantially in the United States after the vaccine was licensed in 1967.[5,33] Consequently, exposures to persons with mumps and nosocomial transmission of mumps are rare.[62,63] In 1996, Fischer et al published a report of an outbreak of mumps in which a 3-year old patient, a nurse, and a physical therapist (who was vaccinated) acquired mumps after a 12-year old Mexican girl who was incubating mumps was admitted to the hospital.[63] Neither the patient who acquired mumps nor the physical therapist had direct contact with the index patient. We have had one documented mumps exposure and one possible mumps exposure at the University of Iowa Hospitals and Clinics in the last 10 years. The documented case occurred in a student who received the measles vaccine, not the measles, mumps, rubella (MMR) vaccine, when he entered college. We implemented droplet precautions once the diagnosis was suspected. Several HCWs were exposed but all of them had been immunized with the MMR vaccine. We did not identify any secondary cases of mumps.

As discussed previously, a computerized database that includes the HCWs' immune status for mumps will help infection control personnel if an exposure to mumps occurs in their hospital. If a database is not available, infection control personnel will need to determine whether HCWs have had either mumps or the mumps vaccine. Most adults are immune to mumps, and approximately 90% of adults who have no history of mumps have antibody to the virus.[5] Thus, only a small proportion of HCWs will be susceptible to mumps. For example, Nichol and Olson found that 6.7% of the medical students they studied were nonimmune.[64] Consequently, it might be cost beneficial to assess antibody titers of exposed persons who have no history of mumps and who have not received the mumps vaccine. Only those who are seronegative would be excluded from patient care during the incubation period (days 11 through 26). Table 11-1 provides information necessary to evaluate an exposure to a person with mumps. Nonimmune patients who have been exposed to mumps should be placed on droplet precautions between days 11 and 26 after their exposure.[12] Nonimmune family members and friends who have been exposed to a person with mumps should not come to the hospital during the incubation period.

Parvovirus B19

Erythema infectiosum, or fifth disease, is a common manifestation of acute parvovirus B19 infection. Fifth disease acquired its name because common childhood exanthems were numbered in the late 19th century. The first 3 illnesses were scarlet fever, rubeola, and rubella, and the fourth was a variation of scarlet fever known as Filatov-Dukes disease. Erythema infectiosum was the fifth disease, and roseola infantum was the sixth. Erythema infectiosum is characterized by mild systemic symptoms (fever in 15% to 30%), followed in 1 to 4 days by an erythematous rash on the cheeks, the "slapped cheek" appearance. Subsequently, an asymmetric macular or maculopapular, lace-like erythematous rash can involve the trunk and extremities.

Parvovirus B19 has a predilection for infecting rapidly dividing cells, especially rapidly dividing red blood cells. Thus, persons with sickle cell disease, hereditary spherocytosis, pyruvate kinase deficiency, and other hemolytic anemias can develop transient hemolytic crises. Parvovirus B19 can cause severe chronic anemia associated with red cell aplasia in persons who are on maintenance chemotherapy for acute lymphocytic leukemia, who have congenital immunodeficiencies, or who have acquired immunodeficiency syndrome (AIDS). Parvovirus B19 can also cause hydrops fetalis. However, most parvovirus B19 infections during pregnancy do not affect the fetus adversely. Several studies indicate that the risk of fetal death is less than 10% in infected fetuses.[5]

Parvovirus B19 DNA has been found in the respiratory secretions of viremic patients, but most persons are no longer viremic when the rash appears. In general, HCWs with parvovirus B19 infection do not need to be removed from patient care because they are usually not diagnosed until after the rash appears. Some hospitals might choose to restrict HCWs from caring for patients at high risk of complications until the HCW's symptoms have resolved. Persons with transient hemolytic crises and babies with hydrops fetalis can remain viremic for prolonged periods. These patients can be the source of infection for susceptible patients or HCWs and thus should be placed on droplet precautions while they are hospitalized to prevent spread of parvovirus B19.[12] Lui et al documented nosocomial patient-to-patient transmission of this virus from a renal transplant patient who apparently transmitted the virus many weeks after the onset of symptoms.[65]

Transmission of parvovirus B19 is common in the community.[66] Outbreaks have occurred in day-care centers and in elementary and junior high schools. Secondary spread to susceptible household contacts also is frequent. Documented transmission within hospitals has been uncommon.[67-72] However, when transmission occurs, a high proportion (13% to 50%) of susceptible persons may be infected.[68,69,72,73] We recently were notified by an infectious diseases consultant that she had parvovirus. She had been in the Virology Clinic on several days when she was potentially infectious. Two pregnant HCWs were exposed to this physician, one of whom was immune (ie, she had antibody to the virus). The other woman was susceptible but she did not acquire a compatible illness or develop antibody to parvovirus B19.

Transmission of parvovirus B19 usually requires prolonged, frequent, close contact. Adler and colleagues investigated the rate of seroconversion to this virus among people employed either in schools or hospitals during an endemic period.[74] These investigators found that the risk of seroconversion for persons who had daily contact with school-aged children at home (ages 5 to 11 years) or at work (ages 5 to 18 years) was 5 times higher than that for other study participants. The overall rate of seroconversion was 5.2% for primary-school employees, 2.4% for other school employees, and 0% to 0.5% for hospital employees.[74]

In general, routine infection control precautions should minimize nosocomial transmission of this virus.[75] A study by Cartter et al of risk factors for parvovirus B19 infection in pregnant women demonstrated that the rate of infection was highest among nurses who cared for patients before they were isolated.[76] These results suggest that isolation precautions can prevent nosocomial spread of this virus from infected patients. Ray et al obtained serologies for parvovirus B19 infection from 32 nonimmune HCWs who cared for 2 patients with transient aplastic crisis before they were put in isolation and from 37 nonimmune HCWs who were not exposed.[69] The incidence of serologic evidence of recent parvovirus B19 infection was 3.1% among the exposed HCWs and 8.1% among the HCWs in the comparison group (p = 0.06). On the basis of their data, Ray et al concluded that the risk of nosocomial transmission was low even when isolation precautions are not implemented.[69]

Table 11-1 provides information about how infection control personnel could evaluate an exposure to parvovirus B19.[5] In addition, the article by Crowcroft and colleagues reviews relevant literature and provides recommendations for protecting "at-risk seronegative HCWs" and "at-risk patients."[72]

Hepatitis A Virus

Hepatitis A is transmitted primarily by the fecal-oral route, but, in hospitals, hepatitis A virus also can be transmitted by blood transfusions. Infected persons excrete the highest concentration of virus in their stools during the 2 weeks before their symptoms begin. Most persons are no longer shedding the virus 1 week after they become jaundiced. However, infants can shed the virus in their stools for months.

Nosocomial transmission of hepatitis A is relatively uncommon. Most nosocomial outbreaks have occurred after an infant or a young child has received blood from a viremic but asymptomatic donor. The child often has an asymptomatic infection.[77-83] Occasionally, nosocomial outbreaks have occurred when HCWs cared for an older child or an adult who had vomiting, diarrhea, or fecal incontinence.[84-93]

HCWs who are exposed to the stool of infected patients are at greatest risk for acquiring hepatitis A infection. Occasionally, patients, visitors, and HCWs could be at risk of acquiring hepatitis A if they eat uncooked food prepared by a food handler who is shedding the virus. Several food-related nosocomial epidemics have been reported.[94,95]

To prevent nosocomial transmission of hepatitis A virus, HCWs should wear gowns and gloves whenever they might contaminate their hands or clothes with a patient's stool. HCWs must perform hand hygiene after doing any patient-care activities and after removing their gloves. Adult patients with hepatitis A who are continent do not require private rooms, but diapered or incontinent persons should be placed in private rooms.[12] HCWs who cared for patients with hepatitis A do not need to be restricted from work unless they develop hepatitis because the risk of acquiring hepatitis from a patient is low, and the risk of transmission from infected HCWs to patients also is low. HCWs with hepatitis A infection should not work during the first 7 days of their symptomatic illnesses. Table 11-1 provides information infection control personnel need when evaluating an exposure to hepatitis A.[5]

The *Guideline for Infection Control in Health Care Personnel, 1998* states that "immunoglobulin given within 2 weeks of exposure is greater than 85% effective in preventing hepatitis A virus infection and may be advisable in some outbreaks."[7] The usual dose of immune globulin is 0.02 mg/kg IM when given as postexposure prophylaxis. The hepatitis A vaccine has helped terminate outbreaks in the community, but its role in hospitals has not been determined.

Influenza Virus

Infection control staff members and other HCWs tend to think that transmission of influenza virus occurs primarily in the community, not in the hospital. However, Evans et al identified 17 reports of nosocomial influenza transmission that were published between 1959 and 1994.[96] In 5 of these outbreaks HCWs were implicated in transmitting the virus, and in 12 outbreaks HCWs became infected with influenza virus. We identified 11 reports from 1/1996 through 7/2003 of nosocomial influenza outbreaks, at least 4 of which clearly stated that HCWs were affected. The affected units included neonatal intensive care units (3), a pediatric unit (1), a solid organ transplant unit (1), adult bone marrow transplant unit (1), a unit for cancer patients (1), and an adult pulmonary unit (1). Thus, patients, visitors, and HCWs can spread this virus in HCFs.[96-112] In the outbreak described by Pachucki et al, 118 workers were affected, including 8% of the nurses and 3% to 6% of the doctors.[98] More recently, Everts et al described 2 outbreaks of influenza A affecting wards that treated and rehabilitated elderly patients.[112] The attack rate among patients was 48% on one ward and 58% on the other; 46% of the ill patients had lower respiratory tract

involvement and 7% died. The attack rate among staff was 69% on one ward and 36% on the other.

Nosocomial influenza probably goes unrecognized in many instances. Clinicians and infection control personnel should consider this diagnosis when staff members or hospitalized patients develop symptoms of influenza during the appropriate season. Table 11-1 describes how infection control personnel could manage HCWs who were exposed to influenza.[5] The role of prophylaxis with amantidine, rimantidine, zanamivir, or oseltamivir has not been defined for HCWs who are exposed to influenza in acute care facilities.[113] In our hospital, we usually identify the exposures after the period when prophylaxis would be worthwhile and, thus, we have rarely offered these agents to HCWs. Fortunately, we have not had extensive transmission of influenza in our hospital.

Influenza increases absenteeism among staff and increases the costs associated with sick leave. In addition, the APIC has recommended that physicians, nurses, and other personnel in both inpatient- and outpatient-care settings who have contact with high-risk persons receive the influenza vaccine.[114] Thus, many HCFs offer their employees the influenza vaccine free of charge to protect the staff and to prevent spread of influenza within the HCF. FluMist (MedImmune Vaccines Inc, Gaithersberg, Md), a live influenza virus vaccine, has been released and could cause acute care facilities some difficulties. The package insert states that vaccinated persons should not have close contact with immunocompromised patients for at least 21 days after receiving the vaccine. In addition, the vaccine should be administered before exposure to influenza and the safety of the vaccine has not been demonstrated for the persons at highest risk of complications from influenza. Thus, we think that this vaccine currently is not useful for acute care hospitals especially in the setting of an influenza exposure.

Creutzfeldt-Jakob Agent

Creutzfeldt-Jakob agent, a prion, has been transmitted in the healthcare setting by brain-to-brain inoculation (eg, through contaminated instruments) and by contaminated tissues or tissue extracts. To date, there have been no documented instances of transmission to HCWs, and the incidence of Creutzfeldt-Jakob disease (CJD) is not higher in HCWs than it is in the general population.[115,116] Berger and Noble reported that 24 HCWs have been identified as having CJD.[117] These authors provided 5 case reports of HCWs (1 neurosurgeon, 1 pathologist, 1 internist who did autopsies for 1 year during his training, and 2 histopathology technicians) who developed CJD.[117] However, none of these persons had documented exposures to the agent.

Criteria for defining exposures to the Creutzfeldt-Jakob agent have not been developed. The WHO categorizes the following tissues as having high infectivity: brain, spinal cord, and eye.[118] WHO categorizes the following tissues or fluids as having low infectivity: cerebrospinal fluid, kidney, liver, lung, lymph nodes, spleen, and placenta.[118] WHO categorizes the following tissues or fluids as having no detectable infectivity: adipose, adrenal gland, gingival, heart muscle, intestine, peripheral nerve, prostate, skeletal muscle, testis, thyroid gland, tears, nasal mucous, saliva, sweat, serous exudates, milk, semen, urine, and feces.[118] The WHO also classifies blood as "no detectable infectivity" despite the fact that blood and its components have been found to have very low levels of infectivity in experimental models. WHO classified blood in this way because the epidemiologic evidence indicates that blood has never transmitted the CJD prion to humans.[118]

The highest risk injuries involve high-risk tissues and needle-stick injuries with inoculation. Exposures via mucous membranes have the "theoretical risk of transmitting the CJC prion." WHO recommends the following procedures if an exposure occurs:

➤ Wash exposed unbroken skin with detergent and abundant quantities of warm water (avoid scrubbing). Then rinse and dry the affected area. Brief (1-minute) exposure to 0.1 N NaOH or a 1:10 bleach solution can be used for maximum safety.

➤ After a needle stick or laceration, gently encourage bleeding, wash (avoid scrubbing) as described above, rinse, dry, cover with a dressing.

➤ After splashing an eye or mouth, irrigate the affected area with saline (eye) or water (mouth).

➤ Report any exposures to the appropriate department.[117]

If an exposure occurs, infection control personnel should create a list of all exposed staff members, which should be saved indefinitely in case anyone develops the disease. Staff members from infection control and the Employee Health service also should counsel HCWs because they most likely will be very distraught and angry. In addition, the infection control staff should work with the staff from the operating suite and central sterile supply to ensure that, if possible, the reusable surgical instruments used on the index case are recalled and reprocessed properly and that all contaminated equipment in other departments (eg, pathology) is properly cleaned and disinfected.

The best exposure management for Creutzfeldt-Jakob agent is to prevent exposures from occurring. Therefore, infection control staff would be wise to work with persons from the operating suite, the neurosurgery department, the ophthalmology department, the pathology department, the laboratory, central sterile supply, and the morgue to develop policies that prevent exposures. These precautions should be used for all persons who undergo invasive procedures or ophthalmologic exams and who are known to have CJD or a progressive dementia; or who have a family history of prion disease, CJD, fatal familial insomnia, or Gerstmann-Sträussler-Scheinker disease.[118,119] The precautions also should be used for patients who have received gonadotropin or human growth hormone extracted from cadaveric pituitary glands.[119]

At the University of Iowa Hospitals and Clinics, we developed and implemented a Creutzfeldt-Jakob policy. The first policy covered only patients with known CJD. Soon after we implemented this policy, a patient who had a progressive dementia underwent a diagnostic brain biopsy. The clinicians were surprised and dismayed when the histopathology revealed spongiform degeneration. The subsequent exposure workup involved 62 personnel from the Department of Pathology, the operating suite, and central sterile supply. In addition, personnel in the Department of Pathology spent numerous hours and approximately $1200 disinfecting the laboratory and equipment that might have been contaminated by the tissues. Thereafter, we expanded our policy to include the conditions, treatments, and family histories listed above.

Infection control personnel who are developing these policies should review recommendations written by Steelman[119,120] and by Rutala.[121] These documents recommend methods for protecting the staff from exposure to potentially infectious tissues, limiting contamination of equipment and the environment, and effectively eradicating the organism from surgical equipment. The guidelines on the care of surgical equipment are extremely important because the Creutzfeldt-Jakob agent is not killed by routine chemical and physical means of sterilization, including routine steam sterilization, ethylene oxide sterilization, and dry heat sterilization; processes using peracetic acid, hydrogen peroxide, ultraviolet light, radiation, freezing, drying, or hot bead glass; and any level of cleaning and disinfection with glutaraldehyde, dry heat radiation, detergents, or formaldehyde. Notably, some of the recommendations differ between the documents developed by Steelman and Rutala.

Variant CJC, or vCJD, has become an important issue in the United Kingdom and Europe.[122-124] One case has been identified in the United States.[123] The patient had lived in the United States for 22 years but was originally from the United Kingdom. vCJD is thought to be transmitted from beef infected with the agent of bovine spongiform encephalopathy (BSE). The United States has not identified BSE as a problem, and thus, many people in this country are not concerned about vCJD. However, given the ease with which people travel, the presence of chronic wasting disease (another spongiform encephalopathy) in cervids in the United States, and the lax regulation of the rendering industry, we think that infection control personnel cannot ignore vCJD.

Unlike the CJD prion, the vCJD prion infects the lymphoreticular tissues. Thus, a tonsilar biopsy is the preferred diagnostic test. Thus, a wider variety of tissues may be able to transmit this agent. The Department of Health in the United Kingdom has mandated that decontamination facilities be upgraded and that all adenotonsillectomy procedures must be performed using disposable instruments.[124] In addition, decontamination and sterilization of equipment is different for vCJD than for CJD.[125,126] Given that lymphoreticular tissue is affected and that infected persons may not show symptoms or signs of the disease for years, many hospitals in Europe have changed their general decontamination and sterilization such that vCJD will be killed.

Bacterial Diseases

Mycobacterium tuberculosis

M. tuberculosis is an acid-fast bacillus that is spread through the air. This organism causes a primary infection, which in normal hosts usually is not manifested as clinical disease, and recrudescent pulmonary or disseminated disease. Persons who are infected with *M. tuberculosis* have positive tuberculin skin tests but are not contagious. Those who have active pulmonary disease are infectious and are the persons who cause most nosocomial exposures. On occasion, patients who have active infections at other sites can also cause exposures. For example, a patient with a large soft-tissue abscess underwent incision, drainage, and irrigation in an operating suite.[127] Because he continued to have copious drainage, the wound was cleaned with a pressurized irrigation system. Subsequently, 59 employees were identified who converted their tuberculin skin tests, and 9 persons acquired active tuberculosis (5 employees, 2 patients, and 2 family members of the index patient). More recently, Matlow et al reported that 111 HCWs were exposed to tuberculosis while caring for an infant with peritoneal tuberculosis.[128] Two (5%) of 39 primary care nurses but no doctors or housekeepers had skin test conversions.

Persons are considered exposed to *M. tuberculosis* if they were not wearing an N95 or better respirator and they shared air space with a patient who had active pulmonary tuberculosis or who had an extrapulmonary site of infection from which *M. tuberculosis* was aerosolized. During outbreaks, a large proportion (3.6% to 100%) of exposed persons may become tuberculin skin-test positive.[127,129-131] In general, approximately 30% of persons will become infected when they are exposed to a patient whose sputum contains acid-fast bacilli, whereas only 10% of persons will become infected when they are exposed to an infected patient whose sputum does not contain visible acid-fast bacilli.[132]

As with the other airborne infections—measles and chicken pox—it is best to prevent exposures by screening patients in clinics and on admission for symptoms and signs of tuberculosis. However, screening can be difficult because some patients present with atypical signs or symptoms and others do not answer truthfully to screening questions designed to identify patients who might have tuberculosis so that they can be isolated before they expose persons in the healthcare setting. In 2003, a high school student who immigrated to the United States from another country came to our emergency room. The patient and her uncle said that she had been diagnosed with pneumonia at another hospital but they denied that she had symptoms consistent with tuberculosis. She was later found to have cavitary tuberculosis. Because the patient did not answer the questions truthfully, 5 HCWs and 38 patients and visitors were exposed. We are currently assessing whether any of them became tuberculin skin-test positive.

Moreover some patients present with tuberculosis at unusual sites and immunocompromised patients can have atypical signs and symptoms. For example, during a 2-month period in 1993, 2 patients were seen at the University of Iowa Hospitals and Clinics who had unusual presentations of tuberculosis. One patient was a 28-year-old man who had a testicular mass that was found to be an abscess during an operation. Subsequently, drainage from the abscess, his urine, and lung tissue all were found to contain *M. tuberculosis*. The second patient was a 57-year-old woman whose tuberculin skin test was negative before she underwent a bilateral lung transplant. The patient was seen several times after the transplant for complaints of decreasing exercise tolerance, fever, and right shoulder pain. Twelve weeks after the transplant, she was admitted with fever, continued right shoulder pain, and cavitary lesions in her lungs.[133] Material from a lung cavity contained acid-fast bacilli, and she was begun on isoniazid, ethambutol, and pyrazinamide. However, she developed renal failure, progressive liver-function abnormalities, a coagulopathy, and respiratory distress. Despite receiving supportive care, including mechanical ventilation, the patient died. An autopsy identified an ill-defined abscess of the subcapularis muscle and numerous abscesses caused by *M. tuberculosis* in the lungs, liver, spleen, pancreas, and small intestine. During the course of their care, the 2 patients described above exposed 150 persons (48 and 102, respectively). Five employees (3.3%) became tuberculin skin-test positive, including 2 persons in the Department of Pathology who had handled tissues from the patients.

In 2003, a patient, who years previously immigrated to the United States from Cambodia, underwent a mastoidectomy for what was felt to be routine chronic mastoiditis. However, during the operation the surgeon remarked that the tissue looked like the patient had tuberculosis! Indeed, *M. tuberculosis* grew from the tissue obtained during the operation. Subsequently, the patient had a chest radiograph that revealed a right upper lobe cavity and his sputum cultures also grew *M. tuberculosis*. Twenty-two HCWs and 78 patients were exposed to this patient.

HCWs still acquire *M. tuberculosis* through occupational exposures.[134-144] In countries where tuberculosis is common, HCWs may be at considerable risk of acquiring tuberculosis.[141-145] A prospective study done in Thailand found that the number of pulmonary tuberculosis cases increased from 102 in 1990 to 356 in 1999; the annual rate of active tuberculosis during 1995 to 1999 was 536/100,000 HCWs.[141] The tuberculin skin test conversion rate decreased from 9.3% (95% confidence interval [CI95], 3.3-15) per 100 person-years during 1995 to 1997 to 2.2 (CI95, 0.0-5.1) per 100 person-years in 1999 after control measures were implemented in 1996. Eyob et al reported that the incidence of tuberculosis among HCWs increased significantly from 1695/100,000 person years in 1989 to 5556/100,000 person years in 1998.[145] The incidence of tuberculosis was 3 times higher among HCWs than in the general population.

In addition as suggested by some of the cases described above, persons who move from countries with high incidences of tuberculosis to countries with low incidences can cause substantial exposures in HCFs.[146,147] In addition, studies done in Canada indicate that delays in diagnosis,[148] inadequate ventilation (<2 air exchanges per hour) in general patient rooms, the type of work (nursing, respiratory therapy, physical therapy, and housekeeping) and the duration of work all increase the risk of transmission.[135]

The goal of an exposure workup is to identify all patients, visitors, and HCWs who were exposed, so that those who become infected can be treated with antimicrobial agents. This task can be very difficult if, before being diagnosed, the infectious person visited many clinics and diagnostic laboratories or was hospitalized in an open bay of an intensive care unit. All persons who meet the criteria for exposure should have baseline tuberculin skin testing if they have not had a recent skin test (within 6 weeks in a high-prevalence area or 1 year in a low-prevalence area). HCWs should be seen in the employee health service. Patients and visitors should be notified about the exposure and told to contact their own physician or should be offered the opportunity to have their skin tests done at the medical facility where the exposure occurred. In addition, the patients' primary physicians should receive letters informing them of the exposure. Twelve weeks after the exposure, exposed persons should have another skin test. If the first skin test is negative and the second skin test is positive, the exposed person should receive treatment.[130]

Neisseria meningitidis

N. meningitidis is a gram-negative diplococcus that causes meningitis and septicemia. Household contacts of persons with invasive meningococcal disease are at 500 to 800 times greater risk of acquiring meningococcal infection than are members of the general public.[148] Other semiclosed or closed populations, such as persons living in college dormitories, chronic-care hospitals, nursery schools, and military barracks, are also at high risk of infection.[149] Despite caring for patients with meningococcal infection, HCWs are not at higher risk than members of the general population for acquiring this infection.[13]

N. meningitidis is transmitted by respiratory droplets. Thus, patients with meningococcal infections should be placed on droplet precautions for the first 24 hours of treatment.[12] Nosocomial transmission of *N. meningitidis*, which has occurred rarely, may be more likely to occur from patients who have meningococcal pneumonia than from patients with meningitis or septicemia.[150,151] We conducted a computerized literature search of reports published between 1975 and 2003 and identified only 5 papers reporting HCWs who acquired meningococcal infection after nosocomial exposure.[150-154] Four of the 6 affected HCWs did mouth-to-mouth resuscitation on patients with meningococcal disease,[148] one was a pediatrician who did not wear protective gear while intubating a child who was thought to have a "meningoencephalitis,"[153] and one was a nurse who did not receive a prophylactic antimicrobial agent after she helped intubate and suction an infected patient.[152]

Persons are considered exposed to *N. meningitidis* if they did not wear a mask and had either prolonged close contact with a person who had meningococcal disease or had contact with the patient's respiratory secretions. Exposed persons should begin prophylactic treatment within 24 hours of their exposure.[5] Thus, immediately upon identifying a patient with meningococcal disease, infection control personnel must determine whether any HCWs met the criteria for exposure. Staff who met criteria for exposure must be sent to the employee health service at once to receive a prescription for an appropriate antimicrobial agent. If the employee health service is not open, infection control staff members should ensure that the HCWs receive the prophylactic agent.

Despite the very low risk of transmission to HCWs, staff members often react irrationally when they learn that a patient with meningococcal disease has been admitted to their unit. Staff members who do not meet the criteria for exposure frequently demand prescriptions for prophylactic antimicrobial agents. If infection control personnel refuse to oblige them, these staff members often have another physician write a prescription for them. However, prophylactic treatment is not without complications. In fact, one of the authors investigated an exposure to *N. meningitidis* in which the hospital had to replace 2 sets of contact lenses because rifampin turned them orange. In addition, a nurse at our hospital experienced an anaphylactic reaction when she took ciprofloxacin as prophylaxis after an exposure.

Bordetella pertussis

The whole-cell pertussis vaccines dramatically altered the epidemiology of pertussis. Before the vaccines were introduced, most adults were immune to pertussis because they had the disease during childhood and their immunity was probably boosted by frequent exposures to infected persons. However, most adults are now susceptible to pertussis because vaccine-induced immunity disappears within 12 years after the last vaccination.[155] Consequently, the incidence of pertussis in adults is now increasing,[156-160] and adolescents and adults have become the primary source of infection for susceptible young children.[159] In the United States the proportion of persons over 10 years of age who acquire pertussis increased from 7.2% during 1992 to 1994 to over 50% during 1997 to 2000.[161]

Pertussis has been transmitted in the hospital by patients, visitors, and HCWs.[162-171] In 1 nosocomial outbreak, a nurse's aide suggested that a pediatric resident might have pertussis, but the physicians discounted her astute diagnosis.[162] Outbreaks also have occurred in other healthcare institutions, including homes for handicapped persons[172-174] and a nursing home.[160] During the outbreak in the nursing home, 11 (10%) of 107 residents and 17 (14%) of 116 employees developed clinical or laboratory-confirmed pertussis infection.[160] The mean age of persons with clinical infection was 75 years for residents and 34 years for employees. Recently, Wright et al reported the results of a study in which they followed 106 resident physicians and 39 emergency room physicians over time to see if their antibody levels to pertussis toxin and filamentous hemagglutinin increased 50% (diagnostic of pertussis infection) over a 1- to 3-year follow-up period.[171] Two residents (1.3%; CI95, 0% to 3.5%) and 3 emergency physicians (3.6% CI95, 0% to 9.6%) had serologic evidence of recent pertussis infection. Only 2 of these 5 physicians had symptomatic illnesses.

Most adults with pertussis have persistent and perhaps severe cough. These adults frequently are diagnosed as having bronchitis. Thus, many exposures are not identified. Several studies indicate that erythromycin treatment early in the course of illness decreases the frequency of secondary spread.[173-175] However, physicians rarely see adult patients early in their illness.

Several communities have experienced outbreaks of pertussis in the last few years.[174,176] Patients involved in these outbreaks have caused exposures when they were evaluated in clinics or were admitted to a hospital. We think that nosocomial outbreaks will occur in the future unless a pertussis vaccine for adults becomes available. Table 11-1 illustrates how infection control personnel could evaluate an exposure to a person with whooping cough.[5,177]

Group A Streptococcus

Although not typically considered a disease warranting postexposure intervention, there have been 3 recent reports of outbreaks that affected HCWs.[178-180] These outbreaks demonstrate that group A streptococcus can spread quickly to both patients and HCWs. To our knowledge there are no guidelines for treating HCWs who have been exposed to patients with streptococcal infections. However, given that group A streptococcus is on occasion transmitted to HCWs, we think that prophylaxis may be appropriate under some circumstances.

Ectoparasites

Infection control personnel also must investigate exposures to ectoparasites such as lice and scabies.[181] We have found that HCWs often react more hysterically to these exposures than they do to exposures involving infectious agents. In fact, HCWs frequently demand prophylactic treatment when it is not necessary. One of the authors remembers a nurse who did not meet the criteria for exposure to lice. When infection control personnel refused to recommend a pediculicide, the nurse had her private physician prescribe Kwell (Reedco, Inc, Humacao, Puerto Rico). The nurse subsequently developed a severe cutaneous allergic reaction that took weeks to resolve.

Lice

Pediculus humanus capitis, *Pediculus humanus corporis*, and *Phthirus pubis* are found not infrequently on patients who have been admitted to HCFs. These ectoparasites are transmitted by direct contact with infested persons or their clothing. Persons infested with lice should be placed on contact precautions until they have been treated.[12,182] All clothing, bedding, hats, and other personal-care items should be washed in hot water and dried on the hot cycle because lice and their eggs cannot survive temperatures above 53.5°C.[9] Clothes that cannot be washed should be dry cleaned or placed in a plastic bag for 2 weeks.[9] Brushes and combs should be soaked in a pediculicide shampoo.[5] HCWs who have had direct contact with the patient's head (head lice) or clothes (body lice) should be evaluated by personnel in the employee health clinic. Because the risk of acquiring lice in a HCF is very low, only staff members who become infested should be treated with a pediculicide.

Scabies

In contrast to lice, *Sarcoptes scabiei* can be transmitted easily within HCFs, especially if the index case has crusted (Norwegian) scabies.[183-198] Van Vliet et al identified 34 reports of 44 scabies outbreaks published between 1976 and 1996, [190] and we identified 9 articles published between 1996 and 2002.[191-198] Of note, 4 of the 8 outbreaks that we identified occurred because patients with human immunodeficiency syndrome and unrecognized Norwegian (crusted or keratotic) scabies were admitted without the necessary precautions.[187,192,195,197]

Such exposures can be quite expensive. For example, an outbreak of scabies occurred in an extended-care unit that was attached to an acute-care hospital. To terminate the outbreak, 78 residents and over 100 staff and family members were treated at a cost of more than $20,000.[189] Scabies spread within the unit, in part because the protocol for control of this ectoparasite was inadequate. The policy was based on the assumption that all staff members would know what to do because they would have had previous experience with scabies exposures.[189] The outbreak described by Obasanjo et al was enormous (773 HCWs and 204 patients were exposed) and was not terminated until precautions beyond those recommended by CDC were implemented.[193] These precautions included early identification of infested patients, prophylactic topical treatment of all exposed HCWs, 2 treatments for patients with Norwegian scabies, barrier isolation precautions until 24 hours after the second treatment, and oral ivermectin treatment for patients who failed conventional therapy. van Vliet et al identified 6 reasons for spread of scabies in HCFs: (1) many patients who have scabies are at risk of developing Norwegian scabies, (2) many people have contact with these patients, (3) diagnosis is often delayed, (4) the epidemiologic evaluation is often inadequate, (5) treatment failures occur, and (6) follow-up is often inadequate.[190]

Persons with scabies should be placed on contact isolation precautions until they are treated.[12] Personnel who have cared for patients with Norwegian scabies or during outbreaks of scabies when transmission continues to occur should be evaluated in the employee health clinic, and those who had contact with the patient's skin should be treated. In "routine" cases of scabies (ie, noncrusted scabies and non-outbreak situation), exposed HCWs should be treated only if they acquire scabies. If 2 or more persons who live or work in a LTCF acquire scabies, all residents and employees should be treated to prevent further spread. Persons receiving effective therapy may have pruritus for up to 2 weeks after therapy. Thus, infection control personnel should not interpret pruritus occurring during this time period as treatment failure.

The index patient's bedding and clothes that contacted the patient's skin should be washed in hot water and dried on the hot cycle.[5] Clothes that cannot be washed can be stored in a plastic bag for several days to a week, because the mite cannot survive more than 3 to 4 days in the environment.[5]

Emerging Pathogens

Just when it seems that we in infection control have survived one crisis and are ready to restore some normalcy, a new disease emerges and upsets our fragile equilibrium. We anticipate that more organisms of epidemiologic import within HCFs will emerge as the global population continues to grow and as world travel remains rapid and common. We chose to discuss 3 viral diseases in this category because infection control staff in the United States have had to spend considerable time dealing with each of them in the last few months.

Smallpox

Smallpox is a serious, contagious, and sometimes fatal infectious disease. Although smallpox was declared globally eradicated in 1980, many people are concerned that smallpox virus may be used for bioterrorism. There is no specific treatment for smallpox disease and the only prevention is vaccination. The smallpox vaccine, which was routinely administered to Americans until 1972, is highly effective in protecting against the disease when given before or shortly after exposure to the virus. Though protection by the live vaccinia virus is long lived and may prevent death from illness in those who were vaccinated over 2 decades ago, all children and most adults are now considered susceptible unless they were recently vaccinated.[199,200] Because of concerns that smallpox could be used as a bioweapon, a program of pre-event vaccination took place in many hospitals in early 2003.[201-204] This allows for recently vaccinated personnel to care for smallpox patients (or patients with suspected smallpox) and to vaccinate other HCWs.

If smallpox virus was released into the community, one would expect transmission to occur as an infected person's fever peaks and the skin rash starts. Persons with smallpox are occasionally contagious during the prodrome phase but they become more contagious with the onset of the rash. Fever usually begins 10 to 14 days after the initial infection (range 7 to 19 days) and the rash typically occurs about 2 to 4 days later.[199,200] Infectious particles are released when oropharyngeal lesions are sloughed (approximately 1 week duration). Transmission via contact with material from the smallpox pustules or crusted scabs can also occur; however, scabs are much less infectious than respiratory secretions. Generally, direct and fairly prolonged face-to-face contact is required to spread smallpox virus from one person to another. Smallpox also can be spread through direct contact with infected bodily fluids or contaminated objects such as bedding or clothing. Rarely, smallpox has been spread by airborne route in enclosed settings such as buildings, buses, and trains.

A HCW would be considered exposed to smallpox if he or she had unprotected contact with an infected case (no N-95 respirator worn within 7 feet and/or no gloves for contact with lesions). Follow-up would include monitoring the HCW's temperature twice daily for 17 days following last exposure date (including vaccination days). It is likely that HCWs exposed to a case of smallpox would be quarantined and that infection control guidelines created by public health officials at the time will direct management of smallpox exposures. At present, infection control and public health personnel disagree about whether HCWs who have had the smallpox vaccine should be restricted from patient care. The official guidelines do not recommend special precautions but many infection control experts disagree.

Severe Acute Respiratory Syndrome

Worldwide, numerous HCWs and patients acquired SARS in HCFs.[205] In fact, HCFs amplified transmission beyond that seen in the community. In general, transmission appears to have occurred after close contact with symptomatic individuals before infection control measures were implemented or if breaches in infection control practices were noted. Studies indicate that appropriate use of masks or respirators, gowns, and hand hygiene significantly decreased the risk of acquiring SARS while caring for patients with SARS[206]; however, some HCWs did acquire SARS despite wearing appropriate protective equipment (gown, mask, goggles or face shield, and gloves) while helping intubate patients with SARS.[207]

The incubation period for SARS ranges from 2 to 10 days, but most patients develop symptoms around day 4 or 5.[208,209] To manage SARS exposures, infection control staff need mechanisms for monitoring healthcare personnel for fever and respiratory symptoms, managing asymptomatic exposed HCWs, symptomatic exposed HCWs, and symptomatic exposed visitors.[210] The definition of a SARS exposure will likely continue to change. Thus, infection control personnel should check the CDC's Web site for current definitions if they think an exposure may have occurred. During the first SARS outbreak in 2003, CDC did not recommend work restrictions for asymptomatic exposed persons unless they had unprotected high-risk exposures. CDC did recommend that exposed HCWs be monitored for respiratory symptoms and fever (ie, check temperature twice daily) for 10 days following their last exposure. If fever or respiratory symptoms develop, the HCW should notify their healthcare provider, restrict their movements outside their home, and reassess the situation in 72 hours. However, a number of hospitals took a more restrictive approach, such as placing HCWs who have unprotected exposure to SARS on leave for 10 days from the last date of exposure.

CDC recommended that HCWs who have unprotected high-risk exposures should be excluded from duty for 10 days following the exposure. An unprotected high-risk exposure is defined as being present in the room when a probable SARS patient underwent an aerosol-generating procedure without complying with the recommended infection control precautions. Symptomatic exposed HCWs who develop either fever or respiratory symptoms within 10 days following exposure should be excluded from duty and should be evaluated in a manner that does not expose other persons to the SARS virus. If symptoms improve or resolve in 72 hours after onset of symptoms, the person may be allowed to return to duty after consultation with infection control and local public health staff. For persons who progress to meet the case definition of SARS, infection control precautions should be continued until 10 days after fever and respiratory symptoms have resolved.

To prevent exposures within HCFs, the infection control staff should consider designing a process for screening HCWs who traveled to areas where the SARS virus is being transmitted. In addition, symptomatic exposed visitors should not be allowed to visit their family member or friend but should be evaluated to determine whether they may have SARS. Thus, infection control personnel must design a way to identify visitors who might have been exposed and to screen them for symptoms and signs of SARS. To prevent transmission within exposed HCW's homes, infection control personnel should counsel exposed persons to avoid contact with members of their household members (ie, avoid physical contact, stay in a separate part of the house, avoid eating together, and use separate bathrooms) or to find alternative living arrangements for household members during the 10 days following exposure.

Monkeypox

Monkeypox is a rare viral disease that occurs mostly in central and western Africa. The monkeypox virus belongs to a group of viruses that includes the smallpox virus (variola), the virus used in the smallpox vaccine (vaccinia), and the cowpox virus. In early June 2003, monkeypox was identified in the United States among persons who had contact with ill pet prairie dogs.[211,212] This is the first time that there has been an outbreak of monkeypox in the United States. People can get monkeypox from an animal with monkeypox if they are bitten or if they touch the animal's blood, body fluids, or skin rash. Person-to-person transmission is believed to occur primarily through direct contact with lesions and also by respiratory droplet spread.

CDC's current recommendations do not restrict the activities of HCWs who have unprotected exposures (ie, were not wearing personal protective equipment) to patients with monkeypox. However, these HCWs should measure their temperatures at least twice daily for 21 days following the exposure. Before reporting for duty each day, exposed HCWs should be interviewed to determine whether they have fever or rash. HCWs who have cared for patients with monkeypox and who adhered to recommended infection control precautions do not need to be monitored. HCWs who cared for a patient with monkeypox should monitor themselves for symptoms suggestive of monkeypox for 21 days after they last had contact with a patient who had monkeypox. HCWs who note concerning symptoms should notify staff in infection control and/or employee health and should be evaluated. CDC is updating previous interim guidelines concerning infection control precautions and exposure management in the healthcare and community settings. Interested infection control staff members should consult the CDC Web site for the most current recommendations.

CONCLUSION

Exposure workups are an important responsibility for infection control personnel. If they evaluate exposures promptly and effectively, infection control staff can prevent transmission of infectious agents or ectoparasites to numerous HCWs, patients, and visitors. Exposure workups consume much time and money. In addition, many exposures could be averted if HCWs were immune to vaccine-preventable infections and if staff used isolation precautions. Thus, wise infection control staff members learn from their own experience and develop policies and procedures to limit the number of exposures in their institutions.

ACKNOWLEDGEMENTS

The authors thank Sandra Von Behren, Stacy Coffman, and Daniel Diekema for reviewing the chapter proofs.

TABLE 11-1. BASIC INFORMATION REGARDING AGENTS THAT CAUSE MOST NOSOCOMIAL EXPOSURES

Etiologic Agent	Incubation Period	Diagnostic Criteria	Exposure Criteria	Period of Communicability	Employee Health	Work Restrictions	Prophylaxis
Varicella zoster virus	▲ Usually 14 to 16 days ▲ Range 10 to 21 days ▲ Up to 28 days in persons who received VZIG	▲ Fever and vesicular rash (chickenpox) or grouped vesicular lesions (shingles) ▲ May consult dermatology	_Chickenpox or disseminated zoster_ ▲ Continuous household contact ▲ ≥ 5 minutes face-to-face contact with infected person without wearing a respirator ▲ Direct contact with vesicle fluid without wearing gloves _Shingles_ ▲ Direct contact with vesicle fluid without wearing gloves	_Chickenpox_ ▲ Most contagious 1 to 2 days before and shortly after rash appears ▲ Transmission can occur until all lesions are crusted ▲ Immunocompromised persons may be contagious as long as new lesions are appearing _Shingles_ ▲ 24 hours before the 1st lesion appears and until all lesions are crusted	▲ Assess immunity ▲ HCW susceptible unless: ➢ Has history of chickenpox ➢ Has serologic evidence of immunity ▲ Consider obtaining varicella IgG antibody titer to determine immune status before HCW is exposed	_Exposed_ ▲ Day 1 to 7 no restrictions ▲ Day 8 to 21 for a single exposure or day 8 of 1st exposure through day 21 of last exposure HCW must: ➢ Not work, or ➢ Have no direct patient contact and work only with immune persons away from patient-care areas ▲ Restrict HCW who received VZIG through day 28 _Infected_ ▲ May return to work after all lesions are crusted	▲ Consider giving VZIG to nonimmune, immunocompromised persons within 96 hours of exposure ▲ Consider giving susceptible HCW varicella virus vaccine within 3 days of exposure to prevent or modify infection. Giving the vaccine does not change the work restrictions

TABLE 11-1. BASIC INFORMATION REGARDING AGENTS THAT CAUSE MOST NOSOCOMIAL EXPOSURES (CONTINUED)

Etiologic Agent	Incubation Period	Diagnostic Criteria	Exposure Criteria	Period of Communicability	Employee Health	Work Restrictions	Prophylaxis

Measles virus	➤ Usually 8 to 12 days
	➤ Range 7 to 18 days
		➤ Fever and rash with positive measles IgM antibody titer
		➤ May consult Dermatology
			➤ Spent time in a room with an infected person without wearing a respirator
			➤ If air is recirculated, spent time in the area supplied by the air handling system while infected person was present or within 1 hour after the person's departure
			➤ Contact with nasal or oral secretions from an infected person or items contaminated with these secretions without wearing gloves
				➤ 3 to 5 days before rash to 4 to 7 days after rash appears, but transmission is minimal 2 to 4 days after rash appears
				➤ Immunocompromised persons may be contagious for the duration of the illness
					➤ Assess immunity
					➤ HCW susceptible unless:
					  ➢ Born before 1957*
					  ➢ Provides serologic evidence of immunity
					  ➢ Has 2 documented doses of measles vaccine
					➤ Obtain blood for IgG antibody titers as needed
						Exposed
						➤ Day 1 to 4 no restrictions
						➤ Day 5 to 21 for a single exposure or day 5 of first exposure through day 21 of last exposure exclude HCW from work setting
						Infected
						➤ May return to work 4 days after developing rash
							➤ For staff who haven't received 2 doses of measles vaccine, consider giving MMR within 3 days of exposure to modify infection
							➤ Vaccine or IG given after exposure does not change work restrictions

* A small percentage of HCWs born before 1957 will not be immune to measles.[45] Infection control personnel should determine whether this criterion is appropriate for the staff in their hospital.

TABLE 11-1. BASIC INFORMATION REGARDING AGENTS THAT CAUSE MOST NOSOCOMIAL EXPOSURES (CONTINUED)

Etiologic Agent	Incubation Period	Diagnostic Criteria	Exposure Criteria	Period of Communicability	Employee Health	Work Restrictions	Prophylaxis
Rubella virus	▲ Usually 16 to 18 days ▲ Range 14 to 21 days	▲ Mild febrile exanthem and positive rubella IgM antibody titer ▲ May consult Dermatology	▲ Contact within 3 feet of infected person without wearing a mask ▲ Contact with nasopharyngeal secretions from an infected person or items contaminated with these secretions without wearing gloves ▲ Contact with nasopharyngeal secretions or urine from infant with congenital rubella without wearing gloves	▲ 7 days before rash to 7 days after rash appears ▲ Up to 1 year for infants with congenital rubella	▲ Assess immunity ▲ HCW susceptible unless: ➢ Born before 1957 ➢ Provide serologic evidence of immunity ➢ Has 1 documented dose of rubella vaccine ▲ Obtain blood for IgG antibody titers as needed	<u>Exposed</u> ▲ Day 1 to 6 no restrictions ▲ Day 7 to 21 for a single exposure or day 7 of first exposure through day 21 of last exposure HCW must: ➢ Not work, or ➢ Have no direct patient contact and work only with immune persons away from patient-care areas <u>Infected</u> ▲ May return to work 7 days after developing rash	▲ None ➢ Rubella vaccine does not prevent infection after exposure ➢ IG does not prevent infection

TABLE 11-1. BASIC INFORMATION REGARDING AGENTS THAT CAUSE MOST NOSOCOMIAL EXPOSURES (CONTINUED)

Etiologic Agent	Incubation Period	Diagnostic Criteria	Exposure Criteria	Period of Communicability	Employee Health	Work Restrictions	Prophylaxis
Mumps virus	▲ Usually 16 to 18 days ▲ Range 12 to 25 days	▲ Fever with swelling and tenderness of the salivary glands or testes and positive mumps IgM antibody titer	▲ Contact within 3 feet of infected person without wearing a mask ▲ Contact with saliva or items contaminated with saliva from an infected person without wearing gloves	▲ Most communicable 48 hours before onset of illness, but may begin as early as 7 days before onset of overt parotitis and/or orchitis and continue 5 to 9 days thereafter (average 5)	▲ Assess immunity ▲ HCW susceptible unless: ➤ Born before 1957 ➤ Provide serologic evidence of immunity ➤ Has 1 documented dose of mumps vaccine ▲ Obtain blood for IgG antibody titers as needed	_Exposed_ ▲ Day 1 to 10 no restrictions ▲ Day 11 to 26 for a single exposure or day 11 of first exposure through day 26 of last exposure HCW must: ➤ Not work, or ➤ Have no direct patient contact and work only with immune persons away from patient-care areas _Infected_ ▲ May return to work 9 days after onset of parotid gland swelling	▲ None ➤ Mumps vaccine not proven to prevent infection after exposure ➤ Mumps IG does not prevent infection
Parvovirus B19	▲ Usually 4 to 14 days ▲ Range up to 21 days ▲ Rash and joint symptoms occur 2 to 3 weeks after infection	▲ "Slapped cheek" rash and positive serum parvovirus B19 IgM antibody titer	▲ Criteria have not been defined but probably include: ➤ Close person-to-person contact (within 3 feet) with infected person without wearing a mask ➤ Contact with respiratory secretions from an infected person or items contaminated with these secretions without wearing gloves	▲ Persons are unlikely to be infectious after the onset of rash ▲ Immunocompromised persons can have chronic infections and can shed virus for prolonged periods ▲ Refer a pregnant HCW to her obstetrician	▲ Assess immunity ▲ Obtain blood for IgG antibody titers as needed ▲ Describe signs and symptoms and inform exposed HCWs that they should not work if these symptoms occur	▲ Not necessary	▲ None

TABLE 11-1. BASIC INFORMATION REGARDING AGENTS THAT CAUSE MOST NOSOCOMIAL EXPOSURES (CONTINUED)[9]

Etiologic Agent	Incubation Period	Diagnostic Criteria	Exposure Criteria	Period of Communicability	Employee Health	Work Restrictions	Prophylaxis
Hepatitis A virus	▲ Usually 25 to 30 days ▲ Range 15 to 50 days	▲ Positive hepatitis A IgM antibody	▲ Contact with stool of infected person without wearing gloves ▲ Consuming uncooked food prepared by an infected person	▲ Viral shedding in stool lasts 1 to 3 weeks ▲ Highest viral titers are found in stool 1 to 2 weeks before onset of symptoms ▲ Risk of transmission is minimal 1 week after onset of symptoms	▲ Assess immunity ▲ Obtain blood for IgG antibody titers as needed ▲ Describe signs and symptoms and ask exposed HCW to return to employee health if these occur	_Exposed_ ▲ None _Infected_ ▲ May return to work 7 days after onset of jaundice or other clinical symptoms	▲ Consider giving exposed HCW IG within 2 weeks of exposure
Influenza virus	▲ Usually 1 to 3 days	▲ Influenza-like illness between October and April ▲ Positive diagnostic test for influenza	▲ Contact within 3 feet of infected person without wearing a mask ▲ Direct contact with secretions from respiratory tract of infected person or items contaminated with these secretions without wearing gloves	▲ Most infectious 24 hours before onset of symptoms ▲ Viral shedding usually ceases within 7 days but can persist longer in children	▲ Assess immunization status ▲ Discuss risks and benefits of chemoprophylaxis ▲ Describe signs and symptoms and inform HCWs that they should not work if these symptoms occur	_Exposed_ ▲ Have not been defined for nonimmune HCW exposed to persons with influenza _Infected_ ▲ Ill HCW should not work	▲ Consider vaccinating exposed nonimmune HCW ▲ Amantidine or rimantadine 100 mg twice per day for adults exposed to influenza A only ▲ Oseltamivir 75 mg twice daily for adults exposed to influenza A or B

TABLE 11-1. BASIC INFORMATION REGARDING AGENTS THAT CAUSE MOST NOSOCOMIAL EXPOSURES (CONTINUED)

Etiologic Agent	Incubation Period	Diagnostic Criteria	Exposure Criteria	Period of Communicability	Employee Health	Work Restrictions	Prophylaxis
Creutzfeldt-Jakob agent[†‡]	▲ 15 months to > 30 years	▲ Progressive dementia ▲ Recipient cadaver-derived-pituitary hormones ▲ Family history of prion disease	▲ Criteria have not been defined but probably include the following if source patient is diagnosed with CJD or has risk factors for CJD: ‡ ➢ Puncture or cut with instruments contaminated with patient's blood or cerebrospinal fluid ➢ Handling cerebrospinal fluid or tissue from brain, spinal cord, or eye without gloves ➢ HCWs working in the operating room, autopsy suite, ophthalmology department, pathology laboratory, or microbiology laboratory have the highest risk of exposure ▲ Routine patient care poses a very low risk to HCW	▲ Unknown, but probably during symptomatic illness and an undetermined period before symptoms appear	▲ Educate employee about CJD and risk of transmission ▲ Counsel employee using data from the literature indicating that the risk of transmission is very low	▲ None	▲ None

† These precautions should be used for persons who have CJD; progressive dementia; or a family history of prion disease, CJD, Gerstmann-Sträussler-Scheinker syndrome, or fatal familial insomnia.

‡ Data from a study with mice suggest that prions might be transmitted by contact of infected blood or CSF with mucous membranes.213 No data are available with humans to support or refute the data from mice.

TABLE 11-1. BASIC INFORMATION REGARDING AGENTS THAT CAUSE MOST NOSOCOMIAL EXPOSURES (CONTINUED)

Etiologic Agent	Incubation Period	Diagnostic Criteria	Exposure Criteria	Period of Communicability	Employee Health	Work Restrictions	Prophylaxis
M. tuberculosis	▲ 2 to 12 weeks from exposure to detection of positive TST ▲ Risk of developing active disease is greatest in first 2 years after infection	▲ MTB or AFB found in respiratory secretions or wound drainage	▲ Spent time in a room with a person who has active disease without wearing a respirator ▲ Packing or irrigating wounds infected with *M. tuberculosis* without wearing a respirator	▲ Persons are considered infectious if they: ➤ Are coughing ➤ Are undergoing cough-inducing or aerosol-generating procedures ➤ Have sputum smears that are positive for acid-fast bacilli ➤ Are not receiving therapy ➤ Have just started therapy ➤ Have poor clinical response to therapy ▲ Persons are considered infectious until they are on effective antituberculosis chemotherapy, respond to therapy, and have 3 consecutive negative sputum smears ▲ Children with primary pulmonary TB are rarely contagious	▲ Obtain baseline TST within 2 weeks of exposure if HCW previously negative ▲ Perform postexposure TST at 12 weeks ▲ Prescribe treatment if postexposure TST is positive	*Exposed* ▲ None for persons whose TST becomes positive *Infected* ▲ Restrict HCWs with active TB until they are on effective antituberculosis chemotherapy, respond to therapy, and have 3 consecutive negative sputum smears	▲ Isoniazid 300 mg daily for 9 mos Pyridoxine 25 to 50 mg daily may be added for persons with conditions in which neuropathy is common ▲ Refer to CDC's Core Curriculum on Tuberculosis for alternative treatment options

TABLE 11-1. BASIC INFORMATION REGARDING AGENTS THAT CAUSE MOST NOSOCOMIAL EXPOSURES (CONTINUED)

Etiologic Agent	Incubation Period	Diagnostic Criteria	Exposure Criteria	Period of Communicability	Employee Health	Work Restrictions	Prophylaxis
N. meningitidis	▲ Usually <4 days ▲ Range 1 to 10 days	▲ Clinical signs of sepsis, meningitis, or pneumonia, and gram-negative diplococci in blood, CSF, or sputum	▲ Extensive contact with respiratory secretions from an infected person without wearing a mask, particularly during ≻ Suctioning ≻ Resuscitation ≻ Intubation ≻ Extensive oral or pharyngeal exam	▲ Persons are infectious until they have taken 24 hours of effective antibiotic therapy	▲ Prescribe prophylaxis ▲ Educate exposed HCW about signs and symptoms of meningitis	<u>Exposed</u> ▲ None	1 of the following: ▲ Ciprofloxacin 500 mg, single dose (contraindicated in pregnancy) ▲ Rifampin 600 mg every 12 hours for 2 days (contraindicated in pregnancy) ▲ Ceftriaxone 250 mg IM, single dose (safe during pregnancy)
Bordetella pertussis	▲ Usually 7 to 10 days ▲ Range 6 to 20 days	▲ Paroxysmal cough, other respiratory symptoms, or inspiratory whoop with positive DFA, culture, PCR, or serology for *B. pertussis*	▲ Contact within 3 feet of infected person without wearing a mask ▲ Direct contact with respiratory tract secretions from infected persons or items contaminated with these secretions without wearing gloves	▲ Most contagious during the catarrhal state ▲ Communicability diminishes rapidly after onset of cough, but can persist as long as 3 weeks	▲ If HCW has no symptoms, begin prophylaxis and return to work ▲ If HCW symptomatic, begin therapy and relieve from work	<u>Exposed</u> ▲ No restrictions <u>Infected</u> ▲ HCW may return to work after taking at least 5 days of therapy	▲ Recommended drug is erythromycin 40 mg/kg/day in 4 divided doses (maximum 2 gm/day) for 14 days (estolate preparation preferred) ▲ Azithromycin 500 mg per day for 5 days may be tolerated better than erythromycin

TABLE 11-1. BASIC INFORMATION REGARDING AGENTS THAT CAUSE MOST NOSOCOMIAL EXPOSURES (CONTINUED)

Etiologic Agent	Incubation Period	Diagnostic Criteria	Exposure Criteria	Period of Communicability	Employee Health	Work Restrictions	Prophylaxis
Lice	▲ 6 to 10 days	▲ Live lice or nits (eggs) on hair shaft <0.5" from skin ▲ May consult Dermatology	▲ Head lice: Hair-to-hair contact with infested person ▲ Body lice: Contact with linen or clothes of infested person without wearing gloves ▲ Pubic lice: Sexual contact	▲ As long as lice or eggs remain alive on infested person, clothing, or personal items ▲ Survival time for lice away from the host ➢ 10 days for head lice ➢ 10 days for body lice ➢ 2 days for pubic lice ▲ Nits ≥10 mm from scalp have been present ≥2 weeks and may not be viable	▲ Treat HCW only if infested	_Exposed_ ▲ No restrictions _Infested_ ▲ Immediate restriction until 24 hours after treatment	▲ Not recommended
Scabies	▲ 4 to 5 weeks if no previous infestation ▲ 1 to 4 days if previous infestation	▲ Burrows or papular lesions in classic body sites and intense itching at night ▲ May consult Dermatology	▲ Prolonged, close personal contact ▲ Minimal direct contact with crusted scabies (Norwegian) can result in transmission	▲ Transmission can occur before the onset of symptoms ▲ Person remains contagious until treated	▲ Prescribe scabicide for all HCWs exposed to persons with crusted scabies ▲ Pregnant women should not use lindane	_Exposed_ ▲ No restriction _Infested_ ▲ Immediate restriction until 24 hours after treatment	▲ Drug of choice: ➢ 5% Permethrin ▲ Alternative drugs: ➢ Lindane ➢ 10% Crotamiton

Abbreviations: VZIG, Varicella-Zoster Immune Globulin; HCW, HCW; IgG, immunoglobulin G; MMR, measles, mumps, and rubella vaccine; IG, immune globulin; CJD, Creutzfeldt-Jakob disease; TST, tuberculin skin test; AFB, acid-fast bacilli; TB, tuberculosis; IM, intramuscular

Adapted from Mandell GL, Bennett JE, Dolin R, eds. *Principles and Practice of Infectious Diseases.* 5th ed. New York, NY: Churchill Livingstone; 2000.

REFERENCES

1. Weltman AC, DiFerdinando GT, Washko R, Lipsky WM. A death associated with therapy for nosocomially acquired multidrug-resistant tuberculosis. *Chest*. 1996;110:279-281.

2. Weber DJ, Rutala WA, Parham C. Impact and costs of varicella prevention in a university hospital. *Am J Public Health*. 1988;78:19-23.

3. Faoagali JL, Darcy R. Chicken pox outbreak among the staff of a large, urban adult hospital: costs of monitoring and control. *Am J Infect Control*. 1995;23:247-250.

4. Christie CDC, Glover AM, Willke MJ, Marx ML, Reising SF, Hutchinson NM. Containment of pertussis in the regional pediatric hospital during the greater Cincinnati epidemic of 1993. *Infect Control Hosp Epidemiol*. 1995;16:556-563.

5. Committee on Infectious Diseases, American Academy of Pediatrics. *2000 Red Book: Report of the Committee on Infectious Diseases*. 25th ed. Elk Grove Village, Ill: American Academy of Pediatrics; 2000.

6. Chin J. *Control of Communicable Diseases Manual*. 17th ed. Washington, DC: American Public Health Association; 2000.

7. Bolyard EA, Tablan OC, Williams WW, et al. Guideline for infection control in health care personnel, 1998. *Infect Control Hosp Epidemiol*. 1998;19:407-463.

8. The Advisory Committee on Immunization Practices. Recommended adult immunization schedule United States, 2002-2003 and Recommended immunizations for adults with medical conditions United States, 2002-2003. *MMWR*. 2002;51:904-908.

9. Mandell GL, Bennett JE, Dolin R, eds. *Principles and Practice of Infectious Diseases*. 5th ed. New York, NY: Churchill Livingstone; 2000.

10. Valenti WM. Employee work restrictions for infection control. *Infect Control*. 1984;5:583-584.

11. Meyers MG, Rasley DA, Hierholzer WJ. Hospital infection control for varicella-zoster virus infection. *Pediatrics*. 1982;70:199-202.

12. Garner JS. Hospital Infection Control Practices Advisory Committee. Guideline for isolation precautions in hospitals. *Infect Control Hosp Epidemiol*. 1996;17:53-80.

13. Sepkowitz KA. Occupationally acquired infections in HCWs. Part I. *Ann Intern Med*. 1996;125:826-834.

14. McKinney WP, Horowitz MM, Battiola RJ. Susceptibility of hospital-based health care personnel to varicella-zoster virus infections. *Am J Infect Control*. 1989;17:26-30.

15. Zimmerman L, Fajardo M, Seward J, Ludwig S, Johnson J, Wharton M. Varicella susceptibility and validity of history among US Coast Guard recruits: an outbreak-based study. *Military Medicine*. 2003;168:404-407.

16. Haiduven DJ, Hench CP, Stevens DA. Postexposure varicella management of nonimmune personnel: an alternative approach. *Infect Control Hosp Epidemiol*. 1994;15:329-334.

17. Hayden GF, Meyers JD, Dixon RE. Nosocomial varicella. part II: suggested guidelines for management. *West J Med*. 1979;130:300-303.

18. Galil K, Lee B, Strine T, et al. Outbreak of varicella at a day-care center despite vaccination. *N Engl J Med*. 2002;347:1909-1915.

19. Galil K, Fair E, Mountcastle N, Britz P, Seward J. Younger age at vaccination may increase risk of varicella vaccine failure. *J Infect Dis*. 2002;186:102-105.

20. Saiman L, LaRussa P, Steinberg SP, et al. Persistence of immunity to varicella-zoster virus after vaccination of HCWs. *Infect Control Hosp Epidemiol*. 2001;22:279-283.

21. Wurtz R, Check IJ. Breakthrough varicella infection in a HCW despite immunity after varicella vaccination. *Infect Control Hosp Epidemiol*. 1999;20:561-562.

22. Richard VS, John TJ, Kenneth J, Ramaprabha P, Kuruvilla PJ, Chandy GM. Should health care workers in the tropics be immunized against varicella? *J Hosp Infect*. 2001;47:243-245.

23. Weinstock DM, Rogers M, Lim S, Eagan J, Sepkowitz KA. Seroconversion rates in HCWs using a latex agglutination assay after varicella virus vaccination. *Infect Control Hosp Epidemiol*. 1999;20:504-507.

24. Nettleman MD, Schmid M. Controlling varicella in the healthcare setting: the cost effectiveness of using varicella vaccine in HCWs. *Infect Control Hosp Epidemiol*. 1997;18:504-508.

25. Tennenberg AM, Brassard JE, Van Lieu J, Drusin LM. Varicella vaccination for HCWs at a university hospital: an analysis of costs and benefits. *Infect Control Hosp Epidemiol*. 1997;18:405-411.

26. Howell MR, Lee T, Gaydos CA, Nang RN. The cost-effectiveness of varicella screening and vaccination in US Army recruits. *Mil Med*. 2000;165:309-315.

27. Weitekamp MR, Schan P, Aber RC. An algorithm for the control of nosocomial varicella-zoster virus infection. *Am J Infect Control*. 1985;13:193-198.

28. Bloch AB, Orenstein WA, Ewing WM, et al. Measles outbreak in a pediatric practice: airborne transmission in an office setting. *Pediatrics*. 1985;75:676-683.

29. Remington PL, Hall WN, Davis IH, Herald A, Gunn RA. Airborne transmission of measles in a physician's office. *JAMA*. 1985;253:1574-1577.

30. Seo SK, Malak SF, Lim S, Eagan J, Sepkowitz KA. Prevalence of measles antibody among young adult HCWs in a cancer hospital: 1980s versus 1998-1999. *Infect Control Hosp Epidemiol*. 2002;23:276-278.

31. Davis RM, Orenstein WA, Frank JA, et al. Transmission of measles in medical settings. 1980 through 1984. *JAMA*. 1986;255:1295-1298.

32. Istre GR, McKee PA, West GR, et al. Measles spread in medical settings: an important focus of disease transmission? *Pediatrics*. 1987;79:356-358.

33. Williams WW, Atkinson WL, Holmes SJ, Orenstein WA. Nosocomial measles, mumps, rubella, and other viral infections. In: Mayhall CG, ed. *Hospital Epidemiology and Infection Control*. Baltimore, Md: Williams & Wilkins; 1996:523-535.

34. Edmonson MB, Addiss DG, McPherson Berg JL, Circo SR, Davis JP. Mild measles and secondary vaccine failure during a sustained outbreak in a highly vaccinated population. *JAMA*. 1990;263:2467-2471.

35. Atkinson WL, Markowitz LE, Adams NC, Seastrom GR. Transmission of measles in medical settings-United States, 1985-1989. *Am J Med*. 1991;91:320S-324S.

36. Raad II, Sherertz RJ, Rains CS, et al. The importance of nosocomial transmission of measles in the propagation of a community outbreak. *Infect Control Hosp Epidemiol*. 1989;10:161-166.

37. Sienko DG, Friedman C, McGee, et al. A measles outbreak at university medical settings involving health care providers. *Am J Public Health*. 1987;77:1222-1224.

38. Rivera ME, Mason WH, Ross LA, Wright HT. Nosocomial measles infection in a pediatric hospital during a community-wide epidemic. *J Pediatr*. 1991;119:183-186.

39. Rank EL, Brettman L, Katz-Pollack H, DeHertogh D, Neville D. Chronology of a hospital-wide measles outbreak: lessons learned and shared from an extraordinary week in late March 1989. *Am J Infect Control*. 1992;20:315-318.

40. Farizo KM, Stehr-Green PA, Simpson DM, Markowitz LE. Pediatric emergency room visits: a risk factor for acquiring measles. *Pediatrics*. 1991;87:74-79.

41. Weber DJ, Rutala WA, Orenstein WA. Prevention of mumps, measles and rubella among hospital personnel. *J Pediatr*. 1991;119:322-326.

42. Subbarao EK, Andrews-Mann L, Amin S, Greenberg J, Kumar ML. Postexposure prophylaxis for measles in a neonatal intensive care unit. *J Pediatr*. 1990;117:782-785.

43. Ammari LK, Bell LM, Hodinka RL. Secondary measles vaccine failure in HCWs exposed to infected patients. *Infect Control Hosp Epidemiol*. 1993;14:81-86.

44. Enguidanos R, Mascola L, Frederick P. A survey of hospital infection control policies and employee measles cases during Los Angeles County's measles epidemic, 1987 to 1989. *Am J Infect Control*. 1992;20:301-304.

45. Wright LJ, Carlquist JF. Measles immunity in employees of a multihospital healthcare provider. *Infect Control Hosp Epidemiol*. 1994;15:8-11.

46. de Swart RL, Wertheim-van Dillen PM, van Binnendijk RS, Muller CP, Frenkel J, Osterhaus AD. Measles in a Dutch hospital introduced by an immuno-compromised infant from Indonesia infected with a new virus genotype. *Lancet*. 2000;355:201-202.

47. Steingart KR, Thomas AR, Dykewicz CA, Redd SC. Transmission of measles virus in healthcare settings during a community-wide outbreak. *Infect Control Hosp Epidemiol*. 1999;20:115-119.

48. Marshall TM, Hlatswayo D, Schoub B. Nosocomial outbreaks—a potential threat to the elimination of measles? *J Infect Dis*. 2003;187:S97-S101.

49. Kelly HA, Riddell MA, Andrews RM. Measles transmission in healthcare settings in Australia. *Med J Aust*. 2002;176:50-51.

50. Greaves WL, Orenstein WA, Stetler HC, Preblud SR, Hinnman AR, Bart KJ. Prevention of rubella transmission in medical facilities. *JAMA*. 1982;248:861-864.

51. Polk BF, White JA, DeGirolami PC, Modlin JF. An outbreak of rubella among hospital personnel. *N Engl J Med*. 1980;303:541-545.

52. Centers for Disease Control and Prevention. Rubella in hospitals—California. *MMWR*. 1983;32:37-39.

53. Poland GA, Nichol KL. Medical students as sources of rubella and measles outbreaks. *Arch Intern Med*. 1990;150:44-46.

54. Storch GA, Gruber C, Benz B, Beaudoin J, Hayes J. A rubella outbreak among dental students: description of the outbreak and analysis of control measures. *Infect Control*. 1985;6:150-156.

55. Strassburg MA, Stephenson TG, Habel LA, Fannin SL. Rubella in hospital employees. *Infect Control*. 1984;5:123-126.

56. Fliegel PE, Weinstein WM. Rubella outbreak in a prenatal clinic: management and prevention. *Am J Infect Control*. 1982;10:29-33.

57. Strassburg MA, Imagawa DT, Fannin SL, et al. Rubella outbreak among hospital employees. *Obstet Gynecol*. 1981;57:283-288.

58. Gladstone JL, Millian SJ. Rubella exposure in an obstetric clinic. *Obstet Gynecol*. 1981;57:182-186.

59. Reef SE, Frey TK, Theall K, et al. The changing epidemiology of rubella in the 1990s: on the verge of elimination and new challenges for control and prevention. *JAMA*. 2002;287:464-472.

60. Anonymous. Control and prevention of rubella: evaluation and management of suspected outbreaks, rubella in pregnant women, and surveillance for congenital rubella syndrome. *MMWR*. 2001;50:1-23.

61. Sheridan E, Aitken C, Jeffries D, Hird M, Thayalasekaran P. Congenital rubella syndrome: a risk in immigrant populations. *Lancet*. 2002;359:674-675.

62. Wharton M, Cochi SL, Hutcheson RH, Schaffner W. Mumps transmission in hospitals. *Arch Intern Med*. 1990;150:47-49.

63. Fischer PR, Brunetti C, Welch V, Christenson JC. Nosocomial mumps: report of an outbreak and its control. *Am J Infect Control*. 1996;24:13-18.

64. Nichol KL, Olson R. Medical students' exposure and immunity to vaccine-preventable diseases. *Arch Intern Med*. 1993;153:1913-1916.

65. Lui SL, Luk WK, Cheung CY, Chan TM, Lai KN, Peiris JS. Nosocomial outbreak of parvovirus B19 infection in a renal transplant unit. *Transplantation*. 2001;71:59-64.

66. Dowell SF, Torok TJ, Thorp JA, et al. Parvovirus B19 infection in hospital workers: community or hospital acquisition? *J Infect Dis*. 1995;172:1076-1079.

67. Bell LM, Naides SJ, Stoffman P, Hodinka RL, Plotkin SA. Human parvovirus B19 infection among hospital staff members after contact with infected patients. *N Engl J Med*. 1989;321:485-491.

68. Seng C, Watkins P, Morse D, et al. Parvovirus B19 outbreak on an adult ward. *Epidemiol Infect*. 1994;113:345-353.

69. Ray SM, Erdman DD, Berschling JD, Cooper JE, Torok TJ, Blumberg HM. Nosocomial exposure to parvovirus B19: low risk of transmission to HCWs. *Infect Control Hosp Epidemiol*. 1997;18:109-114.

70. Shishiba T, Matsunaga Y. An outbreak of erythema infectiosum among hospital staff members including a patient with pleural fluid and pericardial effusion. *J Am Acad Dermatol*. 1993;29:265-267.

71. Miyamoto K, Ogami M, Takahashi Y, et al. Outbreak of human parvovirus B19 in hospital workers. *J Hosp Infect*. 2000;45:238-241.

72. Crowcroft NS, Roth CE, Cohen BJ, Miller E. Guidance for control of parvovirus B19 infection in healthcare settings and the community. *J Public Health Med*. 1999;21:439-446.

73. Lohiya GS, Stewart K, Perot K, Widman R. Parvovirus B19 outbreak in a developmental center. *Am J Infect Control*. 1995;23:373-376.

74. Adler SP, Manganello AM, Koch WC, Hempfling SH, Best AM. Risk of human parvovirus B19 infections among school and hospital employees during endemic periods. *J Infect Dis*. 1993;168:361-368.

75. Centers for Disease Control and Prevention. Risks associated with human parvovirus B19 infection. *MMWR*. 1989;38:81-88, 93-97.

76. Cartter ML, Farley TA, Rosengren S, et al. Occupational risk factors for infection with parvovirus B19 among pregnant women. *J Infect Dis*. 1991;163:282-285.

77. Noble RC, Kane MA, Reeves SA, Roeckel I. Posttransfusion hepatitis A in a neonatal intensive care unit. *JAMA*. 1984;252:2711-2715.

78. Azimi PH, Roberto RR, Guralnik J, et al. Transfusion-acquired hepatitis A in a premature infant with secondary nosocomial spread in an intensive care nursery. *Am J Dis Child*. 1986;140:23-27.

79. Giacoia GP, Kasprisin DO. Transfusion-acquired hepatitis A. *South Med J*. 1989;82:1357-1360.

80. Seeberg S, Brandberg A, Hermodsson S, Larsson P, Lundgren S. Hospital outbreak of hepatitis A secondary to blood exchange in a baby. *Lancet*. 1981;1:1155-1156.

81. Klein BS, Michaels JA, Rytel MW, Berg KG, Davis JP. Nosocomial hepatitis A. A multinursery outbreak in Wisconsin. *JAMA*. 1984;252:2716-2721.

82. Rosenblum LS, Villarino ME, Nainan OV, et al. Hepatitis A outbreak in a neonatal intensive care unit: risk factors for transmission and evidence of prolonged viral excretion among preterm infants. *J Infect Dis*. 1991;164:476-482.

83. Burkholder BT, Coronado VG, Brown J, et al. Nosocomial transmission of hepatitis A in a pediatric hospital traced to an anti-hepatitis A virus-negative patient with immunodeficiency. *Pediatr Infect Dis J*. 1995;14:261-266.

84. Drusin LM, Sohmer M, Groshen SL, Spiritos MD, Senterfit LB, Christenson WN. Nosocomial hepatitis A infection in a pediatric intensive care unit. *Arch Dis Child*. 1987;62:690-695.

85. Reed CM, Gustafson TL, Siegel J, Duer P. Nosocomial transmission of hepatitis A from a hospital-acquired case. *Pediatr Infect Dis J*. 1984;3:300-303.

86. Krober MS, Bass JW, Brown JD, Lemon SM, Rupert KJ. Hospital outbreak of hepatitis A: risk factors for spread. *Pediatr Infect Dis J*. 1984;3:296-299.

87. Orenstein WA, Wu E, Wilkins J, et al. Hospital-acquired hepatitis A: report of an outbreak. *Pediatrics*. 1981;67:494-497.

88. Edgar WM, Campbell AD. Nosocomial infection with hepatitis A. *J Infect*. 1985;10:43-47.

89. Goodman RA, Carder CC, Allen JR, Orenstein WA, Finton RJ. Nosocomial hepatitis A transmission by an adult patient with diarrhea. *Am J Med*. 1982;73:220-226.

90. Petrosillo N, Raffaele B, Martini L, et al. A nosocomial and occupational cluster of hepatitis A virus infection in a pediatric ward. *Infect Control Hosp Epidemiol*. 2002;23:343-345.

91. Jensenius M, Ringertz SH, Berild D, Bell H, Espinoza R, Grinde B. Prolonged nosomial outbreak of hepatitis A arising from an alcoholic with pneumonia. *Scand J Infect Dis*. 1998;30:119-123.

92. Hanna JN, Loewenthal MR, Negel P, Wenck DJ. An outbreak of hepatitis A in an intensive care unit. *Anaesth Intensive Care*. 1996;24:440-444.

93. Doebbeling BN, Li N, Wenzel RP. An outbreak of hepatitis A among health care workers: risk factors for transmission. *Am J Public Health*. 1993;83:1679-1684.

94. Eisenstein AB, Aach RD, Jacobsohn W, Goldman A. An epidemic of infectious hepatitis in a general hospital: probable transmission by contaminated orange juice. *JAMA*. 1963;185:171-174.

95. Meyers JD, Romm FJ, Tihen WS, Bryan JA. Food-borne hepatitis A in a general hospital: epidemiologic study of an outbreak attributed to sandwiches. *JAMA*. 1975;231:1049-1053.

96. Evans ME, Hall KL, Berry SE. Influenza control in acute care hospitals. *Am J Infect Control*. 1997;25:357-362.

97. Weingarten S, Friedlander M, Rascon D, Ault M, Morgan M, Meyer RD. Influenza surveillance in an acute-care hospital. *Arch Intern Med*. 1988;148:113-116.

98. Pachucki CT, Pappas SA, Fuller GF, Krause SL, Lentino JR, Schaaff DM. Influenza A among hospital personnel and patients. Implications for recognition, prevention, and control. *Arch Intern Med*. 1989;149:77-80.

99. Berlinberg CD, Weingarten SR, Bolton LB, Waterman SH. Occupational exposure to influenza-introduction of an index case to a hospital. *Infect Control Hosp Epidemiol*. 1989;10:70-73.

100. Centers for Disease Control and Prevention. Suspected nosocomial influenza cases in an intensive care unit. *MMWR*. 1988;37:3-4, 9.

101. Adal KA, Flowers RH, Anglim AM. Prevention of nosocomial influenza. *Infect Control Hosp Epidemiol*. 1996;17:641-648.

102. Horcajada JP, Pumarola T, Martinez JA, et al. A nosocomial outbreak of influenza during a period without influenza epidemic activity. *Eur Respir J*. 2003;21:303-307.

103. Berg HF, Van Gendt J, Rimmelzwaan GF, Peeters MF, Van Keulen P. Nosocomial influenza infection among post-influenza-vaccinated patients with severe pulmonary diseases. *J Infect*. 2003;46:129-132.

104. Slinger R, Dennis P. Nosocomial influenza at a Canadian pediatric hospital from 1995 to 1999: opportunities for prevention. *Infect Control Hosp Epidemiol*. 2002;23:627-629.

105. Hirji Z, O'Grady S, Bonham J, et al. Utility of zanamivir for chemoprophylaxis of concomitant influenza A and B in a complex continuing care population. *Infect Control Hosp Epidemiol*. 2002;23:604-608.

106. Sagrera X, Ginovart G, Raspall F, et al. Outbreaks of influenza A virus infection in neonatal intensive care units. *Pediatr Infect Dis J*. 2002;21:196-200.

107. Malavaud S, Malavaud B, Sandres K, et al. Nosocomial outbreak of influenza virus A (H3N2) infection in a solid organ transplant department. *Transplantation*. 2001;72:535-537.

108. Weinstock DM, Eagan J, Malak SA, et al. Control of influenza A on a bone marrow transplant unit. *Infect Control Hosp Epidemiol*. 2000;21:730-732.

109. Cunney RJ, Bialachowski A, Thornley D, Smaill FM, Pennie RA. An outbreak of influenza A in a neonatal intensive care unit. *Infect Control Hosp Epidemiol*. 2000;21:449-454.

110. Munoz FM, Campbell JR, Atmar RL, et al. Influenza A virus outbreak in a neonatal intensive care unit. *Pediatr Infect Dis J*. 1999;18:811-815.

111. Schepetiuk S, Papanaoum K, Qiao M. Spread of influenza A virus infection in hospitalised patients with cancer. *Aust N Z J Med*. 1998;28:475-476.

112. Everts RJ, Hanger HC, Jennings LC, Hawkins A, Sainsbury R. Outbreaks of influenza A among elderly hospital inpatients. *N Z Med J*. 1996;109:272-274.

113. Salgado CD, Farr BM, Hall KK, Hayden FG. Influenza in the acute hospital setting. *Lancet Infect Dis*. 2002;2:145-155.

114. Centers for Disease Control and Prevention. Prevention and control of influenza: recommendations of the Immunization Practices Advisory Committee (ACIP). *MMWR*. 1992;41:1-14.

115. Will RG. Epidemiology of Creutzfeldt-Jakob disease. *Br Med Bull*. 1993;49:960-970.

116. Harries-Jones R, Knight R, Will RG, Cousens S, Smith PG, Matthews WB. Creutzfeldt-Jakob disease in England and Wales, 1980-1984: a case-control study of potential risk factors. *J Neurol Neurosurg Psychiatry*. 1988;51:1113-1119.

117. Berger JR, Noble JD. Creutzfeldt-Jakob disease in a physician: a review of the disorder in health care workers. *Neurology*. 1993;43:205-206.

118. WHO. WHO infection control guidelines for transmissible spongiform encephalopathies. Report of a WHO consultation Geneva, Switzerland, 23-26 March 1999. http://www.who.int/emc.

119. Steelman VM. Creutzfeldt-Jakob disease: recommendations for infection control. *Am J Infect Control*. 1994;22:312-318.

120. Steelman VM. Creutzfeldt-Jakob disease: decontamination issues. *Infection Control and Sterilization Technology*. 1996;2:32-39.

121. Rutala WA. APIC guideline for selection and use of disinfectants. *Am J Infect Control*. 1996;24:313-342.

122. Irani DN, Johnson RT. Diagnosis and prevention of bovine spongiform encephalopathy and variant Creutzfeldt-Jakob disease. *Annu Rev Med*. 2003;54:305-319.

123. Centers for Disease Control and Prevention. Probable variant Creutzfeldt-Jakob disease in a U.S. resident-Florida, 2002. *MMWR*. 2002;51:927-929.

124. Frosh A, Rachel J, Johnson A. Iatrogenic vCJD from surgical instruments: the risk is unknown, but improved decontamination will help reduce the risk. [editorial]. *Brit Med J*. 2001;322:1558-1559.

125. Spencer RC, Ridgway GL, vCJD Consensus Group. Sterilization issues in vCJD-towards a consensus: meeting between the Central Sterilizing Club and Hospital Infection Society. 12th September 2000. *J Hosp Infect*. 2002;51:168-174.

126. Axon AT, Beilenhoff U, Bramble MG, et al. Variant Creutzfeldt-Jakob disease (vCJD) and gastrointestinal endoscopy. *Endoscopy*. 2001;33:1070-1080.

127. Hutton MD, Stead WW, Cauthen GM, Block AB, Ewig WM. Nosocomial transmission of tuberculosis associated with a draining abscess. *J Infect Dis*. 1990;161:286-295.

128. Matlow AG, Harrison A, Monteath A, Roach P, Balfe JW. Nosocimal transmission of tuberculosis (TB) associated with care of an infant with peritoneal TB. *Infect Control Hosp Epidemiol*. 2000;21:222-223.

129. Bowden KM, McDiarmid MA. Occupationally acquired tuberculosis: what's known. *J Occup Med*. 1994;36:320-325.

130. Stead WW. Management of health care workers after inadvertent exposure to tuberculosis: a guide for the use of preventive therapy. *Ann Intern Med*. 1995;122:906-912.

131. Templeton GL, Illing LA, Young L, Cave D, Stead WW, Bates JH. The risk for transmission of Mycobacterium tuberculosis at the bedside and during autopsy. *Ann Intern Med*. 1995;122:922-925.

132. Sepkowitz KA, Raffalli J, Riley L, Kiehn TE, Armstrong D. Tuberculosis in the AIDS era. *Clin Microbiol Rev*. 1995;8:180-199.

133. Miller RA, Lanza LA, Kline JN, Geist LJ. *Mycobacterium. tuberculosis* in lung transplant recipients. *Am J Respir Crit Care Med*. 1995;152:374-376.

134. Conover C, Ridzon R, Valway S, et al. Outbreak of multidrug-resistant tuberculosis at a methadone treatment program. *Int J Tuberc Lung Dis*. 2001;5:59-64.

135. Menzies D, Fanning A, Yuan L, FitzGerald JM. Hospital ventilation and risk for tuberculous infection in Canadian health care workers. Canadian Collaborative Group in Nosocomial Transmission of TB. *Ann Intern Med*. 2000;133:779-789.

136. Suzuki K, Onozaki I, Shimura A. Tuberculosis infection control practice in hospitals from the viewpoint of occupational health. *Kekkaku*. 1999;74:413-420.

137. Nakasone T. Tuberculosis among health care workers in Okinawa Prefecture. *Kekkaku*. 1999;74:389-395.

138. Schoch OD, Graf-Deuel E, Knoblauch A. Tuberculin testing of hospital personnel: large investment with little impact. *Schweiz Med Wochenschr*. 1999;129:217-224.

139. Ridzon R, Kenyon T, Luskin-Hawk R, Schultz C, Valway S, Onorato IM. Nosocomial transmission of human immunodeficiency virus and subsequent transmission of multidrug-resistant tuberculosis in a HCW. *Infect Control Hosp Epidemiol*. 1997;18:422-423.

140. Anonymous. Multidrug-resistant tuberculosis outbreak on an HIV ward-Madrid, Spain, 1991-1995. *MMWR*. 1996;45:330-333.

141. Yanai H, Limpakarnjanarat K, Uthaivoravit W, Mastro TD, Mori T, Tappero JW. Risk of *Mycobacterium tuberculosis* infection and disease among health care workers, Chiang Rai, Thailand. *Int J Tuberc Lung Dis*. 2003;7:36-45.

142. Uyamadu N, Ahkee S, Carrico R, Tolentino A, Wojda B, Ramirez J. Reduction in tuberculin skin-test conversion rate after improved adherence to tuberculosis isolation. *Infect Control Hosp Epidemiol*. 1997;18:575-579.

143. Silva VM, Cunha AJ, Oliveira JR, et al. Medical students at risk of Nosocomial transmission of *Mycobacterium tuberculosis*. *Int J Tuberc Lung Dis*. 2000;4:420-426.

144. Kilinc O, Ucan ES, Cakan MD, et al. Risk of tuberculosis among HCWs: can tuberculosis be considered as an occupational disease? *Respir Med*. 2002;96:506-510.

145. Eyob G, Gebeyhu M, Goshu S, Girma M, Lemma E, Fontanet A. Increase in tuberculosis incidence among the staff working at the Tuberculosis Demonstration and Training Centre in Addis Ababa, Ethiopia: a retrospective cohort study (1989-1998). *Int J Tuberc Lung Dis*. 2002;6:85-88.

146. Moore DA, Lightstone L, Javid B, Friedland JS. High rates of tuberculosis in end-stage renal failure: the impact of international migration. *Emerg Infect Dis*. 2002;8:77-78.

147. Greenaway C, Menzies D, Fanning A, et al. Delay in diagnosis among hospitalized patients with active tuberculosis-predictors and outcomes. *Am J Respir Crit Care Med*. 2002;165:927-933.

148. The Meningococcal Disease Surveillance Group. Analysis of endemic meningococcal disease by serogroup and evaluation of chemoprophylaxis. *J Infect Dis*. 1976;134:201-204.

149. Apicella MA. Neisseria meningitidis. In: Mandell GL, Douglas RG, Bennett JE, eds. *Principles and Practice of Infectious Diseases*. 3rd ed. New York, NY: Churchill Livingstone; 1990:1896-1909.

150. Rose HD, Lenz IE, Sheth NK. Meningococcal pneumonia. A source of nosocomial infection. *Arch Intern Med*. 1981;141:575-577.

151. Cohen MS, Steere AC, Baltimore R, et al. Possible nosocomial transmission of group Y *Neisseria meningitidis* among oncology patients. *Ann Intern Med*. 1979;91:7-12.

152. Centers for Disease Control. Nosocomial meningococcemia—Wisconsin. *MMWR*. 1978;27:358,363.

153. Gehanno JF, Kohen-Couderc L, Lemeland JF, Leroy J. Nosocomial meningococcemia in a physician. *Infect Control Hosp Epidemiol*. 1999;20(8):564-565.

154. Feldman HA. Some recollections of the meningococcal diseases. *JAMA*. 1972;220:1107-1112.

155. Lambert HJ. Epidemiology of a small pertussis outbreak in Kent County, Michigan. *Public Health Rep*. 1965;80:365-369.

156. Bass JW, Stephenson SR. The return of pertussis. *Pediatr Infect Dis J*. 1987;6:141-144.

157. Mortimer EA Jr. Pertussis and its prevention: a family affair. *J Infect Dis*. 1990;161:473-479.

158. Mink CM, Cherry J, Christenson P. A search for B pertussis infection in college students. *Clin Infect Dis*. 1992;14:464-471.

159. Nelson JD. The changing epidemiology of pertussis in young infants: the role of adults as reservoirs of infection. *Am J Dis Child*. 1978;132:371-373.

160. Addiss DG, Davis JP, Meade BD, et al. A pertussis outbreak in a nursing home. *J Infect Dis*. 1991;164:704-710.

161. Robbins JB. Pertussis in adults: introduction. *Clin Infect Dis*. 1999;28:S91-S93.

162. Linnemann CC Jr, Nasenbeny J. Pertussis in the adult. *Annu Rev Med*. 1977;28:179-185.

163. Kurt TL, Yeager AS, Guenette S, Dunlop S. Spread of pertussis by hospital staff. *JAMA*. 1972;221:264-267.

164. Linnemann CC Jr, Ramundo N, Perlstein PH, et al. Use of pertussis vaccine in an epidemic involving hospital staff. *Lancet*. 1975;2:540-543.

165. Valenti WM, Pincus PH, Messner MK. Nosocomial pertussis: possible spread by a hospital visitor. *Am J Dis Child*. 1980;134:520-521.

166. Martinez SM, Kemper CA, Haiduven D, Cody SH, Deresinski SC. Azithromycin prophylaxis during a hospitalwide outbreak of a pertussis-like illness. *Infect Control Hosp Epidemiol*. 2001;22:781-783.

167. Spearing NM, Horvath RL, McCormack JG. Pertussis: adults as a source in healthcare settings. *Med J Aust*. 2002;177:568-569.

168. Karino T, Osaki K, Nakano E, Okimoto N. A pertussis outbreak in a ward for severely retarded. *Kansenshogaku Zasshi*. 2001;75:916-922.

169. Gehanno JF, Pestel-Caron M, Nouvellon M, Caillard JF. Nosocomial pertussis in HCWs from a pediatric emergency unit in France. *Infect Control Hosp Epidemiol*. 1999;20:549-552.

170. Matlow AG, Nelson S, Wray R, Cox P. Nosocomial acquisition of pertussis diagnosed by polymerase chain reaction. *Infect Control Hosp Epidemiol*. 1997;18:715-716.

171. Wright SW, Decker MD, Edwards KM. Incidence of pertussis infection in HCWs. *Infect Control Hosp Epidemiol*. 1999;20:120-123.

172. Steketee RW, Burstyn DG, Wassilak SGF, et al. A comparison of laboratory and clinical methods for diagnosing pertussis in an outbreak in a facility for the developmentally disabled. *J Infect Dis*. 1988;157:441-449.

173. Steketee RW, Wassilak SGF, Adkins WN, et al. Evidence for a high attack rate and efficacy of erythromycin prophylaxis in a pertussis outbreak in a facility for the developmentally disabled. *J Infect Dis*. 1988;157:434-440.

174. Fisher MC, Long SS, McGowan KL, Kaselis E, Smith DG. Outbreak of pertussis in a residential facility for handicapped people. *J Pediatr*. 1989;114:934-939.

175. Biellik RJ, Patriarca PA, Mullen JR, et al. Risk factors for community- and household-acquired pertussis during a large-scale outbreak in central Wisconsin. *J Infect Dis*. 1988;157:1134-1141.

176. Christie CD, Marx ML, Marchant CD, Reising SF. The 1993 epidemic of pertussis in Cincinnati. Resurgence of disease in a highly immunized population of children. *N Engl J Med*. 1994;331:16-21.

177. Weber DJ, Rutala WA. Management of HCWs exposed to pertussis. *Infect Control Hosp Epidemiol*. 1994;15:411-415.

178. Kakis A, Gibbs L, Eguia J, et al. An outbreak of group A streptococcal infection among health care workers. *Clin Infect Dis*. 2002;35:1353-1359.

179. Ramage L, Green K, Pyskir D, Simor AE. An outbreak of fatal nosocomial infections due to group A streptococcus on a medical ward. *Infect Control Hosp Epidemiol*. 1996;17:429-431.

180. Hagberg C, Radulescu A, Rex JH. Necrotizing fasciitis due to group A streptococcus after an accidental needle-stick injury. [Letter] *New Engl J Med*. 1997;337:1699.

181. Lettau LA. Nosocomial transmission and infection control aspects of parasitic and ectoparasitic diseases, part III: ectoparasites/summary and conclusions. *Infect Control Hosp Epidemiol*. 1991;12:179-185.

182. Meinking TL, Taplin D, Kalter DC, Eberle MW. Comparative efficacy of treatments for Pediculosis capitis infestations. *Arch Dermatol*. 1986;122:267-271.

183. Degelau J. Scabies in long-term care facilities. *Infect Control Hosp Epidemiol*. 1992;13:421-425.

184. Pasternak J, Richtmann R, Ganme APP, et al. Scabies epidemic: price and prejudice. *Infect Control Hosp Epidemiol*. 1994;15:540-542.

185. Yonkosky D, Ladia L, Gackenheimer L, Schultz MW. Scabies in nursing homes: an eradication program with permethrin 5% cream. *J Am Acad Dermatol*. 1990;23:1133-1136.

186. Clark J, Friesen DL, Williams WA. Management of an outbreak of Norwegian scabies. *Am J Infect Control*. 1992;20:217-220.

187. Corbett EL, Crossley I, Holton J, Levell N, Miller R, De Cock KM. Crusted ("Norwegian") scabies in a specialist HIV unit: successful use of ivermectin and failure to prevent nosocomial transmission. *Genitourin Med*. 1996;72:115-117.

188. Sirera G, Rius F, Romeu J, et al. Hospital outbreak of scabies stemming from two AIDS patients with Norwegian scabies. *Lancet*. 1990;335:1227.

189. Jack M. Scabies outbreak in an extended care unit—a positive outcome. *J Infect Control*. 1993;8:11-13.

190. van Vliet JA, Samsom M, van Steenbergen JE. Causes of spread and return of scabies in health care institutues; literature analysis of 44 epidemics. *Ned Tijdschr Geneeskd*. 1998;142:354-357.

191. Meltzer E. Ivermectin and the treatment of outbreaks of scabies in medical facilities. *Harefuah*. 2002;141:948-952, 1011.

192. Portu JJ, Santamaria JM, Zubero Z, Almeida-Llamas MV, Aldamiz-Etxebarria San Sebastian M, Gutierrez AR. Atypical scabies in HIV-positive patients. *J Am Acad Dermatol*. 1996;34:915-917.

193. Obasanjo OO, Wu P, Conlon M, et al. An outbreak of scabies in a teaching hospital: lessons learned. *Infect Control Hosp Epidemiol*. 2001;22:13-18.

194. Deabate MC, Calitri V, Licata C, et al. Scabies in a dialysis unit. Mystery and prejudice. *Minerva Urol Nefrol*. 2001;53:69-73.

195. Zafar AB, Beidas SO, Sylvester LK. Control of transmission of Norwegian scabies. *Infect Control Hosp Epidemiol*. 2002;23:278-279.

196. Robles Garcia M, de la Lama Lopez-Areal J, Avellaneda Martinez C, Gimenez Garcia R, Cortejoso Gonzalo B, Vaquero Puerta JL. *Revista Clinica Espanola*. 2000;200:538-42.

197. Boix V, Sanchez-Paya J, Portilla J, Merino E. Nosocomial outbreak of scabies clinically resistant to lindane. [Letter] *Infect Control Hosp Epidemiol*. 1997;18:677.

198. Nandwani R, Pozniak AL, Fuller LC, Wade J. Crusted ("Norwegian") scabies in a specialist HIV unit. [Comment. Letter] *Genitourin Med*. 1996;72:453.

199. Centers for Disease Control and Prevention. Clinicians smallpox disease overview. Available at: http://www.bt.cdc.gov/agent/smallpox/index.asp. Accessed June 29, 2004.

200. Notice to readers: smallpox: what every clinician should know—a self-study course. *MMWR*. 2002;51:352.

201. Recommendations for Using Smallpox Vaccine in a Pre-Event Vaccination Program: Supplemental Recommendations of the Advisory Committee on Immunization Practices (ACIP) and the Healthcare Infection Control Practices Advisory Committee (HIC-PAC). *MMWR*. 2003;52(RR07):1-16.

202. Committee on Smallpox Vaccination Program Implementation, Board on Health Promotion and Disease Prevention, Institute of Medicine. Review of the Centers for Disease Control and Prevention's smallpox vaccination program implementation, letter report #4.

203. Notice to Readers: Supplemental Recommendations on Adverse Events Following Smallpox Vaccine in the Pre-Event Vaccination Program: Recommendations of the Advisory Committee on Immunization Practices. *MMWR*. 2003;52:282-284.

204. Update: Adverse Events Following Civilian Smallpox Vaccination—United States, 2003. *MMWR*. 2003;52:819-820.

205. Update: Severe Acute Respiratory Syndrome--Worldwide and United States, 2003. *MMWR*. 2003;52:664-665.

206. Seto WH, Tsang D, Yung RW, et al. Effectiveness of precautions against droplets and contact in prevention of nosocomial transmission of severe acute respiratory syndrome (SARS). *Lancet*. 2003;361:1519-1520.

207. Cluster of Severe Acute Respiratory Syndrome Cases Among Protected Health-Care Workers—Toronto, Canada, April 2003. *MMWR*. 2003;52:433-436.

208. Centers for Disease Control and Prevention. In the absence of SARS-CoV transmission worldwide: Guidance for surveillance, clinical and laboratory evaluation, and reporting. Version 2. Available at: http://www.cdc.gov/ncidod/sars. Accessed June 29, 2004.

209. World Health Organization. Preliminary clinical description of severe acute respiration syndrome. Available at: http://www.who.int/csr/sars/en. Accessed June 292, 2004.

210. Use of Quarantine to Prevent Transmission of Severe Acute Respiratory Syndrome—Taiwan, 2003. *MMWR*. 2003;52:680-683.

211. Update: Multistate Outbreak of Monkeypox-Illinois, Indiana, Kansas, Missouri, Ohio, and Wisconsin, 2003. *MMWR*. 2003; 52 (27); 642-646.

212. Update: Multistate Outbreak of Monkeypox-Illinois, Indiana, and Wisconsin, 2003. MMWR. 2003;52(23):537-540. Available at: Ohttp://www.cdc.gov/ncidod/monkey-pox. Accessed June 29, 2004.

213. Scott JR, Foster JD, Fraser H. Conjunctival instillation of scrapie in mice can produce disease. *Vet Microbiol*. 1993;34:305-309.

CHAPTER TWELVE

ISOLATION

Gonzalo M. L. Bearman, MD, MPH and Michael Edmond, MD, MPH, MPA

INTRODUCTION

The goal of isolation is to prevent transmission of microorganisms from infected or colonized patients to other patients, hospital visitors, and HCWs. Personal protective equipment (eg, masks, eyewear, gloves, and gowns) and specific room requirements help to accomplish this goal.

The importance of appropriate isolation cannot be overstated. The medical literature is replete with examples of nosocomial outbreaks of influenza, tuberculosis, varicella, SARS, and even hepatitis A, all of which could have been prevented if isolation techniques had been optimal. Isolation efforts may be costly, but the direct and indirect costs of nosocomial outbreaks are often substantial. Appropriate isolation remains the cornerstone of infection control and is assuming greater importance as the prevalence of multiply antibiotic-resistant organisms increases.

The ideal isolation system is described in Table 12-1. While no system meets all of these standards, infection control personnel should consider these ideals when designing and implementing a system.

In assessing appropriate infection control for any IDs, one needs to know the mode of transmission (airborne, droplet, contact, via blood and body fluids, or a combination of any of these). Moreover, it is necessary to also know the onset and the termination of infectivity because the patient may be infectious before and after the symptomatic period. The emergence of SARS demonstrated the difficulties of implementing appropriate infection control measures when the mode of transmission and infective period are unclear.

The CDC has led the effort to formalize guidelines for isolation. They published their first guidelines in 1970. Subsequently, the CDC has modified and streamlined these guidelines several times to address emerging problems in IDs, such as multidrug-resistant *M. tuberculosis* and VRE, and to incorporate an increased understanding about the mechanisms of transmission for some diseases.

The CDC and the HICPAC issued a guideline in 1996 for a new system of isolation. This system replaced the previous category and disease-specific systems and integrated universal precautions and body substance isolation. Still, individual healthcare institutions may find it necessary to modify these basic guidelines.

This chapter presents an overview of isolation so that infection control personnel can implement an appropriate system. Infection control personnel should also consult the detailed guidelines for implementing isolation precautions that are referenced at the end of this chapter.

CURRENT CDC GUIDELINES

The CDC and HICPAC developed a system for isolation that has 2 levels of precautions: standard precautions, which apply to all patients, and transmission-based precautions, employed for patients with documented or suspected colonization or infection with certain microorganisms.

Standard Precautions

Standard precautions apply to blood; all body fluids, secretions, excretions except sweat, whether or not they are visibly bloody; nonintact skin; and mucous membranes. The intent of standard precautions is primarily to protect the HCW from pathogens transmitted via blood and body fluids. Requirements for standard precautions are outlined in Table 12-2.

Transmission-Based Precautions

While standard precautions apply to all patients, transmission-based precautions apply to selected patients, based on either a suspected or confirmed clinical syn-

---

TABLE 12-1. CHARACTERISTICS OF THE IDEAL ISOLATION SYSTEM

➤ Uses current understanding of the mechanisms of transmission of infectious pathogens
➤ Requires isolation precautions for all patients with infectious diseases that may be nosocomially transmitted (ie, eliminates transmission of infection in the hospital)
➤ Avoids isolation of patients who do not require it ("over-isolation")
➤ Easily understood by all members of the healthcare team
➤ Easily implemented
➤ Encourages compliance
➤ Avoids unnecessary use of disposable products
➤ Inexpensive
➤ Interferes minimally with patient care
➤ Minimizes patient discomfort

TABLE 12-2. REQUIREMENTS FOR STANDARD PRECAUTIONS[1]

Hand hygiene	➤ After touching blood, body fluids, secretions, excretions, contaminated items ➤ Immediately after gloves removed ➤ Between patient contacts
Gloves	➤ For touching blood, body fluids, secretions, excretions, contaminated items ➤ For touching mucous membranes, nonintact skin
Mask, eye protection, face shield	➤ To protect mucous membranes of the eyes, nose, and mouth during procedures and patient care activities likely to generate splashes or sprays of blood, body fluids, secretions, and excretions
Gown	➤ To protect skin and prevent soiling of clothing during procedures and patient-care activities likely to generate splashes or sprays of blood, body fluids, secretions, excretions
Patient-care equipment	➤ Soiled patient-care equipment should be handled in a manner to prevent skin and mucous membrane exposures, contamination of clothing, and transfer of microorganisms to other patients and environments ➤ Reusable equipment must be cleaned and reprocessed before used in the care of another patient
Environmental control	➤ Requires procedures for routine care, cleaning and disinfection of patient furniture, and the environment
Linen	➤ Soiled linen should be handled in a manner to prevent skin and mucous membrane exposures, contamination of clothing, and transfer of microorganisms to other patients and environments
Sharps	➤ Avoid recapping used needles ➤ Avoid removing used needles from disposable syringes by hand ➤ Avoid bending, breaking, or manipulating used needles by hand ➤ Place used sharps in puncture-resistant containers
Patient resuscitation	➤ Use mouthpieces, resuscitation bags, or other ventilation devices to avoid mouth-to-mouth resuscitation
Patient placement	➤ Patients who contaminate the environment or cannot maintain appropriate hygiene should be placed in a private room

drome or specific diagnosis.[2] Transmission-based precautions (Table 12-3) are divided into 3 categories that reflect the major modes of transmission of infectious agents within the healthcare setting: airborne, droplet, and contact. Some diseases require more than one isolation category.

Airborne Precautions

Airborne precautions prevent diseases transmitted by droplet nuclei or contaminated dust particles.[2] Droplet nuclei are less than 5 μm in size and may remain suspended in the air, allowing them to migrate for long periods of time. Patients with suspected or confirmed tuberculosis (pulmonary or laryngeal), measles, varicella, or disseminated zoster should be placed on airborne precautions. In addition, human immunodeficiency virus-infected patients with cough, fever, and unexplained pulmonary infiltrates in any location should be placed empirically on airborne precautions until tuberculosis can be ruled out. Appropriate isolation requires a private room with negative air pressure and at least 6 air exchanges per hour. Air from the room should be exhausted directly to the outside or through a high-efficiency filter. The door to the room must be kept closed at all times.

If the patient must be transported from the isolation room to another area of the hospital, the patient should put on a standard surgical mask before leaving the isolation room. All people entering the room should wear respirators. The respirator must meet the following CDC performance criteria:

➤ Filters 1-μm particles with an efficiency of at least 95%.

➤ Fits different facial sizes and characteristics.

➤ Can be fit tested to obtain a leakage of less than 10%.

➤ Can be checked for fit each time the HCW puts on the mask.[3]

There are numerous products available that are certified by the National Institute for Occupational Safety and Health as meeting the N-95 standard.

Patients with suspected or confirmed tuberculosis should be instructed to cover their mouths and noses with a tissue when coughing or sneezing. Those with suspected tuberculosis should remain in isolation until tuberculosis can be ruled out. Patients with confirmed tuberculosis who are receiving effective anti-tuberculous treatment can be moved out of the negative-pressure rooms when they have received at least 2 weeks of adequate therapy, when they are improving clinically, and when 3 consecutive sputum smears collected on separate days have no detectable acid-fast bacilli. Some hospitals have more stringent criteria (see Chapter 22). Patients with MDR tuberculosis may need to be isolated for the duration of their hospital stay.

If the patient has suspected or confirmed measles, varicella, or disseminated zoster, nonimmune individuals should not enter the room. If a nonimmune HCW must enter the room, he or she should wear a respirator (described above). People who are immune to measles or varicella do not need to wear a respirator when entering the room.

Droplet Precautions

Droplet precautions prevent the transmission of microorganisms by particles larger than 5 μm.[2] These droplets are produced when the patient talks, coughs, or sneezes. Droplets also may be produced during some procedures. Some illnesses that require droplet precautions include bacterial diseases, such as invasive *H. influenzae* type B infections, meningococcal infections, MDR pneumococcal disease, pharyngeal diphtheria, *Mycoplasma pneumonia*, and pertussis. Some viral diseases, including influenza, mumps, rubella, and parvovirus infection, also require these precautions.

Droplet precautions require patients to be placed in private rooms or cohorted with other patients who are infected with the same organism. The door to the room may remain open. HCWs should wear masks when within 3 feet of the patient; some hospitals may require HCWs to wear a mask when entering the room. When transported out of the isolation room, the patient should wear a mask.

Contact Precautions

Contact precautions prevent transmission of epidemiologically important organisms from an infected or colonized patient through direct (touching the patient) or indirect (touching surfaces or objects in the patient's environment) contact.[2] Contact precautions require patients to be placed in private rooms or cohorted with other patients who are infected with the same organism. HCWs should wear gloves when entering the room. They should change the gloves while caring for the patient if they touch materials containing high concentrations of microorganisms. While still in the isolation room, HCWs should remove their gloves and wash their hands with a medicated handwashing agent; they must take care not to contaminate their hands before leaving the room. HCWs should wear gowns if they may have substantial contact with the patient or the patient's environment. They should also wear gowns in situations where there is an increased risk of contact with potentially infective material (eg, the patient is incontinent, has diarrhea, has a colostomy, has an ileostomy, or has wound drainage that is not contained by a dressing). HCWs should remove gowns while in the isolation room, and they should avoid contaminating their clothing before leaving the room. Noncritical patient care items (eg, stethoscopes, bedside commodes) that are used for the patients in contact isolation should not be used for other patients. If such items must be shared, they should be cleaned and disinfected before reuse. Patients should leave the isolation room infrequently.

Contact isolation is indicated for patients infected or colonized with MDR bacteria (eg, methicillin-resistant *S.*

TABLE 12-3. TRANSMISSION-BASED PRECAUTIONS

	Airborne Precautions	Droplet Precautions	Contact Precautions
Room	Negative pressure, private room, 6 or more air changes/hour, exhaust to outside or high-efficiency filter, door kept closed	Private room (may cohort if necessary); door may remain open	Private room (may cohort if necessary); dedicate use of noncritical patient-care items to a single patient (or cohort colonized/infected with the same organism)
Masks	N95 mask for entering room	Standard surgical mask within 3 feet of patient or when entering the room	
Gowns			If clothing will contact patient, surfaces, items in room; if patient has diarrhea, ileostomy, colostomy, uncontained wound drainage
Gloves			When entering room
Diseases/ Pathogens	Measles Monkeypox* Tuberculosis, pulmonary or laryngeal SARS* Smallpox* Varicella* Viral hemorrhagic fevers* Zoster (disseminated or immunocompromised)*	Adenovirus (infants, children)* Diphtheria, pharyngeal Group A streptococcal pharyngitis, pneumonia, scarlet fever (infants/young children) H. influenzae meningitis, epiglottitis H. influenzae pneumonia (infants, children) Influenza Meningococcal infections Mumps Mycoplasma pneumonia Parvovirus B19 Pertussis Plague, pneumonic Rubella	Adenovirus (infants, children)* Clostridium difficile diarrhea Congenital rubella Diphtheria, cutaneous E. coli O157:H7 colitis (diapered/incontinent) Enteroviral infections (infants, young children) Furunculosis (infants, young children) Group A streptococcal major skin, burn or wound infection Hepatitis A (diapered/incontinent) Herpes simplex (neonatal; disseminated; severe primary mucocutaneous) Impetigo Major (noncontained) abscess, cellulitis, decubiti MDR bacteria (eg, MRSA, VRE) infection/colonization Monkeypox* Parainfluenza infection (infants, children) Pediculosis, scabies Rotavirus (diapered/incontinent) RSV infection (infants, children, immunocompromised) SARS* S. aureus major skin, wound or burn infection Shigella (diapered/incontinent) Smallpox* Varicella* Viral conjunctivitis Viral hemorrhagic fevers* Zoster (disseminated or immunocompromised)*

*Condition requires 2 types of precautions.

Modified from Garner JS, Hospital Infection Control Practices Advisory Committee. Guideline for isolation precautions in hospitals. *Infect Control Hosp Epidemiol. 1996;*17:53-80.

TABLE 12-4. CLINICAL SCENARIOS REQUIRING ASSIGNMENT OF EMPIRIC ISOLATION PRECAUTIONS

Airborne Precautions	Droplet Precautions	Contact Precautions
Vesicular rash*	Meningitis	Acute diarrhea with likely infectious etiology, patient incontinent or diapered
Maculopapular rash with coryza and fever	Petechial/ecchymotic rash with fever	Diarrhea in an adult with a history of recent antibiotic use
Cough/fever/upper lobe pulmonary infiltrate	Paroxysmal or severe persistent cough during periods of pertussis activity	Vesicular rash*
Cough/fever/pulmonary infiltrate in any location in a HIV-infected patient (or patient at risk for HIV infection)	Symptoms of respiratory illness with fever (especially during influenza/respiratory viral season)	Respiratory infections, particularly bronchiolitis and croup, in infants/young children
Fever, respiratory symptoms in a person with recent contact with SARS patient, or recent travel to area with SARS transmission*		History of infection or colonization with MDR organisms
		Skin, wound, or UTI in a patient with a recent hospital or nursing home stay in a facility where MDR organisms are prevalent
		Abscess or draining wound that cannot be covered
		Fever, respiratory symptoms in a person with recent contact with SARS patient or recent travel to area with SARS transmission*

*Condition requires 2 types of precautions.

Modified from Garner JS, Hospital Infection Control Practices Advisory Committee. Guideline for isolation precautions in hospitals. *Infect Control Hosp Epidemiol.* 1996;17:53-80.

aureus and VRE). It also is indicated for patients with *C. difficile* enteritis and for patients who have other agents transmitted by the oral-fecal route (eg, *E. coli* O157:H7, *Shigella*, rotavirus, and hepatitis A) and who are diapered or incontinent. Infants and young children with respiratory syncytial virus, parainfluenza, or enteroviral infections also require contact isolation, as do patients with impetigo, scabies, pediculosis, and significant herpes simplex virus infections (ie, neonatal, disseminated, or severe primary mucocutaneous disease). Patients with varicella or disseminated zoster infections require both contact and airborne precautions. Infants and children with adenovirus infection require both contact and droplet precautions.

INSTITUTING EMPIRIC ISOLATION PRECAUTIONS

Frequently, patients are admitted to the hospital without a definitive diagnosis. However, they may have an infectious process that may place other patients and HCWs at risk. Therefore, patients with certain clinical syndromes should be isolated while a definitive diagnosis is pending. Table 12-4 delineates appropriate empiric iso-

lation precautions for various clinical syndromes based on the potential mechanisms of transmission.

Because many respiratory diseases are spread by the droplet route (including influenza), the CDC has begun to suggest that HCFs emphasize "respiratory hygiene," especially during the winter respiratory viral season. This includes posting signs and offering masks (eg, simple procedure masks) to patients in waiting areas who are coughing. Droplet precautions should be used for patients with symptoms of a respiratory infection, particularly if fever is present, until it is known that their illness is not one that requires continuation of precautions (http://www.cdc.gov/flu/professionals/infectioncontrol/resphygiene.htm).

SPECIAL CONSIDERATIONS FOR VANCOMYCIN-RESISTANT ORGANISMS

During the past several years, VRE have become important nosocomial pathogens. Appropriate isolation for patients colonized or infected with VRE can be implemented by following the guidelines for contact isolation.[1,3] To date, 3 patients with VRSA have been described.

TABLE 12-5. ISOLATION PRECAUTIONS FOR PATIENTS INFECTED OR COLONIZED WITH VANCOMYCIN-RESISTANT *S. AUREUS*[4]

1. Standard and contact precautions apply.
2. After gloves are removed, handwashing with 4% chlorhexidine or 60% isopropyl alcohol is required.
3. Consider placing a monitor at the door to the patient's room 24 hours per day to prevent unauthorized access and to assess compliance with handwashing and barrier precautions.
4. The names of all people entering the room should be recorded for future use if obtaining nasal surveillance cultures become necessary.
5. Patients with VRSA pneumonia requiring mechanical ventilation should have a filter or condensate trap placed on the expiratory phase tubing of the mechanical-ventilator circuit.
6. If oxygen therapy by nasal cannula is required, a standard surgical mask should be worn by all people entering the room.
7. If the patient is colonized in the nares, decolonization with mupirocin should be attempted.
8. Infectious disease consultants should review the patient's antimicrobial therapy. Every effort to reduce the selection of VRSA by eliminating or substituting antibiotics should be made.
9. An effort should be made to limit the number of HCWs who come into contact with the VRSA-infected or colonized patient. To the greatest extent possible, care of the patient should be limited to 1 nurse and 1 physician per shift. Phlebotomy and other ancillary services should be performed by the primary nurse or primary physician whenever possible.
10. Until more is learned about the epidemiology of VRSA, all HCWs caring for the patient should have nasal surveillance cultures for VRSA performed every 2 weeks.
11. Healthcare workers known to be at higher risk for staphylococcal colonization (eg, those with exfoliative dermatitides or diabetes mellitus requiring treatment with insulin) should not care for patients with VRSA colonization or infection.
12. Housekeeping personnel should be instructed to cleanse all horizontal surfaces in the patient's immediate vicinity on a daily basis with a quaternary ammonium compound. Cleaning cloths used in the room should not be used to clean other patients' rooms and equipment. Used cleaning cloths should be carefully discarded.
13. Isolation precautions must continue for the duration of the hospital stay.
14. After the infected/colonized patient is discharged and housekeeping has completed terminal disinfection of the room, environmental cultures should be obtained. The room should remain closed to new admissions until negative cultures have been reported. All equipment used in the room must be disinfected.
15. Prior to discharge, an epidemiology alert sticker should be affixed to the cover of the patient's chart, and a notation should be made in the hospital's information system.
16. If a patient with previous VRSA infection or colonization is readmitted, the patient should be placed into isolation immediately. The patient should remain in isolation until surveillance cultures of the nares and any previously infected, open site have been obtained and are negative.
17. If nosocomial transmission is documented on a hospital unit, the unit should be closed to new admissions. Should a previously uninfected patient from the unit require transfer to another hospital unit, the patient should be placed in isolation in the receiving unit until 2 nasal cultures separated by 48 hours are negative.
18. Diagnostic and therapeutic procedures that require the patient to leave the isolation room should be postponed when possible.
19. When testing is done at the bedside (eg, portable radiography, electrocardiography), equipment should be wiped down with a disinfectant when the test is complete.
20. Collection of microbiologic and other specimens for clinical testing should be done in the patient's room.
21. Clinical specimens from colonized or infected patients should be kept in a leakproof plastic bag for transport. Laboratory forms should not be placed in the bag with the specimen. Care must be taken to prevent contamination of the outside of the bag. The specimen should be taken to the laboratory immediately; it should not be sent through a pneumatic tube system.

Adapted from Edmond MB, Wenzel RP, Pasculle AW. Vancomycin-resistant *Staphylococcus aureus*: perspectives on measures needed for control. *Ann Intern Med. 1996*;124:329-334.

Given the virulence of this organism, every effort must be made to avoid nosocomial spread. Guidelines for controlling VRSA have been proposed based on knowledge regarding transmission and control of *S. aureus* (Table 12-5).[4,5]

TABLE 12-6. ISOLATION PRECAUTIONS FOR BIOTERRORISM-ASSOCIATED DISEASES

| Agent | Precautions | | | |
	Standard	Airborne	Droplet	Contact
Category A				
Anthrax (*Bacillus anthracis*)	X			
Botulism (*Clostridium botulinum* toxin)	X			
Plague (*Yersinia pestis*)	X		X	
Smallpox (variola)	X	X		X
Tularemia (*Francisella tularensis*)	X			
Viral hemorrhagic fevers (filo-, arenaviruses)	X	X		X

SPECIAL CONSIDERATIONS FOR BIOTERRORISM AGENTS

The anthrax attack in 2001 raised concern regarding the future use of bioterrorism agents. HCWs, law enforcement officials, and public health authorities will need to collaboratively work on the control and containment of any future bioterrorism outbreak. A key member of this team will be the hospital epidemiologist with a major role to ensure that appropriate isolation measures are implemented for suspected or confirmed cases of disease due to agents of bioterrorism (see Chapter 20).

Although a review of all potential bioterrorism agents is beyond the scope of this chapter, a listing of CDC category A bioterrorism agents and their corresponding isolation precautions is contained in Table 12-6. Category A agents include pathogens that are rarely seen in the United States. These high-priority agents pose a significant risk to national security as they can be easily disseminated or transmitted from person to person. Also, these agents result in high mortality rates and have the potential for major public health impact.[6]

Some diseases in category A require transmission-based precautions. Because of their ability to cause secondary transmission through inhalation and direct contact, smallpox and viral hemorrhagic fevers require both airborne and contact isolation.[7,8] Pneumonic plague, caused by *Yersinia pestis*, can also be transmitted from person to person. As pneumonic plague can be secondarily transmitted in the healthcare setting by the inhalation of respiratory droplets, droplet precautions are warranted.[9]

SPECIAL CONSIDERATIONS FOR SEVERE ACUTE RESPIRATORY SYNDROME

In late 2002, a new respiratory disease, SARS, emerged in southern China and spread rapidly to other continents. It is characterized by fever, constitutional symptoms, cough, pulmonary infiltrates, and, in some cases, respiratory failure.[10] The causative pathogen has been shown to be a novel coronavirus. The illness is highly contagious, and many cases have been due to nosocomial transmission.[11]

At the present time, it appears that the disease is spread by droplets and possibly through airborne aerosols. Environmental contamination has been documented; thus, transmission via fomites is also suspected. The virus has been detected in stool, blood, and urine of infected individuals. It is not known when infected people become contagious, nor is the duration of infectivity known. Based on the current state of knowledge, patients with documented or suspected SARS should be placed in airborne and contact precautions, with strict adherence to standard precautions, including eye protection. Additional protections (eg, positive pressure respirators) may be needed in certain high-risk situations (eg, intubation). As more is learned about the transmission of SARS, these recommendations may change.

REFERENCES

1. Garner JS, Hospital Infection Control Practices Advisory Committee. Guideline for isolation precautions in hospitals. *Infect Control Hosp Epidemiol.* 1996;17:53-80.

2. Centers for Disease Control and Prevention. Guidelines for preventing the transmission of Mycobacterium tuberculosis in health-care facilities, 1994. *MMWR.* 1994; 43(RR-13):1-132.

3. Hospital Infection Control Practices Advisory Committee. Recommendations for preventing the spread of vancomycin resistance. *Infect Control Hosp Epidemiol.* 1995;16:105-113.

4. Edmond MB, Wenzel RP, Pasculle AW. Vancomycin-resistant *Staphylococcus aureus*: perspectives on measures needed for control. *Ann Intern Med.* 1996;124:329-334.

5. Centers for Disease Control and Prevention. Interim guidelines for prevention and control of staphylococcal infection associated with reduced susceptibility to vancomycin. *MMWR.* 1997;46:626-628, 635.

6. Centers for Disease Control and Prevention. Public Health Emergency Preparedness and Response. Biological agents/Diseases. Available at: http://www.bt.cdc.gov/agent/agentlist-category.asp#a. Accessed July 6, 2003.

7. Henderson DA, Inglesby TV, Bartlett JG, et al. Smallpox as a biological weapon: medical and public health management. *JAMA.* 1999;281:2127-2137.

8. Borio L, Inglesby T, Peters CJ, et al. Hemorrhagic fever viruses as biological weapons: medical and public health management. *JAMA.* 2002;287:2391-2405.

9. Inglesby TV, Dennis DT, Henderson DA, et al. Plague as a biological weapon: medical and public health management. *JAMA.* 2000;283:2281-2290.

10. Poutanen SM, Low DE, Henry B, et al. Identification of severe acute respiratory syndrome in Canada. *New Engl J Med.* 2003;348:1995-2005.

11. Lee N, Hui D, Wu A, et al. A major outbreak of severe acute respiratory syndrome in Hong Kong. *N Engl J Med.* 2003;348:1986-1994.

SUGGESTED READING

American Academy of Pediatrics. In: Pickering LK, ed. *2003 Red Book: Report of the Committee on Infectious Diseases.* 26th ed. Elk Grove Village, Ill: American Academy of Pediatrics; 2003.

Centers for Disease Control and Prevention. Guidelines for environmental infection control in health-care facilities: recommendations of CDC and the Healthcare Infection Control Practices Advisory Committee (HICPAC). *MMWR.* 2003;52(RR10):1-42.

Centers for Disease Control and Prevention. Guideline for hand hygiene in health-care settings: recommendations of the Healthcare Infection Control Practices Advisory Committee and the HICPAC/SHEA/ APIC/IDSA Hand Hygiene Task Force. *MMWR.* 2002:51(RR16);1-44.

Centers for Disease Control and Prevention. Public Health Emergency Preparedness and Response Web Site. Available at http://www.bt.cdc.gov/. Accessed July 6, 2003.

Centers for Disease Control and Prevention. Severe Acute Respiratory Syndrome Web Site. Available at http://www.cdc.gov/ncidod/sars/. Accessed July 6, 2003.

Mayhall CG. *Hospital Epidemiology and Infection Control.* 2nd ed. Philadelphia, Pa: Lippincott, Williams & Wilkins; 1999.

Wenzel RP. *Prevention and Control of Nosocomial Infections.* 4th ed. Philadelphia, Pa: Lippincott, Williams & Wilkins; 2003.

SUPPORT FUNCTIONS

CHAPTER THIRTEEN

CLINICAL MICROBIOLOGY LABORATORY SUPPORT FOR HEALTHCARE EPIDEMIOLOGY

Lance R. Peterson, MD and Patrick A. Hymel, MD

INTRODUCTION

The clinical microbiology laboratory has a long and useful history in the support of infection control activities that reduce risks to patients and improve the overall quality of healthcare. One of the first recognized achievements that microbiologists are credited with is documenting the role of microbial contamination within the operating room environment that resulted from surgeons' normal conversations. This led to the standard practice of personnel wearing masks during surgery.[1] Modern hospital epidemiology is less than half a century old,[2] and during these past 50 years, the clinical microbiology laboratory progressively adopted critical roles for ongoing management and control of healthcare-associated IDs. Increasingly recognized is the fact that surveillance from the laboratory can measure organization-wide (hospital and outpatient) occurrences from a single, central data collection point. The optimal approach for managing healthcare-associated infections is gathering the broadest surveillance data that is achievable, as originally recommended by the CDC.[3] The principal hindrance to achieving this goal has been that manually attempting universal surveillance is very resource intensive and the amount of data collected is overwhelming, even with any traditional computer analysis.[4] The best estimates are that using 20th century approaches to analyzing laboratory data will detect no more than two-thirds of nosocomial infections.[5] However, many now believe that the use of laboratory data will prove the most cost-effective, comprehensive surveillance approach once sufficient analytical tools are available.[6]

A 1998 consensus report set the current standard for required microbiology laboratory services as part of a comprehensive infection control program.[7] The final report indicated that the necessary contribution from the laboratory included surveillance (eg, providing for a systematic observance and measurement of disease) as well as molecular typing of microbial pathogens.[7] In only 5 years since that report, we now recognize even more is required. Present and future needs for laboratory-based surveillance will require reliable detection of new pathogens that emerge as causes of important healthcare-associated infections, which implies accurate identification of microbial organisms; recognition of new or emerging antimicrobial agent resistance; and participation in active surveillance for outbreaks, including preparation of specialized growth media as well as molecular typing.[8] This evolving role dictates a strong collaboration between the hospital epidemiologist and the clinical microbiologist, with a consequent positive impact on both the infection control program and the diagnostic laboratory.[9]

Regulatory agencies are also changing what they expect from the laboratory in its contribution to the infection control program. In July 2003, the JCAHO issued a new set of proposed standards for infection control in hospitals and laboratories.[10,11] These new standards, to be applied beginning in 2005, will require laboratories to formally address their infection control activities. A summary of the necessary contributions from clinical laboratory operations is in Table 13-1. These range from developing a formal departmental plan to providing traditional microbial identification and susceptibility testing to incorporating sophisticated molecular typing and data analysis systems for detection, tracking, and monitoring of healthcare-associated infections for the entire organization. Each of these elements will be addressed in the following sections of this chapter.

TABLE 13-1. NECESSARY FUNCTIONS FOR CLINICAL LABORATORY SUPPORT OF INFECTION CONTROL AND PREVENTION

Element	Description
Infection control plan	Organization-wide and laboratory-specific
Qualified personnel	Knowledge/training in infection prevention/control and data analysis
Data collection	Detect and track rates/trends in infection for organization
Routine surveillance	Reporting that permits surveillance of nosocomial infections
Transmission of infections	Detect pathogens and implement precautions for in-hospital transmission and emerging pathogens in the community
Outbreak investigation	Resources for outbreak investigation should be available (surveillance cultures, molecular typing, species identification, expanded susceptibility testing, and other needs that arise)
Interventions	Prioritize, implement, and evaluate intervention results
Reporting systems	Within the organization and to public health officials
Monitor outcome	Determine if program goals are met; modify interventions if necessary to meet goals
Communicating infection prevention	Infection Control Committee, seminars, personal interactions, newsletters
Coordinated program	Specific Committee or minutes in departmental meetings

Adapted from Scheckler WE, Brimhall D, Buck AS, et al. Requirements for infrastructure and essential activities of infection control and epidemiology in hospitals: a consensus panel report. *Infect Control Hosp Epidemiol.* 1998;19:114-124; and JCAHO. Joint Commission on Accreditation of Healthcare Organizations. Proposed Standards Prevention and Control of Infection: Laboratory. Available at: http://www.jcaho.org/accredited+organizations/accredited+organizations+.htm. Accessed July 30, 2003.

DEVELOPMENT OF AN INFECTION CONTROL PROGRAM

The Pathology and Laboratory Medicine Department should have a written infection control and prevention plan for preventing the transmission of infections that is consistent with the plan for the entire organization. The plan should identify the likely hazards faced by the department and identify risk-reduction strategies to be implemented. Within the departmental plan, there should be specific named individual(s) who are responsible for developing, implementing, and updating the plan. Systems for reporting of appropriate information, both to the key personnel in the organization as well as to local, state, and federal public health officials as legally required, need to be included. The departmental plan should also delineate activities for patients, workers, and trainees who are required to reduce the transmission of infections; facilitate hand hygiene; address screening for pathogen exposure and assess immunity to such potential exposures;

minimize the risk from handling of medical devices; outline the management of infected personnel who may pose a risk to other; and describe the availability and use of personal protective equipment. The proper handling, maintenance, disinfection, and storage of equipment used in the department should be described. Importantly, the plan should include a description of how staff and trainees will receive information about infection prevention and management. All policies, procedures, and activities in the departmental plan should be based upon accepted guidelines and practices demonstrated to be successful.

PERSONNEL

Qualified personnel who are knowledgeable, either through experience or training, in infection prevention and control as well as data analysis are required for the laboratory program. Experience can be gained from the recognized need for microbiology participation in the organizational infection control program.[9,12] Recognized training and certification, either in medical microbiology or in infection control, can be obtained from several resources. Postdoctoral training with specialty certification in medical microbiology is available from the American Board of Pathology[13] and the American Academy for Medical Microbiology.[14] Specialty courses with certification in infection control can be obtained through the SHEA[15] and the APIC.[16] The extent of experience and/or training needed to support the laboratory's infection control plan will be dictated by the size of the healthcare organization and the complexity of the patients being cared for within the system.

DATA COLLECTION FROM MEDICAL MICROBIOLOGY

A cornerstone of managing the spread of infections is surveillance that can detect outbreaks and unfavorable trends. Because all material that is obtained for culture of potentially infected people is sent to the clinical microbiology laboratory for processing, this information resource is critical to an effective infection prevention program. The basic requirement for the microbiology laboratory's participation in the infection control and prevention program is the accurate determination of microbial identification and susceptibility testing.[17,18] For today's laboratory, this has been simplified by the availability of many semiautomated instruments that reliably perform these functions. Also, there are reliable reference texts that provide direction to the clinical laboratory in specimen processing, pathogen detection, and antimicrobial agent susceptibility determination. However, one must be aware of the limitations of instruments and test methods,[18] which are placing ever-growing challenges on the laboratory as new pathogens emerge and antimicrobial resistance disseminates. Particular importance should be focused on accurate species identification of nonfermentative gram-negative bacilli as well as drug-resistant streptococci (eg, enterococci) and detection of methicillin resistance in staphylococci. Additional challenges are accurate detection of vancomycin nonsusceptible staphylococci and enterococci, along with accurate delineation of multidrug-resistant Enterobacteriaceae (MDRE), such as extended-spectrum ß-lactamase producing *E. coli* and *Klebsiella* species or AmpC enzyme containing Enterobacteriaceae with inducible cephalosporinases. It is these very organisms that can pose difficulties for both identification[19,20] and susceptibility testing[21-23] by the automated systems and usually require manual confirmation methods be available for use in clinical laboratories.[24]

A crucial role of the laboratory is that of an "early warning center" for infection control problems arising in the organization.[17] Thus, once the laboratory generates the diagnostic data, the next step is to organize it into useful information that facilitates outbreak detection and tracking of infection trends throughout the healthcare organization. Some of the semiautomated identification and susceptibility testing systems have available surveillance programs to aid in infection control activities, but these have not been well studied and are not widely used. They also require input of any information gathered that is not generated by the identification and susceptibility testing they perform. Use of all the data in the microbiology laboratory information system is the ideal, as it has the potential for monitoring changes in antimicrobial susceptibility as well as detecting infection trends and alerting the infection control program to the appearance of new pathogens. A pilot study analyzing these data using simple algorithms reported the capacity for detecting clonal outbreaks of infection with only a fraction (2%) of the personnel resources needed by traditional infection control surveillance.[25]

The ability to use computer-generated information for determination of infection "rates" to compare current practice against past performance or national "standards" may also be desirable, but this remains problematic as there is yet no mechanism for doing this in a validated way using readily collected data that are reliable as a basis for comparison within or between organizations.

SURVEILLANCE

Perhaps the most important phase in an epidemiologic investigation is the initial step of realizing that a problem exists. Surveillance should be used to identify potential problems, prospectively monitor trends, and assess the quality of care in a critical area of patient safety—preventing healthcare-associated infectious diseases. To optimally do this requires high-quality laboratory data that are timely, accessible, and easily searched so that relevant information can be obtained.[26] Typically, microbiology data are reviewed daily in paper form by the institution's infection control professionals. However, the identification of important patterns relies on establishing associations between results that may be separated in time by weeks or months or nursing units or hospitals. Other factors that must be taken into consideration are isolate details such as susceptibility phenotype, source of the specimen, or admitting service; and all must be put into context with the historical data for each facility. Occasionally, the laboratory personnel may recognize a problem exists and notify infection control. However, planned use of the data generated by the microbiology laboratory information system will be the most efficient and effective approach to ensure the broadest monitoring for potential infection control issues. Complicating this approach is the fact that during the past 20 years, the volume of electronic data managed by laboratory staff has increased exponentially. In the 1980s and 1990s, the challenge faced by laboratorians was one of workflow, data entry, access, and physical storage. Today, the challenge is to unlock the tremendous potential of the vast electronic data sets our clinical efforts create and provide added value to our patients and their healthcare facilities.

To effectively use the microbiology data for infection control and prevention management, an effective computerized approach is needed (see Chapter 15). Currently, there are 2 data management concepts being developed for application to the microbiology laboratory information system: data presentation and data mining. The key differentiating factor between data presentation and data mining is that the former requires the analyst to first ask a question or design a query. The user of the data presentation tool is then presented with the results of the "question" asked. This type of hypothesis-driven process works well for low-dimensional data over limited periods of time, and even can be very sophisticated if a high number of the "right" questions are posed. However, there are trillions of potential surveillance patterns of interest within clinical data, and often the key to identifying an important trend requires the identification of complex, subtle, or unexpected relationships that emerge over time. Data mining systems can incorporate artificially intelligent algorithms that consider billions of possible combinations over multiple historical data timeframes and data fields and do not require that the user specify criteria in order for important patterns to be recognized. When properly designed, the data mining system will add patient location tracking information to the microbiology result data so that an elegant computer analysis can place patients with pathogens of importance together geographically and temporally in ways that are not possible with any type of manual surveillance approach.

The potential of this new data analysis technology to assist and expand traditional infection control surveillance has been demonstrated in initial assessments[27,28] and offers an opportunity to enhance healthcare-associated infection surveillance in the immediate future.[29] For laboratories that serve a large number of community physician offices, the use of technology that effectively screens the microbiology laboratory information system database can also detect infection pattern trends in the patients cared for in the community offices and alert their healthcare organization to the emergence of infections presenting in their outpatient population (eg, influenza virus, *Campylobacter* spp., rotavirus). Postdischarge infections that are detected only in the physician's office can also be monitored in such a setting, assuming cultures are taken in the practices when one of these infections develops. Similarly, clinical laboratories that service residents of LTCFs and have sophisticated monitoring of their information system data can play an important disease surveillance, outbreak detection, and antimicrobial resistance monitoring role in this major part of the healthcare sys-

tem, whose infection control and prevention needs are only beginning to be recognized.[30]

The laboratory leadership must also be aware of the potential of laboratory-acquired infections[17] and provide for the safety of workers through the provision of safe practices, appropriate personal protective equipment, education regarding effective hand hygiene, and offering of effective vaccines. These practices need to be updated whenever new issues relating to laboratory safety are recognized.[31]

Detecting Infection Transmission

Just as genetic testing has allowed microbiologists to rename and reclassify pathogens, new advances in the analysis of clinical laboratory data have exposed trends that may herald the need for the revision of what comprises an "outbreak." Traditionally, a microbiology result must be combined with clinical confirmation of active, symptomatic infection before a case can be entered into a formal surveillance system. This approach is time consuming, requiring ongoing chart review and clinical examination by ICPs. While an established practice, it can severely limit the scope, sensitivity, and timeliness of traditional surveillance. As a result, opportunities to intervene proactively on the underlying process failures that cause preventable nosocomial infections may be missed.[32] Importantly, recent clinical studies illustrate the need to consider tracking increased colonization as a harbinger for impending infections.[33,34]

The clinical microbiology laboratory that makes good use of its electronic data sources as a resource for infection control and prevention is in the best position to report accurate, objective rates and help focus infection prevention interventions.[35] They can monitor for outcomes beyond strictly symptomatic patients, discovering quality issues that may not have yet resulted in poor clinical outcomes. This will be critical as we strive for zero-tolerance of preventable hospital-associated infections.[27]

Outbreak Investigation

The clinical microbiology laboratory needs to have the capacity (either internally or through a reference laboratory) for effective outbreak investigation. A component of this that may not be immediately apparent is the requirement for ongoing services relating to outbreak investigation once an intervention is initiated by the infection control department and there is a need for monitoring of the results following the intervention. In addition to the information needed for effective surveillance described earlier, the laboratory should have the capacity for performance of subspecies identification (fingerprinting) that can aide the infection control professionals in the outbreak investigation.[36] Subspecies identification for determination of microbial clonality can rapidly focus the infection control professional's attention as to the cause of an outbreak during the initial investigation. For example, transmission of microbes from patient-to-patient is likely if strains are identical or closely related. In this event, enhancement and/or retraining in the appropriate infection control practices are needed. This scenario is less likely if strains are unrelated at the subspecies level. Causes of outbreaks due to unrelated strains are often found to be changes in antimicrobial prescribing or breaks in standard nursing practice techniques, and a focus on these factors often can rapidly resolve the outbreak.[36,37] Figure 13-1 provides an example of an epidemiologic typing report from the laboratory.

There are several methods for the laboratory determination of subspecies relatedness, often referred to as DNA fingerprinting,[38] which are discussed in detail in Chapter 14. The important issue to consider when choosing a system is to inquire if it has been validated against clinical epidemiologic information. To date, the most information regarding clinical validation supports the utility of pulsed-field gel electrophoresis (PFGE) and genomic restriction endonuclease analysis (REA). Both typing systems have been validated using organisms from documented outbreak scenarios,[39,40] and PFGE is available as a commercial product. An automated ribotyping system is also commercially available, but the clinical epidemiologic utility of this system has not been consistently confirmed.[41,42] The decade of the 1990s saw the introduction of this technology as a powerful tool for outbreak investigation, and the accessibility of subspecies identification is now widespread.[43,44] For a laboratory to adequately support the infection control program in this aspect of outbreak investigation, all potentially relevant microbial isolates need to be saved for a period of time so that they can be recovered from storage in case molecular typing is needed once a potential outbreak is recognized. With an active program of surveillance of the microbiology laboratory information system data that typically detects potential outbreaks on a monthly basis, we have found it sufficient to store any bacterial isolate that had undergone susceptibility testing for a total of 2 months. This 2-month time period for storage has facilitated retrospective DNA fingerprint analysis whenever needed and has not unnecessarily burdened the laboratory personnel resources or storage (space) capacity. Storage for 2 months can be accomplished for most organisms using primary purity plate cultures held at room or refrigerator temperature, after which the organisms and media can be safely discarded by following the established local and federal regulations for disposal of biohazardous material.

Another important role for the clinical laboratory during outbreak investigation and infection control management is supporting active surveillance to detect carriers of the pathogen(s) of concern. This capacity has increased during the past 10 years, rising from 51.7% of clinical laboratories providing this service in 1993 to a full 94.8% having this ability in 2003.[44] The most frequently encountered organisms where active surveillance cultures are recommended are MRSA and VRE.[45-52] However, in an outbreak setting, special media and recovery techniques may be required to detect a wide range of bacteria encompassing Enterobacteriaceae,[47,51,52] *P. aeruginosa*,[53] *A. baumannii*,[54] and *C. difficile*,[55] as a few examples. Here, the laboratory's role ranges from preparing special screening media to rapid detection of the target organisms and reporting the findings to the infection control professionals.

A new, developing technology will expand the role of active surveillance and the participation of the clinical laboratory in effective infection control and prevention. Application of the polymerase chain reaction (PCR) to surveillance activities has great potential as it can quickly detect specific resistance determinants and unique virulence factors that are markers for the presence of pathogenic bacteria of importance to the management of healthcare-associated infections. Paule and colleagues have developed a PCR test for VRE that permits perianal sampling with PCR yielding results as sensitive as intrarectal culture,[56] thus making surveillance for VRE less invasive. The new technology of real-time PCR (R-PCR) has been applied to surveillance for *S. aureus*. This test can be completed in as little as 2 hours from the time of patient sampling, with initial reports finding the PCR test performed directly on an anterior nares swab nearly as sensitive as culture.[57] Using a novel enhancement for this test, Paule and colleagues have developed a R-PCR assay for *S. aureus* that is more sensitive than screening culture and validated its performance in both adults and neonates.[58] Technology such as this has the potential to revolutionize active surveillance screening followed by isolation or decolonization of important pathogens to limit spread of nosocomially acquired bacteria in ways not previously attempted. PCR has been suggested in the past as a means for reliable detection of *C. difficile* infection by targeting its pathogenic toxin genes.[59] R-PCR has the potential for rapidly detecting this microbe as well and may offer the opportunity for improved management of this nosocomial infection of worldwide importance.

Additional resource needs may be required from the clinical microbiology laboratory when an outbreak investigation and intervention are underway. These can vary from the relatively simple task of performing some additional susceptibility testing to more complex tasks such as airborne or environmental pathogen detection. Whenever such additional tasks are considered, the protocols should

The Healthcare Organization   MICROBIOLOGY EPIDEMIOLOGY REPORT
2050 Main Ave   DEPARTMENT OF PATHOLOGY AND LABORATORY MEDICINE
Largeville, DC   METROPOLITAN HEALTHCARE

Request: Typing MRSA Isolates from Northside Hospital
Requested by: Dr. Jones, Infection Control
Date requested: 1/31/2004

Method: MRSA isolates were typed by PFGE of genomic DNA. The DNA was digested
                                     with *SmaI* restriction enzyme resulting in fragments ranging from 50 to 500 kb.

Method of interpretation: The resulting DNA banding patterns of each isolate were visually compared to
                                     one another to determine if they were genetically related.

Interpretation	Visual Analysis
Identical	0 Band Difference
Closely related	1-3 Band Differences
Possibly related	4-6 Band Differences
Unrelated	≥7 Band Differences

PFGE is used to supplement an epidemiological investigation. In general, common source or cross transmission of strains is likely if strains are identical and probable if strains are closely related. Common source of cross transmission is less likely if strains are possibly related and improbable if strains are unrelated. Causes of outbreaks due to unrelated strains are often changes in antimicrobial prescribing or breaks in standard nursing practice techniques.

Results: Gel: A07212

Lane	Isolate	Patient Number	Type
1	Control	1	NH-A0
2	Blood	5	NH-F0
3	Fluid	12	NH-B2
4	Blood	15	NH-B0
5	Sputum	16	NH-D1
6	Catheter	23	NH-D0
7	Urine	24	NH-G0
8	Surveillance	25	NH-C0
9	Blood	33	NH-E0

The DNA banding patterns of the MRSA isolates received from Northside Hospital (NH) were compared to one another and to all previous MRSA isolates from NH sent to Metropolitan Hospital for PFGE Typing. The DNA banding patterns of the MRSA isolates from patient number 12 were closely related to Type NH-B0 and were designated Type NH-B2. The DNA banding pattern of the MRSA isolate from patient number 16 was distantly (6 bands in common) related to Type NH-D0 and was designated Type NH-D1. The DNA banding pattern of the MRSA isolate from patient number 24 was unrelated to all other MRSA isolates and was designated Type NH-G0.

The preliminary results were phoned to Dr. Jones in NH Infection Control on January 4, 2004.

Interpretation (by Dr. Smith): These results suggest ongoing transmission of several clonal MRSA strains within the nursing unit and that a clinical epidemiological investigation with intervention is warranted. Also, because there continues to be introduction of new, unrelated strain types into the nursing unit, it appears worthwhile to consider implementing an ongoing screening program with the objective of early recognition and isolation of patients newly colonized with MRSA.

Figure 13-1. Example of a molecular typing report from the clinical microbiology laboratory.

be developed jointly between the clinical laboratory and the infection control staff. It is important to not overuse the resources of the clinical laboratory, which is best accomplished through careful planning of what is needed and how the goals are to be accomplished before the surveillance project begins. A good example of this is in the area of environmental sampling. Such testing is not generally recommended because some microorganisms are always recovered; however, it can be invaluable when the source of a clonal outbreak involving many different patients is thought to be something in the healthcare environment. When such sampling is considered, it is imperative to carefully define ahead of time what pathogen(s) are being sought and then to confine the search to detect only those organisms predefined before the surveillance cultures were obtained. When such advanced planning is not done, many resources are wasted, both in the laboratory through culture and identification of a wide array of recovered species and on the part of the infection control professionals in trying to determine the meaning and impact of the recovered microbes.

INTERVENTIONS

Interventions to limit the spread of healthcare-associated infections and antimicrobial resistance are among the most critical activities of the infection control and prevention program and are carried out by the infection control professionals. Interventions are most successful if there is a thorough understanding of the problem being confronted and knowledge of what has been useful for past management of similar occurrences. Because modern healthcare is increasingly complex and the nature of any given problem is often unclear, frequent meetings between the key infection control stakeholders,[36,37,60] typically the Infection Control Department, Clinical Microbiology, and Infectious Diseases, facilitates interpretation of microbial trend, outbreak, and antibiotic resistance information. When an intervention is designed and ready for implementation, a monitoring system, usually based upon the same surveillance methods that initially detected the problem, must be in place so that the outcome of the intervention is tracked to measure the effectiveness of the effort.

REPORTING SYSTEMS

The clinical laboratory has many requirements for effectively transmitting the information it generates and collects. In addition to the direct patient care reporting that is its traditional role, the clinical laboratory needs to effectively report relevant information to the infection control professionals responsible for infection manage-

ment and prevention within the organization. Beyond this, the entire United States communicable disease surveillance system depends on the reporting of clinical and public health laboratories.[61] Both the CDC as well as local public health departments set regulations for reportable diseases, and the clinical microbiology laboratory must work closely with the infection control professionals of their organization to make sure the reporting system is well organized and ensures that all required reports are efficiently transmitted. The reporting requirements are the same for healthcare organizations regardless of whether their microbiology testing is done on-site or at a referral laboratory, and this must be taken into account whenever the system for implementing infection control notification is designed.

MONITORING OUTCOME

Tracking the medical and economic benefits of a comprehensive infection management and prevention program is perhaps one of the most difficult tasks faced by the program, but it is critical if adequate long-term resources are to be provided for all necessary aspects of this important patient safety effort.[62] We have found, using global hospital nosocomial infection data, that enhancing an existing program by adding new laboratory resources reduced patient care costs by $5.00 for each additional dollar spent in the laboratory support of infection control.[36] Additional work in health economics research suggests that enhanced surveillance also reduces morbidity, mortality, and cost.[63] Finally, as computer systems for monitoring the microbiology laboratory information system data mature, they will enable the laboratory to provide various types of outcome analysis information as a routine function and further document the medical and economic benefits of the infection control program.

COMMUNICATING INFECTION PREVENTION

The need for ongoing, continuing education is a well-recognized requirement for an effective infection control and prevention program.[7] The laboratory contributes to this through formal participation in the organization's infection control committee[9] and through active involvement in the departmental infection control plan.[11] In a less formal manner, the laboratory can help in the ongoing education of healthcare personnel through daily interpersonal interactions while reporting patient laboratory results, by presenting healthcare infection information at conferences and seminars, and through highlighting the activities of the organizations' infection control and prevention activities in newsletters throughout the year. Such ongoing communication of the many aspects of the infection control program is necessary and beneficial and is an expected contribution of the clinical microbiology laboratory for improving patient care.

THE COORDINATED PROGRAM

Infection control and prevention as an important aspect of high-quality medical care cannot be underestimated. It requires continued effort not only in the performance of myriad managerial and technical activities, but also in the effort required to maintain effective interactions between all the personnel and departments involved in the organization's program. Two critical elements of this interactive management plan are the infection control and clinical microbiology professionals who must work closely together and collaborate for the patients' benefit.[64] The collaboration takes place in formal committee meetings as well as in informal daily discussions of infection control-related activities.

CONCLUSIONS

The 21st century is beginning with increased opportunities for the diagnostic clinical microbiology laboratory to impact the effectiveness of the healthcare organization's infection control and prevention program. Traditional requirements for accurate and timely microbial identification and susceptibility testing remain as key pillars for supporting infection control professionals. However, emerging technologies now permit even more opportunities for lowering the risk of a patient developing a healthcare-associated infection if fully implemented by the diagnostic laboratory. Molecular technology is readily available that can quickly determine the presence of microbial clonality and focus the direction of an epidemiologic investigation so that the proper intervention can be applied more quickly. Soon, molecular tests also may provide real-time active surveillance to effectively limit spread of important healthcare pathogens more quickly than ever possible before. Novel informatics such as data mining with artificial intelligence now offer the capacity to track trends and detect outbreaks ranging from community settings over a wide geographic area to transmission of a healthcare pathogen between 2 or 3 people on a single nursing ward. Once widely applied, they can even alert us to sentinel events indicating new antimicrobial resistance, and perhaps the emergence of novel, previously unrecognized infectious diseases. The future is very

bright for an ever-strengthening partnership between the infection control and clinical microbiology professional as a team to lower healthcare infections, enhance patient safety, and improve the quality of care.

REFERENCES

1. Wangensteen OH, Wangensteen SD. *The Rise of Surgery*. Minneapolis, Minn: University of Minnesota Press; 1978.

2. LaForce FM. The control of infections in hospitals: 1750-1950. In: Wenzel RP, ed. *Prevention and Control of Nosocomial Infections*. 3rd ed. Baltimore, Md: Williams & Wilkins; 1997:1-32.

3. Emori TG, Culver DH, Horan TC, et al. National nosocomial infections surveillance system (NNIS): Description of surveillance methods. *Am J Infect Control*. 1991;19:19-35.

4. Haley RW, Aber RC, Bennett JV. Surveillance of nosocomial infections. In: Bennett JV, Brachman PS, eds. *Hospital Infections*. New York, NY: Little, Brown & Company; 1986:51-71.

5. Gross PA, Beaugard A, Van Antwerpen C. Surveillance for nosocomial infections: can the sources of data be reduced? *Infect Control*. 1980;1:233-236.

6. Haley RW, Schaberg DR, McClish DK, et al. The accuracy of retrospective chart review in measuring nosocomial infection rates. *Am J Epidemiol*. 1980;111:516-533.

7. Scheckler WE, Brimhall D, Buck AS, et al. Requirements for infrastructure and essential activities of infection control and epidemiology in hospitals: a consensus panel report. *Infect Control Hosp Epidemiol*. 1998;19:114-124.

8. Pfaller MA, Cormican MG. Microbiology: the role of the clinical laboratory. In: Wenzel RP, ed. *Prevention and Control of Nosocomial Infections*. 3rd ed. Baltimore, Md: Williams & Wilkins; 1997:95-118.

9. Peterson LR, Hamilton JD, Baron EJ, et al. Role of clinical microbiology laboratories in the management and control of infectious diseases and the delivery of healthcare. *Clin Infect Dis*. 2001;32:605-610.

10. JCAHO. Joint Commission on Accreditation of Healthcare Organizations. Proposed Standards Prevention and Control of Infection: Hospital Program. Available at: http://www.jcaho.org/accredited+organizations/accredited+organizations+.htm. Accessed July 30, 2003.

11. JCAHO. Joint Commission on Accreditation of Healthcare Organizations. Proposed Standards Prevention and Control of Infection: Laboratory. Available at: http://www.jcaho.org/accredited+organizations/accredited+organizations+.htm. Accessed July 30, 2003.

12. JCAHO. Joint Commission on Accreditation of Healthcare Organizations 2005 Laboratory Surveillance, Prevention, and Control of Infection Standards. http://www.jcaho.org/accredited+organizations/laboratory+services/standards/pre-publication/prepub_standards.htm. Accessed June 19, 2004.

13. Accreditation Council for Graduate Medical Education. Program Requirements for Residency Education in Medical Microbiology. Available at: http://www.acgme.org/. Accessed August 7, 2003.

14. The American College of Microbiology. Microbiology Training Standards. Available at: http://www.asm.org/Academy/index.asp?bid=2253. Accessed August 7, 2003.

15. The Society for Healthcare Epidemiology of America, Inc. SHEA/CDC Training Course in Healthcare Epidemiology. Available at: http://www.shea-online.org/Courses.html. Accessed August 7, 2003.

16. Association for Professionals in Infection Control and Epidemiology, Inc. Infection Control Education. Available at: http://www.apic.org/educ/. Accessed August 7, 2003.

17. Weinstein RA, Mallison GF. The role of the microbiology laboratory in surveillance and control of nosocomial infections. *Am J Clin Pathol*. 1978;69:130-136.

18. Diekema DJ, Pfaller MA. Infection control epidemiology and clinical microbiology. In: Murray PR, Baron EJ, Jorgensen JH, Pfaller MA, Yolken RH, eds. *Manual of Clinical Microbiology*. 8th ed. Washington, DC: American Society for Microbiology Press; 2003:129-138.

19. Warren JR, Farmer JJ III, Dewhirst FE, et al. Outbreak of nosocomial infections due to extended spectrum b-lactamase-producing strains of Enteric Group 137: a new Enterobacteriaceae closely related to *Citrobacter farmeri* and *Citrobacter amalonaticus. J Clin Microbiol*. 2000;38:3946-3952.

20. Gavin PJ, Warren JR, Obias AA, Collins SM, Peterson LR. Evaluation of the Vitek 2 system for rapid identification of clinical isolates of gram-negative bacilli and members of the family Streptococcaceae. *Eur J Clin Microbiol Infect Dis*. 2002;21:869-874.

21. Ender PT, Durning SJ, Woelk WK, et al. Pseudo-outbreak of methicillin-resistant *Staphylococcus aureus. Mayo Clin Proc*. 1999;74:855-859.

22. Tsakris A, Pantazi A, Pournaras S, Maniatis A, Polyzou A, Sofianou D. Pseudo-outbreak of imipenem-resistant Acinetobacter baumannii resulting from false susceptibility testing by a rapid automated system. *J Clin Microbiol*. 2000;38:3505-3507.

23. Steward CD, Mohammed JM, Swenson JM, et al. Antimicrobial susceptibility testing of carbapenems: multicenter validity testing and accuracy levels of five antimicrobial test methods for detecting resistance in Enterobacteriaceae and *Pseudomonas aeruginosa* isolates. *J Clin Microbiol*. 2003;41:351-358.

24. Swenson JM, Hindler J, Peterson LR. Special phenotypic methods for detecting antibacterial resistance. In: Murray PR, Baron EJ, Jorgensen JH, Pfaller MA, Tenover FC, Yolken RH, eds. *Manual of Clinical Microbiology*. 7th ed. Washington, DC: American Society for Microbiology Press; 1999:1563-1577.

25. Hacek DM, Cordell RL, Noskin GA, Peterson LR. Computer-assisted surveillance for detecting clonal outbreaks of nosocomial infection. *J Clin Microbiol*. 2004;42:1170-1175.

26. Emori TG, Gaynes RP. An overview of nosocomial infections, including the role of the microbiology laboratory. *Clin Microbiol Rev*. 1993;6:428-442.

27. Gerberding JL. Hospital-onset infections: a patient safety issue. *Annals of Internal Medicine*. 2002;137:665-670. new

28. Brossette SE, Sprague AP, Jones WT, Moser SA. A data mining system for infection control surveillance. *Meth Informatics Med*. 2000;39:303-310.

29. Hacek D, Vescio T, Thomson R, Paule S, Brossette S, Peterson L. Initial experience with data mining surveillance service (DMSS®) as part of an enhanced infection control program. Program and Abstracts of the Forty-First Annual Meeting of the Infectious Diseases Society of America, October 9-12, 2003 San Diego, Calif. Abstract #908.

30. Simor AE. The role of the laboratory in infection prevention and control programs in long-term-care facilities for the elderly. *Infect Control Hosp Epidemiol*. 2001;7:459-463.

31. Centers for Disease Control and Prevention. Laboratory-acquired meningococcal disease—United States, 2000. *MMWR*. 2002;51:141-144.

32. Price CS, Hacek DM, Noskin GA, Peterson LR. Outbreak of bloodstream infections in an outpatient hemodialysis center. *Infect Control Hosp Epidem*. 2002;23:725-729.

33. Settle CD, Wilcox MH, Fawley WN, Corrado OJ, Hawkey PM. Prospective study of the risk of *Clostridium difficile* diarrhea in elderly patients following treatment with cefotaxime or piperacillin-tazobactam. *Aliment Pharmacol Ther*. 1998;12:1217-1223.

34. Bradley SJ, Wilson AL, Allen MC, Sher HA, Goldstone AH, Scott GM. The control of hyperendemic glycopeptide-resistant Enterococcus spp. on a haematology unit by changing antibiotic usage. *J Antimicrob Chemother*. 1999;43:261-266.

35. Wright MO, Perencevich EN, Novak C, Hebden JN, Standiford HC, Harris AD. Preliminary assessment of an automated surveillance system for infection control. *Infect Control Hosp Epidemiol*. 2004;25:325-332.

36. Peterson LR, Noskin GA. New technology for detecting multidrug-resistant pathogens in the clinical microbiology laboratory. *Emerg Infect Dis*. 2001;7:306-311.

37. Hacek DM, Suriano T, Noskin GA, Kruszynski J, Reisberg B, Peterson LR. Medical and economic benefit of a comprehensive infection control program that includes routine determination of microbial clonality. *Am J Clin Pathol*. 1999;111:647-654.

38. Soll DR, Lockhart SR, Pujol C. Laboratory procedures for the epidemiological analysis of microorganisms. In: Murray PR, Baron EJ, Jorgensen JH, Pfaller MA, Yolken RH, eds. *Manual of Clinical Microbiology*. 8th ed. Washington, DC: American Society for Microbiology Press; 2003:139-161.

39. Clabots CR, Johnson S, Bettin KM, et al. Development of a rapid and efficient restriction endonuclease analysis (REA) typing system for Clostridium difficile and correlation with other typing systems. *J Clin Microbiol*. 1993;31:1870-1875.

40. Savor C, Pfaller MA, Kruszynski JA, Hollis RJ, Noskin GA, Peterson LR. Genomic methods for differentiating strains of *Enterococcus faecium*: an assessment using clinical epidemiologic data. *J Clin Microbiol*. 1998;36:3327-3331.

41. Price CS, Huynh H, Paule S, et al. Comparison of an automated ribotyping system to restriction endonuclease analysis and pulsed-field gel electrophoresis for differentiating vancomycin-resistant *Enterococcus faecium*. *J Clin Microbiol*. 2002;40:1858-1861.

42. Fontana J, Stout A, Bolstorff B, Timperi R. Automated ribotyping and pulsed-field gel electrophoresis for rapid identification of multidrug-resistant Salmonella serotype Newport. *Emerg Infect Dis*. 2003;9:496-499.

43. McGowan JE Jr. New laboratory techniques for hospital infection control. *Am J Med*. 1991;91(3B):S245-S251.

44. Peterson L, Miller JM. ClinMicroNet. Microbiology directors' forum (a worldwide electronic information network of leading clinical microbiology laboratory directors; not available to general public). *ClinMicroNet*. February, 2003.

45. Muto CA, Jernigan JA, Ostrowsky BE, et al. SHEA guideline for preventing nosocomial transmission of multidrug-resistant strains of *Staphylococcus aureus* and *enterococcus*. *Infect Control Hosp Epidemiol*. 2003;24: 362-386.

46. Noskin GA, Bednarz P, Suriano T, Reiner S, Peterson LR. Persistent contamination of fabric-covered furniture by vancomycin-resistant enterococci: implications for upholstery selection in hospitals. *Am J Infect Control*. 2000;28:311-313.

47. Collins SM, Hacek DM, Degan LA, Wright MO, Noskin GA, Peterson LR. Contamination of the clinical microbiology laboratory with vancomycin-resistant enterococci and multidrug-resistant Enterobacteriaceae: implications for hospital and laboratory workers. *J Clin Microbiol*. 2001;39:3772-3774.

48. Trick WE, Temple RS, Chen D, Wright MO, Solomon SL, Peterson LR. Patient colonization and environmental contamination by vancomycin-resistant enterococci in a rehabilitation facility. *Arch Phys Med Rehabil*. 2002;83: 899-902.

49. Singh K, Gavin PJ, Vescio T, et al. Microbiologic surveillance using nasal cultures alone is sufficient for detection of methicillin-resistant *Staphylococcus aureus* isolates in neonates. *J Clin Microbiol*. 2003;41:2755-2757.

50. Price CS, Paule S, Noskin GA, Peterson LR. Active surveillance reduces the incidence of vancomycin-resistant enterococcal bacteremia. *Clin Infect Dis*. 2003;37:921-928.

51. Hacek DM, Trick WE, Collins SM, Noskin GA, Peterson LR. Comparison of the RODAC imprint method with selective enrichment broth for the recovery of vancomycin-resistant enterococci and drug resistant Enterobacteriaceae from environmental surfaces. *J Clin Microbiol*. 2000;38: 4646-4648.

52. Hacek DM, Bednarz P, Noskin GA. Zembower T, Peterson LR. Yield of vancomycin-resistant enterococci (VRE) and multidrug-resistant Enterobacteriaceae (MDRE) from stool submitted for *Clostridium difficile* testing compared to results from a focused surveillance program. *J Clin Microbiol*. 2001;39:1152-1154.

53. Sorin M, Segal-Maurer S, Mariano N, Urban C, Combest A, Rahal JJ. Nosocomial transmission of imipenem-resistant *Pseudomonas aeruginosa* following bronchoscopy associated with improper connection to the Steris System 1 processor. *Infect Control Hosp Epidemiol*. 2001;22:409-413.

54. Urban C, Segal-Maurer S, Rahal JJ. Considerations in control and treatment of nosocomial infections due to multidrug-resistant *Acinetobacter baumannii*. *Clin Infect Dis*. 2003;36:1268-1274.

55. Clabots CE, Bettin KM, Peterson, LR, Gerding DN. Evaluation of cycloserine-cefoxitin-fructose agar and cycloserine-cefoxitin-fructose broth for recovery of *Clostridium difficile* from environmental sites. *J Clin Microbiol*. 1991;29:2633-2635.

56. Paule SM, Trick WE, Tenover FC, et al. Comparison of polymerase chain reaction to culture for surveillance detection of vancomycin-resistant enterococci. *J Clin Microbiol*. 2003;41:4805-4807.

57. Shrestha NK, Shermock KM, Gordon SM, et al. Predictive value and cost-effectiveness analysis of a rapid polymerase chain reaction for preoperative detection of nasal carriage of *Staphylococcus aureus*. *Infect Control Hosp Epidemiol*. 2003;24:327-333.

58. Paule SM, Pasquariello AC, Hacek DM, Fisher AG, Thomson RB Jr, Kaul KL,. Peterson LR. Direct detection of *Staphylococcus aureus* from adult and neonate nasal swab specimens using real-time polymerase chain reaction. *J Molec Diag*. In press.

59. Tang YJ, Gumerlock PH, Weiss JB, Silva J Jr. Specific detection of *Clostridium difficile* toxin A gene sequences in clinical isolates. *Mol Cell Probes*. 1994;8:463-467.

60. Kolmos HJ. Role of the clinical microbiology laboratory in infection control—a Danish perspective. *J Hosp Infect*. 2001;48(Suppl A):S50-S54.

61. Skeels MR. Laboratories and disease surveillance. *Military Med*. 2000;165(7 Suppl 2):16-19.

62. Roberts RR, Scott RD II, Cordell R, et al. The use of economic modeling to determine the hospital costs associated with nosocomial infections. *Clin Infect Dis*. 2003;36:1424-1432.

63. Lee TA, Hacek DM, Stroupe KT, Collins SM, Peterson LR. Three surveillance strategies for vancomycin-resistant enterococci in hospitalized patients: Detection of colonization efficiency and a cost effectiveness model. *Infect Control Hosp Epidemiol*. In press.

64. Pfaller MA, Herwaldt LA. The clinical microbiology laboratory and infection control: emerging pathogens, antimicrobial resistance, and new technology. *Clin Infect Dis*. 1997;25:858-870.

CHAPTER FOURTEEN

MOLECULAR TYPING SYSTEMS

Carolyn V. Gould, MD and Joel Maslow, MD, PhD

INTRODUCTION

The hospital epidemiologist is frequently presented with situations that suggest that multiple patients may be infected with genetically identical organisms representing an outbreak situation. While many of these cases are clearly due to a common source exposure, being limited by time and place, other events are not as obvious. For the latter cases, it is helpful to be able to determine whether groups of organisms are the same or different (ie, represent a common source outbreak or not).

Molecular typing methods have become increasingly powerful tools for epidemiologic investigations of nosocomial infections.[1] When used properly as adjuncts to classical epidemiologic studies, these methods can greatly facilitate the job of the hospital epidemiologist. Infection control professionals must be familiar with the ever-expanding number of typing methods along with the limitations, costs, and applicability of the various techniques in order to choose the most appropriate method for a given purpose. A major caveat in this field is that results of molecular typing should never be interpreted in the absence of data from sound clinical epidemiologic studies. Molecular studies can prove or disprove epidemiologic hypothesis; however, when used inappropriately, incorrect conclusions may be drawn and laboratory resources wasted.

When used in conjunction with epidemiological data, molecular typing systems are valuable tools for investigating potential outbreaks of infection. The goal of strain typing is to provide laboratory evidence that epidemiologically related isolates implicated in an outbreak are also genetically related and therefore are the same strain, presumably transmitted by a common source of exposure or from patient to patient.[2] For this to be put into practice, a sec-

ond caveat is given: isolates must be saved prospectively for later comparison.

In addition to aiding in outbreak investigations, molecular techniques have been increasingly employed to detect slow-growing or fastidious organisms such as *Bartonella henselae, M. tuberculosis*, and uncultivatable viruses. A more recent use has been the rapid detection of organisms carrying antibiotic resistance genes such as those that encode for methicillin and vancomycin resistance and detection of antibiotic resistance among slow-growing organisms such as *M. tuberculosis*. These techniques offer advantages in infection control and timelier, appropriate treatment for patients.[3] Thus, there is considerable overlap between molecular diagnostics and molecular epidemiology.

BASIC BIOLOGICAL PRINCIPLES

Three assumptions are generally made in using molecular typing for the purpose of epidemiologic studies of microorganisms: (1) isolates responsible for an outbreak are the recent progeny of a common ancestor, (2) these isolates have the same genotype, and (3) epidemiologically unrelated strains have different genotypes.[1,2] The concept of clonality is a fundamental principle in strain typing. Microbial isolates recovered from different sources are considered to be "clones" if they have "so many identical phenotypic and genetic traits that the most likely explanation for this identity is a common origin."[4] Therefore, the determination of clonality cannot be made with absolute certainty, but instead represents a statistical likelihood of identity among a group of independently isolated organisms.[5] The better the discriminatory power of the technique used to identify the isolate, the more likely clonality can be ensured. However, because of the inherent instability of phenotypic traits in all organisms, especially in the presence of environmental selective pressure, clonality must be considered in a relative rather than an absolute sense.[5] Because of natural genetic drift, it is important to consider the length of time over which isolates have been collected when interpreting results. In general, isolates from a potential outbreak spanning 1 to 3 months are appropriate for strain typing analyses.[1] The rate of genetic drift will determine the likelihood that clonally derived progeny maintain similarity when analyzed over prolonged periods of time.

In most cases, wide genetic variability within a bacterial species usually allows for the differentiation of unrelated strains using a number of different techniques.[1] However, because the most virulent bacterial strains often are clonally restricted (ie, represent only a small fraction of the number of clones within a species[6]), bacteria that are most likely to cause infection may have little genetic diversity, making them difficult to differentiate. An example of this uniformity is MRSA isolates, which are derived from a small number of clones.[7]

EPIDEMIOLOGIC ANALYSIS: OUTBREAK INVESTIGATION VERSUS SURVEILLANCE

There are 2 major epidemiologic reasons for doing strain typing: (1) conducting outbreak investigations, and (2) performing long-term prospective surveillance for the purpose of detecting and monitoring emerging or reemerging pathogens. Outbreak investigations typically involve the analysis of a limited number of isolates collected over a relatively short period of time.[8] Results of these comparative typing systems are usually applicable only to a particular local problem. In contrast, monitoring the prevalence and geographic spread of epidemic and endemic clones in a population over longer periods of time requires the development of typing "libraries" and mandates the use of typing systems that are standardized, highly reproducible, and uniform in nomenclature.[8] Many potentially useful techniques include genome restriction fragment length polymorphism (RFLP) analysis, repetitive elements PCR spacer typing, PCR-sequencing, and high-density DNA probe assays (DNA chip technology).[8]

DIAGNOSIS

The rapid expansion of sequence-based techniques has opened up potentially limitless opportunities to diagnose infectious diseases and simultaneously to differentiate

individual strains. Specific PCR assays now exist for a wide variety of fastidious, slow-growing, or uncultivatable organisms, and broad-range PCR techniques can be used to diagnose previously unrecognized pathogens.[9] For example, broad range bacterial 16S rDNA amplification and sequencing was used to detect the uncultivatable Whipple bacillus, *Tropheryma whippelii*.[10] PCR testing for *Herpes simplex* virus has supplanted brain biopsy as the gold standard for diagnosing *H. simplex* encephalitis.[11] Molecular methods are also valuable tools in cases where conventional culture fails because of previous antibiotic use or specimen mishandling or formalin preservation.

MOLECULAR METHODS: AN OVERVIEW

The most useful typing methods fulfill 3 criteria: (1) *typeability*—the ability of the technique to give an unambiguous result (type) for each isolate; (2) *reproducibility*—the capacity of the method to give the same result upon repeat testing; and (3) *discriminatory power*—the ability of the system to differentiate among epidemiologically unrelated strains.[1,12,13] Choosing a typing method depends not only on the strengths of the particular method in each of these areas, but on the organism in question. Also, the *ease of performance* in terms of the technical complexity and the costs of reagents and equipment as well as *ease of interpretation* are important criteria for choosing a typing system.[1,13]

Phenotypic Methods

Phenotypic methods were the original techniques used for epidemiologic purposes. They detect characteristics expressed by microorganisms, such as enzymatic products or cell surface proteins and include biotyping, serotyping, bacteriophage susceptibility, antimicrobial susceptibility, and bacteriocin production. Biotyping and antibiotic susceptibilities are routinely automated as part of the routine workup of clinical specimens. The remaining techniques have ceased to be routinely available and are now relegated to certain research labs. Because many phenotypic traits are particularly susceptible to environmental pressure, phenotypic methods are limited in their discriminatory power and reproducibility.

Genotypic Methods

Genotypic methods involve direct DNA-based analyses of chromosomal or extra-chromosomal genetic elements. The introduction of DNA-based methods in molecular typing has vastly improved the ability of investigators to distinguish among different strains within a species. The techniques offer improved typeability, reproducibility, and discriminatory power as compared to phenotypic meth-

TABLE 14-1. PHENOTYPIC AND GENOTYPIC TYPING METHODS*

Phenotypic Methods	*Genotypic Methods*
Biotyping	Plasmid fingerprinting, with or without REA
Antimicrobial susceptibility testing	
Serotyping	Chromosomal restriction enzyme analysis with conventional electrophoresis
Bacteriophage typing	Genome RFLP
Bacteriocin typing	Insertion sequence (IS) probe fingerprinting
Multilocus enzyme electrophoresis (MLEE)	Ribotyping
	PFGE
	PCR
	Arbitrarily primed PCR (AP-PCR)
	PCR of repetitive chromosomal elements (Rep-PCR)
	Polymerase chain reaction-restriction fragment length polymorphism (PCR-RFLP)

*List not comprehensive

ods. Genotypic methods are also less affected by natural variation in a population, although changes such as insertions or deletions of DNA into the chromosome, the gain or loss of extrachromosomal DNA, or random mutations may introduce difficulties in interpretation.[1]

Phenotypic and genotypic methods commonly used for epidemiologic typing of microorganisms are listed in Table 14-1.

CHOOSING CONTROLS

In all typing systems, well-characterized control strains should be analyzed together with the clinical isolates in question. This ensures that all steps in the protocol are working and that the results of the procedure are reproducible from run to run within the laboratory and are consistent with those obtained by other investigators for the same strain.[2] The use of reference strains provides for consistency between analyses performed at different times. Such strains may also be used to provide molecular weight information.

Reference strains should not, however, be the sole source of controls. It is also important when investigating a potential outbreak of nosocomial infections to include epidemiologically unrelated strains to ensure that the procedure is able to differentiate between epidemic and endemic strains.[1,2] Typically, such strains should be similar geographically and temporally to the strains of interest. This is particularly important for strains with limited genetic variability such as MRSA because it may not be possible to discriminate easily between outbreak and nonoutbreak strains by any molecular typing method.[7] Thus,

it may appear that groups of patients are infected with the same strain. If, however, most MRSA from that hospital are of the same pattern regardless of epidemiology, then a common source exposure cannot be determined by molecular methods.

The use of appropriate controls is critical for PCR-based methodologies as well. Amplification of a highly conserved region or gene may give the appearance that unrelated organisms are in fact related. Alternatively, amplification of hypervariable targets may yield differences due to rapid genetic drift (such as with some viral antigens) and obscure genetic relatedness between strains. Thus, the choice of control strains or regions should be considered carefully.

PHENOTYPIC METHODS

Colony Morphology

Certainly for the microbiologist, the most immediate and obvious difference that exists between colonies on a culture plate is colony morphology. While colonial variants of the same species frequently represent distinct strains, this is not the case universally.

Biotyping

Organisms can be identified to the genus and species level using a panel of biochemical reagents to determine the pattern of activity of cellular metabolic enzymes.[14] This information is routinely obtained in clinical microbiology laboratories using automated systems and is relatively inexpensive. While biotyping methods do not discriminate between strains of the same species, identification of multiple isolates of an unusual species or unusual biotype (eg, hydrogen sulfide-producing strains of *E. coli*) can suggest a common source outbreak.[1,12] One limitation is that variation in gene expression in the same strain may lead to different biochemical reactions.[14,15]

Antimicrobial Susceptibility Testing

Antimicrobial susceptibilities (antibiograms) are also routinely performed by clinical microbiology laboratories for most bacterial isolates. Manual and automated systems are widely available, easy to use, and relatively inexpensive. Because many nosocomial pathogens such as VRE demonstrate little variability in their antimicrobial susceptibility patterns, antibiograms have relatively poor discriminatory power. In addition, spontaneous phenotypic variation can lead to rapidly changing susceptibility patterns. Antibiotic selective pressure in hospitals further drives these changes, often mediated by plasmids and other mobile genetic elements.[16] For example, during an outbreak, acquisition of the same plasmid may result in unrelated strains exhibiting identical antibiograms.[1] Despite these limitations, detection of a cluster of pathogens with a new or unusual pattern of resistance may raise suspicion of an outbreak, leading to further epidemiologic and molecular evaluations.

Serotyping and Phage Typing

Serotyping is a classic strain typing technique that uses antibodies to detect antigenic determinants on the bacterial cell surface. It remains an important method for typing organisms such as *Salmonella*, *Shigella*, and pneumococci.[1] Some virulence factors and clinical syndromes are linked to specific serotypes within a species, such as Shiga-toxin producing *E. coli* 0157:H7 and the hemolytic-uremic syndrome. Thus, serotyping remains a valuable technique.[17] Its limitations in epidemiological studies include poor discriminatory power, lack of typeability by many organisms, and the burden of maintaining stocks of typing sera for each species.

Bacteriophage typing involves characterization of isolates by their susceptibility to a panel of lytic bacteriophages. Like serotyping, this method also lacks typeability and discriminatory power. It is technically difficult and available through reference labs only. Bacteriocin typing tests susceptibilities of isolates to bacterial toxins and has similar limitations to phage typing.

Multilocus Enzyme Electrophoresis

Multilocus enzyme electrophoresis (MLEE) detects differences in electrophoretic mobilities of individual soluble metabolic enzymes, which are highly polymorphic in bacterial populations.[5] Cellular proteins are separated by starch gel electrophoresis with individual enzymes detected by use of specific substrates. Variations in mobility typically reflect amino acid substitutions that alter the charge of the protein.[14] MLEE is limited less in stability than other phenotypic methods because the genes encoding the enzymes used are relatively unaltered by environmental pressures.[5] The strength of MLEE has been its use in population genetics with its ability to group genetically similar isolates.[18] MLEE has not been as useful for outbreak investigations because of its technical complexity.

GENOTYPIC METHODS

Plasmid Restriction Endonuclease Analysis

This technique uses plasmids, extrachromosomal DNA elements that are present in most bacteria. Plasmid fingerprinting is the process by which plasmids are extracted from bacteria by cell lysis and separated by agarose gel electrophoresis. The pattern of banding is detected by staining the gel with ethidium bromide and photographing it under UV light. In REA, restriction endonucleases, enzymes that digest (cleave) DNA at particular sequences, are used to cleave the plasmids prior to separating them on a gel, and the numbers and sizes of the fragments are compared. The use of restriction enzymes improves the discriminatory power of plasmid analysis, particularly in the case of large plasmids, and prevents the problem of undigested plasmids running at different rates on the gel depending on whether they are in circular or linear forms.

Plasmid REA is the simplest of the DNA-based methods and is relatively inexpensive. It is limited by the fact that plasmids can be spread to multiple species ("plasmid outbreak"), lost spontaneously, or altered by mobile genetic elements that they frequently carry. The strong selective pressure of the hospital environment for organisms to carry antibiotic resistance or virulence factors can also drive these changes. Plasmid REA is generally most effective in analyzing whether the presence of antibiotic resistance elements that may be carried by genetically distinct strains results from the dissemination of resistance plasmids.[19]

Chromosomal REA

In this technique, restriction enzymes cleave bacterial chromosomal DNA at particular sequences that may be repeated multiple times in the genome, generating numerous fragments that can be separated using agarose gel electrophoresis. Different strains of the same bacterial species have different REA profiles because of variations in DNA sequences that alter the frequency and distribution of restriction sites. The advantage of this technique is that all isolates are typeable by REA. The disadvantage, however, is the difficulty in interpreting complex profiles that may contain hundreds of unresolved and overlapping bands. REA patterns may also be confounded by the presence of contaminating plasmids. Currently, the primary use of chromosomal REA is as an alternative technique for evaluating *C. difficile*.[1,17]

Southern Blot Analysis of Chromosomal DNA

In this method, the restriction fragments separated by conventional agarose gel electrophoresis described above are transferred onto a nitrocellulose or nylon membrane, and a chemically or radioactively labeled fragment of DNA or RNA is used as a probe to detect fragment(s) containing sequences (loci) homologous to the probe. Variations in the number and size of these fragments are called RFLPs. While this technique is generally too laborious and time-consuming for typing most hospital pathogens, RFLP analysis remains the method of choice for typing *M. tuberculosis* isolates using the DNA insertion element IS*6110*, a mobile sequence present in virtually all strains of *M. tuberculosis*.[17,20] In addition, RFLP analysis of mec (the gene encoding methicillin resistance) and Tn*554* (which carries the gene encoding erythromycin resistance) has been used for typing *S. aureus*.[7]

Ribotyping is a variation of this method, using a ribosomal RNA probe for detecting DNA sequences that encode rRNA loci.[21] All bacterial isolates can be typed using this method because they all have at least one chromosomal rRNA operon and the sequences are highly conserved. While ribotyping has only moderate discriminatory power in relation to the number of ribosomal operons, its use as a tool to group phylogenetically related organisms is excellent.[22]

Pulsed-Field Gel Electrophoresis

This technique, first described in 1984 as a way of evaluating chromosomal DNA in yeast,[23] has proven to be an excellent typing method that has been successfully used for a wide variety of bacterial species.[13,24,25] In contrast to REA, the restriction enzymes used in PFGE have fewer recognition sites in the bacterial chromosomal DNA, yielding a smaller number (10 to 30) of restriction fragments. The fragments are separated in agarose gel using a specialized chamber with 3 sets of electrodes arranged around the gel in a hexagon that apply alternating pulses of electric current in different directions. This technique allows for a higher level of band resolution than with conventional electrophoresis. PFGE is highly discriminatory and reproducible and can be used for numerous bacterial species. A notable exception is that certain strains of *C. difficile* are not typeable using PFGE because of spontaneous degradation of chromosomal DNA during the protocol.[26]

Major limitations of PFGE include the need for technical expertise and the initial costs of the equipment, although many laboratories are skilled in this technique. While commercial products exist for DNA preparation, these are not universally used. On the other hand, interpretation of restriction profiles produced by PFGE is more straightforward than those of chromosomal REA, and guidelines with criteria for strain typing with PFGE have been published.[2]

Polymerase Chain Reaction

PCR is a powerful molecular method that has been adapted for use as a typing tool for epidemiologic investigations.[27] Amplification of minute quantities of microbial DNA present in a sample allows for detection and identification of microbes and can generate a "molecular fingerprint" for each organism based on its unique sequences of DNA (or RNA). The PCR reaction involves the denaturation of an organism's genomic DNA, followed by the hybridization of specific oligonucleotide probes (primers) to the complementary DNA strands, and replication of the DNA template by DNA polymerase in the region between the 2 primers. Twenty to 30 cycles of this process are performed, resulting in exponential amplification of the DNA.

Compared to other methods, PCR offers the advantage of speed (minutes to hours) and is unrivaled in sensitivity.[9] PCR can also be extremely specific depending on the assay. Specific PCR assays use primers that are complementary to unique DNA sequences in a particular microbe's genome, while broad-range PCR assays are designed to amplify conserved regions of microbial DNA in order to detect a wider variety of organisms. Unique sequences of DNA within these conserved regions may then be used to identify specific microbes by sequencing enzyme analysis or REA. For example, the bacterial 16S rRNA gene is a useful gene for both broad-range and organism-specific PCR.[9]

The high sensitivity of PCR can lead to its greatest limitation, in that false positive results can occur due to amplification of contaminating DNA that may be present in a sample. Therefore, PCR should be performed only by personnel trained for the technique in a laboratory specifically set up for the procedure, and negative controls must always be used. Numerous automated, closed systems have been developed and are commercially available, eliminating or limiting many of the technical problems associated with DNA purification and cross-contamination.

Several modifications of PCR useful for epidemiological purposes are outlined below.

Arbitrarily Primed PCR

Arbitrarily primed PCR, also know as randomly amplified polymorphic DNA assay (RAPD), has expanded the use of PCR for epidemiological purposes. In this technique, short primers that are not directed toward a known genetic sequence randomly hybridize to areas in the genome. When 2 primers hybridize to opposite strands of DNA in proximity to one another, the segment in between is amplified, and multiple fragments produced in this manner can be analyzed by agarose gel electrophoresis. This method has the advantage of wide applicability to many bacterial as well as eukaryotic species[27] and is more rapid than other typing systems. However, because of substantial variations in results that occur with only slight changes in reaction conditions, it is often difficult to obtain reproducible patterns from experiment to experiment and between different laboratories.[28] Therefore, the most reliable results are obtained when testing a set of isolates in a single experiment. In addition, standardized guidelines have not yet been developed for interpreting data from AP-PCR.[1]

PCR of Repetitive Chromosomal Elements

With PCR of repetitive chromosomal elements (REP-PCR), primers are designed to hybridize to repetitive chromosomal elements that are often present in more than one copy in the genome, producing several bands of different sizes when separated by gel electrophoresis. Examples of these repetitive elements are IS*6110* in *M. tuberculosis* and ERIC sequences in other bacteria. Again, related organisms have similar banding patterns. This technique has been used to type higher organisms such as fungi and amoeba.[12] For organisms such as *E. coli*, individual primer sets may yield only minimal discrimination between strains, necessitating the use of multiple different primer sets to achieve higher discriminatory power.[29] This technique may, however, yield phylogenetic information similar to MLEE.[29]

Polymerase Chain Reaction-Restriction Fragment Length Polymorphism

PCR-RFLP involves digesting DNA segments amplified by PCR with a restriction enzyme and separating the resulting fragments by agarose gel electrophoresis. Patterns of different organisms can be compared to determine relatedness. This method has been useful in subtyping fastidious bacteria such as *B. henselae* and *N. meningitidis* as well as viruses such as cytomegalovirus and *H. simplex* virus.[12] It is limited by the fact that PCR products must be large enough to be digested, and the method lacks discriminatory power compared to other PCR techniques.[12]

Preferred strain typing techniques for particular microorganisms are presented in Table 14-2.

Antibiotic Resistance Genotyping

Nucleic acid-based molecular techniques can rapidly and accurately detect genetic determinants of antimicrobial resistance.[30] For example, methicillin resistance in S. aureus is mediated by the *mec* A gene, which encodes a unique penicillin-binding protein (pbp 2), while van-

comycin resistance in enterococci is conferred by one of several genes (*van A, B, C, or D*) (Table 14-3). The rapid detection of these organisms as well as others, such as multidrug-resistant *M. tuberculosis* and extended-spectrum beta-lactamase (ESBL) producing Enterobacteriaceae, is vital for patient management and infection control programs and may assist in outbreak investigations and detection of spread of resistance genes.[3,31] Assays have been described that detect resistance determinants in bacteria directly from clinical specimens such as blood cultures.[32]

CONCLUSION

Molecular methods have gained in utility as adjunctive to classical epidemiologic studies. In this chapter, we have reviewed the various techniques now available. In addition to classical outbreak analysis, molecular techniques have been employed to answer questions related to pathogenesis, phylogeny, and disease progression. The two most important caveats to the use of molecular methods involve the use of appropriate controls and the need to save isolates prospectively for later comparison.

ACKNOWLEDGMENT

Supported in part by AI 450008, AI 32783, and AI 12849.

REFERENCES

1. Tenover FC, Arbeit RD, Goering RV, and the Molecular Typing Working Group of the Society for Healthcare Epidemiology of America. How to select and interpret molecular strain typing methods for epidemiological studies of bacterial infections: a review for healthcare epidemiologists. *Infect Control Hosp Epidemiol.* 1997;18: 426-439.
2. Tenover FC, Arbeit RD, Goering RV, et al. Interpreting chromosomal DNA restriction patterns produced by pulsed-field gel electrophoresis: criteria for bacterial strain typing. *J Clin Microbiol.* 1995;33:2233-2239.
3. Pfaller MA, Herwaldt LA. The clinical microbiology laboratory and infection control: emerging pathogens, antimicrobial resistance, and new technology. *Clin Infect Dis.* 1997;25:858-870.
4. Orskov F, Orskov I. From the National Institutes of Health. Summary of a workshop on the clone concept in the epidemiology, taxonomy, and evolution of the enterobacteriaceae and other bacteria. *J Infect Dis.* 1983;148:346-357.
5. Eisenstein BI. New molecular techniques for microbial epidemiology and the diagnosis of infectious diseases. *J Infect Dis.* 1990;161:595-602.

TABLE 14-2. PREFERRED STRAIN TYPING TECHNIQUES FOR NOSOCOMIAL AND COMMUNITY-ACQUIRED PATHOGENS

Species	Reference Method	Alternative Methods
S. aureus	PFGE	AP-PCR, PF
Coagulase-negative staphylococci	PFGE	PF
S. pneumoniae	PFGE	Serotyping
Enterococci	PFGE	—
E. coli[†], Citrobacter, Proteus, Providencia	PFGE	AP-PCR
Klebsiella, Enterobacter, Serratia	PFGE	PF
Salmonella, Shigella	Serotyping	PFGE
P. aeruginosa	PFGE	—
Burkholderia, Stenotrophomonas, Acinetobacter	PFGE	—
C. difficile	AP-PCR	REA, PFGE[§]
M. tuberculosis	IS6110 RFLP	REP-PCR
Mycobacteria other than TB	PFGE	—

Abbreviations: PFGE, pulsed-field gel electrophoresis; AP-PCR, arbitrarily primed polymerase chain reaction; PF, plasmid fingerprinting (with or without restriction analysis); REA, restriction endonuclease analysis of chromosomal DNA using conventional electrophoresis; RFLP, restriction fragment-length polymorphism typing using IS6110; REP-PCR, repetitive-element polymerase chain reaction.
[†] E. coli 0157:H7 must be identified by serotyping.
[§] Many strains of C. difficile are nontypeable by PFGE due to DNA degradation.

Adapted from Tenover FC, Arbeit RD, Goering RV, and the Molecular Typing Working Group of the Society for Healthcare Epidemiology of America. How to select and interpret molecular strain typing methods for epidemiological studies of bacterial infections: a review for healthcare epidemiologists. *Infect Control Hosp Epidemiol.* 1997;18:426-439.

TABLE 14-3. PCR-BASED DETECTION OF ANTIMICROBIAL RESISTANCE USED IN EPIDEMIOLOGIC STUDIES*

Organism	Antimicrobial Resistance	Target Gene
Staphylococcus spp.	Methicillin/oxacillin	mec A
Enterococcus spp.	Glycopeptides	van A, B, C, D
S. pneumoniae	ß-lactams	pbp 1A, 2B, 2X
Enterobacteriaceae	Extended-spectrum penicillins and cephalosporins	tem, shv, other ß-lactamase genes
M. tuberculosis	Rifampin	rpo B
	Isoniazid	kat G, inh A, ahp C

* Note: list is not all-inclusive

Adapted from Pfaller MA, Herwaldt LA. The clinical microbiology laboratory and infection control: emerging pathogens, antimicrobial resistance, and new technology. *Clin Infect Dis.* 1997;25:858-870; and Louie M, Louie L, Simor AE. The role of DNA amplification technology in the diagnosis of infectious diseases. *CMAJ Canadian Medical Association Journal.* 2000;163:301-309.

6. Musser JM. Molecular population genetic analysis of emerging bacterial pathogens: selected insights. *Emerg Infect Dis*. 1996;2:1-17.

7. Kreiswirth B, Kornblum J, Arbeit RD, et al. Evidence for a clonal origin of methicillin resistance in *Staphylococcus aureus*. *Science*. 1993;259:227-230.

8. Struelens MJ, De Gheldre Y, Deplano A. Comparative and library epidemiological typing systems: outbreak investigations versus surveillance systems. *Infect Control Hosp Epidemiol*. 1998;19:565-569.

9. Fredricks DN, Relman DA. Application of polymerase chain reaction to the diagnosis of infectious diseases. *Clin Infect Dis*. 1999;29:475-488.

10. Relman DA, Schmidt TM, MacDermott RP, Falkow S. Identification of the uncultured bacillus of Whipple's disease. *N Engl J Med*. 1992;327:293-301.

11. Lakeman FD, Whitley RJ, and Group tNIoAaIDCAS. Diagnosis of *herpes simplex* encephalitis: application of polymerase chain reaction to cerebrospinal fluid from brain-biopsied patients and correlation with disease. *J Infect Dis*. 1995;171:857-863.

12. Weber S, Pfaller MA, Herwaldt LA. Role of molecular epidemiology in infection control. *Infect Dis Clin North Am*. 1997;11:257-278.

13. Arbeit RD. *Laboratory Procedures for the Epidemiologic Analysis of Microorganisms*. 6th ed. Washington, DC: American Society for Microbiology; 1995.

14. Maslow JN, Mulligan ME, Arbeit R. Molecular epidemiology: application of contemporary techniques to the typing of microorganisms. *Clin Infect Dis*. 1993;17:153-164.

15. Maslow JN, Brecher SM, Adams KS, Durbin A, Loring S, Arbeit RD. The relationship between indole production and differentiation of *Klebsiella* species: indole-positive and -negative isolates of *Klebsiella* determined to be clonal. *J Clin Microbiol*. 1993;31:2000-2003.

16. Davies J. Inactivation of antibiotics and the dissemination of resistance genes. *Science*. 1994;264:375-382.

17. Maslow JN, Mulligan ME. Epidemiologic typing systems. *Infect Control Hosp Epidemiol*. 1996;17:595-604.

18. Selander RK, Musser JM, Caugant DA, Gilmour MN, Whittam TS. Population genetics of pathogenic bacteria. *Microb Pathol*. 1987;3:1-7.

19. Lautenbach E, Patel JB, Bilker WB, Edelstein PH, Fishman NO. Extended-spectrum beta-lactamase-producing *Escherichia coli* and *Klebsiella pneumoniae*: risk factors for infection and impact of resistance on outcomes. *Clin Infect Dis*. 2001;32:1162-1171.

20. van Embden JDA, Cave MD, Crawford JT, et al. Strain identification of *Mycobacterium tuberculosis* by DNA fingerprinting: recommendations for a standardized methodology. *J Clin Microbiol*. 1993;31:406-409.

21. Stull TL, LiPuma JJ, Edlind TD. A broad-spectrum probe for molecular epidemiology of bacteria: ribosomal RNA. *J Infect Dis*. 1988;157:280-286.

22. Maslow JN, Whittam TS, Gilks CF, et al. Clonal relationship among bloodstream isolates of *Escherichia coli*. *Infect Immunol*. 1995;63:2409-2417.

23. Schwartz DC, Cantor CR. Separation of yeast chromosome-sized DNAs by pulsed-field gel electrophoresis. *Cell*. 1984;37:67-75.

24. Maslow JN, Slutsky AM, Arbeit RD. *The Application of Pulsed Field Gel Electrophoresis to Molecular Epidemiology*. Washington, DC: American Society for Microbiology; 1993.

25. Goering RV. Molecular epidemiology of nosocomial infection: analysis of chromosomal restriction fragment patterns by pulsed-field gel electrophoresis. *Infect Control Hosp Epidemiol*. 1993;14:595-600.

26. Kato H, Kato N, Watanabe K, et al. Application of typing by pulsed-field gel electrophoresis to the study of Clostridium difficile in a neonatal intensive care unit. *J Clin Microbiol*. 1994;32:2067-2070.

27. Van Belkum A. DNA fingerprinting of medically important microorganisms by use of PCR. *Clin Microbiol Rev*. 1994;7:174-184.

28. Van Belkum A, Kluytmans J, van Leeuwen W, et al. Multicenter evaluation of arbitrarily primed PCR for typing of *Staphylococcus aureus* strains. *J Clin Microbiol*. 1995;33:1537-1547.

29. Johnson CE, Maslow JN, Fattlar DC, Adams KS, Arbeit RD. The role of bacterial adhesins in the outcome of childhood urinary tract infections. *Am J Dis Child*. 1993;147:1090-1093.

30. Fluit AC, Visser MR, Schmitz FJ. Molecular detection of antimicrobial resistance. *Clin Microbiol Rev*. 2001;14:836-871.

31. Pfaller MA. Molecular epidemiology in the care of patients. *Arch Pathol Lab Med*. 1999;123:1007-1010.

32. Maes N, Magdalena J, Rottiers S, De Gheldre Y, Struelens MJ. Evaluation of a triplex PCR assay to discriminate *Staphylococcus aureus* from coagulase-negative staphylococci and determine methicillin resistance from blood cultures. *J Clin Microbiol*. 2002;40:1514-1517.

CHAPTER FIFTEEN

COMPUTERS FOR HEALTHCARE EPIDEMIOLOGY

Keith Woeltje, MD, PhD

COMPUTER HARDWARE

Computers have become ubiquitous tools in modern offices. Unfortunately, because infection control programs are not themselves revenue generating, they are typically not first in line for the most modern equipment. Fortunately, most applications used by healthcare epidemiologists do not require new top-of-the-line computers, and equipping an infection control office can be done on a relatively small budget. If there is an opportunity to get new equipment, a few considerations are in order. Because things like processor speed and hard-disk capacity change so quickly, definitive suggestions quickly become dated, but a few general observations can be made.

Before choosing computer hardware, one must consider what operating system (OS) is going to be used. An OS is a computer program that controls the underlying details of the computer hardware. Popular examples include Microsoft Windows XP (Microsoft Corp, Redmond, Wash) and Apple Macintosh OS X (ten) (Apple Computer Inc., Cupertino, Calif). An OS called Linux has become very popular for servers (computers that provide infrastructure services like e-mail and Web sites); it can be used for desktop computers, but to do so requires a fair amount of expertise. Linux is an example of an "open source" project (http://www.opensource.org), in which computer programmers from around the globe voluntarily work on developing software, with the understanding that anyone who wants to distribute or modify the program can do so. As such, Linux is available from a wide number of sources, not just one company. Programs written to run under one OS typically do not work on a computer running a different OS. Some programs have different versions that run on different OSs (eg, Microsoft Office), but in this case the Windows version could not run on a Macintosh, and vice-versa. The largest exception to this general rule is that programs written in a computer language called "Java" can often have the very same version of a program run on different systems. The reason for discussing any of this is that with the exception of computer professionals and avid hobbyists, most people do not care what OS they are using, but they do care about what programs they are using. Software is discussed in more detail below. Most basic software (eg, word processing, spreadsheets) is available for almost all OSs. However, many specialty programs (eg, statistical packages) may only be available for one OS. Thus, the choice of OS is driven by the choice of software you would like to use. Your hospital's information technology (IT) department may also mandate that a particular OS be used; however, if you can make a compelling case that a different OS is needed to run necessary software, often exceptions will be made.

Once the OS is chosen, then the computer hardware can be chosen. OS X runs only on hardware from Apple Computer. Windows XP (and other versions of Microsoft Windows) runs on hardware that comes from many manufacturers. When choosing computer hardware, decisions have to be made in a few key areas: the form factor, the processor, memory, hard-disk storage, optical media, ports, networking, graphics, and sound (Table 15-1). Your hospital's IT department may have set standards for new computers regarding basic hardware configuration. This minimum may be adequate, but some components may need to be upgraded to suit the needs of the healthcare epidemiologist.

The largest decision regarding the form factor is whether to purchase a laptop or a desktop computer. In the past, one of the advantages of a desktop computer was that it provided more options for internal expansion. Spaces were available for adding additional drives of various types. In addition, most of the connections to external components were handled by add-on cards that fit into

TABLE 15-1. SUGGESTED MINIMUM HARDWARE CONFIGURATION FOR HEALTHCARE EPIDEMIOLOGY USE

CPU:	Several speed steps behind the most current processor
Memory:	At least 256 MB (consider doubling hospital recommended minimum)
Hard drive:	40 GB (or hospital recommended minimum)
Optical drives:	DVD-ROM and CD-RW (or combination drive)
Video:	Enough to support DVD video playback
Ports:	Multiple USB ports (most recent version)
Networking:	Ethernet card
Audio:	Sound card and external speakers

expansion slots on the computer's main board (also called the motherboard—the large circuit board that contains the processor, the memory, and additional chips that allow the computer to communicate with other components). This allowed individual components to be upgraded without upgrading the whole computer. But now many desktop computers come in small cases with limited expansion ability, and many of the connections are now included on the main board, eliminating the need for extra cards. Also, the performance differential between desktop and laptop computers has largely been eliminated. All of the components discussed below are now available in a laptop computer. However, for any given level of performance, a laptop computer will be somewhat more expensive than an equivalent desktop computer. Still, a high-end laptop alone is less expensive than purchasing a desktop computer and having a laptop for travel. More and more people are choosing a laptop as their sole computer.

The processor (or central processing unit [CPU]) is the most hyped component of a computer, but may actually be one of the least important. You often pay a significant premium for the latest processor; a CPU 1 or 2 steps down (in terms of chip speed) from the top of the line may be significantly less expensive with only slightly less performance. If your IT department has some recommended minimum, this may be completely adequate for your needs. The one caveat is that some manufacturers make an "economy" line of CPUs with slightly impaired performance compared with their primary line (eg, the Intel Celeron [Santa Clara, Calif] compared with the Pentium 4). This difference involves the internal architecture of the CPU and not just the speed of the processor. While for routine office tasks the economy line is a good choice, for some computationally intensive applications (eg, complex statistical calculations), the difference in performance may be more noticeable. Thus, a CPU from the primary line of processors may be preferable. Likewise, regarding computer memory (aka RAM, for Random Access Memory), the IT minimum standard is likely aimed at routine office use. Adding RAM is an inexpensive way to improve performance. Consider doubling the IT mini-

mum in order to better handle large datasets for statistical analysis, and to have several programs running at the same time. Two hundred fifty-six megabytes (MB) of RAM should be considered a bare minimum, with 512 MB or even 1 gigabyte (GB) being reasonable at this time.

Hard disks have gotten very large. However, most files used by healthcare epidemiologists will consist of text and numbers and will typically not be very large. The IT suggested minimum (40 GB is about the smallest you will find now) should be adequate unless you work a lot with graphics or large datasets. You should also include a CD-RW drive that can store data on blank CDs. This provides a convenient way to share information because almost all computers now have at least a CD-ROM drive that can read CDs. It also provides a good way to back up your data; as reliable as computer hardware has become, making copies of important files on a regular basis is imperative. Your computer should also come equipped with a DVD-ROM drive that can read DVDs. Some large computer programs and databases now come on DVD rather than multiple CDs. In addition, some training information now comes on DVD rather than videocassette, so being able to play these disks on your computer is not just a luxury. Drives are available to record DVD disks. Currently, however, there is no single accepted standard, and the drives and disks are expensive. Inevitably prices will fall, and such recordable DVD drives will become common, replacing CD-RW drives.

For routine office use, a top of the line 3-D graphics card is not needed (these are designed primarily for games and other advanced graphics applications). Basic graphics may be built into the computer's main board and not require a separate card per se. As long as it will support video playback from the DVD drive, it will be adequate for your needs. If you do want to view training DVDs, you will also need an audio card (this also may be included on the computer's main board) and external speakers (the speaker inside a desktop computer is only good for warning beeps. However, laptop computers do usually have acceptable speakers built in). The IT suggested minimum configuration is probably acceptable for video and audio if it will support DVD playback. Otherwise, the minimum required for the DVD drive will do.

Typically you will want to connect additional peripherals to your computer, like a printer. Although computers previously had multiple different connectors for different purposes, today the Universal Serial Bus (USB) connector can be used for many different kinds of accessories. The latest iteration (USB 2.0 at the time of this writing) can transfer data faster than older versions. In addition to printers, external hard drives (for additional data storage or back-ups), digital cameras, and many other devices can be connected via USB. The more USB ports available on your computer, the better, as these will likely be the primary connection for peripherals for at least the next few years (external adapters are available to increase the number of ports should the need arise). A variety of other connection ports (some of which are faster than USB 2.0) are available; whether you will need any of these depends on whether the peripherals you plan on using require such connectors.

The usefulness of a computer is increased tremendously if it can be connected to other computers. For this reason, your computer should have some means of connecting to a computer network. This is now almost always done with what is called an "Ethernet port," or more correctly, an RJ-45 jack. This looks like an oversized telephone jack. Most computers now come with this routinely, but check to make sure. There are various speeds of Ethernet, but your IT department's minimum will be adequate. If you do not currently have access to an Ethernet network and choose not to get an Ethernet port, an inexpensive card can be added later if your computer has internal expansion slots. If you do not have access to an Ethernet network, consider getting a telephone modem for the computer so that you can connect to the Internet using a dial-up connection.

As the performance of computer hardware improves, we are seeing computers that have very reasonable performance (exceeding the minimums outlined above) for under $1000.

COMPUTER SOFTWARE

Basic Software

Computers are only as useful as the software that runs on them. If CD-RW and DVD drives are included in the computer, software that allows the use of these drives typically comes with the computer. If the computer has a connection to the Internet, then email and Web browser software is needed (and usually comes with the computer).

Two essential programs for getting work done are a word processing program and a spreadsheet program. Typically such software comes packaged in "suites"—collections of multiple programs. Other useful programs may be included, such as programs for making presentations and programs for generating graphics. Such suites may come with the computer. Microsoft Office is currently the most popular such suite of programs. Because of their popularity, the file formats used by the Office programs have become *de facto* standards. Other office suites usually have the ability to read and write files using the same formats. This allows users of different programs, in theory, to exchange documents that look the same (in practice, small formatting differences often become apparent). Recently the office suite OpenOffice.org has garnered significant attention because it is available for free from the project's Web site (http://www.openoffice.org/). Open Office.org is another open source project.

Word processors (eg, Microsoft Word, OpenOffice.org Writer) allow the user to generate attractive documents for dissemination. Their utility is somewhat obvious, and will not be discussed further. Likewise presentation programs (such as Microsoft PowerPoint or Apple Keynote) will not be discussed.

Spreadsheets (eg, Microsoft Excel, OpenOffice.org Calc) were originally developed for working with financial data, but work well with any numerical data. Spreadsheets are essentially large tables, organized by columns and rows. Information can be entered into some of the cells. In other cells the user can enter formulas that take data from designated cells and calculate a result. The result then appears in the cell into which the formula was entered. If any of the numbers in the source cells change, then the result will change to reflect that. Spreadsheets typically make it easy to copy formulas from one cell to another, so that repetitive calculations can be done without having to enter long formulas repeatedly. Spreadsheets are thus ideal for many applications in healthcare epidemiology. You can enter data on the number of surgeries done and the number of SSIs and have the spreadsheet calculate the rates, for example. Spreadsheet software typically also will allow the user to generate graphs relatively easily. Some basic statistics (eg, means, standard deviations) can also be done with many spreadsheets, but more complicated statistics are better handled by dedicated statistics programs (see below). Spreadsheets can also be used as simple databases, such as for a line list during an outbreak (see Chapter 10). However, as data collection needs become more complicated, actual database programs make a better choice for storing data.

Actual database programs (eg, Microsoft Access, FileMaker Pro [FileMaker Inc, Santa Clara, Calif]) are not included with most office suites. They are also intrinsically somewhat more complicated than word processors or spreadsheets. For these reasons, many computer users are unfamiliar with them. Their utility becomes apparent when trying to collect and save complex information. Consider a surgical site infection outbreak investigation.

A given patient may have had several nurses involved in the surgery and more than one surgeon. There is no really good way to collect this data in tabular form on a spreadsheet. You could put several names in one cell under the column "Surgeon" or "Nurse," but this would limit your ability to search the information or tally it appropriately. You could have several columns "Surgeon1," "Surgeon2," "Nurse1," "Nurse2," "Nurse3," etc. However, if you wanted to find all the cases a particular surgeon or nurse was involved in, you would have to search in several different columns. In addition, you'd have to allow enough columns to accommodate the patient with the most surgeons or nurses. Most patients would have many empty cells in their records. Alternatively, you could have each surgeon and nurse listed by name at the top of each column, with "yes" or "no" indicated in the column to indicate involvement. Data entry would be tedious, and patterns would be difficult to spot. However, a true database program can handle such problems very easily by storing different kinds of information in different tables, which have a defined relationship to one another. Many commercial desktop database programs have tutorials (often called "wizards") to simplify setting up a basic database. The greatest payback will come from spending a modest amount of time learning about the underlying design of these databases. A number of excellent references are available in print and on-line. One good general introduction that is not specific to any one program is *Database Design for Mere Mortals* by Hernandez.[1]

General Statistical Software

Although counts and some basic statistics can be done using spreadsheet software, even modestly advanced statistics (see Chapter 5) will require actual statistical software. Some basic programs frequently come bundled with introductory statistical texts. These programs will often handle basic needs (such as chi-square and simple analysis of variance). Epidemiologists who require more advanced statistics may need to use one of the many advanced statistical packages that are available such as SPSS (SPSS Inc., Chicago, Ill), SAS (SAS Institute, Cary, NC), or STATA (Stata Corporation, College Station, Tex). These programs are extremely versatile, but have significant learning curves and are more than most healthcare epidemiologists need.

Specialty Infection Control Software

A number of software packages for personal computers are available that are specifically designed for infection control programs. Such software is not as versatile as a general statistics package, but can provide fairly sophisticated statistical analysis and graphing with very little set up. Such packages are particularly useful for those with

limited computer skills or those who would prefer not to spend a lot of time using spreadsheets and statistics programs to maintain routine data. Well-known packages include AICE (ICPA, Austin, Tex), EpiQuest (EpiQuest LLC, Key Largo, Fla), and ClinTrac Infection Control Manager (SoftMed Systems, Folsom, Calif); other packages are available.

All of these programs have different features and options, and additional features are added with some frequency. Software vendors usually make demonstration software available so that you can get a feel for a program's features and its ease of use. The vendors should also be able to provide you with a list of current users so that you can discuss how they use the software, and perhaps arrange for a site visit to see the product in actual use.

Epi Info

Epi Info is a computer program designed by the CDC, and is available as a free download from the CDC Web site (http://www.cdc.gov/epiinfo/). Epi Info is only available for Microsoft Windows (older versions ran on Microsoft MS-DOS). Epi Info was originally designed as a program for field epidemiologists but has become versatile enough for myriad uses. It sits somewhere between a general purpose statistical package and a specialized infection control package in its scope.

Epi Info consists of a number of modules. One, NutStat, is designed for nutritional anthropometry, and is of limited use to most healthcare epidemiologists. During program installation you can choose which modules to install, so you can elect not to install this component. The other modules are MakeView, Enter, Analysis, and EpiMap. A number of small utility programs are also included, including a program to quickly calculate 2x2 contingency table statistics and a program to password protect files that might contain sensitive information.

MakeView allows the user to create data entry screens. These screens are then used by another program, Enter, as we'll see. The screens can be laid out to simplify data entry by making them attractive and by grouping similar information. During the design, constraints can be placed on the various data entry fields so that only appropriate answers can be entered (eg, only "Y" or "N" would be allowed for a yes/no question—the data entry person could be prevented from entering a different letter or a number). The user can also specify whether a particular field can be left blank. Epi Info was built on top of the Microsoft Access database program (the user need not have Access installed to use Epi Info). Because a true database stores the data, data entry forms can be designed that avoid the "doctor1, doctor2,..." problem discussed previously. Once the data entry screens are designed, the Enter program can be used to enter data into Epi Info. Data entry can be done at various times. It is even possible to allow different people to enter data on their own computers and then consolidate the data later. Data can also be updated or changed once it has been entered.

Analysis provides statistical analysis of the data. In addition to analyzing data collected using MakeView and Enter, Analysis can also read files created by some other programs, including Microsoft Excel and older versions of Epi Info. Analysis can perform basic statistics such as frequencies, chi-square (and Fisher's exact test), and analysis of variance. Advanced statistics include logistic regression and Kaplan-Meier survival curves. Within Analysis, the user can create new variables and can recode variables to simplify analysis (for example, if you were investigating an SSI outbreak and had a list of surgeons for each patient, you could create a new variable "DrSmith," and then code it as either "Y" or "N" depending on whether the patient had Dr. Smith as a surgeon. This would allow you to do a 2x2 contingency table). This facility can greatly simplify analysis, and allows the user not to have to guess when designing the data entry screens at all of the possible analyses that will eventually be wanted.

EpiMap allows the user to link data in Epi Info files to maps. Maps for all US states and many countries are available from the CDC's Epi Info Web site. The site also has links to other resources for finding pre-existing maps. Commercial tools are available for creating maps in the appropriate format. It would be possible, for example, to create a map of a hospital and display color-coded rates of MRSA, for example.

Other Software

A variety of other programs are available that are useful to healthcare epidemiologists. Some of these are smaller programs that are more suitable for "quick-and-dirty" calculations than full-fledged statistics packages. Epi Info comes with a program StatCalc that allows for quick entry of 2x2 tables and for calculations of sample size needed to reach designated statistical power. A similar (and more versatile) program is EpiCalc (by Mark Myatt, available from http://www.myatt.demon.co.uk/; this site also has links to other useful small programs).

AUTOMATED SURVEILLANCE

Personal computers (PCs) can serve as very useful tools for healthcare epidemiologists by allowing them to organize and analyze data more efficiently than by hand. Shortly after personal computers became widely available, they were adopted for this purpose.[2] However, as more clinical information is available on computers, and as computers become networked together (allowing data to be transferred from one computer to another relatively easily), then even more automation could occur. Considerable thought has gone in to what would make an ideal automated surveillance system.[3] Unfortunately, actual imple-

mentation of such systems has occurred in relatively few settings. A few examples are given to provide an idea of the scope and abilities of various systems that have been implemented.

A system based on automated review of microbiology data has been in place at Barnes-Jewish Hospital in St. Louis since 1993. Called GermWatcher, the system takes positive culture results from the microbiology lab and subjects them to analysis based on a series of computerized rules. The system is used for surveillance of a number of nosocomial infections. Error rates for detection of nosocomial bacteremia have been reported to be as low as 3.5%. Reports generated by the system allow infection control practitioners to more readily spot patterns in nosocomial infections.[4-6] Systems using laboratory data (and sometimes other information, like pharmacy data) have been implemented at other institutions as well.[7-16]

Although these systems have been largely developed at the institutions themselves, software with similar function is now becoming available commercially. At least 3 companies (Cereplex, Gaithersburg, Md; MedMined, Birmingham, Ala; and TheraDoc, Salt Lake City, Utah) offer software products that take data from hospital laboratory systems (and other systems) and generate some form of automated report. MedMined and Cereplex both download data in a secure manner over the Internet. Analysis is done on computers at the company, which then makes reports readily available via a Web browser (using a secure connection). They use very different internal methods to evaluate the data, but both have been shown to be effective at assisting with nosocomial infection surveillance.[17-19]

The Brigham and Women's Hospital and Harvard Pilgrim Healthcare in Boston have developed a system that goes beyond using hospital data to do automated surveillance for nosocomial infection. They include HMO data as well (including outpatient visit diagnoses codes and antibiotic prescription information) to assist with surgical site infection surveillance.[20-22]

In addition to nosocomial infection surveillance, automated systems can also assist with other tasks important to the healthcare epidemiologist. One such task is timely isolation of patients with contagious diseases. Columbia-Presbyterian Medical Center in New York City implemented an automated clinical decision support for the prompt isolation of patients who might have TB.[23] This worked by using computer analysis of dictated chest x-ray reports, as well as using laboratory and pharmacy information.

CONCLUSION

A personal computer is an essential tool for the healthcare epidemiologist. A relatively modest computer with a few well-chosen programs can serve most of the needs of the healthcare epidemiologist in terms of manipulating epidemiologic data and generating reports. As computers are networked together, and as hospitals shift to having more clinical data available on computers, data gathering and analysis should become more automated. A few institutions already have examples in place. These tools promise not to replace healthcare epidemiologists, but to provide them with better information and to free them from tedious data gathering and entry chores. This was well put by John Burke, an early leader in this field, in a recent editorial,[24] "We can expect that such efforts and automation will create the need for more, not fewer, infection control professionals. Time saved by automating surveillance will lead to the need for more human work, not less, to manage still more data and answer yet more questions."

REFERENCES

1. Hernandez MJ, Viescas JL. *SQL Queries for Mere Mortals*. Boston, Mass: Addison-Wesley; 2000.

2. Schifman RB, Palmer RA. Surveillance of nosocomial infections by computer analysis of positive culture rates. *J Clin Microbiol*. 1985;21:493-495.

3. Mertens R, Ceusters W. Quality assurance, infection surveillance, and hospital information systems: avoiding the Bermuda Triangle. *Infect Control Hosp Epidemiol*. 1994;15:203-9.

4. Kahn MG, Steib SA, Fraser VJ, Dunagan WC. An expert system for culture-based infection control surveillance. *Proceedings—the Annual Symposium on Computer Applications in Medical Care*. 1993;171-75.

5. Kahn MG, Steib SA, Dunagan WC, Fraser VJ. Monitoring expert system performance using continuous user feedback. *J Am Med Inform Assoc*. 1996;3:216-223.

6. Kahn MG, Bailey TC, Steib SA, Fraser VJ, Dunagan WC. Statistical process control methods for expert system performance monitoring. *J Am Med Inform Assoc*. 1996;3:258-269.

7. Yokoe DS, Anderson J, Chambers R, et al. Simplified surveillance for nosocomial bloodstream infections. *Infect Control Hosp Epidemiol*. 1998;19:657-60.

8. Evans RS, Gardner RM, Bush AR, et al. Development of a computerized infectious disease monitor (CIDM). *Comput Biomed Res*. 1985;18:103-113.

9. Evans RS, Larsen RA, Burke JP, et al. Computer surveillance of hospital-acquired infections and antibiotic use. *JAMA*. 1986;256:1007-1011.

10. Burke JP, Classen DC, Pestotnik SL, Evans RS, Stevens LE. The HELP system and its application to infection control. *J Hosp Infect*. 1991;18 Suppl A:424-431.

11. Classen DC, Burke JP, Pestotnik SL, Evans RS, Stevens LE. Surveillance for quality assessment: IV. Surveillance using a hospital information system. *Infect Control Hosp Epidemiol*. 1991;12:239-244.

12. Rocha BH, Christenson JC, Evans RS, Gardner RM. Clinicians' response to computerized detection of infections. *J Am Med Inform Assoc*. 2001;8:117-125.

13. Samore MH, Schaecher B, Yih R, Christofferson K, Carroll KC. Prospective, real-time molecular typing study using clinical computer systems and automated ribotyping. Abstract, 40th Annual ICAAC, Toronto, Canada. 2000.

14. Hirschhorn LR, Currier JS, Platt R. Electronic surveillance of antibiotic exposure and coded discharge diagnoses as indicators of postoperative infection and other quality assurance measures. *Infect Control Hosp Epidemiol*. 1993;14:21-28.

15. Trick WE, Zagorski BM, Tokars JI, et al. Comparison of Computer Algorithms (CA) to Traditional Surveillance (TS) to Calculate Bloodstream Infection (BSI) Rates at Three Healthcare Facilities. Abstract, IDSA 40th Annual Meeting, Chicago, Ill; October 2002.

16. Bouam S, Girou E, Brun-Buisson C, Karadimas H, Lepage E. An intranet-based automated system for the surveillance of nosocomial infections: prospective validation compared with physicians' self-reports. *Infect Control Hosp Epidemiol*. 2003;24:51-55.

17. Brossette SE, Sprague AP, Hardin JM, Waites KB, Jones WT, Moser SA. Association rules and data mining in hospital infection control and public health surveillance. *J Am Med Inform Assoc*. 1998;5:373-381.

18. Hymel PA, Brossette SE. Data mining-enhanced infection control surveillance: sensitivity and specificity. Abstract, Society for Healthcare Epidemiology of America (SHEA) Annual Meeting, Toronto, Canada. 2001.

19. Wright MO, Perencevich EN, Novak C, Hebden JN, Standiford HC, Harris AD. Assessment of an Automated Surveillance System for Infection Control. *Infect Control Hospital Epidemiol*. In press.

20. Platt R, Yokoe DS, Sands KE, CDC Eastern Massachusetts Prevention Epicenter Investigators. Automated methods for surveillance of surgical site infections. *Emerg Infect Dis*. 2001;7:212-216.

21. Sands K, Vineyard G, Platt R. Surgical site infections occurring after hospital discharge. *J Infect Dis*. 1996;173:963-970.

22. Sands K, Vineyard G, Livingston J. Efficient identification of postdischarge surgical site infections using automated medical records. *J Infect Dis*. 1999;179:434-441.

23. Knirsch CA, Jain NL, Pablos-Mendez A, Friedman C, Hripcsak G. Respiratory isolation of tuberculosis patients using clinical guidelines and an automated clinical decision support system. *Infect Control Hosp Epidemiol*. 1998;19:94-100.

24. Burke JP. Surveillance, reporting, automation, and interventional epidemiology. *Infect Control Hosp Epidemiol*. 2003;24:10-12.

ANTIMICROBIAL RESISTANCE

CHAPTER SIXTEEN

CONTROL OF GRAM-POSITIVE MULTIDRUG-RESISTANT PATHOGENS

Mark E. Rupp, MD

INTRODUCTION

Antimicrobial-resistant pathogens are a significant and increasingly important threat to human health. Approximately 70% of nosocomial infections are caused by antibiotic-resistant pathogens.[1] The costs related to the treatment of infections due to antibiotic-resistant pathogens have been estimated to exceed $4 billion annually.[2] Healthcare settings are crucial pivot points in the initial development of antimicrobial resistance traits and the clonal expansion of antibiotic-resistant pathogens via person-to-person transmission. Healthcare epidemiologists are increasingly involved in programs to make more prudent use of antimicrobial agents and to control epidemic and endemic transmission of multidrug-resistant pathogens.

Multidrug resistent pathogens are defined as pathogens that are resistant to more than one class of antimicrobial agents. Although the names of the most common MDROs imply resistance to only one antibiotic, such as MRSA or VRE, these pathogens are often resistant to all but a few available antimicrobial agents.

PREVALENCE AND SIGNIFICANCE

Unfortunately, the prevalence of MDROs is increasing dramatically (Figure 16-1). For example, MRSA was observed in Europe approximately 40 years ago concomitant with the introduction of anti-staphylococcal penicillins. During the 1970s and 1980s, outbreaks of MRSA occurred primarily in hospitals throughout the world. More recently, infections due to community-acquired MRSA have been documented. The CDC reported that from 1998 through 2002, 51.3% of *S. aureus* isolates recovered from patients in ICUs were MRSA.[3] For the same time period, non-ICU inpatient areas and outpatient areas were associated with MRSA rates of 41.4% and 25.7%, respectively.[3] VRE made up 12.8% of enterococcal isolates from ICU patients, 12% from non-ICU patients, and 4.7% from outpatient areas.[3] Although penicillin-resistant pneumococci satisfy the definition for classification as a gram-positive MDRO and approximately one-third of United States isolates are nonsusceptible to penicillin,[4] they rarely result in nosocomial infections and will not be considered further in this chapter.

Increasing data indicate that antibiotic resistance is associated with less favorable clinical outcomes. Kollef and colleagues found that among ICU patients who received inadequate initial antimicrobial treatment, frequently due to antibiotic resistance, infection-related mortality was 2.37 times more likely (p<0.001) than for patients who received antibiotics to which the causative pathogen was susceptible.[5] With regard to gram-positive MDROs, numerous investigators have documented their clinical significance. Compared to patients with infections due to MSSA, those with infections due to MRSA have significantly increased mortality, increased length of hospital stay, and greater economic cost.[6-10] For example, Engemann et al studied staphylococcal surgical site infections and found that patients infected with MRSA were 3.4 times more likely to die than patients infected with MSSA.[6] Excess hospital charges attributed to MRSA were $13,901 per infection.[6] Although similar observations have been made regarding the significance of VRE, conclusions are less clear cut due to multiple confounding variables that often exist in patients infected with VRE. Edmond and colleagues observed a 37% attributable mortality and a risk ratio for mortality of 2.3 in comparing patients with VRE bacteremia to matched controls.[11]

Linden and colleagues observed an enterococcus-associated mortality rate of 46% for patients with VRE bacteremia versus 25% for patients with VSE bacteremia on a liver transplant service.[12] In a prospective, multi-center study, Vergis and colleagues noted that vancomycin resistance was an independent predictor of mortality in patients with enterococcal bacteremia.[13] In similar studies, several investigators have noted that vancomycin resistance is not associated with differences in outcomes in various patient cohorts.[14-16] However, all agree that antimicrobial-resistant pathogens are problematic due to the limitation of therapeutic choices, need for utilization of more costly and potentially more toxic antimicrobial agents, and the increased cost associated with surveillance cultures and patient isolation.

MECHANISMS OF RESISTANCE AND RESERVOIRS FOR TRANSMISSION

Methicillin-Resistant Staphylococcus aureus

Methicillin resistance in *S. aureus* is due to the production of an alternate penicillin-binding protein (PBP2a) that has a low affinity for all ß-lactam antibiotics and generates stable peptidoglycan products in the presence of inhibitory concentrations of ß-lactam antibiotics.[17] The genetic element encoding methicillin-resistance is carried on the staphylococcal chromosome cassette *mec* (SCC*mec*), which is a large chromosomal element containing the *mec*A gene, regulators, and usually a variety of other resistance genes. Genetic transfer of SCC*mec* from strain to strain is a very rare event, and thus, the worldwide spread of MRSA is thought to be almost exclusively due to clonal expansion of a few genetic background strains via person-to-person spread. Transmission of MRSA has traditionally been associated with the healthcare system, and almost all subjects colonized or infected with MRSA can be traced back to contact with the healthcare system (eg, inpatient care, hemodialysis, long-term care settings, home infusion therapy).[18] More recently, community-acquired MRSA has been defined in people without other risk factors for acquisition of MRSA. Preliminary data indicate that these strains of MRSA involve a smaller, perhaps more mobile, SCC*mec*-type IV.[19] In the future, community-acquired MRSA mediated by type IV SCC*mec* may radically alter the epidemiology of MRSA and influence containment practices. However, at the present time, the reservoir for MRSA consists primarily of patients with significant contact with the healthcare system, and spread is via healthcare workers, and to a lesser extent via medical fomites such as stethoscopes, blood

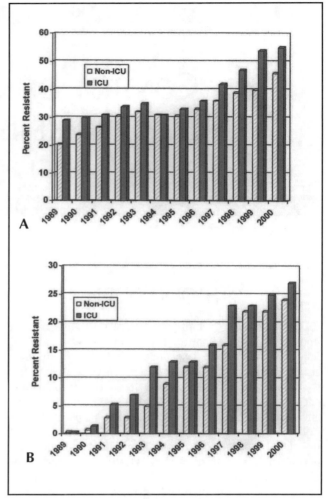

Figure 16-1. Prevalence of (A) MRSA and (B) VRE among isolates causing nosocomial infections in the United States. The lighter bar indicates isolates from infections occurring in ICU patients; the darker bar indicates isolates from infections occurring in other hospitalized patients. (Adapted from Center for Disease Control and Prevention. NNIS system. Available at: www.cdc.gov/drugresistance/healthcare/default.htm. Accessed July 13, 2004.)

pressure cuffs, and thermometers, and environmental surfaces such as bed rails and tables. It should be emphasized that the majority of carriers of MRSA are patients with asymptomatic colonization. The natural ecologic niche for MRSA is human skin and mucosal membranes, and they are readily recovered from the anterior nares of colonized subjects.

VRE

Vancomycin resistance in *Enterococcus faecalis* and *E. faecium* is primarily due to the acquisition of *van*A or *van*B gene clusters, which encode enzymes responsible for the production of peptidoglycan precursors that bind to glycopeptides with reduced affinity. The resistance genes are carried on mobile genetic elements that are readily transferable between enterococcal strains.

In the United States, VRE are almost always linked to people with significant contact with the healthcare system. The transmission of VRE in the United States is similar to that of MRSA—via healthcare workers and medical fomites. In Europe, the epidemiology of VRE is somewhat different. Until 1997, avoparcin, a glycopeptide, was widely used as a growth promoter in farm animals. It appears that a significant proportion of VRE acquisition was due to transmission by food products. However, this mode of acquisition appears to have diminished dramatically in response to the prohibition of avoparcin as a growth promoter.[20] The natural ecologic niche of enterococci is the gut, and VRE can be readily recovered from rectal swabs or stool cultures of colonized people.

CONTROL MEASURES

Infection control efforts to limit the spread of gram-positive MDROs must be considered in the larger context and should be part of a comprehensive, system-wide program directed at antimicrobial resistance. It must be recognized that the major driving factor in the emergence of antimicrobial resistance is the overuse and inappropriate use of antimicrobial agents.[21] Antimicrobial use within hospitals and in other areas of the healthcare system is only one, albeit quite important, part of the overall equation. Efforts to reduce selective pressure through more prudent antimicrobial use should be coupled with primary efforts to prevent infection such as vaccination programs and efforts to prevent nosocomial infections.[22] Finally, the chain of contagion must be broken by identifying people infected or colonized with MDROs and preventing transmission through rigorous use of standard precautions and contact isolation procedures.

Two comprehensive statements from the SHEA and the CDC's HICPAC regarding control of gram-positive MDROs have recently been promulgated.[23,24] The HICPAC document, which covers control considerations for a broad range of potential pathogens, including gram-positive MDROs, is in draft form and is available at www.cdc.gov/ncidod/hip/isoguide.htm as noted in the Federal Register 69:33034, 2004. Although these papers differ in a number of areas, they are in agreement in many respects. Key issues in a comprehensive program to limit the spread of gram-positive MDROs are discussed below and summarized in Table 16-1.

Surveillance

As previously mentioned, the majority of patients harboring MRSA or VRE are asymptomatically colonized. Therefore, case finding based solely on detection of gram-positive MDROs from routinely submitted clinical specimens will not detect the majority of asymptomatic carriers.[23,25] For example, Giroe and colleagues noted that approximately one-half of MRSA-colonized or -infected patients admitted to an ICU were discovered only by screening cultures.[26] Similarly, Franchi and colleagues noted that only 16% of VRE-colonized subjects were identified through routine clinical specimens.[27]

Both the SHEA guideline and the draft HICPAC statement recognize the significance of patients asymptomatically colonized with gram-positive MDROs. The 2 statements differ somewhat with regard to how aggressively colonized patients should be sought. The SHEA guideline recommends that surveillance cultures should be performed at the time of admission and then weekly (or other periodic timeframe) for high-risk, hospitalized patients. They also recommend surveillance cultures be performed throughout the healthcare system (long-term care, dialysis, etc.) with the goal of identifying all colonized patients.[23] The draft CDC HICPAC statement recommends that institutions define a threshold prevalence of MDROs or nosocomial transmission incidence that would trigger additional preventive measures based upon institutional priorities and resources. These measures could include active surveillance cultures in target populations or care units.[24] A full description of laboratory methods to detect gram-positive MDROs and the role of the clinical microbiology laboratory in infection control efforts is beyond the scope of this chapter, and the interested reader is referred to recent reviews.[28,29]

Isolation Precautions

Standard Precautions

Standard precautions should be used in all patient encounters. The draft HICPAC guidelines recommend that all patients should be considered as possibly colonized with an MDRO and emphasize the role of standard precautions.[24] Hand hygiene is a cornerstone of standard precautions. HCWs should be encouraged to use an approved alcohol-based hand rub for routine hand disinfection and to wash their hands with soap and water whenever their hands are visibly soiled with blood or body fluids.[30] The guideline on hand hygiene is available via the internet at www.cdc.gov/handhygiene.

Contact Isolation

Patients known or strongly suspected of harboring a gram-positive MDRO should be cared for under contact isolation precautions. Patients should be housed to provide spatial separation in order to reduce the risk of trans-

TABLE 16-1. MEASURES TO PREVENT THE TRANSMISSION OF GRAM-POSITIVE MDROs

Recommendation	Strength of Evidence*
Administrative Measures	
Prevention of transmission of GP-MDROs should be an institutional priority and should be part of the institutional patient safety program.	II
GP-MDRO prevention issues should be considered in institutional decisions regarding facility design and construction, personnel staffing, laboratory support, and overall allocation of institutional resources.	IB
Education	
Education and training regarding GP-MDROs should be conducted with all healthcare workers.	IB
HCWs should receive feedback on institutional and unit rates of GP-MDRO prevalence and rates of adherence to preventive measures (hand hygiene compliance, etc).	IB
Antimicrobial Use	
Physicians should be instructed in appropriate prescribing and stewardship of antimicrobial agents.	IB
Antimicrobial usage patterns should be monitored, and antimicrobials should be used in ways to minimize selective pressure.	IB
Surveillance	
Laboratory-based protocols should be devised to promptly identify GP-MDROs and notify appropriate HCWs.	IB/IC
Surveillance should be conducted to identify nosocomial infections due to GP-MDROs.	IA
Active surveillance cultures should be obtained to identify asymptomatically colonized individuals, particularly in high-risk patients or institutions with significant nosocomial transmission of GP-MDROs. Cultures should be performed at appropriate periodic intervals.	IB
Isolation Precautions	
Standard precautions should be employed in the care of all patients and should include meticulous hand hygiene, appropriate use of gloves and gowns, mucous membrane protection, and appropriate cleansing and disinfection of patient care equipment and the environment of care.	IA
Contact isolation should be employed in caring for patients colonized or infected with GP-MDROs.	IB
House patients in order to provide maximal spatial separation, preferably in private room with private bath.	IB
Gloves and gowns should be worn when caring for a patient colonized or infected with GP-MDROs.	IB
Masks should be worn when caring for patients colonized or infected with MRSA, VISA, or VRSA whenever droplet aerosols may be encountered (respiratory suctioning, wound irrigation, etc.). SHEA guideline recommends wearing masks at all times when caring for MRSA, VISA, or VRSA patients.	IB
Noncritical equipment should be patient dedicated.	IB
Patient transportation out of the room should be limited as much as possible and should be conducted with appropriate contact isolation practices.	II
Recommendations for discontinuation of contact isolation are not available.	Unresolved issue
Recommendations for appropriate use of surveillance cultures and contact isolation precautions in home care setting and some ambulatory care settings are not available.	Unresolved issue

TABLE 16-1. MEASURES TO PREVENT THE TRANSMISSION OF GRAM-POSITIVE MDROs (CONTINUED)

Recommendation	Strength of Evidence*
Patient Care Environment	
Environmental disinfection should be conducted with an emphasis on "high-touch" areas.	IB
Effectiveness of cleaning procedures can be enhanced through use of dedicated individuals.	II
Environmental cultures should be obtained when there is epidemiologic evidence of an environmental source for patient transmission.	IB
Decolonization	
HCWs colonized with MRSA should be decolonized if they are implicated in on-going transmission.	IB
Decolonization of patients colonized with MRSA should be considered as an adjunctive measure in special circumstances. Consultation with experts in infectious diseases/infection control is recommended on a case-by-case basis. Consideration of susceptibility and resistance issues is required.	II

*Adapted from the CDC/HICPAC method for evaluating quality of scientific evidence. IA = strongly recommended for implementation and strongly supported by well-designed experimental, clinical, or epidemiologic studies; IB = strongly recommended for implementation and supported by some experimental, clinical, or epidemiological studies, and a strong theoretical rationale; IC = required for implementation as mandated by federal or state regulation or standard; II=suggested for implementation and supported by suggestive clinical or epidemiologic studies or a theoretical rationale.

GP-MDRO = gram-positive multidrug-resistant organisms, HCW = healthcare worker, MRSA = methicillin-resistant *S. aureus*, VISA = vancomycin-intermediate susceptible *S. aureus*, VRSA = vancomycin-resistant *S. aureus*.

Adapted from the SHEA *Guideline for Preventing Nosocomial Transmission of Multidrug-Resistant Strains of* Staphylococcus aureus *and* Enterococcus[23] and the CDC HICPAC *Draft Guideline to Prevent Transmission of Infectious Agents in Healthcare Settings.*[24]

mission. The most effective means of accomplishing this goal is to mandate private rooms for people infected or colonized with gram-positive MDROs. When this is not practical, patients harboring the same species of gram-positive MDRO may be cohorted with one another in order to provide physical barriers between colonized or infected patients and those who do not harbor MDROs.

Gloves

Gloves should be worn as part of standard precautions whenever it can be reasonably anticipated that contact with blood, mucous membranes, potentially infectious material, or colonized skin will occur.[31] The use of gloves is uniformly recommended when caring for a person infected or colonized with a gram-positive MDRO. It should be stressed to HCWs that gloves should be changed between patients and between tasks when a contamination-prone task (eg, repositioning a patient, changing diapers, or emptying a bedpan) is followed by a task involving a clean site (eg, manipulation of an IV catheter, intramuscular injection).[30] In addition, use of gloves does not obviate the need for hand hygiene, and hands should be disinfected following removal of gloves.[30]

Gowns

Gowns should be worn as part of standard precautions to protect uncovered skin and prevent soiling of clothing during patient care activities that are likely to generate splashes or sprays of blood or body fluids.[31] However, many HCWs question the use of gowns in the routine care of patients asymptomatically colonized with gram-positive MDROs. Several issues should be noted in this regard.

First, patients colonized or infected with gram-positive MDROs often result in widespread contamination of the environment.[32-34] Furthermore, it has been demonstrated that HCWs readily contaminate their clothing in the routine care of patients colonized with gram-positive MDROs and that gowns prevent such contamination.[32,35,36] Last, most studies examining the role of gowns in the prevention of transmission of gram-positive MDROs have indicated better control of transmission when gowns are in use.[23,37,38]

Masks

The SHEA statement and the draft HICPAC guidelines differ somewhat on the routine use of masks in prevention of gram-positive MDRO transmission. The SHEA guideline relates that masks should be worn when entering the room of a patient colonized with MRSA, vancomycin-intermediate susceptible S. aureus (VISA), or VRSA to decrease nasal acquisition.[23] The draft HICPAC document relates that masks are not recommended for routine use, but should be used during interactions that may result in the production of droplet aerosols.[24]

Equipment

Numerous studies have documented that equipment items such as stethoscopes, thermometers, tourniquets, and glucose monitors become contaminated with gram-positive MDROs during patient care activities.[39-42] Furthermore, some investigators have linked contaminated equipment with transmission of gram-positive MDROs to patients.[41,42] Therefore, noncritical patient care equipment should be dedicated to a single patient. If use of common equipment items is unavoidable, they should be carefully cleaned and disinfected between patients.

Environmental Measures

As previously mentioned, patients harboring gram-positive MDROs can result in widespread contamination of the patient care environment, including such items as bed clothes, linens, bedrails, wheelchairs, bedside tables, patient care equipment, door knobs, faucet handles, telephone hand sets, and computer keyboards.[23,24,37,43-45] In addition, gram-positive MDROs are quite hardy, resist desiccation, and remain viable on inanimate surfaces for days to months.[34,46,47] Therefore, it is important to include environmental services in a comprehensive program to combat the spread of gram-positive MDROs. Environmental service workers should be educated, and procedures should be implemented to ensure consistent cleaning and disinfection, particularly of "high touch" surfaces such as bedrails, doorknobs, and faucet handles.[24] MRSA and VRE are rapidly killed by standard, low-level disinfectants.[48] Cleaning and disinfection must be performed with careful attention to the adequacy of cleaning, disinfectant dilution, and contact time.[49] Environmental cleaning can be enhanced by dedicating consistent individuals to perform cleaning and disinfection services.[24] Environmental cultures are recommended only when there is epidemiologic evidence suggesting that an environmental source is responsible for transmission.[24]

Discontinuation of Contact Isolation Precautions

Indications for the discontinuation of contact isolation precautions are controversial. For example, although guidelines from the CDC recommend discontinuing contact isolation for VRE when 3 stool cultures, obtained at weekly intervals, are negative,[50] more recent experience has indicated that such screening may not detect people with low-level colonization that may persist indefinitely.[51-53] Similarly, colonization with MRSA may be persistent and may be difficult to detect in people with low-level colonization or intermittent shedding.[54-56] The draft HICPAC guideline for prevention of transmission of infectious agents regards this as an unresolved issue awaiting more definitive studies.[20] A prudent compromise measure may be to regard these patients as persistently colonized in the short term and manage them accordingly. In the longer term, their colonization status could be evaluated after an arbitrary period of time (6 to 12 months), during which they remain free of hospitalization and antimicrobial therapy.

Practice Settings

Consensus exists regarding patients in acute-care settings (eg, ICU, burn units, inpatient wards): They are at high risk for the development of nosocomial infections, and comprehensive measures should be implemented to prevent nosocomial acquisition and transmission of gram-positive MDROs.[23,24] However, it is less clear as to what measures should be practiced in ambulatory care, long-term care, or home care settings. One view, espoused in the SHEA guidelines, persuasively argues that transmission of gram-positive MDROs can occur in any healthcare setting and that to be most effective and have long-term effects, widespread application of surveillance cultures and strict adherence to contact isolation precautions should be employed throughout the healthcare system.[23] Alternatively, the draft HICPAC guideline emphasizes standard precautions and points out that risk factors for infection differ markedly in various care settings and among different patient populations and that application of surveillance cultures and isolation precautions should be influenced by individual patient risk factors, institutional priorities, and resources, and should be implemented with some degree of flexibility.[24]

Decolonization

In general, decolonization is not recommended as a standard measure to prevent the transmission of gram-positive MDROs. Suppression of carriage has been used as an adjunctive measure to control the spread of MRSA.[23] However, suppression of MRSA colonization is often transient and at times complicated by the emergence of resistance to agents used in the decolonization scheme.[57,58] Decolonization of HCWs colonized with MRSA should be limited to instances where HCWs have been implicated epidemiologically to transmission. The efficacy of decolonization regimens of VRE has not been established, and they should not, at this time, be routinely employed.

CONCLUSION

Antimicrobial resistance is a significant and growing problem among gram-positive pathogens. The fearful specter of a "post-antibiotic era" in which drug development does not keep pace with the emergence of antimicrobial resistance is a realistic possibility. Therefore, efforts to control the spread of gram-positive MDROs are of paramount importance. Infection control efforts should be part of a comprehensive program that includes antimicrobial stewardship and primary infection prevention measures.

The foundation of infection control programs directed at the prevention of transmission of gram-positive MDROs is the uniform application of standard precautions and hand hygiene. In addition, patients asymptomatically colonized with VRE or MRSA should be actively sought through surveillance cultures, and appropriate contact isolation precautions should be employed in people colonized with gram-positive MDROs. These measures are particularly important to prevent infection in high-risk populations, but should be employed as broadly as possible and practical.

Challenges for the future will include the changing epidemiology of MRSA in the form of community-acquired MRSA and in defining the most cost-effective means to prevent transmission of gram-positive MDROs. There remain major gaps in our knowledge regarding the pathogenesis of disease and factors that influence colonization and infection by gram-positive MDROs. The most pressing immediate needs include an affordable, rapid, and sensitive means to detect colonization and more effective means to eliminate or block gram-positive MDRO colonization.

REFERENCES

1. Centers for Disease Control and Prevention. Division of Healthcare Quality Promotion. Antimicrobial resistance: A growing threat to public healthcare. Available at: http://www.cdc.gov/ncidod/hip/Aresist/am_res.htm. Accessed June 16, 2004.

2. Task force on antibiotic resistance. Report of the ASM task force on antibiotic resistance. *Antimicrob Agents Chemoth*. 1995;Supplement:1-23.

3. National Nosocomial Infections Surveillance (NNIS) System Report, data summary from January 1992 to June 2002, issued August 2002. *Am J Infect Control*. 2002;30:458-475.

4. Sahm DF, Thornsberry C, Jones ME, et al. Correlations of antimicrobial resistance among Streptococcus pneumoniae in the U.S.: 2001-2002 TRUST surveillance. From abstracts of the 42nd Interscience Conference on Antimicrobial Agents and Chemotherapy; September 2002; San Diego, CA. Abstract C2-1640.

5. Kollef MH, Sherman G, Ward S, Fraser VJ. Inadequate antimicrobial treatment of infections: a risk factor for hospital mortality among critically ill patients. *Chest*. 1999;115:462-474.

6. Engemann JJ, Carmeli Y, Cosgrove SE, et al. Adverse clinical and economic outcomes attributable to methicillin resistance among patients with *Staphylococcus aureus* surgical site infection. *Clin Infect Dis*. 2003;36:592-598.

7. Abramson MA, Sexton DJ. Nosocomial methicillin-resistant and methicillin-susceptible *Staphylococcus aureus* primary bacteremia: at what costs? *Infect Control Hosp Epidemiol*. 1999;20:408-411.

8. Cosgrove SE, Sakoulas G, Perencevich EN, Schwaber J, Karchmer AW, Carmeli Y. Comparison of mortality associated with methicillin-resistant and methicillin-susceptible *Staphylococcus aureus* bacteremia: a meta-analysis. *Clin Infect Dis*. 2003;36:53-59.

9. Romero-Vivas J, Ruio M, Fernandez C, Picazo JJ. Mortality associated with nosocomial bacteremia due to methicillin-resistant *Staphylococcus aureus*. *Clin Infect Dis*. 1995;21:1417-1423.

10. Rubin RJ, Harrington CA, Poon A, Dietrich K, Greene JA, Moiduddin A. The economic impact of *Staphylococcus aureus* infection in New York city hospitals. *Emerg Infect Dis*. 1999;5:9-17.

11. Edmond MB, Ober JF, Dawson JD, Weinbaum DL, Wenzel RP. Vancomycin-resistant enterococcal bacteremia: natural history and attributable mortality. *Clin Infect Dis*. 1996;23:1234-1239.

12. Linden PK, Pasculle AW, Manez R, et al. Differences in outcomes for patients with bacteremia due to vancomycin-resistant *Enterococcus faecium* or vancomycin-susceptible *E. faecium*. *Clin Infect Dis*. 1996;22:663-670.

13. Vergis EN, Hayden MK, Chow JW, et al. Determinants of vancomycin resistance and mortality rates in enterococcal bacteremia. *Ann Intern Med*. 2001;135:484-492.

14. Shay DK, Maloney SA, Montecalvo M, et al. Epidemiology and mortality risk of vancomycin-resistant enterococcal bloodstream infections. *J Infect Dis*. 1995;172:993-1000.

15. Stroud L, Edwards J, Danzig L, Culver D, Gaynes R. Risk factors for mortality associated with enterococcal bloodstream infections. *Infect Control Hosp Epidemiol*. 1996;17:576-580.

16. Garbutt JM, Ventrapragada M, Littenberg B, Mundy LM. Association between resistance to vancomycin and death in cases of *Enterococcus faecium* bacteremia. *Clin Infect Dis*. 2000;30:466-472.

17. Chambers HF. Methicillin-resistant Staphylococci. *Clin Microbiol Rev*. 1988;1:173-186.

18. Salgado CD, Farr BM, Calfee DP. Community-acquired methicillin-resistant *Staphylococcus aureus*: a meta-analysis of prevalence and risk factors. *Clin Infect Dis*. 2003;36:131-139.

19. Said-Salim B, Mathema B, Kreiswirth BN. Community-acquired methicillin-resistant *Staphylococcus aureus*: an emerging pathogen. *Infect Control Hosp Epidemiol*. 2003;24:451-455.

20. Wegener HK. Ending the use of antimicrobial growth promoters is making a difference. *ASM News*. 2003;69:443-448.

21. World Health Organization. Department of Communicable Disease Surveillance and Response. WHO global strategy for containment of antimicrobial resistance. 2001;1-105. Available at http://www.who.int/csr/resources/publications/drugresist/EGlobal_Strat.pdf.

22. Centers for Disease Control and Prevention. Prevent antimicrobial resistance in healthcare settings: twelve steps to prevent antimicrobial resistance among hospitalized adults. Available at http://www.cdc.gov/drugresistance/healthcare/ha/12steps_HA.htm. Accessed June 16, 2004.

23. Muto CA, Jernigan JA, Ostrowsky BE, et al. SHEA guideline for preventing nosocomial transmission of multidrug-resistant strains of *Staphylococcus aureus* and Enterococcus. *Infect Control Hosp Epidemiol*. 2003;24: 362-386.

24. Centers for Disease Control and Prevention. Healthcare Infection Control Practices Advisory Committee. Draft guideline to prevent transmission of infectious agents in healthcare settings 2003. Available at: http://www.cdc.gov/ncidod/hip/isoguide.htm. Accessed July 13, 2004.

25. Warren DK, Fraser VJ. Infection control measures to limit antimicrobial resistance. *Crit Care Med*. 2001;29(suppl 4):128-134.

26. Girou E, Pujade G, Legrand P, Cizeau F, Brun-Buisson C. Selective screening of carriers for control of methicillin-resistant *Staphylococcus aureus* (MRSA) in high-risk hospital areas with a high level of endemic MRSA. *Clin Infect Dis*. 1998;27:543-550.

27. Franchi D, Climo MW, Wong AHM, Edmond MB, Wenzel RP. Seeking vancomycin resistant *Staphylococcus aureus* among patients with vancomycin-resistant enterococci. *Clin Infect Dis*. 1999;29:1556-1558.

28. Pfaller MA, Herwaldt LA. The clinical microbiology laboratory and infection control: emerging pathogens, antimicrobial resistance, and new technology. *Clin Infect Dis*. 1997;25:858-870.

29. Willey BM, Jones RN, McGeer A, et al. Practical approach to the identification of clinically relevant *Enterococcus* species. *Diag Microbiol Infect Dis*. 1999;34:165-171.

30. Centers for Disease Control and Prevention. Guideline for hand hygiene in health-care settings: recommendations of the healthcare infection control practices advisory committee and the HICPAC/SHEA/APIC/IDSA hand hygiene task force. *MMWR*. 2002;51:1-45.

31. Occupational exposure to bloodborne pathogens-OSHA. Final Rule. *Fed Regist*. 1991;56:64004-64182.

32. Boyce JM, Potter-Bynoe G, Chenevert C, King T. Environmental contamination due to methicillin-resistant *Staphylococcus aureus*: possible infection control implications. *Infect Control Hosp Epidemiol*. 1997;18: 622-627.

33. Rutala W, Katz E, Sherertz R Sarubbi F. Environmental study of methicillin-resistant *Staphylococcus aureus* epidemic in a burn unit. *J Clin Microbiol*. 1983;18:683-688.

34. Falk PS, Winnike J, Woodmansee C, Desai M, Mayhall CG. Outbreak due to vancomycin-resistant enterococci (VRE) in a burn unit. *Infect Control Hosp Epidemiol*. 2000;21: 575-582.

35. Smith TL, Iwen PC, Olson SB, Rupp ME. Environmental contamination with vancomycin-resistant enterococci in an outpatient setting. *Infect Control Hosp Epidemiol*. 1998;19:515-518.

36. Boyce JM, Chenevert C. Isolation gowns prevent health care workers (HCWs) from contaminating their clothing, and possibly their hands, with methicillin-resistant *Staphylococcus aureus* (MRSA) and resistant enterococci. Eighth Annual Meeting of the Society for Healthcare Epidemiology of America; April 5-7, 1998; Orlando, Fla. Abstract S74:52.

37. Puzniak LA, Leet T, Mayfield J, Kollef M, Mundy LM. To gown or not to gown: the effect on acquisition of vancomycin resistant enterococci. *Clin Infect Dis*. 2002;35: 18-25.

38. Srinivasan A, Song X, Bower R, et al. A prospective study to determine whether cover gowns in addition to gloves decrease nosocomial transmission of vancomycin-resistant enterococci in an ICU. *Infect Control Hosp Epidemiol*. 2002;23:424-428.

39. Bernard L, Kereveur A, Durand D, et al. Bacterial contamination of hospital physicians' stethoscopes. *Infect Control Hosp Epidemiol*. 1999;20:626-628.

40. Cohen HA, Amir J, Matalon A, et al. Stethoscopes and otoscopes: a potential vector of infection? *Fam Pract*. 1997;14:446-449.

41. Livornese LL, Dias S, Romanowski B, et al. Hospital-acquired infection with vancomycin-resistant *Enterococcus faecium* transmitted by electronic thermometers. *Ann Intern Med*. 1992;117:112-116.

42. Brooks S, Khan A, Stoica D, Griffith J. Reduction in vancomycin-resistant *Enterococcus* and *Clostridium difficile* infections following change to tympanic thermometers. *Infect Control Hosp Epidemiol*. 1998;19:333-336.

43. Boyce JM, Potter-Bynoe G, Chenevert C, King T. Environmental contamination due to methicillin-resistant *Staphylococcus aureus*: possible infection control implications. *Infect Control Hosp Epidemiol*. 1997;18: 622-627.

44. Noskin GA, Peterson L, Warren J. *Enterococcus faecium* and *Enterococcus faecalis* bacteremia: acquisition and outcome. *Clin Infect Dis*. 1995;20:296-301.

45. Rutula W, Katz E, Sherertz R, Sarubbi F. Environmental study of methicillin-resistant *Staphylococcus aureus* epidemic in a burn unit. *J Clin Microbiol*. 1983;18:683-688.

46. Neely AN, Maley MP. Survival of enterococci and staphylococci on hospital fabrics and plastics. *J Clin Microbiol*. 2000;38:724-726.

47. Wendt C, Wiesenthal B, Dietz E, Ruden H. Survival of vancomycin-resistant and vancomycin-susceptible enterococci on dry surfaces. *J Clin Microbiol*. 1998;36:3734-3736.

48. Ayliffe GAJ. Control of *Staphylococcus aureus* and enterococcal infections. In: Block SS, ed. *Disinfection, Sterilization, and Preservation*. 5th ed. Philadelphia, Pa: Lippincott, Williams & Wilkins; 2001:491-504.

49. Centers for Disease Control and Prevention. Healthcare Infection Control Practices Advisory Committee (HICPAC). Guidelines for environmental infection control in health-care facilities. *MMWR*. 2003;52:1-44.

50. Centers for Disease Control and Prevention. Healthcare Infection Control Practices Advisory Committee (HICPAC). Recommendations for preventing the spread of vancomycin resistance. *MMWR*. 1995;44(RR12):1-13.

51. Bonten MJ, Slaughter S, Ambergen AW, et al. The role of "colonization pressure" in the spread of vancomycin-resistant enterococci: an important infection control variable. *Arch Intern Med*. 1998;158:1127-1132.

52. Donskey CJ, Hoyen CK, Das SM, Helfand MS, Hecker MT. Recurrence of vancomycin-resistant *Enterococcus* stool colonization during antibiotic therapy. *Infect Control Hosp Epidemiol*. 2002;23:436-440.

53. D'Agata EM. Antimicrobial-resistant gram-positive bacteria among patients undergoing chronic hemodialysis. *Clin Infect Dis*. 2002;35:1212-1218.

54. Scanvic A, Denic L, Gaillon S, Giry P, Andremont A, Lucet JC. Duration of colonization by methicillin-resistant *Staphylococcus aureus* after hospital discharge and risk factors for prolonged carriage. *Clin Infect Dis*. 2001;32: 1393-1398.

55. Hachem R, Raad I. Failure of oral antimicrobial agents in eradicating gastrointestinal colonization with vancomycin-resistant enterococci. *Infect Control Hosp Epidemiol*. 2002;23:43-44.

56. Harbarth S, Liassine N, Dharan S, Herrault P, Auckenthaler R, Pittet D. Risk factors for persistent carriage of methicillin-resistant *Staphylococcus aureus*. *Clin Infect Dis*. 2000;31:1380-1385.

57. Doebbeling BN, Regan DR, Pfaller MA, Houston AK, Hollis RJ, Wenzel RP. Long-term efficacy of intranasal mupirocin ointment: a prospective cohort study of *Staphylococcus aureus* carriage. *Arch Intern Med*. 1994;154:1505-1508.

58. Miller MA, Dascal A, Portnory J, Medelson J. Development of mupirocin resistance among methicillin-resistant *Staphylococcus aureus* after widespread use of nasal mupirocin ointment. *Infect Control Hosp Epidemiol*. 1996;17:811-813.

CHAPTER SEVENTEEN

ANTIBIOTIC-RESISTANT GRAM-NEGATIVE INFECTIONS

David L. Paterson, MBBS, FRACP and Mesut Yilmaz, MD

INTRODUCTION

During the past 10 years, considerable attention has been paid to antibiotic resistance in gram-positive cocci. MRSA, VRE, and most recently VRSA have become well known to hospital epidemiologists and infection control practitioners. In response to the threat of these organisms, pharmaceutical manufacturers have developed a considerable armamentarium active against the resistant gram-positive cocci—linezolid, quinupristin/dalfopristin, and daptomycin are the first of a significant pipeline of antibiotics active against vancomycin-resistant gram-positive cocci.

In contrast, virtually no new antibiotics have become available against antibiotic-resistant gram-negative bacilli (GNB). Furthermore, trends in resistance of GNB have been toward multiple antibiotic resistance and, in some instances, resistance to all commercially available antibiotics. Given this development, control of spread of antibiotic-resistant GNB has become a significant infection control problem. The purpose of this chapter is to briefly review the mechanisms of antibiotic resistance in GNB before discussing in detail potential strategies for the control of such organisms in a hospital environment.

MICROBIOLOGY AND EPIDEMIOLOGY OF THE GRAM-NEGATIVE BACILLI TYPICALLY FOUND IN HOSPITALIZED PATIENTS

The most clinically relevant classification of the common GNB is to distinguish between the Enterobacteri-aceae (which ferment, rather than oxidize D-glucose and other sugars) and the nonfermentative GNB, which usually degrade glucose oxidatively (Table 17-1). Although some pathogenic species are not adequately covered by this distinction, the vast majority of aerobic GNB encountered in hospitals will be.

The Enterobacteriaceae

The members of the Enterobacteriaceae are GNB that are usually resident in the GI tract. Examples of such organisms include *E. coli*, *Klebsiella pneumoniae*, *Enterobacter cloacae*, and *Citrobacter freundii* (see Table 17-1). In one study, the Enterobacteriaceae accounted for 29% of ICU-acquired pneumonia, 28% of ICU-acquired UTIs, and 12% of ICU-acquired bloodstream infections.[1] The risk of such infections is high in patients with intra-abdominal pathology. Spillage of enteric organisms into the peritoneal cavity in such patients may lead to intra-abdominal abscess formation. UTIs with the Enterobacteriaceae may occur in both catheterized and noncatheterized patients because of the proximity of the urethral meatus to the anus. Finally, patients who have been in the hospital for a prolonged period of time may develop skin and upper respiratory tract colonization with GI tract flora. Therefore, central venous line-related infections and ventilator-associated pneumonia may occur due to the Enterobacteriaceae.

Unfortunately, during the past decade, increasing antibiotic resistance has been observed in the Enterobacteriaceae. The NNIS System has provided useful data on the extent of antibiotic resistance in the United States for the time period January 1998 to June 2002.[2] Of more than 4000 *Enterobacter* isolates from 101 ICUs in the United States, 26.3% of isolates were resistant to third-generation cephalosporin antibiotics.[2] In Europe, depending on the country, between 23% and 51% of ICU-acquired *Enterobacter* isolates were resistant to piperacillin/

tazobactam, and in some countries more than 30% of such isolates were resistant to ciprofloxacin.[3] In the United States, 6.1% of more than 6000 *K. pneumoniae* isolates were resistant to third-generation cephalosporins.[2] However, notably, in more than 10% of ICUs, more than 25% of *K. pneumoniae* isolates were resistant to third-generation cephalosporins. In Latin America, Eastern Europe, and Asia, rates of resistance may be much greater.

In general, rates of antibiotic resistance in the Enterobacteriaceae are much higher in ICUs than in other areas of the hospital. However, quinolone resistance may be one area in which these divergences are less pronounced. NNIS data show that 5.8% of *E. coli* isolates from ICUs in the period 1998 to 2002 were resistant to quinolone antibiotics, whereas 5.3% of *E. coli* isolates from non-ICU inpatient areas were quinolone resistant.[2] Additionally, in LTCFs,[4] and in certain specialized units of acute-care hospitals, rates of resistance to many antibiotics may parallel those seen in ICUs.

It should be noted that resistance of the Enterobacteriaceae to the carbapenems, whether it be occurring in ICU or non-ICU settings, remains an exceedingly rare event. We recommend that the occurrence of carbapenem-resistant *E. coli*, *K. pneumoniae*, *Serratia marcescens*, or *Enterobacter* spp. should be investigated by the healthcare epidemiology team.

THE NONFERMENTATIVE GRAM-NEGATIVE BACILLI

Examples of nonfermentative GNB include *P. aeruginosa*, *Acinetobacter* spp., and *Stenotrophomonas maltophilia*. *P. aeruginosa* and other *Pseudomonas* spp. (for example, *P. fluorescens*, *P. putida*, and *P. stutzeri*) have a predilection for water. They have been found in a variety of aqueous solutions in the hospital, including irrigation fluids, soaps, disinfectants, eye drops, and dialysis fluids.[5] *P. aeruginosa* has classically been regarded as the most common cause of ventilator-associated pneumonia; *Acinetobacter* spp. and *S. maltophilia* may also cause this infection. It should be noted, however, that these organisms may colonize the respiratory tract as well as cause true pneumonia. *P. aeruginosa* is also a potent cause of bloodstream infection (classically in neutropenic patients) and postprocedure cholangitis.

Antibiotic resistance is also a considerable concern in the nonfermentative GNB. NNIS data from ICUs in the United States from 1998 to 2002 show that the mean percentage of *P. aeruginosa* isolates resistant to commonly used anti pseudomonal antibiotics was levofloxacin 37.8%, ciprofloxacin 36.3%, imipenem 19.6%, piperacillin 17.5%, and ceftazidime 13.9%.[2] As with the

TABLE 17-1. COMMONLY ENCOUNTERED GRAM-NEGATIVE BACILLI IN THE HOSPITAL SETTING

Enterobacteriaceae (Glucose Fermenters)
Klebsiellae
    K. pneumoniae
    K. oxytoca
E. coli
Enterobacter spp.
    E. cloacae
    E. aerogenes
S. marcescens
Morganella morganii
Citrobacter spp.
    C. freundii
    C. diversus
Proteus spp.
    P. mirabilis
    P. vulgaris
Providencia stuartii

Nonfermentative Bacteria (Do Not Ferment Glucose)
P. aeruginosa
Acinetobacter spp.
S. maltophilia

Enterobacteriaceae, resistance was more frequent in ICUs than in other areas of the hospital. A most disturbing problem with the nonfermentative GNB has been the advent of resistance to multiple antibiotics simultaneously. Given the lack of availability of new antibiotics active against organisms such as *P. aeruginosa*, it is likely that multidrug resistance will be as great a problem as VRE was in the 1990s.

MECHANISMS OF RESISTANCE OF COMMON GRAM-NEGATIVE BACILLI

Resistance to Cephalosporins

The predominant mechanism of resistance of the common GNB to cephalosporins is beta-lactamase production. More than 300 different beta-lactamases have been described. They have been classified in a variety of differ-

TABLE 17-2. COMMON MECHANISMS OF RESISTANCE IN GRAM-NEGATIVE BACILLI

Resistance to Third-Generation Cephalosporins

Extended-spectrum beta-lactamases (ESBLs)
AmpC type beta-lactamases
Carbapenemases
Efflux pumps

Resistance to Piperacillin/Tazobactam and Other Beta-Lactam/Beta-Lactamase Inhibitor Combinations

Hyperproduction of beta-lactamases
Outer membrane protein deficiencies
Efflux pumps

Resistance to Carbapenems

Outer membrane protein deficiencies
Carbapenemases

Resistance to Quinolones

Target mutations
Efflux pumps

ent ways. However, the most commonly used classifications are based on molecular structure (classified as classes A through D) or functional characteristics such as substrate and inhibitor profile (classified as groups 1 through 4).[6] The beta-lactamases inactivate cephalosporins by splitting the amide bond of the antibiotic's beta-lactam ring.

Most strains of *P. aeruginosa*, *Enterobacter* spp., *Citrobacter* spp., *Providencia* spp., *M. morganii*, and *Serratia* spp. resistant to third-generation cephalosporins produce a functional Group 1 (molecular class C) beta-lactamase. A representative of this class is the AmpC enzyme. Characteristically, this beta-lactamase can inactivate first- and second-generation cephalosporins (including the cephamycins such as cefoxitin and cefotetan) and third-generation cephalosporins (Table 17-2). These beta-lactamases are not inhibited by beta-lactamase inhibitors such as clavulanic acid. An important characteristic of this group of beta-lactamases is that their production can be increased by exposure of the bacteria to certain antibiotics. This phenomenon is known as induction. The amount of beta-lactamase production depends on the concentration of the antibiotic and the time of exposure. Penicillin, ampicillin, most first-generation cephalosporins, cefoxitin, and imipenem are strong inducers. All

of these antibiotics but imipenem will be inactivated by the Group 1 beta-lactamases.

In most populations of organisms such as *Enterobacter* spp., mutants exist that permanently hyperproduce Group 1 beta-lactamases.[7] These mutants usually occur at frequencies of 10^{-5} to 10^{-8}. Their presence at this low frequency is not enough to result in frank resistance to antibiotics such as the third-generation cephalosporins. However, there are important clinical implications of these mutants. Antibiotic therapy with agents that are not inducers of transient beta-lactamase production (for example, third-generation cephalosporins) will kill all organisms in the colony except the permanently hyperproducing mutants. These mutants, therefore, become the dominant population at a site of infection and lead to frank resistance to third-generation cephalosporins. This can result in emergence of resistance during therapy.[8,9]

Organisms such as *K. pneumoniae*, *E. coli*, or *P. mirabilis* do not characteristically hyperproduce Group 1 beta-lactamases. Occasionally, they may acquire plasmid-mediated Group 1 beta-lactamases. However, much more commonly, they may acquire plasmid-mediated beta-lactamases of Group 2be, known as ESBLs. These beta-lactamases have important differences compared with Group 1 beta-lactamases. These differences have significant clinical implications.

ESBLs were first described in 1983.[10] Importantly, these beta-lactamases were not found prior to the introduction of third-generation cephalosporins into clinical practice. The gene encoding the first ESBL showed a mutation of a single nucleotide compared to the gene encoding SHV-1, a beta-lactamase produced by more than 95% of *K. pneumoniae* isolates.[10] Production of SHV-1 produces resistance to ampicillin and first-generation cephalosporins, but not to third-generation cephalosporins. The ESBL derivative of SHV-1 was now resistant to the third-generation cephalosporins. Other ESBLs were soon discovered that were closely related to TEM-1 and TEM-2, beta-lactamases that were commonly produced by *E. coli*, resulting in resistance of the organism to ampicillin. Again, the ESBL derivative of TEM-1 or TEM-2 was able to confer resistance to the extended-spectrum cephalosporins.[11]

Because these new beta-lactamases had an extended spectrum of activity compared to their parent enzymes, they were coined the ESBLs. It is not appropriate to designate Group 1 beta-lactamases as ESBLs because they do not have an extended spectrum of activity compared to any parent enzyme. The ESBLs also differ from Group 1 beta-lactamases in that they are not able to inactivate the cephamycins (eg, cefoxitin or cefotetan) and because they are inactivated in vitro by the beta-lactamase inhibitor clavulanic acid.

Worse still, the genes encoding ESBLs are carried on plasmids. This enables transfer of genetic material from organism to organism. Furthermore, genes encoding resistance mechanisms for other antibiotics (eg, aminoglycosides, trimethoprim/sulfamethoxazole) are carried on the same plasmids as ESBLs. This means that ESBL-producing organisms are truly multidrug resistant. Unfortunately, many clinical microbiology laboratories do not use specialized detection methods for ESBLs, so in many cases the presence of ESBLs goes unnoticed.

Resistance to Beta-Lactam/Beta-Lactamase Inhibitor Combinations

Piperacillin/tazobactam, ticarcillin/clavulanate, and ampicillin/sulbactam are examples of the combination of a beta-lactam with a beta-lactamase inhibitor. The theoretical advantage of addition of a beta-lactamase inhibitor is that this protects the beta-lactam antibiotic from the destructive effects of the beta-lactamase. The beta-lactamase inhibitors in current use are active against the beta-lactamases produced by anaerobic organisms such as *Bacteroides fragilis*, as well as the TEM-1 and SHV-1 beta-lactamases commonly produced by *E. coli* and *K. pneumoniae*, and the penicillinases produced by *S. aureus*.

Unfortunately, multiple mechanisms of resistance may work together in producing resistance to the beta-lactam/beta-lactamase inhibitor combinations. The entry of any beta-lactam antibiotics into the bacterial cell is via outer membrane proteins, which function as channels through which the antibiotics pass. These proteins may be lost, contributing to decreased entry of the antibiotic and decreased antimicrobial activity. In some sites of infection with high organism load (eg, intra-abdominal abscesses or severe cases of ventilator-associated pneumonia), the sheer weight of beta-lactamase production by a high inoculum of organisms may overcome the effects of beta-lactamase inhibitors.[12] Finally, as noted above, Group 1 beta-lactamases (produced by organisms such as *Enterobacter* spp.) are not susceptible to the effects of beta-lactamase inhibitors and, therefore, may be inherently resistant to beta-lactam/beta-lactamase inhibitor combinations.

Resistance to Quinolones

There is an increased probability of resistance of ESBL-producing organisms to quinolones compared to non-ESBL-producing organisms of the same species.[13,14] The reasons for this co-resistance are not entirely clear. Plasmid-mediated quinolone resistance, although reported,[15] appears not yet to be widespread. It appears more likely that seriously ill patients are subject to multiple antibiotic exposures. If third-generation cephalosporins and quinolones are used in the same patient, ESBL pro-

duction and quinolone resistance may be selected by independent mechanisms.

One mechanism of resistance to quinolones is mutation of the genes that encode the target enzymes (DNA gyrase and topoisomerase IV) for quinolones. Stepwise increasing resistance occurs if there are mutations in one and then 2 of the genes encoding these enzymes.

Alterations in outer membrane proteins coupled with active efflux pumps (which pump antibiotics out of the bacterial cell) appear to be important additional mechanisms of bacterial resistance to quinolones, especially in *P. aeruginosa*. Most of the common pump systems in *P. aeruginosa* remove multiple antibiotic classes—for example, quinolones, penicillins, and cephalosporins. This makes them potent causes of multidrug resistance.[16]

Resistance to Carbapenems

Carbapenems are often used as drugs of last resort in treatment of serious infections due to GNB, but are increasingly used empirically in hospitals where multidrug resistance abounds. In *P. aeruginosa*, imipenem resistance may arise via loss of OprD, an outer membrane protein that is accessible to carbapenems but not other antibiotics. Some efflux mechanisms result in reduced susceptibility to meropenem.[16] *S. maltophilia* has been known for many years to be carbapenem resistant by way of production of class B beta-lactamases known as metalloenzymes. A variety of metalloenzymes have also been detected in *P. aeruginosa*, *Acinetobacter*, and even members of the Enterobacteriaceae. Of concern, many of these are transferable from one bacterial genus to others. Thus far, these enzymes are extremely rare in *Enterobacteriaceae*. The usual mechanism of carbapenem resistance in these organisms is the combination of outer membrane protein deficiency coupled with production of beta-lactamases.[11]

OPTIONS FOR CONTROL OF MULTIPLY RESISTANT GRAM-NEGATIVE BACILLI IN THE HOSPITAL

Investigation for a Common Environmental Source of Infection

A common environmental source of multiply resistant gram-negative organisms always needs to be considered when an apparent outbreak is detected. Nonfermentative bacteria, in particular (but not exclusively), have been linked to water reservoirs in the hospital.[17] Examples of such sources include faucets and faucet aerators and immersion or whirlpool baths. Potable water itself may be a source, although *P. aeruginosa* isolates from potable water are rarely multidrug resistant unless faucets or faucet aerators are contaminated in a healthcare setting. As has been well documented in recent years, improperly cleaned bronchoscopes may be an important source of multidrug-resistant *P. aeruginosa*.[18]

Bronchoscopes have also been implicated in an outbreak of ESBL-producing *Klebsiellae*,[19] as has ultrasonography coupling gel[20] and glass thermometers (used in axillary measurement of temperature).[21] Outbreaks of infection with *E. cloacae* and *S. marcescens* have been associated with unintentionally contaminated medications or human albumin solutions.[22,23] HCWs wearing artificial nails have been linked to nosocomial outbreaks of infection due to *P. aeruginosa* and *S. marcescens*.[24-26]

Cockroaches have been implicated as possible vectors of infection; in one recent study, ESBL-producing *K. pneumoniae* isolated from cockroaches was indistinguishable from that infecting patients.[27] ESBL-producing organisms have been isolated from patients' soap, sink basins, and babies' baths, but the contribution of this environmental contamination to infection was impossible to determine.

In response to an outbreak of multiply resistant GNB, a reasonable approach complementing the traditional outbreak investigation would be to perform molecular epidemiologic typing of the implicated organisms (Figure 17-1). If genotypically identical or similar isolates are found, culturing of environmental sites would be prudent. Discovery of a removable environmental focus that harbored genotypically related isolates to the outbreak strain should obviously lead to an investigation as to how that object became contaminated and removal of the focus from the ward involved.

Three examples of such an intervention have been described in the context of controlling outbreaks of infection with ESBL-producing organisms. Gaillot et al found that contaminated gel used for ultrasonography was contaminated with ESBL-producing organisms.[20] Replacement of this gel quickly curtailed the outbreak. Branger et al found that a poorly maintained bronchoscope was colonized with ESBL-producing organisms and could be linked to respiratory tract infections with the same strain.[19] Repair and proper maintenance of the bronchoscope stopped nosocomial transmission of the organism. Finally, Rogues et al found colonization of four of 12 glass mercury thermometers with ESBL-producing *K. pneumoniae* and axillary colonization with the same strain in 2 patients.[21] Disinfection of the thermometers curtailed the outbreak.

Person-to-Person Transmission Via the Hands

Many infection control practitioners use active surveillance cultures and stringent contact isolation precautions as a means of preventing spread of MRSA or VRE.[28] However, the need for such measures in the control of multiply resistant GNB has not been as widely expressed. There is a widespread belief that multiply resistant GNB are selected primarily by antibiotic use or result from exposure to a contaminated environmental source rather than passed from person to person. Yet, there is ample evidence of nosocomial transmission of ESBL-producing GNB and carbapenemase-producing *P. aeruginosa*. A review of more than 50 studies that used molecular epidemiologic techniques to analyze outbreaks of ESBL-producing organisms found that in all cases at least 2 patients in each hospital shared genotypically similar strains, implying person-to-person spread of the organism.[29] In fewer than 10% of these outbreaks were environmental foci discovered. Several recent studies have demonstrated clonal spread of carbapenemase-producing *K. pneumoniae* or *P. aeruginosa*.[30-32] No longer should multiply resistant GNB be regarded as selected by antibiotic use to the exclusion of the possibility of person-to-person transmission by the hands of HCWs.

Hand carriage of resistant GNB has been documented by most, but not all, investigators who have sought it.[33,34] In these instances, the hand isolates were genotypically identical to isolates that caused infection in patients. Hand carriage by HCWs is usually eliminated by hand hygiene with chlorhexidine or alcohol-based antiseptics. However, the authors know of one example of prolonged, persistent skin carriage in a nurse with chronic dermatitis. GI tract carriage has been documented in HCWs, but is astonishingly rare and seldom prolonged, except with ESBL-producing *Salmonella* species.

The hands of HCWs are presumably colonized by contact with the skin of patients with cutaneous colonization of the organism. It is important to recognize that many patients may have asymptomatic colonization with multiply resistant gram-negative organisms without overt signs of infection. These patients represent an important reservoir of organisms. For every patient with clinically significant infection with an ESBL-producing organism, for example, at least one other patient exists in the same unit with GI tract colonization with an ESBL producer. In some hyperendemic ICUs and transplants units, 30% to 70% of patients have GI tract colonization with ESBL producers at any one time.[35]

Because GI tract colonization with GNB occurs in every person, selective media must be used to assess the carriage of resistant organisms. This can be readily achieved by addition of appropriate concentrations of antibiotics in the media, in order to select for organisms with the resistance profile in question. Prior GI carriage of ESBL-producing organisms is an independent variable associated with infection with ESBL producers and may sometimes occur with multiply resistant *P. aeruginosa*. At least 80% of patients with infection with ESBL-producing *K. pneumo-*

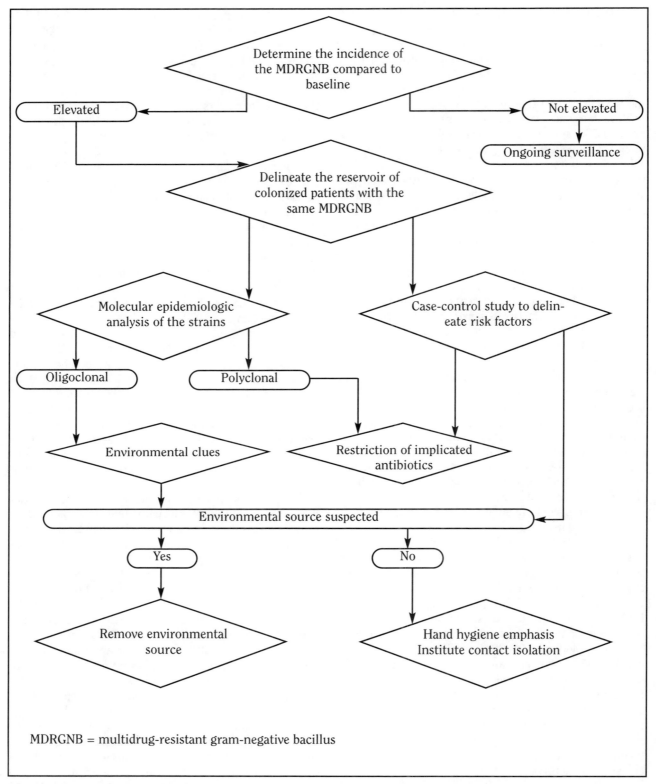

MDRGNB = multidrug-resistant gram-negative bacillus

Figure 17-1. Algorithm for investigation and control of multidrug-resistant GNB.

niae can be documented to have prior GI tract carriage.[36] Patients who develop infection usually do so within days to weeks of acquiring GI tract colonization.

Control of an initial outbreak of multiply resistant gram-negative organisms in a hospital, or specialized unit of a hospital, is of critical importance. The initial stages of the infection control program in a hospital or unit that has not previously been affected by organisms with the resistance profile in question should include (1) performance of rectal swabs to delineate patients colonized (but not infected) with the resistant organism; (2) evaluation for the presence of a common environmental source of infection; (3) molecular epidemiologic analysis; (4) a campaign to improve hand hygiene; and (5) introduction of contact isolation for those patients found to be colonized or infected, if there is molecular evidence of spread of related organisms and no common environmental source was found (see Figure 17-1).

Contact isolation implies use of gloves and gowns when contacting the patient. Several studies have documented that this practice alone can lead to reduction in horizontal spread of ESBL-producing organisms.[29] However, compliance with these precautions needs to be high to maximize the effectiveness of these precautions.[37] Furthermore, we recommend that patients who have GI tract colonization as well as those with frank infection should undergo contact isolation. It has been noted that standard methods of hand hygiene, screening for colonization, and patient isolation may not always be effective in controlling outbreaks of ESBL-producing organisms. In some situations, temporary ward closure is necessary to adequately control an outbreak that had been unresponsive to conventional measures.[38]

ANTIBIOTIC MANAGEMENT AND MULTIPLY RESISTANT GRAM-NEGATIVE BACILLI

In settings where molecular epidemiologic evidence is not supportive of patient-to-patient transmission of multiply-resistant organisms, antibiotic management may play an important role. Examples of strategies used in antibiotic management include modification of prescribing patterns by education or by "front-end" restriction of availability of certain antibiotics, "downstream" streamlining of antibiotic therapy, antibiotic cycling, and use of selective digestive tract decolonization. Well-designed case-control studies examining which antibiotics provide a risk for the multiply resistant GNB under question are a necessary prerequisite. Obviously, prescribers need to be informed of the results of these studies. If exposure to a certain antibiotic is clearly implicated in subsequent

infection with a multidrug-resistant organism, use of that antibiotic may be restricted by the need for a prior telephone call by the prescriber to the hospital's antibiotic management program. Careful attention needs to be paid to ensuring that the appropriateness of antibiotic therapy for serious infections is not compromised by restriction of antibiotic choice. Alteration in the availability of multiple antibiotic classes, by way of a telephone preapproval program, has been successfully used in the context of an outbreak of infection with multiply resistant *Acinetobacter* spp.[39]

Elimination of overly broad antibiotic therapy, once culture results are available, is a practical way of reducing the burden of "antibiotic pressure" on selection of multiply-resistant organisms. The value of such streamlining may seem intuitive to ID physicians and infection control practitioners, but for many other physicians, an attitude of "don't change a winning team" is pervasive. Furthermore, in some situations, cultures are negative, yet an infection is clinically present, or in other situations, cultures are positive but indicate the presence of colonization rather than true infection. There are thus some practical issues to the practice of streamlining.

There is currently little information on the optimal duration of antibiotic therapy for many commonly encountered conditions. Studies comparing different durations of antibiotic regimens are currently underway for infections such as ventilator-associated pneumonia and will likely show that shorter course regimens are just as effective as long course regimens but with lower risk of superinfection with resistant organisms. Use of invasive testing strategies (such as quantitative culture of bronchoscopically obtained respiratory specimens) may allow differentiation of colonization from true infection and may also promote more appropriate antibiotic use.[40] Use of clinical scoring systems in differentiating infection from noninfectious etiologies of clinical or radiologic signs may also yield a reduction in antibiotic use and antibiotic-resistant superinfections.[41]

Another consideration is whether particular antibiotic classes should be avoided as "workhorse" therapy because of an intrinsic high risk of promoting multidrug resistance.

It is increasingly evident that third-generation cephalosporins may be linked to the emergence of many multidrug-resistant organisms and, therefore, may be particularly useful as targets in an antibiotic restriction campaign.[42] It is noteworthy that in a survey of 15 different hospitals, an association existed between cephalosporin and aztreonam usage at each hospital and the isolation rate of ESBL-producing organisms and multiply resistant *Acinetobacter* and *P. aeruginosa* at each hospital.[43,44] Reduction in use of extended-spectrum cephalosporins is the common theme underlying many successful interventions in outbreaks with ESBL-producers.[45] However, it must also be noted that drugs with antianaerobic activity, by interfering with GI tract flora,[46,47] and fluoro-quinolones, by upregulating efflux pumps,[16,48] may also be potential culprits in selecting for multidrug resistance and, therefore, may be targets for restriction as empiric therapy.

Although restriction of availability of certain antibiotic classes is of demonstrable value in an outbreak situation, mathematical modeling studies suggest the most likely way to reduce selection pressure leading to antibiotic resistance is to use a variety of antibiotics (that is, to create a setting of antibiotic heterogeneity).[49] In such a scenario, antibiotics are used in equal amounts during the same time period. For example, equal availability of fluoroquinolones, aminoglyco-sides, anti-pseudomonal penicillins, β-lactam/β-lactamase inhibitor combinations, cephalosporins with anti-pseudomonal activity, and carbapenems would exist for empirical antibiotic therapy for suspected gram-negative bacterial infections in a given ICU. To our knowledge, a study evaluating an unrestricted ICU armamentarium ver-sus a restricted ICU armamentarium has never been per-formed. It should also be noted that the usefulness of antibi-otic heterogeneity in a given ICU depends on the baseline susceptibility to the various compounds.[50]

Scheduled rotation of antibiotics (antibiotic cycling) is in some respects conceptually attractive. It is theorized that withdrawal of an antibiotic from use for a defined period of time will limit antibiotic pressure as a stimulus for antibiotic resistance. Early experience with rotating amikacin and gentamicin use supported this concept.[51] However, examples also exist whereby resistance does not disappear in the absence of antibiotic use. For example, while streptomycin was virtually never used at a large teaching hospital, 20% of isolates of Enterobacteriaceae were resistant to this antibiotic.[52] Furthermore, mathe-matical models suggest that cycling is inferior even to a situation where just 2 antibiotics are used simultaneously in the same population.[49]

Thus far, studies that have examined antibiotic cycling have yielded positive results, but have been mired with potential confounders to the positive outcomes they have observed.[53,54] It can be argued that a reliance on antibiotic cycling to reduce or prevent the emergence of resistance is naïve given our detailed understanding of the molecular genetics of antibiotic resistance and known associations between antimicrobial usage and resistance. The existence of multi-resistance plasmids (some ESBL plasmids carry more than a dozen resistance genes) and common resist-ance associations (such as ESBLs with fluoroquinolone resistance) make the choices of empirical rotation regimens quite problematic. Practical problems also exist. In a recent report, "off cycle" antibiotics were necessary in nearly 50% of patients requiring antibiotics.[55]

A number of groups have previously attempted SDD as a means of reducing colonization with resistant GNB. A large randomized controlled trial performed in the Netherlands has shown that SDD resulted in a significant decrease in colonization with resistant GNB and reduced mortality in the ICU.[56] It is important to note that this study was performed in a setting of low prevalence of VRE and MRSA, making extrapolation of these results difficult to hospitals where these organisms are endemic. SDD has been used as a means of interrupting transmission of ESBL-producing organisms. Successfully applied regi-mens have included polymyxin, neomycin and nalidixic acid, colistin and tobramycin, or norfloxacin.[57] It should be noted that in many hospitals at least 15% to 30% of ESBL-producing organisms are quinolone resistant[13,58] and, therefore, are unlikely to be suppressed by use of nor-floxacin prophylaxis. Additionally, MDR isolates are unlikely to respond to SDD using aminoglycosides.

An alternative approach to digestive tract decoloniza-tion has been decolonization of the nasopharynx. A recent study has used a nasal spray with povidone-iodine as a means of decolonizing the upper respiratory tract.[59] In this study (performed in a neurologic rehabilitation unit), only 1 of 10 patients had GI carriage with an ESBL-producing organism, but all had nasotracheal coloniza-tion. Upper airway decolonization led to management of an outbreak.

CONCLUSION

It appears safe to say that multiresistant GNB will be with us for many years to come. The likely shortage of new antibi-otics to cope with these organisms will place a spotlight on their epidemiology within hospitals and the ability of efforts to control their spread. This will require a multipronged approach, including an understanding of their mechanisms of resistance, application of molecular epidemiologic tech-niques, and case-control studies. Efforts to reduce environ-mental contamination, patient-to-patient transmission, and antibiotic misuse will be of great importance.

REFERENCES

1. Richards MJ, Edwards JR, Culver DH, Gaynes RP. Nosocomial infections in medical intensive care units in the United States. National Nosocomial Infections Surveillance System. *Crit Care Med.* 1999;27:887-892.

2. NNIS. National Nosocomial Infections Surveillance (NNIS) System Report, data summary from January 1992 to June 2002, issued August 2002. *Am J Infect Control.* 2002;30:458-475.

3. Hanberger H, Garcia-Rodriguez JA, Gobernado M, Goossens H, Nilsson LE, Struelens MJ. Antibiotic suscep-tibility among aerobic gram-negative bacilli in intensive care units in 5 European countries. French and Portuguese ICU Study Groups. *JAMA.* 1999;281:67-71.

4. Wiener J, Quinn JP, Bradford PA, et al. Multiple antibiotic-resistant *Klebsiella* and *Escherichia coli* in nursing homes. *JAMA*. 1999;281:517-523.

5. Morrison AJ Jr., Wenzel RP. Epidemiology of infections due to *Pseudomonas aeruginosa*. *Rev Infect Dis*. 1984;6 Suppl 3:S627-S642.

6. Bush K, Jacoby GA, Medeiros AA. A functional classification scheme for beta-lactamases and its correlation with molecular structure. *Antimicrob Agents Chemother*. 1995;39:1211-1233.

7. Livermore DM. Beta-lactamases in laboratory and clinical resistance. *Clin Microbiol Rev*. 1995;8:557-584.

8. Chow JW, Fine MJ, Shlaes DM, et al. *Enterobacter* bacteremia: clinical features and emergence of antibiotic resistance during therapy. *Ann Intern Med*. 1991;115:585-590.

9. Kaye KS, Cosgrove S, Harris A, Eliopoulos GM, Carmeli Y. Risk factors for emergence of resistance to broad-spectrum cephalosporins among *Enterobacter* spp. *Antimicrob Agents Chemother*. 2001;45:2628-2630.

10. Knothe H, Shah P, Krcmery V, Antal M, Mitsuhashi S. Transferable resistance to cefotaxime, cefoxitin, cefamandole and cefuroxime in clinical isolates of *Klebsiella pneumoniae* and *Serratia marcescens*. *Infection*. 1983;11:315-317.

11. Bradford PA. Extended-spectrum beta-lactamases in the 21st century: characterization, epidemiology, and detection of this important resistance threat. *Clin Microbiol Rev*. 2001;14:933-951.

12. Thomson KS, Moland ES. Cefepime, piperacillin-tazobactam, and the inoculum effect in tests with extended-spectrum beta-lactamase-producing Enterobacteriaceae. *Antimicrob Agents Chemother*. 2001;45:3548-3554.

13. Lautenbach E, Strom BL, Bilker WB, Patel JB, Edelstein PH, Fishman NO. Epidemiological investigation of fluoroquinolone resistance in infections due to extended-spectrum beta-lactamase-producing *Escherichia coli* and *Klebsiella pneumoniae*. *Clin Infect Dis*. 2001;33:1288-1294.

14. Paterson DL, Mulazimoglu L, Casellas JM, et al. Epidemiology of ciprofloxacin resistance and its relationship to extended-spectrum beta-lactamase production in *Klebsiella pneumoniae* isolates causing bacteremia. *Clin Infect Dis*. 2000;30:473-478.

15. Martinez-Martinez L, Pascual A, Jacoby GA. Quinolone resistance from a transferable plasmid. *Lancet*. 1998;351:797-799.

16. Livermore DM. Multiple mechanisms of antimicrobial resistance in *Pseudomonas aeruginosa*: our worst nightmare? *Clin Infect Dis*. 2002;34:634-640.

17. Anaissie EJ, Penzak SR, Dignani MC. The hospital water supply as a source of nosocomial infections: a plea for action. *Arch Intern Med*. 2002;162:1483-1492.

18. Srinivasan A, Wolfenden LL, Song X, et al. An outbreak of *Pseudomonas aeruginosa* infections associated with flexible bronchoscopes. *N Engl J Med*. 2003;348:221-227.

19. Branger C, Bruneau B, Lesimple AL, et al. Epidemiological typing of extended-spectrum beta-lactamase-producing *Klebsiella pneumoniae* isolates responsible for five outbreaks in a university hospital. *J Hosp Infect*. 1997;36:23-36.

20. Gaillot O, Maruejouls C, Abachin E, et al. Nosocomial outbreak of *Klebsiella pneumoniae* producing SHV-5 extended-spectrum beta-lactamase, originating from a contaminated ultrasonography coupling gel. *J Clin Microbiol*. 1998;36:1357-1360.

21. Rogues AM, Boulard G, Allery A, et al. Thermometers as a vehicle for transmission of extended-spectrum-beta-lactamase producing *Klebsiella pneumoniae*. *J Hosp Infect*. 2000;45:76-77.

22. Wang SA, Tokars JI, Bianchine PJ, et al. *Enterobacter cloacae* bloodstream infections traced to contaminated human albumin. *Clin Infect Dis*. 2000;30:35-40.

23. Ostrowsky BE, Whitener C, Bredenberg HK, et al. *Serratia marcescens* bacteremia traced to an infused narcotic. *N Engl J Med*. 2002;346:1529-1537.

24. Passaro DJ, Waring L, Armstrong R, et al. Postoperative *Serratia marcescens* wound infections traced to an out-of-hospital source. *J Infect Dis*. 1997;175:992-995.

25. Moolenaar RL, Crutcher JM, San Joaquin VH, et al. A prolonged outbreak of *Pseudomonas aeruginosa* in a neonatal intensive care unit: did staff fingernails play a role in disease transmission? *Infect Control Hosp Epidemiol*. 2000;21:80-85.

26. Foca M, Jakob K, Whittier S, et al. Endemic *Pseudomonas aeruginosa* infection in a neonatal intensive care unit. *N Engl J Med*. 2000;343:695-700.

27. Cotton MF, Wasserman E, Pieper CH, et al. Invasive disease due to extended spectrum beta-lactamase-producing *Klebsiella pneumoniae* in a neonatal unit: the possible role of cockroaches. *J Hosp Infect*. 2000;44:13-17.

28. Muto CA, Jernigan JA, Ostrowsky BE, et al. SHEA guideline for preventing nosocomial transmission of multidrug-resistant strains of *Staphylococcus aureus* and enterococcus. *Infect Control Hosp Epidemiol*. 2003;24:362-386.

29. Paterson DL, Yu VL. Extended-spectrum beta-lactamases: a call for improved detection and control. *Clin Infect Dis*. 1999;29:1419-1422.

30. Cornaglia G, Mazzariol A, Lauretti L, Rossolini GM, Fontana R. Hospital outbreak of carbapenem-resistant *Pseudomonas aeruginosa* producing VIM-1, a novel transferable metallo-beta-lactamase. *Clin Infect Dis*. 2000;31:1119-1125.

31. Yan JJ, Ko WC, Tsai SH, Wu HM, Wu JJ. Outbreak of infection with multidrug-resistant *Klebsiella pneumoniae* carrying bla(IMP-8) in a university medical center in Taiwan. *J Clin Microbiol*. 2001;39:4433-4439.

32. Giakkoupi P, Xanthaki A, Kanelopoulou M, et al. VIM-1 Metallo-beta-lactamase-producing *Klebsiella pneumoniae* strains in Greek hospitals. *J Clin Microbiol*. 2003;41:3893-3896.

33. Royle J, Halasz S, Eagles G, et al. Outbreak of extended spectrum beta lactamase producing *Klebsiella pneumoniae* in a neonatal unit. *Arch Dis Child Fetal Neonatal Ed*. 1999;80:F64-F68.

34. Eisen D, Russell EG, Tymms M, Roper EJ, Grayson ML, Turnidge J. Random amplified polymorphic DNA and plasmid analyses used in investigation of an outbreak of multiresistant *Klebsiella pneumoniae. J Clin Microbiol.* 1995;33:713-717.

35. Green M, Barbadora K. Recovery of ceftazidime-resistant *Klebsiella pneumoniae* from pediatric liver and intestinal transplant recipients. *Pediatr Transplant.* 1998;2:224-230.

36. Pena C, Pujol M, Ardanuy C, et al. Epidemiology and successful control of a large outbreak due to *Klebsiella pneumoniae* producing extended-spectrum beta-lactamases. *Antimicrob Agents Chemother.* 1998;42:53-58.

37. Lucet JC, Decre D, Fichelle A, et al. Control of a prolonged outbreak of extended-spectrum beta-lactamase-producing enterobacteriaceae in a university hospital. *Clin Infect Dis.* 1999;29:1411-1418.

38. Macrae MB, Shannon KP, Rayner DM, Kaiser AM, Hoffman PN, French GL. A simultaneous outbreak on a neonatal unit of two strains of multiply antibiotic resistant *Klebsiella pneumoniae* controllable only by ward closure. *J Hosp Infect.* 2001;49:183-192.

39. White AC Jr., Atmar RL, Wilson J, Cate TR, Stager CE, Greenberg SB. Effects of requiring prior authorization for selected antimicrobials: expenditures, susceptibilities, and clinical outcomes. *Clin Infect Dis.* 1997;25:230-239.

40. Fagon JY, Chastre J, Wolff M, et al. Invasive and noninvasive strategies for management of suspected ventilator-associated pneumonia. A randomized trial. *Ann Intern Med.* 2000;132:621-630.

41. Singh N, Rogers P, Atwood CW, Wagener MM, Yu VL. Short-course empiric antibiotic therapy for patients with pulmonary infiltrates in the intensive care unit. A proposed solution for indiscriminate antibiotic prescription. *Am J Respir Crit Care Med.* 2000;162:505-511.

42. Safdar N, Maki DG. The commonality of risk factors for nosocomial colonization and infection with antimicrobial-resistant *Staphylococcus aureus,* enterococcus, gram-negative bacilli, *Clostridium difficile,* and *Candida. Ann Intern Med.* 2002;136:834-844.

43. Saurina G, Quale JM, Manikal VM, Oydna E, Landman D. Antimicrobial resistance in Enterobacteriaceae in Brooklyn, NY: epidemiology and relation to antibiotic usage patterns. *J Antimicrob Chemother.* 2000;45:895-898.

44. Landman D, Quale JM, Mayorga D, et al. Citywide clonal outbreak of multiresistant *Acinetobacter baumannii* and *Pseudomonas aeruginosa* in Brooklyn, NY: the preantibiotic era has returned. *Arch Intern Med.* 2002;162:1515-1520.

45. Rahal JJ, Urban C, Horn D, et al. Class restriction of cephalosporin use to control total cephalosporin resistance in nosocomial *Klebsiella. JAMA.* 1998;280:1233-1237.

46. Donskey CJ, Chowdhry TK, Hecker MT, et al. Effect of antibiotic therapy on the density of vancomycin-resistant enterococci in the stool of colonized patients. *N Engl J Med.* 2000;343:1925-1932.

47. Hoyen CK, Pultz NJ, Paterson DL, Aron DC, Donskey CJ. Effect of parenteral antibiotic administration on establishment of intestinal colonization in mice by *Klebsiella pneumoniae* strains producing extended-spectrum beta-lactamases. *Antimicrob Agents Chemother.* 2003;47:3610-3612.

48. Villers D, Espaze E, Coste-Burel M, et al. Nosocomial *Acinetobacter baumannii* infections: microbiological and clinical epidemiology. *Ann Intern Med.* 1998;129:182-189.

49. Bonhoeffer S, Lipsitch M, Levin BR. Evaluating treatment protocols to prevent antibiotic resistance. *Proc Natl Acad Sci USA.* 1997;94:12106-12111.

50. Paterson DL, Rice LB. Empirical antibiotic choice for the seriously ill patient: are minimization of selection of resistant organisms and maximization of individual outcome mutually exclusive? *Clin Infect Dis.* 2003;36:1006-1012.

51. Gerding DN, Larson TA. Aminoglycoside resistance in gram-negative bacilli during increased amikacin use. Comparison of experience in 14 United States hospitals with experience in the Minneapolis Veterans Administration Medical Center. *Am J Med.* 1985;79:1-7.

52. Chiew YF, Yeo SF, Hall LM, Livermore DM. Can susceptibility to an antimicrobial be restored by halting its use? The case of streptomycin versus Enterobacteriaceae. *J Antimicrob Chemother.* 1998;41:247-251.

53. Gruson D, Hilbert G, Vargas F, et al. Rotation and restricted use of antibiotics in a medical intensive care unit. Impact on the incidence of ventilator-associated pneumonia caused by antibiotic-resistant gram-negative bacteria. *Am J Respir Crit Care Med.* 2000;162:837-843.

54. Raymond DP, Pelletier SJ, Crabtree TD, et al. Impact of a rotating empiric antibiotic schedule on infectious mortality in an intensive care unit. *Crit Care Med.* 2001;29:1101-1108.

55. Bochorishvili B, Madariaga MG, Pur S, Weinstein RA, Segreti J. Reasons for non-compliance with voluntary cycling of antibiotics. Abstracts of the Infectious Diseases Society of America 40th Annual Meeting 2002.

56. de Jonge E, Schultz MJ, Spanjaard L, et al. Effects of selective decontamination of digestive tract on mortality and acquisition of resistant bacteria in intensive care: a randomised controlled trial. *Lancet.* 2003;362:1011-1016.

57. Paterson DL, Singh N, Rihs JD, Squier C, Rihs BL, Muder RR. Control of an outbreak of infection due to extended-spectrum beta-lactamase-producing *Escherichia coli* in a liver transplantation unit. *Clin Infect Dis.* 2001;33:126-128.

58. Babini GS, Livermore DM. Antimicrobial resistance amongst *Klebsiella* spp. collected from intensive care units in Southern and Western Europe in 1997-1998. *J Antimicrob Chemother.* 2000;45:183-189.

59. Hollander R, Ebke M, Barck H, von Pritzbuer E. Asymptomatic carriage of *Klebsiella pneumoniae* producing extended-spectrum beta-lactamase by patients in a neurological early rehabilitation unit: management of an outbreak. *J Hosp Infect.* 2001;48:207-213.

CHAPTER EIGHTEEN

ANTIMICROBIAL STEWARDSHIP

Robert A. Duncan, MD, MPH and Kenneth R. Lawrence, BS, PharmD

INTRODUCTION

Antibiotics comprise the second most commonly used class of drugs in hospital formularies. Up to 30% of hospitalized patients receive antimicrobial agents,[1] and expenditures for these drugs may comprise 10% to 40% of the hospital pharmacy budget.[1,2] They are unique among pharmaceuticals in that they affect not only individual patients, but the larger environment as well. Nearly all practicing physicians readily prescribe antibiotics, with varying levels of competence.[3] It is estimated that 40% to 50% of antibiotic use in hospitals is inappropriate,[4-6] and hospitals are often where patterns are set for outpatient prescribing practice.[7] Physicians commonly focus on the individual patient and are rarely aware of the ecologic effects of antimicrobial agents on the patient, the hospital, LTCFs, the community, or the world at large.[8]

Excessive use of antibiotics is linked not only to the emergence and spread of resistance,[9,10] but also to adverse drug reactions, the added cost of high-end treatment, and increased infection control efforts required to prevent spread.[11-14] Consequently, there is a growing awareness among hospital administrators and insurers of the clinical and financial benefits of containing antibiotic use and resistant organisms.

Inappropriate use of antimicrobial agents and the resultant increase in resistant organisms have gained national attention (see Chapters 16 and 17). In 1997, a joint committee of the SHEA and the IDSA published *Guidelines for the Prevention of Antimicrobial Resistance in Hospitals.*[15] The CDC, FDA, and WHO have since identified antimicrobial stewardship as an essential component of efforts to prevent and reduce resistance.[16-18] In addition, the JCAHO has now identified prevention of healthcare-acquired infection as one of the National Patient Safety Goals.[19] This combination of economic and regulatory incentives provides a driving force for clinical and ecological reforms that previously concerned a more limited audience.

Antimicrobial stewardship lies at the intersection of ID, infection control, safety and quality improvement, and cost containment. It has been defined as the "appropriate selection, dosing, and duration of antimicrobial therapy to achieve optimal efficacy in managing infections."[15] It is thus an important tool in the effort to reduce inappropriate use of antimicrobials and subsequent development of both resistant microorganisms and drug-related adverse events.[20] Effective antimicrobial stewardship requires the collaboration of many disciplines, including medical and surgical services, nursing, infection control, laboratory, and pharmacy. Monitoring antimicrobial use is an important component of stewardship because of the close relationship between use of antimicrobial agents and the emergence of bacterial resistance.[10,21-24] For example, excessive use of third-generation cephalosporins and of vancomycin has been linked to emergence of several resistant organisms, including MRSA, VRE, and ESBL-producing *E. coli* and *Klebsiella* spp.[22-24]

This chapter describes how to organize an antimicrobial stewardship program, including options for hospitals with a range of resources.

ORGANIZATION AND PERSONNEL

An effective program of antibiotic reform requires a team approach. This starts with formation of an antibiotic utilization committee, chaired by a member of the ID staff or someone with sophisticated knowledge of ID treatment. There should also be representatives from pharmacy, microbiology, and infection control; depending on the size and structure of the hospital, representation from several other departments may be helpful (Table 18-1). Residency staff should be included because they often prescribe most (or all) antibiotics in training hospitals. Direct involvement of a key administrator provides liaison to higher levels of hospital leadership, as well as vital support when reform efforts must be promoted among the medical staff.[25] In addition, collaboration with quality improvement teams may bring substantial administrative resources to bear and facilitates innovation and change. A small working group, including the chair, an ID pharmacist, and (optimally) a data manager, provides most of the effort, with advice from the larger committee.

DATA COLLECTION

Data for monitoring antimicrobial prescribing come from many sources, ranging from pharmacy purchasing records or individual patient records to computerized clinical databases. Pharmacy purchasing data are easily obtainable and may be useful when tracking trends over a period of time, yet have limited utility for epidemiologic analysis. Retrospective or prospective review of a patient's medical record yields actual dispensed doses but is laborious. Computerized systems can provide the time, date, location, prescriber, and dosage of each drug. These data allow calculation of defined drug densities (eg, grams of drug used per 1000 patient days) and cost per hospitalization or per patient-day, as well as density of drug use within specific areas of the hospital (eg, vancomycin use per patient-day in an ICU). This helps to pinpoint areas of misuse/overuse and provides targets for educating clinicians. Finally, summary data from health maintenance organizations (HMOs) and Medicare allow researchers to analyze utilization of antimicrobial agents on a broader scale. Despite availability, national utilization data are difficult to link to practices in local hospitals. Commercial databases used by the pharmaceutical industry may provide detailed prescriber-specific information.

Benchmarking studies have been suggested as a means to compare the use of antimicrobials between hospitals of similar size, acuity, and function, aiming to identify both "best practice" and significant variation in usage patterns.[26] Clearly, the clinical areas in which a hospital specializes will affect the types and patterns of prescribed agents and must be considered when examining the results from such studies.

Drug utilization evaluations (DUEs) identify usage patterns and trends, according to service or hospital unit.[27] This process focuses on a particular drug or class of drugs, assessing optimal prescribing, as defined by local experts (eg, parenteral fluoroquinolone use). Other projects may examine antibiotic therapy for a specific disease, such as community-acquired pneumonia (CAP). A DUE should examine a few questions, rather than attempt a compre-

TABLE 18-1. COMPOSITION OF AN ANTIMICROBIAL UTILIZATION COMMITTEE

Infectious disease staff (Chair)
Pharmacy director
Infectious disease pharmacist
Microbiology director/supervisor
Infection control practitioner(s)
Surgeon
General internist
Pediatrician
Intensivist
Emergency room staff
House staff
Staff nurse
Quality improvement staff
Administrator
Data manager

hensive review. It may also detect variability in practice or identify unrecognized medication errors. Follow-up DUEs give essential feedback to clinicians and document whether reforms were effective. Initial projects might examine the role of antibiotics in emergence of a resistant pathogen (eg, imipenem-resistant *P. aeruginosa*), overutilization of antimicrobial agents, dosing regimens that are ineffective or toxic, or surgical prophylaxis. A list of the pharmacy's "Top 200" expenditures reveals crude patterns of drug use and helps identify targets for intervention[28] (eg, if purchases of a parenteral fluoroquinolone are outpacing oral forms, an aggressive IV-to-PO conversion campaign may be warranted).

The microbiology laboratory is of vital importance in any antimicrobial stewardship program (see Chapter 13). It supplies hospital-wide antimicrobial susceptibility results ("antibiograms") to help in choosing empiric antibiotic therapy, as well as providing separate profiles for ICUs; each must be updated regularly. The laboratory also must inform the committee about emerging problems with resistant organisms and document changes in susceptibility patterns that may be attributable to changes in use of antimicrobial agents.

INTERVENTIONS

Development of Antimicrobial Management Programs

After establishing baseline characteristics of current antimicrobial use and local hospital resistance patterns, the committee should determine what they wish to accomplish and then develop a mission statement.[28,29] When developing programs, the committee should consider several factors, including hospital size, physician make-up (private practice model vs. training program), special patient populations (eg, solid organ or bone marrow transplantation, pediatrics, trauma, or burns), referral resources (eg, rehabilitation or chronic care facilities), and hospital politics.

Initial recommendations and interventions should be limited in scope and should have strong potential to improve patient care, reduce medication errors, and decrease cost, but should also have a high likelihood of success and physician acceptance. Medical staff support is usually strong: in a survey of 490 internal medicine physicians at four Chicago hospitals, almost 90% considered antibiotic resistance to be an important problem and still more felt that inappropriate antimicrobial prescribing was an important contributor.[30] The committee and administrators should agree on formulas to measure the results of its initiatives.

After initial success, the committee may tackle more challenging programs. These could include local adaptation of treatment guidelines, such as a CAP pathway,[31] or joining a national collaborative, like the Surgical Infection Prevention project.[32]

Interventions to improve antimicrobial prescribing, reduce resistance, and decrease cost are listed in Table 18-2 and are discussed below.[1,8,28,33] Caveats are noted in Table 18-3.

Revising the Formulary

Formulary revision is a common and easily implemented method of modulating antimicrobial use.[34,35] Open formularies impose few controls on availability or prescribing of medications by physicians, whereas closed formularies use a systematic process to choose the best 1 or 2 agents among existing drugs in a class and to evaluate new medications. The plethora of available oral and parenteral antimicrobial agents has made selection of an appropriate agent difficult for clinicians, and the committee can help to simplify these choices. Inclusion in the formulary should be based upon clinical efficacy, safety, pharmacokinetic and pharmacodynamic profiles, and dosing convenience. Communication with the microbiology laboratory is important to ensure that susceptibility testing for a new agent does not incur unnecessary cost. If 2 or more drugs within a pharmacologic class are considered therapeutically equivalent, cost often becomes an important factor in the final choice. Negotiation with competing pharmaceutical companies for the best contract can result in substantial savings. The committee should also consider the formularies of referring managed healthcare organizations to ensure continuity of therapy upon hospital discharge, but should ultimately make decisions in the best interest of the hospital and its patients and budget. Periodic review of the formulary avoids therapeutic duplication and eliminates little-used agents or those associated with newly reported adverse events.

One recent but important variable is a manufacturer's shortage of medication.[36] Drug shortages are due to multiple factors, including shortages of raw materials and unsafe manufacturing practices that cause a product to be temporarily unavailable. Medication shortages increasingly affect patient care[36] and may force compensatory alterations of the formulary.

Recently, the benefit of a closed antimicrobial formulary has been challenged. Polk and colleagues demonstrated that centers employing a narrow, closed antibiotic formulary were associated with increased bacterial resistance, compared to facilities with a more varied formulary.[37] These data suggest that heterogeneous antimicrobial prescribing may slow the development of antimicrobial resistance[38] and may raise concerns about the consequences of relatively uniform prescribing in clinical pathways or guidelines.

Reporting Laboratory Data

Susceptibility reporting should include results only for agents available on formulary. Laboratories can influence antibiotic use by reporting susceptibility results for expensive, broad-spectrum agents only when organisms are resistant to narrower spectrum and less expensive drugs.

Educational Programs

To assist physicians in prescribing antimicrobial therapy appropriately, a comprehensive educational program should be developed. This should include formal presentations, such as grand rounds and staff conferences, as well as more informal conferences for resident report and patient care rounds. Presentations should discuss national guidelines, current resistance trends in the hospital, and the importance of appropriate antimicrobial prescribing, with an emphasis on specific problems identified within the hospital. Hospitals with training programs should regularly review basic antimicrobial therapeutics and clinical microbiology with house staff. An audience response system is a useful teaching tool, providing anonymous assessment, comparison with peers, and immediate expert feedback. Newsletters may include emerging resistance issues, lessons from antimicrobial drug utilization evaluations, and reviews of new antimicrobials on the hospital formulary.

Home-grown, pocket-sized guides that contain information on antimicrobial therapy are popular with house staff and attending physicians. Information in the guide may include the hospital antibiogram, usual antimicrobial dosages, drug level monitoring recommendations, adjustments for impaired renal and hepatic function, common

TABLE 18-2. COMPONENTS OF ANTIMICROBIAL STEWARDSHIP AND
COST-CONTAINMENT PROGRAMS

Data Collection and Target Identification
➤ Routine monitoring of pharmacy purchasing volume and costs
➤ Focused, problem-oriented DUEs of individual drugs or practices
➤ Review of "top 200" high-cost formulary agents
➤ Comprehensive review of patterns of antimicrobial usage, with feedback from ID physicians or pharmacists
➤ Computerized DUEs that integrate data from the departments of pharmacy, microbiology, chemistry, and radiology

Formulary Revision
➤ Expert committee selects formulary and limits pharmacy stocks to one or a few optimal drugs within a therapeutic class
➤ Generic substitution of proprietary agents
➤ Competitive contract bidding for similar drugs with equivalent efficacy
➤ Cyclic rotation of formulary agents within a class

Microbiology Testing and Reporting
➤ Routine susceptibility testing done only for formulary agents
➤ Graded susceptibility reporting, based on level of resistance and cost-effectiveness
➤ Regular reporting of susceptibility patterns and empiric drugs of choice, according to ICU, ward, or outpatient isolates
➤ May include level of restriction, usual dosing regimens, renal dose adjustments, and costs

Education
➤ Direct education of healthcare providers by physicians or pharmacists, one-on-one or by group
➤ Use of clinical pathways or guidelines
➤ Counter-detailing of drug information
➤ Concurrent review and advice provided by ID physicians or pharmacists
➤ Computerized decision support of prescribing choices
➤ Feedback to providers
➤ Educate and recruit senior department heads and opinion leaders

Restriction Policies
➤ Open formulary unrestricted but closed ⇒monitored ⇒ID telephone approval required ⇒ID consult required
➤ Limit drugs to clinical scenarios (eg, diabetic foot infections), locations (eg, ICUs), or services
➤ Remove or restrict specific problem agents (eg, habitual antibiotic choices)

Ordering Policies
➤ Antimicrobial agent order forms, including common dosing parameters and educational information
➤ Specified duration of therapy and prophylaxis
➤ Surgical prophylaxis protocols with specified doses and duration
➤ Automatic stop orders for prophylaxis, empiric therapy, and specific therapy, or duration limited without approval
➤ Computerized physician order entry incorporating decision-support tools

Drug Administration
➤ ID pharmacist clinical intervention program
➤ Pharmacokinetic consultation
➤ Revision of standard dosing regimens, based on new pharmacodynamic data
➤ Streamlining of broad-spectrum or multiple-drug antimicrobial regimens
➤ Once-daily aminoglycoside dosing
➤ IV-to-PO or step-down conversion
➤ Home IV therapy

Limiting Contact With Pharmaceutical Representatives
➤ Restrict access of pharmaceutical representatives to clinical care areas
➤ Review "detailing" information and coordinate with representatives
➤ Therapeutic "partnering" with pharmaceutical firms to coordinate education, clinical pathways, and drug selection according to institutionally selected criteria

TABLE 18-3. CAVEATS WHEN IMPLEMENTING AN ANTIMICROBIAL STEWARDSHIP PROGRAM

➤ Provide antimicrobial agent stewardship; don't become a policeman or zealot
➤ Avoid formulary changes for only short-term gain
➤ Financial concerns should not be more important than clinical efficacy and safety
➤ Substitution may alienate devoted users of a specific agent
➤ Formulary changes may necessitate changes in automated susceptibility testing
➤ Don't add to clinicians' paperwork or burden them with collecting your data

drug interactions, antibiotic cost, and approved treatment guidelines. A list of restricted agents and criteria for use of specific antibiotics should be included and updated regularly. For hospitals with internal computer networks, educational information can be posted on the intranet (see Chapter 15).

An effective but labor-intensive form of education is one-on-one or small group discussion, often referred to as "academic counter-detailing."[39] This method uses an evidence-based approach to educate clinicians about appropriate drug therapy in a specific clinical scenario and is often implemented in response to advice from manufacturers' representatives that may be inconsistent with institutional goals.

One-time educational programs have little long-term impact, but, when applied continuously, are essential strategic components of every antibiotic stewardship program.

RESTRICTING AGENTS

One of the most widely used active antibiotic containment strategies is restriction of use. This ranges from open, unrestricted formularies in which any available pharmaceutical may be used, to heavily restricted formularies in which specific drugs may not be prescribed without consultation and approval by the ID service. Options are delineated below, in order of increasing restriction[28]:

1. Open formulary. Physicians may prescribe any available pharmaceutical agent, without restriction.

2. Unrestricted but closed formulary. The formulary is limited to agents approved by the hospital's Pharmacy & Therapeutics Committee, but physicians may prescribe any drug in the formulary without restriction.

3. Monitored drugs. The pharmacy monitors use of particular agents and assesses appropriateness of use. An ID pharmacist or the ID service may be asked to review cases in which antimicrobial agents are used inappropriately.

4. Limited (criteria-based) drugs. Use of some drugs is limited to specific clinical scenarios (eg, diabetic foot infections), locations (eg, ICUs), or services. Any other use is subject to ID approval.

5. Approval required from the ID service. Physicians who wish to use specified antimicrobial agents must discuss the case with the ID service to obtain verbal approval. An initial grace period (eg, 24 hours) is commonly allowed before approval must be obtained.

6. ID consultation is required. Physicians who wish to use a restricted drug must obtain on-site consultation by the ID service before the pharmacy will release the specified drug. An initial grace period may be offered.

Antimicrobial restriction programs have evolved over the decades since their introduction by McGowan and Finland,[40] shifting from simple approval programs administered by ID fellows to educational efforts combined with pre-established criteria for use of broad-spectrum agents.[41-43] In one dramatic example, White and colleagues[44] describe instituting a prior approval system for restricted antibiotics in response to an outbreak of multidrug-resistant Acinetobacter infections. This was administered by ID faculty who were available 24 hours per day and resulted in increased susceptibilities (especially in ICUs), a 32% reduction in expenditures for parenteral antimicrobials, and estimated annual pharmacy budget savings of $863,100, at a cost of less than $150,000.[44] Other more complex programs are described below.

Although commonly used, antimicrobial restriction programs are controversial.

Unrestricted drug access exposes staff to complex choices for which they have neither the time, information, nor expertise required to select drugs appropriately. Indeed, Kunin has argued that "use of high-cost, specialized antimicrobial agents should be a privilege of ID consultants and others trained in their use, just as performance of invasive procedures is limited to those who are qualified."[45] However, excessive antibiotic restriction fosters an adversarial relationship between ID consultants and medical, surgical, and house staff services and can interfere with timely antibiotic administration. Thus, most hospitals maintain graduated levels of monitoring and restriction, depending on the severity of prescribing and resistance problems, potential toxicity, and costs. The most restrictive policies are usually reserved for the most toxic, unfamiliar, or expensive agents (eg, antifungal therapy). ICUs may be the most appropriate sites for active stewardship because of the concentration of severe illness, widespread antimicrobial use, and opportunities for spread of infection and antimicrobial resistance.[46] Yet, tightly restricted formularies are rarely practical outside of large teaching hospitals, where resistance problems are severe enough to provide an impetus and ID fellows can staff 24-hour approval programs. Narrowing rather than restricting options may achieve many of the same goals while maintaining collegial relationships.

ANTIMICROBIAL ORDER FORMS

Antimicrobial order forms may incorporate formalized criteria for use of antimicrobial agents, suggest dosing regimens, and define the duration of use for prophylactic, empiric, or specific therapy.[47] Pharmacies often provide time limits for empiric therapy (eg, for the initial 72 hours). However, such policies must include measures to prevent inadvertent lapses in appropriate therapy. Forms can facilitate antimicrobial audits, yet the quality of information is dependent on those filling out the forms and must be viewed with caution.

SURGICAL PROPHYLAXIS

In 1981, Durbin and colleagues[48] showed that requiring physicians to indicate on a form whether antimicrobial use was prophylactic, empiric, or therapeutic increased the number of patients receiving appropriate prophylactic antibiotics and reduced the duration of surgical prophylaxis by 2 days, from 4.9 to 2.9 days. Two decades later, many centers now use standing order forms for selected surgical procedures that incorporate recommended prophylactic dosing regimens and limit duration to a single preoperative dose or to a 24-hour postoperative period. This standardizes many aspects of preoperative orders, minimizes excessive prophylaxis, and reduces errors.

COMPUTERIZED PHYSICIAN ORDER ENTRY

Computerized physician order entry offers an automated and more versatile version of order forms for those hospitals with adequate computer resources.[49] Software can generate educational pop-up screens in response to requests for restricted or monitored agents or may require prescribers to justify choices before therapy can be dispensed. When designed adequately, these systems also yield prospective, provider-specific utilization data for review without being burdensome and may increase the success of antimicrobial stewardship programs.[49]

COMPUTERIZED DECISION SUPPORT

Researchers at LDS Hospital in Salt Lake City have written extensively on the capabilities of their computer system, which features decision support.[50,51] They developed a computer-assisted management program that provides integrated, real-time data pertaining to treatment of infections, with multiple advantages.

First, the program can evaluate clinical data and alert clinicians that antibiotic therapy is necessary. It then suggests appropriate empiric or therapeutic antimicrobial regimens for individual patients after reviewing diagnoses, vital signs, renal function, and microbiology reports, as well as other data. In an ICU trial, the program significantly reduced medication errors, inappropriate use of antimicrobial therapy, and total hospital and antimicrobial costs.[50] At present, this methodology offers the best hope of integrating clinical, pharmacologic, and epidemiologic data and then generating informed clinical advice at the bedside.

ANTIMICROBIAL CYCLING

Recent proposals to prevent antimicrobial resistance use different classes of antimicrobial agents sequentially,[38] injecting heterogeneity by scheduling changes of empiric antimicrobial regimens.[52] Antibiotic cycling programs typically rotate empiric use of beta-lactam/beta-lactamase inhibitor combinations, fluoroquinolones, carbapenems, and cephalosporins, often in an ICU setting, changing every few months. Pilot studies claim to have reduced antimicrobial resistance, infections due to drug-resistant pathogens, and mortality when compared to historical controls in critically ill ICU patients.[53,54] However, these studies are often confounded by other concurrent interventions, and well-designed, multicenter studies have yet to be published. In addition, some studies have shown that up to half of patients receive off-cycle antimicrobial agents, due to prescriber concerns. These programs do little to foster familiarity or expertise with a selected armamentarium and have an unclear effect on long-term prescribing. Further study is required to determine the impact of cycling programs on resistance and on clinicians' overall knowledge of appropriate antimicrobial use.

INTRAVENOUS-TO-ORAL CONVERSION

Many antimicrobial agents have excellent oral bioavailability, including fluoroquinolones, most azole antifungal agents, linezolid, rifampin, metronidazole, clindamycin, trimethoprim-sulfamethoxazole, azithromycin, doxycycline, valacyclovir, and valganciclovir. Because these oral formulations offer similar clinical efficacy, fewer risks of catheter-associated complications, and the chance to discharge patients sooner, oral therapy should be recommended in place of parenteral therapy for patients who are improving.[55] Furthermore, the cost of oral formulations is often 5- to 10-fold less than the parenteral forms, reaping substantial savings.

In "switch therapy," an oral formulation substitutes for the parenteral form of the same drug (eg, oral ciprofloxacin for IV ciprofloxacin), whereas "step-down therapy" connotes change from one IV agent to a different oral agent with a similar *in vitro* spectrum (eg, IV ceftriaxone changed to oral cefpodoxime or cefdinir). Several controlled trials have demonstrated the safety, efficacy, and significant cost saving associated with IV-to-oral conversion programs.[55,56] In our experience, automatic conversion for selected agents is both appropriate and more efficient than making recommendations that must then be implemented by the clinical services.

ANTIMICROBIAL OPTIMIZATION (STREAMLINING)

Programs that seek to optimize antimicrobial therapy by selecting the most appropriate drug and dosage are increasingly popular. New FDA labeling, scheduled for 2004 for all systemic antibiotics, reflects the time-honored dictum that culture and susceptibility information be considered when selecting and then modifying antibacterial therapy.[17] Antimicrobial therapy should be tailored to provide a narrow spectrum of activity for a specific pathogen, based on *in vitro* susceptibility data.[57] However, it is often difficult to convince clinicians to switch from broad to targeted, narrow spectrum therapy when the patient is responding clinically.[57] Many of the strategies that follow are advocated as ways to minimize selection of resistant organisms while maximizing individual outcomes.[58]

The science of antibacterial pharmacodynamics describes the relationship between serum and tissue concentrations and drug effect, allowing clinicians to optimize antimicrobial therapy, improve clinical efficacy, and reduce the development of antimicrobial resistance.[59]

Recently, investigators have used pharmacodynamic modeling to recommend lower doses of antibiotics that maintain adequate serum and tissue concentrations, providing clinical outcomes similar to those with FDA-approved dosage regimens.[60] These principals also allow less frequent administration of a drug while providing unchanged total daily dosage.[61] Continuous infusion (eg, of beta-lactams) and once-daily aminoglycoside dosing protocols offer improved efficacy but also reduce pharmacy preparation time and nursing administration time, thus reducing cost.

ANTIMICROBIAL ADVISORY TEAMS

In 1988, the IDSA suggested development of antimicrobial advisory teams as a way to improve antibiotic prescribing.[27] Prospective review of antimicrobial regimens by multidisciplinary teams has since proven to be an effective way to improve use of antibiotics.[62,63] Armed with pharmacokinetic and pharmacodynamic data, teams staffed by ID-trained pharmacists and/or physicians recommend changes in dosing amounts and frequency, IV-to-oral conversion, and discontinuance or streamlining of antibiotic therapy. Physicians are notified of team recommendations by notes left in the medical record. Recommendations from these teams have an acceptance rate in most studies of greater than 80%.

COMPREHENSIVE ANTIMICROBIAL MANAGEMENT PROGRAMS

A multifaceted program at the University of Pennsylvania encompasses many of the methods used to alter antimicrobial prescribing.[64] Antimicrobial management began at this hospital in 1993, with the goal of improving the quality of patient care by ensuring the effective use of antibiotics. In collaboration with the Infection Control and Infectious Disease departments, the formulary was reviewed and modified, use of vancomycin and broad-spectrum antibiotics was restricted, and empiric treatment guidelines were initiated. In addition, they developed dosing recommendations based on disease state, pharmacokinetics, and pharmacodynamics, along with antibiotic streamlining, continuous education, and monitoring of antibiotic usage. An ID-trained pharmacist and an ID physician were responsible for approving restricted drugs prior to use. This program increased the appropriate use of restricted antibiotics and demonstrated significant improvements in patient outcomes, as well as reducing antibiotic and total hospital costs, compared to a control group that received advice from ID fellows.[64] This study did not address use of unrestricted antibiotics.

In further work, these researchers studied the effect of antibiotic restriction on resistance. Similar methods were successful in reducing third-generation cephalosporin use by 85.8% but had little durable effect on vancomycin use.[65] Despite dramatic overall changes in antibiotic use, the prevalence of VRE continued to increase. Although disappointing, these efforts may simply have been inadequate to counter widespread burgeoning VRE rates. Given the numerous risk factors selecting for drug resistance and the complexity of "bug-drug" combinations,[22] successful elimination of multiply-resistant organisms will likely require this type of multidisciplinary effort (involving surveillance, infection control, and stewardship) plus collaborative interventions among broad networks of institutions.[25,66] The gains of smaller, local programs may be more difficult to document, despite intrinsic value.

OUTCOMES

Most studies of antimicrobial stewardship programs report reduction of antibiotic costs, and some report significant declines in adverse drug events and errors[50,51] but few have systematically studied the impact of such programs on bacterial resistance or patient outcomes.[34,41,44] In a program instituted in response to increasing bacterial resistance, Rahal and colleagues observed that restricting cephalosporins reduced colonization and infection with ceftazidime-resistant *Klebsiella* spp. by almost 45%.[67] In this study, an 80% reduction in cephalosporin use was observed after restrictions were implemented. However, during the same time period, use of imipenem increased 140%, and there was a hospital-wide increase in imipenem-resistant *P. aeruginosa* isolates,[67] followed by an outbreak of multidrug-resistant *A. baumannii*.[68] These results, an example of "squeezing the balloon,"[69] highlight the capacity to alter resistance problems by changing antimicrobial usage, as well as the complexity of hospital ecologies and the need for careful monitoring of antimicrobial use and bacterial resistance after implementing restriction programs.

FUNDING

It is important to enumerate the many benefits that antimicrobial improvement programs offer to patients and hospitals. Patients receive more efficient antimicrobial therapy, experience fewer adverse events and drug-resistant infections, and often have shorter hospitalizations. Prescribers gain knowledge of appropriate antibiotic use, and the institution reduces its pharmacy and other

expenditures, all while achieving better patient outcomes. Third-party payers, contractors, and other administrators are interested in these improvements as well and may base referral contracts on these indicators of high-quality health care.

In 1987, Woodward and colleagues reported saving $24,620 per month by restricting the formulary and requiring justification for use of restricted agents,[34] spawning numerous subsequent endeavors. In a comprehensive review of cost containment programs, John and Fishman[33] found that a focus on one drug could save several thousand dollars, but multidisciplinary interventional strategies could save as much as $500,000 per year. Estimated costs for salary and benefits for an ID pharmacist and a part-time ID physician were $104,810, suggesting a 5:1 return on investment. As an example, Fishman's group saved an average of $385,000 per year during an initial 3 years of study.[33]

Our experience at Lahey Clinic is similar. Our Antimicrobial Advisory Program is a multidisciplinary effort similar to the University of Pennsylvania program and is funded through an at-risk arrangement with the hospital, based on projected cost savings. In the 10 years since the advent of our program in 1993,[70] pharmacy expenditures for antimicrobial agents initially declined but ultimately increased 41%, whereas the rest of the budget increased 234%. The proportion of the budget spent on antimicrobials decreased from 16.6% to 7.8%, despite substantial increases in the complexity of services provided and in case mix index. Over time, the ID pharmacist position was intermittently diverted to other duties; antimicrobial expenditures decreased substantially while the stewardship program was active but climbed rapidly during inactive periods. Using 3 alternate methods to predict antimicrobial expenditures with and without a stewardship program, we estimate savings ranging from $3.5 to $8.7 million over 10 years, or $347,000 to $871,000 per year, at a cost of less than $110,000 annually. Because the ID pharmacist position was funded and active for about half the decade, this suggests a roughly 5- to 12-fold return on the dollar, based on pharmacy expenditures alone (Robert A. Duncan, unpublished data).

MAINTAINING AND EVALUATING THE SUCCESS OF YOUR PROGRAM

It is essential to make administrators aware of the significance of antimicrobial stewardship efforts[71] and to periodically reinforce the importance of these endeavors. In addition to pharmacy budget savings, the volume and scope of interventions can be tallied, as well as rates of medication errors and adverse events. Antimicrobial usage and resistance patterns should be monitored to document successes and to provide alerts to new problems. Costs associated with specific diagnosis-related groups may drop if targeted programs result in shorter length of hospitalization. These data should be shared with hospital administrators to reinforce the financial and clinical value of the program.

Benefits can be further expressed in measures of prevented morbidity, mortality, resistance, errors, adverse events, wasted medications, and excess length of hospitalization, as well as the "added value" of decreased adverse publicity and liability. Estimates of savings associated with these parameters may be based on published data if cost-measuring databases are unavailable. Collaboration with the institution's financial officers can add sophistication to a business plan and bolster credibility with other members of administration.

CONCLUSIONS

Antimicrobial stewardship is a prominent part of local and national efforts to contain and reverse antimicrobial resistance. A range of intervention options is available to institutions with varying levels of resources and can yield substantial improvements in morbidity, mortality, quality of care, and cost. The cost of delivering such programs is dwarfed by the benefits and provides an opportunity for hospital epidemiologists to garner support. This suggests that antimicrobial management programs belong to the rarefied group of truly cost-saving quality improvement initiatives. Well designed, multicenter studies evaluating this would be welcome.

Future systems promise greater integration and analysis of data, facilitated delivery of information to the clinician, and rapid and expert decision support that will optimize patient outcomes while minimizing antimicrobial resistance. They may also offer our best hope for avoiding an "antibiotic Armageddon."[72]

REFERENCES

1. Bryan CS. Strategies to improve antibiotic use. *Infect Dis Clin North Am.* 1989;3(4):723-734.

2. Salama S, Rotstein C, Mandell L. A multidisciplinary hospital-based antimicrobial use program: impact on hospital pharmacy expenditures and drug use. *Can J Infect Dis.* 1996;7:104-109.

3. Neu HC, Howrey SP. Testing the physician's knowledge of antibiotic use: self-assessment and learning via videotape. *N Engl J Med.* 1975;293:1291-1295.

4. Maki DG, Schuna A. A study of antimicrobial misuse in a university hospital. *Am J Med Sci.* 1987;275:271-282.

5. Hecker MT, Aron DC, Patel NP, et al. Unnecessary use of antimicrobials in hospitalized patients: current patterns of misuse with emphasis on the antianaerobic spectrum of activity. *Arch Intern Med.* 2003;163:972-978.

6. Dunagan WC, Woodward RS, Medoff G, et al. Antimicrobial misuse in patients with positive blood cultures. *Am J Med.* 1989;87:253-259.

7. Owens RC Jr, Prato BS, Lucas FL, Bachman D, Glenski SL. Impact of a hospital's formulary on outpatient antimicrobial prescribing. 41st Annual Meeting of the Infectious Disease Society of America, October 9-12, 2003, San Diego, Calif. Page 55, Abstract 162.

8. Kunin CM. Problems in antibiotic usage. In: Mandell GL, Douglas RG, Bennett JE, eds. *Principles and Practice of Infectious Diseases.* 3rd ed. New York, NY: Churchill Livingstone; 1990:427-434.

9. Neu HC. The crisis in antibiotic resistance. *Science.* 1992;257:1064-1073.

10. McGowan JE Jr. Antimicrobial resistance in hospital organisms and its relation to antibiotic use. *Rev Infect Dis.* 1983;5:1033-1048.

11. Roberts RR, Scott RD, Cordell R, et al. The use of economic modeling to determine the hospital cost associated with nosocomial infections. *Clin Infect Dis.* 2003;36:1424-1432.

12. Burke JP. Infection control: a problem for patient safety. *New Engl J Med.* 2003;348:651-656.

13. Engemann JJ, Carmeli Y, Cosgrove SE, et al. Adverse clinical and economic outcomes attributable to methicillin resistance among patients with *Staphylococcus aureus* surgical site infection. *Clin Infect Dis.* 2003;36:592-598.

14. Cosgrove S, Carmeli Y. The impact of antimicrobial resistance on health and economic outcomes. *Clin Infect Dis.* 2003;36:1433-1437.

15. Shlaes DM, Gerding DN, John JF, et al. Society of Healthcare Epidemiology of America and Infectious Disease Society of America Joint Committee on the Prevention of Antimicrobial Resistance. Guidelines for the prevention of antimicrobial resistance in hospitals. *Clin Infect Dis.* 1997;25:584-599.

16. 12 steps to prevent antimicrobial resistance among hospitalized patients. http://www.cdc.gov/drugresistance/healthcare/ha/12steps_HA.htm. Accessed July 1, 2003.

17. Food and Drug Administration, HHS. Labeling requirements for systemic antibacterial drug products for human use. Federal Register. Feb. 6, 2003;68(25):6062-6081.

18. Global strategy for containment of antimicrobial resistance. Available at: http://www.who.int/csr/resources/publications/drugresist/EGlobal_Strat.pdf. Accessed July 1, 2003.

19. 2004 National Patient Safety Goals. Available at: http://www.jcaho.org/news+room/news+release+archives/npsg_04.htm. Accessed Nov. 26, 2003.

20. Gerding DN. Good antimicrobial stewardship in the hospital setting: fitting, but flagrantly flagging. *Infect Control Hosp Epidemiol.* 2000;21(4):253-255.

21. Austin DJ, Kristinsson KG, Anderson RM. The relationship between the volume of antimicrobial consumption in human communities and the frequency of resistance. *Proc Natl Acad Sci USA*. 1999;96:1152-1156.

22. Safdar N, Maki DG. The commonality of risk factors for nosocomial colonization and infection with antimicrobial-resistant *Staphylococcus aureus*, *Enterococcus*, gram-negative bacilli, *Clostridium difficile*, and *Candida*. *Ann Intern Med*. 2002;136:834-844.

23. Fridkin SK, Edwards JR, Courval JM, et al. The effect of vancomycin and third-generation cephalosporins on prevalence of vancomycin-resistant enterococci in 126 U.S. adult intensive care units. *Ann Intern Med*. 2001;135:175-183.

24. Monnet DL. Methicillin-resistant *Staphylococcus aureus* and its relationship to antimicrobial use: possible implications for control. *Infect Control Hosp Epidemiol*. 1998; 19:552-559.

25. Goldmann DA, Weinstein RA, Wenzel RP, et al. Strategies to prevent and control the emergence and spread of antimicrobial-resistant microorganisms in hospitals; A challenge to hospital leadership. *JAMA*. 1996;275:234-240.

26. Rifenburg RP, Paladino JA, Hanson SC, et al. Benchmark analysis of strategies hospitals use to control antimicrobial expenditures. *Am J Health-Syst Pharm*. 1996;53: 2054-2062.

27. Marr JJ, Moffet HL, Kunin CM. Guidelines for improving the use of antimicrobial agents in hospitals: a statement by the Infectious Disease Society of America. *J Infect Dis*. 1988;157:869-876.

28. Duncan RA. Controlling use of antimicrobial agents. *Infect Control Hosp Epidemiol*. 1997;18:260-266.

29. Fishman NO. Antimicrobial management and cost containment. In: Mandell GL, Bennett JE, Dolin R, eds. *Principles and Practice of Infectious Diseases*, 5th ed. New York, NY: Churchill Livingstone; 2000:539-546.

30. Wester CW. Antibiotic resistance: a survey of physician perceptions. *Arch Intern Med*. 2002;162:2210.

31. Mandell LA, Bartlett JG, Dowell SF, File TM Jr, Musher DM, Whitney C. Update of practice guidelines for the management of community-acquired pneumonia in immunocompetent adults. *Clin Infect Dis*. 2003;37:1405-1433.

32. Medicare Quality Improvement Community. Surgical infection prevention project description. Available at: http://www.medqic.org/content/nationalpriorities/topics/p rojectdes.jsp?topicID=461&pageID=2. Accessed July 13, 2004.

33. John JF, Fishman NO. Programmatic role of the infectious disease physician in controlling antimicrobial cost in the hospital. *Clin Infect Dis*. 1997;24:471-485.

34. Woodward RS, Medoff G, Smith MD, et al. Antimicrobial cost savings from formulary restrictions and physician monitoring in a medical school-affiliated hospital. *Am J Med*. 1987;83:817-823.

35. Klapp DL, Ramphal R. Antibiotic restrictions in hospitals associated with medical schools. *Am J Hosp Pharm*. 1983; 40:1957-1960.

36. Strausbaugh LJ, Jernigan DB, Liedtke LA, et al. National shortages of antimicrobial agents: results of 2 surveys from the Infectious Disease Society of America Emerging Infections Network. *Clin Infect Dis*. 2001;33:1495-1501.

37. Polk RE, Nichols M, Johnson CK. Hospitals with "open" antibiotic formularies may be associated with lower rates of bacterial resistance: from the SCOPE-MMIT Antimicrobial Surveillance Network. 42nd ICAAC Abstracts, American Society for Microbiology, September 27-30, 2002, San Diego, CA, page 327, Abstract K-1352.

38. Bonhoeffer S, Lipsitch M, Levin BR. Evaluating treatment protocols to prevent antibiotic resistance. *Proc Natl Acad Sci USA*. 1997;94:12106-12111.

39. Avorn J, Solomon DH. Cultural and economic factors that (mis)shape antibiotic use: the non-pharmacologic basis of therapeutics. *Ann Intern Med*. 2000;133:128-135.

40. McGowan JE Jr, Finland M. Usage of antibiotics in a general hospital: effect of requiring justification. *J Infect Dis*. 1974;130:165-168.

41. Coleman RW, Rodondi LC, Kaubisch S, et al. Cost-effectiveness of prospective and continuous parenteral antibiotic control: experience at the Palo Alto Veterans Affairs Medical Center from 1987 to 1989. *Am J Med*. 1991; 90:439-444.

42. Ahern JW, Grace CJ. Effectiveness of a criteria-based educational program for appropriate use of antibiotic. *Infect Med*. 2002;19(8):364-374.

43. Regal RE, DePestel DD, VandenBussche HL. The effect of an antimicrobial restriction program on *Pseudomonas aeruginosa* resistance to B-lactams in a large teaching hospital. *Pharmacotherapy*. 2001;23(5):618-624.

44. White AC, Atmar RL, Wilson J, et al. Effects of requiring prior authorization for selected antimicrobials: expenditures, susceptibilities, and clinical outcomes. *Clin Infect Dis*. 1997;25:230-239.

45. Kunin CM. The responsibility of the infectious disease community for the optimal use of antimicrobial agents. *J Infect Dis*. 1985;3:388-398.

46. Paterson DL. Restrictive antibiotic policies are appropriate in intensive care units. *Crit Care Med*. 2003;31(Suppl 1):S25-S28.

47. Lesar TS, Briceland LL. Survey of antibiotic control policies in university-affiliated teaching institutions. *Ann Pharmacother*. 1996;30(1):31-34.

48. Durbin WA, Lapidas B, Goldmann DA. Improved antibiotic usage following introduction of a novel prescription system. *JAMA*. 1981;246:1796-1800.

49. Kaushal R, Shojania K, Bates DW. Effects of computerized physician order entry and clinical decision support systems on medication safety. *Arch Intern Med*. 2003; 163:1409-1416.

50. Evans RS, Pestotnik SL, Classen DC, et al. A computer-assisted management program for antibiotics and other anti-infective agents. *New Engl J Med*. 1998;338:232-238.

51. Pestotnik SL, Classen DL, Evans RS, Burke JP. Implementing antibiotic practice guidelines through computer-assisted decision support: clinical and financial outcomes. *Ann Intern Med*. 1996;124:884-890.

52. Fridkin SK. Routine cycling of antimicrobial agents as an infection control measure. *Clin Infect Dis*. 2003;36:1438-1444.

53. Kollef MH, Vlasnik J, Sharpless L, et al. Scheduled change of antibiotic classes; a strategy to decrease the incidence of ventilator-associated pneumonia. *Am J Respir Crit Care Med*. 1997;156:1040-1048.

54. Gruson D, Hilbert G, Vargas F, et al. Rotation and restricted use of antibiotics in a medical intensive care unit. *Am J Respir Crit Care Med*. 2000;162:837-843.

55. Ramirez JA, Vargas S, Ritter GW, et al. Early switch from intravenous to oral antibiotics and early hospital discharge: a prospective observational study of 200 consecutive patients with community acquired pneumonia. *Arch Intern Med*. 1999;159:2449-2454.

56. Kuti JL, Le TN, Nightingale CH, et al. Pharmacoeconomics of a pharmacist-managed program for automatically converting levofloxacin route from IV to oral. *Am J Health-Syst Pharm*. 2003;59(22):2209-2215.

57. Briceland LL, Nightingale CH, Quintiliani R, et al. Antibiotic streamlining from combination therapy to monotherapy utilizing an interdisciplinary approach. *Arch Intern Med*. 1988;148:2019-2022.

58. Paterson DL, Rice LB. Empirical antibiotic choice for the seriously ill patient: are minimization of selection of resistant organisms and maximization of individual outcome mutually exclusive? *Clin Infect Dis*. 2003;36:1006-1012.

59. Craig WA. Pharmacokinetic/pharmacodynamic parameters: rationale for antibacterial dosing of mice and men. *Clin Infect Dis*. 1998;26:1-12.

60. Kuti JL, Maglio D, Nightingale CH, et al. Economic benefit of a meropenem dosing strategy based on pharmacodynamic concepts. *Am J Health-Syst Pharm*. 2003;60:565-568.

61. Kim MK, Capitano B, Mattoes HM, et al. Pharmacokinetic and pharmacodynamic evaluations of two dosing regimens for piperacillin-tazobactam. *Pharmacotherapy*. 2002;22(5):569-577.

62. Fraser GL, Stogsdill P, Dickens JD, et al. Antibiotic optimization: an evaluation of patient safety and economic outcomes. *Arch Intern Med*. 1997;157:1689-1694.

63. Gums JG, Yancey RW, Hamilton CA, et al. A randomized, prospective study measuring outcomes after antibiotic therapy intervention by a multidisciplinary consult team. *Pharmacotherapy*. 1999;19(12):1369-1377.

64. Gross R, Morgan AS, Kinky DE, et al. Impact of a hospital-based antimicrobial management program on clinical and economic outcomes. *Clin Infect Dis*. 2001;33:289-295.

65. Lautenbach E, LaRosa LA, Marr AM, Nachamkin I, Bilker WB, Fishman NO. Changes in the prevalence of vancomycin-resistant enterococci in response to antimicrobial formulary interventions: impact of progressive restrictions on use of vancomycin and third-generation cephalosporins. *Clin Infect Dis*. 2003;36:440-446.

66. Weinstein RA. Controlling antimicrobial resistance in hospitals: infection control and use of antibiotics. *Emerg Infect Dis*. 2001;7(2):188-192.

67. Rahal JJ, Urban C, Horn D, et al. Class restriction of cephalosporin use to control total cephalosporin resistance in nosocomial *Klebsiella*. *JAMA*. 1998;280:133-137.

68. Rahal JJ, Urban C, Segal-Maurer S. Nosocomial antibiotic resistance in multiple gram-negative species: experience at one hospital with squeezing the resistance balloon at multiple sites. *Clin Infect Dis*. 2002;34:499-503.

69. Burke JP. Antibiotic resistance—squeezing the balloon? *JAMA*. 1998;280:1270.

70. Duncan RA, Segarra M, Anderson ER, Chow LS, Needham C, Jacoby GA. A comprehensive approach to reforming therapeutic antibiotic (Abx) use. *Infect Control Hosp Epidemiol*. 1995;16(suppl):37. Abstract M7.

71. Petrak RM, Sexton DJ, Butera ML, et al. The value of an infectious diseases specialist. *Clin Infect Dis*. 2003;36:1013-1017.

72. Kunin CM. Antibiotic armageddon. *Clin Infect Dis*. 1997;25:240-241.

SPECIAL TOPICS

CHAPTER NINETEEN

IMPROVING HAND HYGIENE
IN HEALTHCARE SETTINGS

John M. Boyce, MD and Didier Pittet, MD, MS

INTRODUCTION

In the mid 1800s, studies by Ignaz Semmelweis in Vienna and by Oliver Wendell Holmes in Boston established that hospital-acquired diseases, now known to be caused by infectious agents, were transmitted via the hands of HCWs. A prospective controlled trial conducted in a hospital nursery setting and investigations conducted during the past 40 years have confirmed the important role that contaminated hands of HCWs play in transmission of healthcare-associated pathogens.[1,2] As a result, for many years, handwashing has been considered one of the most important measures for preventing the spread of pathogens in healthcare settings.[3]

Despite the fact that handwashing guidelines were published by the CDC in 1985 and by the APIC in 1988 and 1995, adherence of HCWs to recommended handwashing procedures remained unacceptably low for decades. Among 34 published observational surveys of hand hygiene adherence among HCWs, rates of adherence ranged from 5% to 81%, with an average of about 40% (Figure 19-1). These low rates of compliance persisted despite the fact that multidrug-resistant pathogens such as MRSA, VRE, and resistant GNB, which have increased in prevalence in recent years, are transmitted primarily on the hands of HCWs. Continued poor handwashing adherence among HCWs and the increasing spread of MDR healthcare-associated pathogens suggested the need to study the causes of poor handwashing practices among HCWs and to develop new strategies for improving them.

In the largest study of its kind, Pittet and colleagues[4] observed more than 2800 opportunities for hand hygiene in a large hospital and used multivariate analysis to determine factors associated with poor compliance among HCWs. Factors associated with poor compliance included a high intensity of care (ie, many opportunities for hand hygiene per hour of patient care), weekdays, working in an ICU, and procedures associated with a high risk of contamination. Poor adherence associated with a high intensity of care suggested that HCWs did not have enough time to wash their hands as frequently as recommended, a complaint registered by nurses in previous studies.

In fact, a study by Voss and Widmer[5] revealed that it took ICU nurses an average of 62 seconds to leave a patient's bedside, find a sink, wash and dry their hands, and return to patient care activities. The authors estimated that in an ICU with 12 nurses on duty each shift, achieving 100% compliance with recommended handwashing practices would require 16 hours of nursing time per shift. In contrast, if bedside dispensers of an alcohol-based hand rub were available, achieving 100% compliance with recommended hand hygiene practices would require only 4 hours of nursing time per shift. This study questioned the practicality of traditional handwashing recommendations. Other factors associated with poor adherence to recommended handwashing practices include irritant contact dermatitis caused by frequent exposure to soap and water, lack of convenient access to handwashing facilities (sinks, paper towels), lack of awareness of HCWs of recommended practices, and lack of administrative concern.[6-9]

Alcohol-based hand rubs (gels, rinses, foam) have characteristics that address a number of the problems associated with washing hands with soap and water. At least 20 published studies have shown that alcohol solutions reduce bacterial counts of the hands of volunteers to a greater degree than washing hands with nonantimicrobial soap and water, and in all but 2 studies, alcohol was more effective than washing hands with antimicrobial soap and water.[10] Several clinical trials involving HCWs have documented that well-formulated alcohol-based hand rubs containing emollients cause less skin irritation and dry-

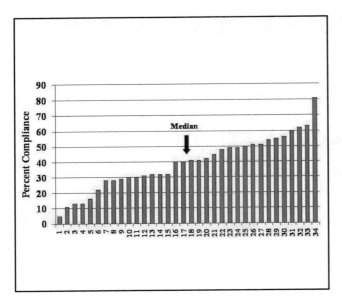

Figure 19-1. Handwashing compliance rates among healthcare workers in 34 observational surveys, 1981-2000. (Adapted from the Hand Hygiene Resource Center [HHRC], http://www.handhygiene.org/, with permission.)

TABLE 19-1. ADVANTAGES OF ALCOHOL-BASED HAND RUBS WHEN COMPARED TO TRADITIONAL SOAP AND WATER HANDWASHING

Compared to traditional soap and water handwashing, alcohol-based hand rubs:
➤ Take less time to use.
➤ Can be made much more accessible because they do not require the use of sinks. They can be made available at many locations in patient care areas and can even be supplied in pocket-sized bottles.
➤ Cause less skin irritation and dryness. Virtually all current products designed for use by HCWs contain emollients that help prevent dry, irritated skin.
➤ Reduce bacterial counts on hands to a greater degree.
➤ Do not require the use of water or paper towels.

ness with repeated use than washing hands with soap and water.[11-13] Also, because alcohol-based hand rubs do not require the use of water, they can be made available at many more locations than handwashing facilities. Finally, making such products readily accessible (near each patient's bedside or in pocket-sized bottles) has been shown to improve adherence of HCWs to recommended hand hygiene practices.[14] In ICUs, where the workload is high, with corresponding elevated numbers of indications for hand hygiene per hour of patient care,[4] preferential use of hand rubs can reduce the impact of time constraints, with subsequent improvement in compliance.[15]

However, making alcohol-based hand rub products available in patient care areas, by itself, is not sufficient to improve hand hygiene practices among HCWs.[16] Several studies have demonstrated that multimodal, multidisciplinary promotional campaigns are needed to achieve long-lasting improvements in hand hygiene compliance. Such programs must include education, feedback to HCWs regarding their performance, innovative motivational material, and appropriate administrative support.[9,10,14,17,18]

To address the issue of poor handwashing compliance, the Board of Directors of the SHEA approved formation of the SHEA Hand Hygiene Task Force in November 1998. Shortly after formation of the SHEA Hand Hygiene Task Force, representatives of APIC and the CDC HICPAC notified SHEA that they were also considering revising their

hand hygiene guidelines and proposed the formation of a multiorganization task force to address the issue. A review of more than 700 articles dealing with various aspects of hand hygiene revealed that alcohol-based hand rubs have a number of advantages over traditional soap and water handwashing (Table 19-1). The literature review also revealed that providing HCWs with feedback regarding their adherence to recommended hand hygiene practices and development of multidisciplinary, multimodal promotional campaigns were necessary to achieve enduring improvements in HCW hand hygiene practices.[10,14] After preparation of multiple drafts, a proposed hand hygiene guideline was published for public comment in November 2001. On the basis of public comments, input from the FDA and further input from HICPAC and representatives from SHEA, APIC, and the IDSA, the final *Guideline for Hand Hygiene in Healthcare Settings* was published in the *Morbidity and Mortality Weekly Report* in October 2002.[10]

GUIDELINE FOR HAND HYGIENE IN HEALTHCARE SETTINGS

The background section of the guideline includes a glossary of terms used throughout the document, several of which are worthy of mention:

➤ Handwashing—washing hands with a nonantimicrobial soap and water

➤ Antiseptic hand wash—washing hands with an antimicrobial soap and water

➤ Antiseptic hand rub—applying a waterless antiseptic agent to all surfaces of the hands to reduce the number of microorganisms present

➤ Hand antisepsis—includes either antiseptic handwash or antiseptic hand rub

➤ Hand hygiene—includes handwashing with either nonantimicrobial or antimicrobial soap and water, or use of a waterless antiseptic agent (ie, alcohol-based hand rub product)

To comply with HICPAC policies for guideline development, each recommendation was categorized on the basis of existing scientific data, theoretical rationale, applicability, and economic impact. Recommendations included in the *Guideline for Hand Hygiene in Healthcare Settings* are summarized in Table 19-2.[10]

IMPLEMENTING A HAND HYGIENE IMPROVEMENT PROGRAM

Administrative Support

To implement an effective hand hygiene promotional campaign, it is imperative to seek support from high-level administrators who can make the necessary resources available. In the past, many administrators and purchasing agents sought to acquire the least expensive soap for use by HCWs, despite the fact that frequent use of such products sometimes causes considerable irritant contact dermatitis. To convince administrators that purchasing alcohol-based hand rub products is worthwhile, it is often helpful to make a presentation to the administration regarding the high cost of healthcare-associated infections.[19] There is no single original scientific study that dealt specifically with the subject of the cost-effectiveness of different hand hygiene products or the exact financial benefit of increased hand hygiene compliance in the hospital setting. A few recent articles roughly estimated some of the financial effects of hand hygiene and described the potential benefits of using alcohol-based hand antisepsis compared with standard handwashing with soap and water. Not surprisingly, the current consensus is that modest increases in costs for alcohol-based hand hygiene products are tiny in comparison to excess hospital costs and years of life lost associated with severe nosocomial infections. According to Boyce, if frequent use of an alcohol-based hand rub by HCWs prevents only a few SSIs

or bloodstream infections per year, the savings accrued by preventing such infections will be greater than the institution's entire annual budget for hand hygiene products.[20] Webster and colleagues[21] reported a cost saving of approximately $17,000 resulting from the reduction in the use of vancomycin following the observed decrease in MRSA incidence in a neonatal intensive care unit during a 7-month period.

The hand hygiene promotion campaign at the University of Geneva Hospitals constitutes the first reported experience of a sustained improvement in compliance with hand hygiene, coinciding with a reduction of nosocomial infections and MRSA transmission.[14] Including both direct costs associated with the intervention and indirect costs associated with healthcare personnel time, costs of the promotion campaign at the University of Geneva Hospitals were less than $2.30 per patient admitted. Total costs of hand hygiene promotion corresponded to less than 1% of costs associated with nosocomial infection over a 7-year period.[22] More studies, ideally in the form of randomized clinical trials that include prospectively collected costing information and concurrent surveillance of nosocomial infections, need to be conducted to provide more evidence of the cost-benefit of hand hygiene promotion strategies. Although refined cost-effectiveness analyses comparing the costs of alternative strategies for achieving a given outcome are needed, it is clear that improvement in hand hygiene compliance is cost effective in most instances, seen from a societal perspective.

Finally, preventing healthcare-associated infections through improved HCW hand hygiene practices can be incorporated into the institution's overall plan to improve patient safety.

FORM A MULTIDISCIPLINARY COMMITTEE

The new hand hygiene guideline strongly recommends that institutions develop a multimodal, multidisciplinary promotional campaign to improve hand hygiene.[10] Such a committee should be comprised of HCWs from various departments and with different job descriptions.[14] To stimulate HCW interest in and commitment to improving hand hygiene practices, it is helpful to engage nurses, physicians, and other caregivers in planning various aspects of a promotional campaign.[14,23,24] This can be done by involving HCWs in selection of a slogan for the promotional campaign, by having them participate in design of motivational materials (brochures, visual reminders of the importance of hand hygiene), and in selection of hand hygiene agents to be used in the institution.[14,23] Another strategy that may be helpful is to make

TABLE 19-2. RECOMMENDATIONS FROM THE *GUIDELINE FOR HAND HYGIENE IN HEALTHCARE SETTINGS*

Note: Each recommendation was categorized on the basis of existing scientific data, theoretical rationale, applicability, and economic impact. The CDC/HICPAC system for categorizing recommendations is as follows:

Category IA.	Strongly recommended for implementation and strongly supported by well-designed experimental, clinical, or epidemiologic studies.
Category IB.	Strongly recommended for implementation and supported by some experimental, clinical, or epidemiologic studies and a strong theoretical rationale.
Category IC.	Required for implementation, as mandated by federal and/or state regulation or standard.
Category II.	Suggested for implementation and supported by suggestive clinical or epidemiologic studies or a theoretical rationale.
No recommendation unresolved issue	Practices for which insufficient evidence or no consensus regarding efficacy exist.

1. Indications for handwashing and hand antisepsis
   A. When hands are visibly dirty or contaminated with proteinaceous material or are visibly soiled with blood or other body fluids, wash hands with either a nonantimicrobial soap and water or an antimicrobial soap and water (IA).
   B. If hands are not visibly soiled, use an alcohol-based hand rub for routinely decontaminating hands in all other clinical situations described in items I.C. through I.J. listed below (IA). Alternatively, wash hands with an antimicrobial soap and water in all clinical situations described in items I.C. through I.J. (IB).
   C. Decontaminate hands before having direct contact with patients (IB).
   D. Decontaminate hands before donning sterile gloves when inserting a central intravascular catheter (IB).
   E. Decontaminate hands before inserting indwelling urinary catheters, peripheral vascular catheters, or other invasive devices that do not require a surgical procedure (IB).
   F. Decontaminate hands after contact with a patient's intact skin (as in taking a pulse or blood pressure or lifting a patient) (IB).
   G. Decontaminate hands after contact with body fluids or excretions, mucous membranes, nonintact skin, or wound dressings, as long as hands are not visibly soiled (IA).
   H. Decontaminate hands if moving from a contaminated body site to a clean body site during patient care (II).
   I. Decontaminate hands after contact with inanimate objects (including medical equipment) in the immediate vicinity of the patient (II).
   J. Decontaminate hands after removing gloves (IB).
   K. Before eating and after using a restroom, wash hands with a nonantimicrobial soap and water or with an antimicrobial soap and water (IB).
   L. Antimicrobial-impregnated wipes (towelettes) may be considered as an alternative to washing hands with nonantimicrobial soap and water. Because they are not as effective as alcohol-based hand rubs or washing hands with an antimicrobial soap and water for reducing bacterial counts on the hands of healthcare personnel, they are not a substitute for using an alcohol-based hand rub or antimicrobial soap (IB).
   M. Wash hands with nonantimicrobial soap and water or with antimicrobial soap and water if exposure to *Bacillus anthracis* (*anthrax bacillus*) is suspected or proven. The physical action of washing and rinsing hands under such circumstances is recommended because alcohols, chlorhexidine, iodophors, and other antiseptic agents have poor activity against spores (II).
   N. No recommendation on routine use of nonalcohol-based hand rubs for hand hygiene in healthcare settings. Unresolved issue.
2. Hand hygiene technique
   ➤ When decontaminating hands with an alcohol-based hand rub, apply product to palm of one hand and rub hands together, covering all surfaces of hands and fingers, until hands are dry (IB). Follow the manufacturer's recommendations on the volume of product to use.

TABLE 19-2. RECOMMENDATIONS FROM THE *GUIDELINE FOR HAND HYGIENE IN HEALTHCARE SETTINGS* (CONTINUED)

➤ When washing hands with soap and water, wet hands first with water, apply an amount of product recommended by the manufacturer to hands, and rub hands together vigorously for at least 15 seconds, covering all surfaces of the hands and fingers. Rinse hands with water and dry thoroughly with a disposable towel. Use towel to turn off the faucet (IB). Avoid using hot water, as repeated exposure to hot water may increase the risk of dermatitis (IB).

➤ Liquid, bar, leaflet, or powdered forms of plain soap are acceptable when washing hands with a non-antimicrobial soap and water. When bar soap is used, soap racks that facilitate drainage and small bars of soap should be used (II).

➤ Multiple-use cloth towels of the hanging or roll type are not recommended for use in healthcare settings (II).

3. Surgical hand antisepsis

➤ Remove rings, watches, and bracelets before beginning the surgical hand scrub (II).

➤ Remove debris from underneath fingernails using a nail cleaner under running water (II).

➤ Surgical hand antisepsis using either an antimicrobial soap or an alcohol-based hand rub with persistent activity is recommended before donning sterile gloves when performing surgical procedures (IB).

➤ When performing surgical hand antisepsis using an antimicrobial soap, scrub hands and forearms for the length of time recommended by the manufacturer, usually 2 to 6 minutes. However, long scrub times (eg, 10 minutes) should not be necessary (IB).

➤ When using an alcohol-based surgical hand scrub product with persistent activity, follow the manufacturer's instructions. Before applying the alcohol solution, pre-wash hands and forearms with a nonantimicrobial soap, and dry hands and forearms completely. After application of the alcohol-based product as recommended, allow hands and forearms to dry thoroughly before donning sterile gloves (IB).

4. Selection of hand hygiene agents

➤ Provide personnel with efficacious hand hygiene products that have low irritancy potential, particularly when used multiple times per shift (IB). This applies to products used for hand antisepsis before and after patient care in clinical areas and to products used for surgical hand antisepsis by surgical personnel.

➤ To maximize acceptance of hand hygiene products by health personnel, solicit input from healthcare personnel regarding the feel, fragrance, and skin tolerance of any products under consideration. The cost of hand hygiene products should not be the primary factor influencing product selection (IB).

➤ When selecting nonantimicrobial soaps, antimicrobial soaps, or alcohol-based hand rubs, solicit information from manufacturers about any known interactions between products used to clean hands, skin care products, and the types of gloves used in the institution (II).

➤ Prior to making purchasing decisions, evaluate the dispenser systems of various product manufacturers or distributors to ensure that dispensers function adequately and deliver an appropriate volume of product (II).

➤ Do not add soap to a partially empty soap dispenser. This practice of "topping off" dispensers may lead to bacterial contamination of soap (IA).

5. Skin care

➤ Provide HCWs with hand lotions or creams to minimize the occurrence of irritant contact dermatitis associated with hand antisepsis or handwashing (IA).

➤ Solicit information from manufacturers regarding any effects that hand lotions, creams, or alcohol-based hand antiseptics may have on the persistent effects of antimicrobial soaps being used in the institution (IB).

6. Other aspects of hand hygiene

➤ Do not wear artificial fingernails or extenders when having direct contact with high-risk patients, such as those in intensive care units or operating rooms (IA).

➤ Keep natural nail tips less than ¼ inch long (II).

➤ Wear gloves when it can be reasonably anticipated that contact with blood or other potentially infectious materials, mucous membranes, and nonintact skin will occur (IC).

TABLE 19-2. RECOMMENDATIONS FROM THE *GUIDELINE FOR HAND HYGIENE IN HEALTHCARE SETTINGS* (CONTINUED)

> Remove gloves after caring for a patient. Do not wear the same pair of gloves for the care of more than one patient, and do not wash gloves between patients (IB).

> Change gloves during patient care if moving from a contaminated body site to a clean body site (II).

> No recommendation on wearing rings in healthcare settings. Unresolved issue.

7. HCW educational and motivational programs

> As part of an overall program to improve hand hygiene practices of HCWs, educate personnel regarding the types of patient care activities that can result in hand contamination and the advantages and disadvantages of various methods used to clean their hands (II).

> Monitor HCWs' adherence with recommended hand hygiene practices and provide personnel with information regarding their performance (IA).

> Encourage patients and their families to remind HCWs to decontaminate their hands (II).

8. Administrative measures

> Make improved hand hygiene adherence an institutional priority and provide appropriate administrative support and financial resources (IB).

> Implement a multidisciplinary program designed to improve adherence of health personnel to recommended hand hygiene practices (IB).

> As part of a multidisciplinary program to improve hand hygiene adherence, provide HCWs with a readily accessible alcohol-based hand rub product (IA).

> To improve hand hygiene adherence among personnel who work in areas where high workloads and high intensity of patient care are anticipated, make an alcohol-based hand rub available at the entrance to the patient's room or at the bedside, in other convenient locations, and in individual pocket-sized containers to be carried by HCWs (IA).

> Store supplies of alcohol-based hand rubs in cabinets or areas approved for flammable materials (IC).

Part III. Outcome or Process Measurements

1. Develop and implement a system for measuring improvements in adherence of HCWs to recommended hand hygiene practices. Examples are listed below.

> Periodically monitor and record adherence as the number of hand hygiene episodes performed by personnel/number of hand hygiene opportunities, by ward, or by service. Provide feedback to personnel regarding their performance.

> Monitor the volume of alcohol-based hand rub (or detergent used for handwashing or hand antisepsis) used/1000 patient-days.

> Monitor adherence to policies dealing with wearing of artificial nails.

> When outbreaks of infection occur, assess the adequacy of HCW hand hygiene.

Adapted from Boyce JM, Pittet D, Healthcare Infection Control Practices Advisory Committee and the HICPAC/SHEA/APIC/IDSA Hand Hygiene Task Force. Guideline for hand hygiene in health-care settings. *MMWR.* 2002;51:1-45.

the improvement of hand hygiene adherence a nursing unit-based quality improvement project.

SELECTING HAND HYGIENE AGENTS FOR USE IN THE FACILITY

Nonantimicrobial soaps, antimicrobial soaps, and alcohol-based hand rubs possess widely differing characteristics that can have a major impact on the acceptance of products by HCWs. Such characteristics include their scent, consistency (feel), ease of application, and propensity to cause irritant contact dermatitis with frequent use.[25,26] In addition, alcohol-based hand rubs are available as rinses (low viscosity), gels, and foams that vary in terms of how they "feel" when applied, the extent to which they cause a "sticky" sensation during or after application (sometimes a major cause of decreased compliance), drying time, likelihood of causing a build-up of emollients after repeated use, in vivo antimicrobial activity, dispenser design, and tendency to interact with powder used in some types of gloves.[24] As a result, it is imperative to involve HCWs from various departments and job descriptions when evaluating hand hygiene products that are being considered for use in a facility. Selection of a product that has one or more undesirable characteristics or that has poorly functioning dispensers can adversely affect the frequency of use by HCWs.[27]

If alcohol-based hand rub products are used for preoperative surgical hand antisepsis, it is important to determine that the product has in vivo activity for an appropriate time period after application. In the United States, the FDA requires that such products maintain bacterial counts on the hands at baseline levels for 6 hours after application.[28] We advise that personnel involved in product selection check with manufacturers to determine if the product(s) under consideration meet this standard. A more in-depth discussion of selecting alcohol-based hand rub products for use in healthcare institutions can be found at the Educational Aides section of www.handhygiene.org.

EDUCATION OF HEALTHCARE WORKERS

Educating HCWs regarding the types of patient care activities that result in hand contamination and in the advantages and disadvantages of soap and water handwashing and alcohol-based hand rubs can be achieved in various ways. It is often helpful to use one or more of the following approaches: conducting small educational sessions on each nursing unit or in each clinical department; giving conferences using audience participation technology; making interactive, computer-based hand hygiene educational modules available on the institution's intranet; having HCWs place their hands on agar plates and showing them the subsequent growth of bacteria on the plate; or using fluorescent powder or liquid to demonstrate the efficacy (or lack thereof) of handwashing or hand antisepsis technique.

MOTIVATIONAL MATERIALS

Successful promotional campaigns have also developed innovative motivational material stressing the importance of good hand hygiene. For example, Pittet and colleagues[14] enlisted the help of a professional cartoonist who met with ward personnel in order to develop a collection of colorful reminders of various aspects of hand hygiene (see www.hopisafe.ch). The posters were placed in specific, designated locations on all wards and in public areas of the hospital, and they were changed by housekeeping personnel every week. A poster that remains on a ward for many months or for an entire year is not likely to be noticed by personnel after a few weeks. Other motivational strategies that might be considered include rewarding HCWs on wards or services with the highest levels of adherence to recommended hand hygiene policies or printing hand hygiene reminders on objects such as ballpoint pens or coffee cups. In one of our facilities, HCWs on wards with the best adherence rates were given coupons that allowed them to receive complimentary food items at the hospital's cafeteria.[23]

OBSERVATIONAL HAND HYGIENE ADHERENCE SURVEYS

Conducting periodic observational surveys of HCWs engaged in patient care activities is currently the "gold standard" for determining hand hygiene adherence rates among personnel. Although such surveys are somewhat time-consuming, they are currently the most reliable method of assessing the adequacy of hand hygiene practices. Developing a structured data collection sheet that includes categories of HCWs observed; whether they cleaned their hands before patient contact, after various types of patient care activities, and after removing gloves; and whether hands were cleaned by washing them with soap and water or by using an alcohol-based hand rub is essential. In general, we do not record the identity of HCWs being observed. Although monitoring the amount of alcohol-based hand rub used, expressed as the number of liters used per 1000 patient-days may be useful and is recommended,[10,14] such measurements cannot at the present time be considered a replacement for observational surveys.

PROVIDING HEALTHCARE WORKERS WITH FEEDBACK REGARDING THEIR PERFORMANCE

Providing HCWs with feedback regarding how well they adhere to recommended patient care practices, including hand hygiene, has been one of the most effective methods for modifying patterns of behavior.[10,14,24] Feedback can be provided during ward-based educational sessions, larger conferences given to HCWs, or posting adherence rates for wards or services in highly visible areas of the facility. We favor giving feedback to groups of HCWs on each ward or service; no attempt is made to single out individuals with the lowest adherence rates.

IMPORTANCE OF DISPENSER DESIGN AND PLACEMENT

Before selecting alcohol-based hand rub products or soaps for use by HCWs, institutions should evaluate the design and reliability of dispensers that will be provided by the manufacturer or vendor. One institution that installed a viscous, alcohol-based hand rinse hospital-wide based on a short trial using table-top pump bottles found that within months of installation of wall-mounted dispensers, HCWs noticed that dispensers often became partly or totally plugged.[27] Partly plugged dispensers often squirted product onto the wall or floor instead of onto the HCW's hand. Constant problems with dispensers probably accounted in part for the low rate of use of the product by personnel.

Placing alcohol-based hand rub dispensers adjacent to patients' beds or making pocket-sized bottles available can ensure that the product is readily available to HCWs.[5,14] Some experts also favor placing dispensers in hallways adjacent to patient room doors, but placement of alcohol-based hand rub dispensers at such locations may not comply with fire safety codes in some geographic areas.[29] Therefore, before installing dispensers in hallways of healthcare institutions, it is important to check with fire safety officials regarding local regulations.

SURGICAL HAND ANTISEPSIS

Surgical hand antisepsis has traditionally been performed by using a brush or a sponge to scrub hands with an antimicrobial soap for 2 to 5 minutes, or even longer. Frequent use of such regimens causes irritant contact dermatitis in some individuals and is time-consuming if longer scrub times are used. Although the new *Guideline for Hand Hygiene in Healthcare Settings* recommends that surgical hand antisepsis be performed by using either an antimicrobial soap or an alcohol-based hand rub product with persistent activity, some surgeons have questioned whether the incidence of SSIs is comparable with the 2 regimens. A recent prospective controlled trial involving several thousand surgical patients revealed that the incidence of SSIs among patients whose surgeons used an alcohol-based hand rub for surgical hand antisepsis was nearly identical to the incidence among patients whose surgeons performed a traditional scrub using an antimicrobial soap.[30] Making surgical personnel aware of this study may allay concerns of the efficacy of alcohol-based hand rubs for surgical hand antisepsis.

OTHER LOGISTIC ISSUES

Because alcohol-based hand rubs are flammable, it is imperative that large stocks of such products are stored in approved areas of the facility and that they be protected from high temperatures or flames. Specific individuals should be assigned the responsibility for transporting the product from bulk storage areas to clinical areas and for checking dispensers on a regular basis to make sure they are not empty. In some institutions, one or more of these individuals can assist with monitoring the amount of product that is used or the amount that is delivered to each ward.

If providing hand hygiene products (soaps and alcohol-based hand rubs) is part of housekeeping functions that are out-sourced to contractors, it is important that managers of such contractors understand the importance of hand hygiene and comply with policies of the HCF. Some facilities belong to large healthcare-associated buying groups that dictate the hand hygiene products that are available to the institution. If evaluation by HCWs of alcohol-based hand rub products available through the buying group reveals that none are acceptable to a majority of personnel, then the institution should examine buying group contracts to determine if preferable products can be purchased from other vendors.

Depending on the consistency of the alcohol-based hand rub product in use and the type of dispensers used, alcohol-containing rinses or gels may sometimes drip from the hands of HCWs during application. At some institutions, this has affected the wax finish on floors underneath dispensers and has required a change in floor care procedures.

Any difficulties in implementing a hand hygiene promotional campaign, as well as evidence of improved hand hygiene compliance that is achieved, should be discussed with high-level administrators and should be presented at appropriate committee meetings and conferences.

REFERENCES

1. Mortimer EA, Lipsitz PJ, Wolinsky E, et al. Transmission of Staphylococci between newborns. *Am J Dis Child.* 1962;104:289-295.

2. Ehrenkranz NJ, Alfonso BC. Failure of bland soap handwash to prevent hand transfer of patient bacteria to urethral catheters. *Infect Control Hosp Epidemiol.* 1991;12:654-662.

3. Larson E. A causal link between handwashing and risk of infection? Examination of the evidence. *Infect Control Hosp Epidemiol.* 1988;9:28-36.

4. Pittet D, Mourouga P, Perneger TV, members of the Infection Control Program. Compliance with handwashing in a teaching hospital. *Ann Intern Med.* 1999;130:126-130.

5. Voss A, Widmer AF. No time for handwashing!? Handwashing versus alcoholic rub: can we afford 100% compliance? *Infect Control Hosp Epidemiol.* 1997;18:205-208.

6. Larson E, Killien M. Factors influencing handwashing behavior of patient care personnel. *Am J Infect Control.* 1982;10:93-99.

7. Larson E, McGeer A, Quraishi A, et al. Effect of an automated sink on handwashing practices and attitudes in high-risk units. *Infect Control Hosp Epidemiol.* 1991;12:422-428.

8. Larson E, Friedman C, Cohran J, Treston-Aurand J, Green S. Prevalence and correlates of skin damage on the hands of nurses. *Heart Lung.* 1997;26:404-412.

9. Pittet D, Boyce JM. Hand hygiene and patient care: pursuing the Semmelweis legacy. *Lancet Infectious Diseases.* 2001;April:9-20.

10. Boyce JM, Pittet D, Healthcare Infection Control Practices Advisory Committee and the HICPAC/SHEA/APIC/IDSA Hand Hygiene Task Force. Guideline for hand hygiene in health-care settings. *MMWR.* 2002;51:1-45.

11. Boyce JM, Kelliher S, Vallande N. Skin irritation and dryness associated with two hand hygiene regimens: soap and water handwashing versus hand antisepsis with an alcoholic hand gel. *Infect Control Hosp Epidemiol.* 2000;21:442-448.

12. Winnefeld M, Richard MA, Drancourt M, Grobb JJ. Skin tolerance and effectiveness of two hand decontamination procedures in everyday hospital use. *Br J Dermatol.* 2000;143:546-550.

13. Larson E, Aiello AE, Heilman JM. Comparison of different regimens for surgical hand preparation. *AORN J.* 2001;73:412-432.

14. Pittet D, Hugonnet S, Harbarth S, Mourouga P, Sauvan V, Touveneau S. Effectiveness of a hospital-wide programme to improve compliance with hand hygiene. *Lancet.* 2000;356:1307-1312.

15. Hugonnet S, Perneger TV, Pittet D. Alcohol-based handrub improves compliance with hand hygiene in intensive care units. *Arch Intern Med.* 2002;162:1037-1043.

16. Muto CA, Sistrom MG, Farr BM. Hand hygiene rates unaffected by installation of dispensers of a rapidly acting hand antiseptic. *Am J Infect Control.* 2000;28:273-276.

17. Larson EL, Early E, Cloonan P, Sugrue S, Parides M. An organizational climate intervention associated with increased handwashing and decreased nosocomial infections. *Behav Med.* 2000;26:14-22.

18. Pittet D. Improving compliance with hand hygiene in hospitals. *Infect Control Hosp Epidemiol.* 2000;21:381-386.

19. Jarvis WR. Selected aspects of the socioeconomic impact of nosocomial infections: morbidity, mortality, cost, and prevention. *Infect Control Hosp Epidemiol.* 1996;17:552-557.

20. Boyce JM. Antiseptic technology: access, affordability and acceptance. *Emerg Infect Diseases.* 2001;7:231-233.

21. Webster J, Faoagali JL, Cartwright D. Elimination of methicillin-resistant *Staphylococcus aureus* from a neonatal intensive care unit after hand washing with triclosan. *J Paediatr Child Health.* 1994;30:59-64.

22. Pittet D, Sax H, Hugonnet S, Harbarth S. Cost implications of successful hand hygiene promotion. *Infect Control Hosp Epidemiol.* 2004;25(3):264-266.

23. Ligi CE, Kohan CA, Dumigan DG, Havill NL, Pittet D, Boyce JM. A multifaceted approach to improving hand hygiene practices among healthcare workers using an alcohol-based hand gel. Presented at the 13th Annual Meeting of the Society for Healthcare Epidemiology of America, Arlington, Va, April 2003.

24. Harbarth S, Grady L, Zawacki A, Potter-Bynoe G, Samore MH, Goldmann DA. Interventional study to evaluate the impact of an alcohol-based hand gel in improving hand hygiene compliance. *Pediatr Infect Dis J.* 2002;21:489-495.

25. Larson E, Leyden JJ, McGinley KJ, Grove GL, Talbot GH. Physiologic and microbiologic changes in skin related to frequent handwashing. *Infect Control.* 1986;7:59-63.

26. Scott D, Barnes A, Lister M, Arkell P. An evaluation of the user acceptability of chlorhexidine handwash formulations. *J Hosp Infect.* 1991;18:51-55.

27. Kohan C, Ligi C, Dumigan DG, Boyce JM. The importance of evaluating product dispensers when selecting alcohol-based handrubs. *Am J Infect Control.* 2002;30(6):373-375.

28. Food and Drug Administration. Tentative final monograph for healthcare antiseptic drug products; proposed rule. Federal Register. 1994:31441-31452.

29. Boyce JM, Pearson ML. Low frequency of fires from alcohol-based hand rub dispensers in healthcare facilities. *Infect Control Hosp Epidemiol*. 2003;24:618-619.

30. Parienti JJ, Thibon P, Heller R, et al. Hand-rubbing with an aqueous alcoholic solution vs. traditional surgical hand-scrubbing and 30-day surgical site infection rates. *JAMA*. 2002;288:722-727.

CHAPTER TWENTY

THE ROLE OF INFECTION CONTROL IN BIOTERRORISM

Mary L. Fornek, BSN, MBA, CIC and Kelly J. Henning, MD

INTRODUCTION

Many biological agents cause illness; however, not all are capable of causing mass casualties, high mortality, or public panic and social disruption. In 1999, the CDC formed a Bioterrorism Preparedness and Response Office as part of a Congressional initiative to upgrade the national public health agency's ability to respond to biological terrorism. On June 3-4, 1999, various experts in ID, public health, representatives from the Department of Health and Human Services, civilian and military intelligence, and law enforcement agencies met to discuss the threat potential of various biological agents.[1,2]

A biological agent was assessed based on the following factors: (1) ability to cause illness and death; (2) ease of deliverability to large populations based on stability of the agent, ability to mass produce and distribute the agent, and potential for person-to-person transmission; (3) the public's awareness of the agent and potential for public panic or fear; and (4) public health preparedness needs such as stockpiles of medication/vaccines, surveillance capabilities, and diagnostic needs. Participants reviewed lists of biological warfare or potential biological threat agents, which included but was not limited to the Biological Weapons Convention list, the WHO Biological Weapons list, the unclassified military list of biological warfare agents, and the Australian Group List of Biological Agents for Export Control. The group selected the agents they felt posed the greatest threat to civilian populations. After the meeting, the CDC evaluated the potential agents based on the general areas noted above and categorized them as Agents A, B, or C for initial public health preparedness (Table 20-1).

INFECTION CONTROL IN THE HOSPITAL BIOTERRORISM RESPONSE PLAN

Development

ICPs, including the hospital epidemiologist, must be involved in the development of the Hospital Response Plan from inception (Table 20-2). It is crucial to meet with and gain the support of those people, such as emergency planners, safety officers, and emergency medicine personnel, who are developing hospital plans around bioterrorism issues. Working with emergency planners *before* an event occurs is critical to the smooth operation of a bioterrorism plan if it is activated.

Planning efforts should draw on the expertise of ICPs and hospital epidemiologists in the areas of surveillance and epidemiology to aide in the development of protocols for identification of an attack and tracking of potential cases. The ICP may assist the emergency department (ED) and ambulatory clinics in development of automated surveillance systems. Collaboration with hospital information specialists and health department surveillance experts is a key component in participating in larger, community-wide surveillance efforts.

Fact sheets containing critical information about infection control protocols for each biological agent, including the types of isolation precautions required and personal protective equipment (PPE) needed for each circumstance, should be developed as part of the Hospital Response Plan. ICPs play a central role in distribution of relevant infection control information via existent channels and additional means identified in the plan.

TABLE 20-1. CENTERS FOR DISEASE CONTROL AND PREVENTION CLASSIFICATION OF BIOLOGICAL AGENTS

_Category A_*		_Category B_†		_Category C_‡	
Biological Agent	_Disease_	_Biological Agent_	_Disease_	_Biological Agent_	_Disease_
Variola major	Smallpox	_Coxiella burnetti_	Q fever	Nipah virus	Encephalitis
B. anthracis	Anthrax	_Brucella_ species	Brucellosis	Hantaviruses	Hantavirus pulmonary syndrome
Y. pestis	Plague	_Burkholderia mallei/pseudo-mallei_	Glanders/ Melioidosis	_M. tuberculosis_	Multidrug-resistant _tuberculosis_
C. botulinum	Botulism	Alphaviruses (Venezuelan, eastern and western equine encephalomyelitis)	Encephalitis		
F. tularensis	Tularemia	Toxins (Ricin, epsilon toxin of _Clostridium perfringens_, _Staphylococcus_ enterotoxin B)	Toxic syndromes		
Filoviridae (Ebola, Marburg) Arenaviridae (Lassa, Machupo), Flaviviridae (Yellow fever)	Hemorrhagic fever viruses	_Chlamydia psittaci_ _Rickettsia prowazekii_ Food-borne or waterborne agents: _Salmonella_ species _Shigella dysenteriae_ _E. coli_ O157:H7 _Vibrio cholerae_ _Cryptosporidium parvum_ Gastroenteritis	Psittacosis Typhus fever		

*Category A diseases/agents are high-priority organisms that pose a risk to national security because they can be easily disseminated or transmitted from person to person; result in high mortality rates and have the potential for major public health impact; might cause public panic and social disruption; and require special action for public health preparedness.

†Category B agents are the second highest priority agents, which are moderately easy to disseminate; result in moderate morbidity rates and low mortality rates; and require specific enhancements of CDC's diagnostic capacity and enhanced disease surveillance.

‡Category C agents are the third highest priority agents, which are emerging pathogens that could be engineered for mass dissemination in the future because of availability; ease of production and dissemination; and potential for high morbidity and mortality rates and major health impact.

Adapted from Centers for Disease Control and Prevention. Biological and chemical terrorism: strategic plan for preparedness and response. Recommendations of the CDC Strategic Planning Workgroup. _MMWR Morbid Mortal Wkly Rep._ 2000;49(RR-4):1-8.

TABLE 20-2. COMPONENTS OF A HOSPITAL BIOTERRORISM RESPONSE PLAN

Institutional Considerations	Review the facility emergency/disaster plan, which should include a section on bioterrorism. Ensure the emergency/ disaster plan includes responding to both incidents of limited and mass casualties.	Determine if the facility has been designated to receive patients in the National Disaster Management System (NDMS).	The emergency/disaster plan must detail the communication plan with the local Emergency Medical Service (EMS) Agencies, local Emergency Management Agency, and the local Health Department.	Each hospital department (ie, Nursing, Security, Mortuary, Radiology, Laboratory, Pharmacy, Pastoral Care) must develop standard operating procedures to reflect how the department will continue to provide services continually in a 24-hour period.
Identification of Authorized Personnel	Designate a person as "Incident Commander (IC)" or disaster coordinator who is available on a 24-hour basis.	Designate a medical commander who is responsible for the hospital's medical responses during the time the plan is activated.	Identify individuals who have a key role in disaster management (ie, nurse executive, safety officer, hospital epidemiologist).	Develop job action sheets or role cards for all personnel involved in disaster response.
Surveillance	Develop a system to contact Infection Control 24 hours a day/7 days a week.	Identify the number and location of negatively ventilated isolation rooms. Information must be available for the IC or disaster coordinator at all times.	The microbiology lab must have the capability to monitor 100% of all microbiology results and stratify according to organism.	Establish an automated baseline of patient visits stratified according to clinical symptoms in the ED and outpatient areas.
Communication of Plan	All individuals expected to implement and use the emergency/disaster plan must be familiar with it.	The facility must establish communication networks with the local EMS Agency, Emergency Management Agency, and local Department of Health.	If the facility's communication system fails/overloads (ie, telephones, cell phones, pagers, and facsimiles), an alternative communication system should be in place (ie, walkie-talkie sets).	Staff members must notify Infection Control Personnel immediately upon identification of exposure/symptoms related to biological agents.
Activation of Plan	The emergency/disaster plan must specify who has the authority to activate/deactivate the plan including nights, weekends, and holidays.	Identify specific circumstances under which the plan may be activated.	Activation stages should be established, and the roles of each individual should be outlined for each stage.	Test the activation plan by initiating a mock bioterrorism event and evaluating the communication component of notifying key departments (ie, pharmacy, sterile, processing department [SPD],).

TABLE 20-2. COMPONENTS OF A HOSPITAL BIOTERRORISM RESPONSE PLAN (CONTINUED)

Response	Review the ventilation/air handling system for the ED and other patient care areas. Determine if the ventilation system could be shut down or isolated.	Identify isolation facilities within the ED and alternative sites to triage infectious patients after ED resources are expended.	Develop a plan for the safe transfer of infectious patients from ED to inpatient wards (eg, designated elevator).	Develop a plan that would enable unaffected facility departments to continue during a biological disaster. Include re-establishment of operations after disaster.
Reception of Casualties/ Victims	Establish a plan to segregate/isolate disaster victims from the rest of the facility if those victims are contaminated.	Develop a procedure to triage patients who are exposed to biological agents to appropriate treatment facilities.	After a disaster is confirmed, provide for the following: 1. Clearance of all nonemergency patients and visitors from the ED. 2. Cancellation of all elective admissions and surgeries. 3. Determination of: - all available or open beds - open areas that can be converted to patient care areas - number of patients who can be transferred or discharged.	A communication method must be established so that communication is established and maintained with the local EMS Agencies, Emergency Management Agency, Federal Bureau of Investigation, and the local Health Department.
	Ensure that sufficient equipment, supplies, and apparatus are readily available to permit prompt and efficient casualty movement. The area must be supplied with electricity either from the facility or by generators.	The following respiratory equipment should be available: HEPA masks (OSHA/NIOSH-approved high-efficiency particulate N-95 respirators) and positive air pressure respirators (PAPRs) for individuals unable to wear N-95 respirators.	All staff members must receive training on selection and use of appropriate PPE. They must simulate patient care while wearing full PPE.	Determine if facility has a patient tracking/identification system. Determine if facility has logistical assets (vehicles capable of patient transport) to transport mass casualties to collection points and/or other facilities if your facility fills to capacity.

TABLE 20-2. COMPONENTS OF A HOSPITAL BIOTERRORISM RESPONSE PLAN (CONTINUED)

Diagnostic Capabilities	Determine the percent of laboratory specimens analyzed in-house and/or by contracted laboratories.	Identify alternative laboratories in the event that your current laboratory is contaminated/inundated or does not meet the biosafety lab requirements.	Ensure there are procedures/protocols in place and all personnel have received education about acquisition, handling, and transportation of suspected laboratory specimens.	Confirm that the telephone numbers for the Public Health Department are posted in your laboratory.
Pharmaceuticals	Determine if the facility's pharmaceutical inventory could support the treatment and provide prophylaxis for mass numbers of patients. Examples include ciprofloxacin, doxycycline, penicillin, chloramphenicol, rifampin, gentamicin.	Verify facility personnel have access to therapies for patients (adult and pediatric) exposed to biological agents. Ensure there is adequate medication-administering equipment available for the on-hand quantities of medication.	Identify an emergency pharmaceutical supply system via local pharmacies and pharmaceutical vendors related to the prophylaxis and treatment for exposure to biological agents.	Designate a staff member(s) to accept deliveries from the National Pharmaceutical Stockpile.
Educational Requirements	Identify internal resources and external organizations that can provide training in emergency preparedness/awareness.	Develop a method for assessing emergency preparedness training and continuing education needs based on the roles/responsibilities of staff members. Include all clinical personnel providing direct patient care and the following personnel in training: ➤ Emergency department ➤ Laboratory workers ➤ Morgue personnel ➤ Mortuary professionals ➤ Pathologists ➤ Security ➤ Environmental workers ➤ Pastoral care ➤ Mental health/social workers	Provide emergency/disaster awareness/preparedness educational material at staff orientation to facilitate staff awareness.	Cross-train personnel with external organizations who are involved in the city's/region's emergency response system.

Adapted from references 2 to 7.

Logistical considerations should be well delineated in the plan. These include identification of isolation areas in the ED, alternative sites to triage infectious cases after ED resources have been expended, and locating areas in the facility that may be used for infectious cases if the negative pressure isolation rooms are occupied. The ICP needs to collaborate with the Central Sterile Supply Department and Pharmacy to establish needed levels of PPE and medications for contained and mass casualty situations.

The Hospital Response Plan should contain a concise framework for notification and coordination within the facility as well state and local health agencies and local emergency services. Based on long-standing relationships between infection control departments and public health departments, specifically in the area of communicable disease reporting, ICPs are ideally suited to establish and maintain communication with relevant agencies. Further communication needs center around interactions with local broadcast media systems and other governmental agencies, such as the Federal Bureau of Investigation (FBI) and the Federal Emergency Management Agency (FEMA).[2]

IMPLEMENTATION

All individuals expected to implement and use the Hospital Response Plan must become familiar with the plan. This can be accomplished through educational sessions, quick reference sheets, videotaped lectures, or intranet/internet-based programs.

If the Hospital Response Plan is activated, the ICP should be notified immediately. The ICP must report all clusters of disease as well as even a single case of an unusual disease to the local or state department of health. The ICP will ensure that cases are isolated appropriately and will act as a resource for HCWs. Members of the infection control department will likely be called upon to provide information to or to directly participate in the Incident Management Center initiated by hospital administration. More specific duties for ICPs may include obtaining and communicating guidance for the acquisition, handling, and transportation of suspected laboratory specimens; providing daily tallies of affected patients and HCWs; and identifying breaks in appropriate infection control procedures. The ICP should be available 24/7 to provide education, guidance, and assistance during the implementation phase of the Hospital Response Plan.

EVALUATION

The Hospital Response Plan should be evaluated biannually for deficiencies/weaknesses and should be revised as appropriate. The following areas should be evaluated:

handling and disposal of waste, space and equipment needs, emergency procedures for exposures, proper use and availability of PPE, transportation of patients and appropriate use of isolation precautions, patient tracking, appropriate segregation of cases from the "worried well," resources for relatives searching for each other, use of the isolation rooms, use of alternative sites if isolation rooms are expended, and the effectiveness of the communication matrix to include testing of the employee call back system. In addition to meetings of hospital emergency response personnel and others involved in the development of the plan, more formal testing of response capabilities should be initiated, such as bioterrorism tabletop exercises or drills.[8]

IDENTIFICATION OF A BIOTERRORISM OUTBREAK

Clinical Clues

The release of biological agents would most likely occur as a covert event, one in which the impact will not be immediately known because of the delay between exposure and onset of illness (eg, incubation period).[1] The first casualties from a covert attack will present to primary care physician offices, ambulatory clinics, or EDs. The first signs and symptoms of most of the Category A agents are nonspecific and resemble a number of viral or respiratory illnesses (Table 20-3). Patients might present with any combination of fever, chills, malaise, headache, and/or cough, which is easily interpreted as a viral syndrome. As the disease progresses, a maculopapular rash may develop (smallpox), the patient may develop hemoptysis (plague), or a hemorrhagic or purpuric rash, epistaxis, hematemesis, hemoptysis, or blood in the stool may occur (hemorrhagic fever viruses). Clinicians must be knowledgeable of the signs and symptoms of the Category A agents to detect a potential outbreak due to a biological agent. Seasonal disparities or illness among unexpected age groups may provide clues to a biological attack. For example, a cluster of patients presenting to the ED or ambulatory clinic in July with complaints of flu-like symptoms should alert clinicians to a possible outbreak. Similarly, if a relatively young patient presents to an ED or ambulatory clinic with pneumonia, which rapidly progresses to death, a biological agent should be considered, and the ICP should be notified immediately.

Surveillance Needs

Early detection of a potential bioterrorism event is essential for ensuring prompt interventions and minimizing casualties.[9] Surveillance is a process for gathering,

TABLE 20-3. CATEGORY A BIOTERRORISM AGENTS

Agent	Symptoms	Incubation Period	Transmission Person to Person	Duration of Illness	Lab Diagnosis*	Fatality Rate
Anthrax	*Inhalation* Fever, chills, fatigue, malaise, dyspnea, cough, headache, nausea, and/or vomiting. Rapid progression to sepsis, respiratory failure, shock. *Cutaneous* Initial macule or papule enlarges to round ulcer by day 2, development of painless, black eschar with local edema, lymphagitis, painful lymphadenopathy.	*Inhalation* 1 to 6 days *Cutaneous* 1 to 10 days	*Inhalation* No *Cutaneous* Potential by direct contact with a draining lesion.	3 to 5 days (inhalational anthrax usually fatal if not treated)	*Inhalation* Blood cultures, sputum from lower respiratory tract, gram stain, PCR, Ag-ELISA *Cutaneous* Gram stain and culture of vesicular fluid. If gram stain negative, obtain a punch biopsy for immunohistochemical staining or PCR. Nasal swab should not be used as a diagnostic test.	*Inhalation* 45% (in US 2001 attack) *Cutaneous* Up to 20% if not treated, rare if treated
Plague	*Pneumonic* Fever, cough, chest pain, tachypnea, dyspnea, and hemoptysis. Gastrointestinal symptoms common (ie, nausea, vomiting, abdominal pain, and diarrhea).	1 to 6 days (most often 2 to 4 days)	Yes	2 to 6 days (usually fatal if not treated)	Bronchial wash/transtracheal aspirate, sputum, or blood: gram stain, Wright, Giemsa, or Wayson stain. Antigen detection, IgM enzyme immuno assay, immunostaining, and PCR available through Public Health laboratories.	High (57%) unless treated within 24 hours of symptoms
Smallpox	High fever, malaise, prostration with headache and backache. A maculopapular rash appears on the mucosa of the mouth, pharynx, face, and forearms, then spreads to the trunk and legs (centrifugal). Rash becomes vesicular followed by pustules that crust and separate, leaving pitted scars.	7 to 17 days	Yes	4 weeks	Electron microscopic examination of vesicular or pustular fluid or scab. Definitive identification requires growth of virus in ell culture or use of PCR and restriction fragment-length polymorphisms. Studies performed only in predesignated laboratories.	30%

TABLE 20-3. CATEGORY A BIOTERRORISM AGENTS (CONTINUED)

Agent	Incubation Symptoms	Transmission Period	Duration of Person to Person	Lab Illness	Fatality Diagnosis*	Rate
Tularemia	Abrupt onset of fever, chills, pharyngitis, headache, and myalgia with cough may progress to hilar lymphadenitis, pleuropneumonitis, and meningitis.	1 to 14 days (usually 3 to 5 days)	No	2 weeks or more	Blood and respiratory cultures, biopsied tissue or scraping of an ulcer, or aspirate of involved tissue: direct fluorescent Ab or immunohistochemical stains. Microscopic fluorescent-labeled Ab testing, Ag detection, and PCR in designated laboratories.	<2%
Botulinum	Symmetric, descending flaccid paralysis with prominent bulbar palsies. Afebrile with clear sensorium, usually accompanied by ptosis, blurred vision, dysarthria, dysphonia, and dysphagia.	_Inhalation_ 72 hours _Foodborne_ 2 hours to 8 days	No	Weeks to months	Blood, stool, gastric aspirate, vomitus, and suspect food (solid or liquid) specimens for mouse bioassay. Obtain samples prior to administering antitoxin. Must coordinate with public health laboratories.	6%
Hemorrhagic Fever Viruses (eg, _Filoviridae_: Ebola, Marburg; _Arenaviridae_: Lassa fever)	Varies with virus origin. Suspect hemorrhagic fever if patient has acute onset of fever of less than 3 weeks' duration, no known predisposing host factors for hemorrhagic symptoms, and any 2 of the following: hemorrhagic or purpuric rash, epistaxis, hemoptysis, hematemesis, bloody stool.	2 to 21 days	Yes	Convalescence may be prolonged	Diagnosis only available at specialized laboratories. Viral isolation, serology, antigen-capture ELISA, and RT-PCR may be used.	Varies depending on virus: <1% to 90%

*Alert laboratory personnel to special diagnostic and safety procedures if caring for patients with suspect bioterrorism agent.
Ag = antigen; Ab = antibody; PCR = polymerase chain reaction; RT-PCR = reverse transcriptase PCR; Ag-ELISA = Antigen-capture enzyme-linked immunosorbent assay; RDT = rapid diagnostic test.

Adapted from references 1 and 10 to 22.

managing, analyzing, and reporting data on events that occur in a specific population. These data enable the ICP to develop baseline rates, detect changes in the rates or distribution of these events, and investigate any changes.[23] This is called diagnosis-based or traditional surveillance and is dependent on the physician's interpretation of symptoms.

Syndromic surveillance is the evaluation of a group of nonspecific signs and symptoms to detect clusters of illness at the earliest time point (eg, before assignment of a specific diagnosis). Syndromic surveillance is designed to look in "real time" for aberrant patterns of disease. Syndromic monitoring may also assist in geographic tracking of an outbreak and may provide reassurance of the absence of a bioterrorism event. This reassurance is useful in settings where an outbreak is occurring in an adjacent region or when suspicion for such an event is high.[24] Syndromic surveillance compares the number of patients in the "signs and symptoms" group with historical data on the number of patients expected in these groups. When the daily number of patients with similar signs and symptoms increases to significantly greater than the number expected, the system triggers an "alarm." Automated systems can be developed to send an e-mail alert to specified individuals, including appropriate personnel at the local department of health. The alert may inform the recipient that a trigger above baseline was detected, may include which bioterrorism agent(s) are potentially involved, and may provide the number of patients identified with the signs and symptoms of concern.[9] Local and state health departments are key participants in the design and implementation of syndromic surveillance in many areas in the United States.[25]

Direct communication with public health departments regarding unusual illness or disease clusters in the hospital environment is the responsibility of all healthcare providers, especially ICPs. This direct reporting, together with the use of diagnosis-based and syndromic surveillance, is critical for early detection of potential bioterrorism events.

Education

In the event of a bioterrorism attack, the first casualties will most likely present to an ambulatory clinic or a physician's office; therefore, clinicians must have basic clinical knowledge about biological agents to appropriately triage, diagnose, and treat. Physicians and nurses should be provided with current information about treatment, immunizations, and prophylactic treatment of contacts (Table 20-4). ICPs can facilitate educating HCWs in their facility by providing annual bioterrorism lectures, updated fact sheets, and/or Web-based programs. All HCWs who are required to implement and use the Hospital Response Plan must receive bioterrorism education.

Management of a Bioterrorism Event

The Suspect Case

Staff personnel/physicians must notify the ICP immediately upon identification of exposure/symptoms related to biological agents. Many primary care, ambulatory care, and ED physicians and other providers may not be aware of this critical "need to notify." The ICP education efforts before a suspect case occurs will be critical to the entire management of such an event. Improving the ease of contacting the infection control program and clear guidance on how to reach such personnel after-hours and on weekends is essential. Once notified of a suspect case, the ICP must immediately notify the local department of public health and all people designated in the Hospital Response Plan. The ICP will ensure that appropriate PPE is being used and that proper isolation precautions are being implemented (Table 20-5).

"Town hall meetings" with employees should be held to provide information about the suspected biological agent and to provide an opportunity for questions. Fact sheets and other up-to-date information should be distributed. The Hospital Response Plan and the responsibilities of each hospital employee should be reviewed. The meetings will ease panic and fear among employees and will provide an opportunity for employees to discuss their fears. Mental health personnel (psychiatrists, psychologists, social workers, counselors, and clergy) should be available to provide support to employees and patients.

Contained Casualty Situation

In a contained casualty setting, clusters of patients would arrive in the ED with similar symptoms over a period of hours to days. Suspect bioterrorism cases should be segregated from the other patients in the ED, ambulatory care areas, and on inpatient floors. Units, predesignated in the Hospital Response Plan for isolating bioterrorism cases, should be notified of the need to prepare for admissions. All departments involved in the Hospital Response Plan need to be informed of a contained casualty situation. The ICP is the initial liaison with the local department of health and should be available to disseminate necessary information to the designated hospital IC who is leading the hospital response. The ICP is responsible for developing a database of all suspect and actual cases, developing an epidemiological curve, and recording mortality rates among the bioterrorism cases. This information must be updated on a continual basis and must be available for the hospital IC, department of public health, and law enforcement agencies. As bioterrorism cases are discharged from the facility, proper cleaning, disinfection, and disposal of

TABLE 20-4. SUMMARY OF TREATMENT, PRE- AND POSTPROPHYLAXIS, AND VACCINE AVAILABILITY*†

Agent	Treatment	Postexposure Duration	Prophylaxis	Vaccine
Anthrax	*Inhalation* Ciprofloxacin, 400 mg IV q 12 h (pediatric: 10 to 15 mg/kg q 12 h[1]) or doxycycline, 100 mg q 12 h (pediatric: 2.5 mg/kg q 12h) *and* 1 or 2 additional antimicrobials.[2] Pregnant women and immunocompromised people: Same *Cutaneous* Ciprofloxacin, 500 mg orally twice daily (pediatric: 10 to 15 mg/kg q 12 h) or doxycycline, 100 mg orally twice daily (pediatric: 2.2 mg/kg q 12 h). Pregnant women and immunocompromised people: Same	IV treatment initially before switching to oral antimicrobial therapy when clinically stable: Ciprofloxacin, 500 mg po twice daily (pediatric: 10 to 15 mg/kg po q 12 h) or doxycycline, 100 mg po twice daily (pediatric: 2.2 mg/kg po twice daily) Total treatment period (IV and po): 60 days	Ciprofloxacin, 500 mg po q 12 h x 60 days (pediatric: 10 to 15mg/kg po q 12h) x 60 days Pregnant women and immunocompromised adults and children: Same Alternative: If strain is susceptible: Doxycycline, 100 mg po q 12 h or amoxicillin, 500 mg po q 8 h (pediatric: if ≥20 kg: amoxicillin, 500 mg po q 8 h, if <20 kg: amoxicillin, 40 mg/kg/d po ÷ tid) x 60 days Immunocompromised adults and children: Same Pregnant women: Amoxicillin, 500 mg po q 8 h	FDA-licensed vaccine: 0.5 mL SC at 0, 2, and 4 weeks and 6, 12, and 18 months, then annual boosters
Plague	Streptomycin, 1 g IM twice daily (pediatrics: 15 mg/kg IM twice daily) or gentamicin, 5 mg/kg IM or IV once daily or 2 mg/kg loading dose followed by 1.7 mg/kg IM or IV 3 times daily (pediatric: 2.5 mg/kg IV 4 times daily). Pregnant women: Gentamicin, 5 mg/kg IM or IV once daily or 2 mg/kg loading dose followed by 1.7 mg/kg IM or IV 3 times daily	10 days	Doxycycline, 100 mg po twice daily (pediatrics: 2.2 mg/kg po twice daily) x 7 days or ciprofloxacin, 500 mg po twice daily (pediatrics: 20 mg/kg po twice daily) x 7 days. Pregnant women: Same as adults	None

TABLE 20-4. SUMMARY OF TREATMENT, PRE- AND POSTPROPHYLAXIS, AND VACCINE AVAILABILITY (CONTINUED)*†

Agent	Treatment	Duration	Postexposure Prophylaxis	Vaccine
Smallpox	Supportive care and antibiotics as indicated for treatment of occasional secondary bacterial infections. Cidofovir (effective in vitro) is investigational. Topical idoxuridine may be considered for treatment of corneal lesions with daily eyewashes to prevent blindness.		Smallpox vaccine administered within 4 days of first exposure; best within 24 hours.	Smallpox vaccine administered by scarification.
Tularemia	Streptomycin, 1 g IM twice daily (pediatric: 15 mg/kg IM twice daily[3]) or gentamicin, 5 mg/kg IM or IV qd (pediatric: 2.5 mg/kg IM or IV 3 times daily) Alternative: Doxycycline, 100 mg IV twice daily (pediatric: 2.2 mg/kg twice daily) or ciprofloxacin 400 mg IV twice daily (pediatric: 15 mg/kg IV twice daily). Pregnant women: Same as adult	10 days for streptomycin, gentamicin, or ciprofloxacin; 14 to 21 days for doxycycline. IV/IM therapy may be switched to oral when clinically indicated.	*Exposed people:* Doxycycline, 100 mg po twice daily (pediatric: 2.2 mg/kg po twice daily) or ciprofloxacin, 500 mg po twice daily (pediatric: 15 mg/kg po twice daily) for 14 days. Pregnant women: Same. People *potentially* exposed should begin a fever watch. People who develop an unexplained fever or flu-like illness within 14 days of presumed exposure should begin antibiotic treatment. *Postexposure prophylaxis is not recommended for close contacts of tularemia patients.*	None
Botulinum	Supportive care and licensed equine trivalent (type A, B, E) antitoxin; administer one 10-mL vial per patient, diluted 1:10 in 0.9% saline solution by slow IV infusion.[4]			(DOD) Pentavalent toxoid vaccine for serotypes A-E for investigational use only

TABLE 20-4. SUMMARY OF TREATMENT, PRE- AND POSTPROPHYLAXIS, AND VACCINE AVAILABILITY (CONTINUED)*†

Agent	Treatment	Duration	Postexposure Prophylaxis	Vaccine
Hemorrhagic Fever Viruses	Supportive therapy and ribavirin, loading dose of 30 mg/kg IV (maximum 2 g) once followed by 16 mg/kg IV (maximum, 1 g per dose) q 6 h for 4 d, followed by 8 mg/kg IV (maximum, 500 mg per dose) q 8 h for 6 d Pediatric: Same as adults)	10 days Ribavirin only active against Lassa fever and select New World Arenaviruses. Decision to continue therapy depends on viral isolation.	High-risk and close contacts should record their temperatures twice daily for 21 days and report any temperatures ≥101°F (38.3°C) to a hospital epidemiologist or public health authority	Licensed vaccine for Yellow Fever only

* Treatment summary for contained situation; refer to federal, state, and local public health recommendations for mass casualty situations.
† If child is >45 kg, give adult dosage.
1 In children, ciprofloxacin dosage should not exceed 1 g/d.
2 Other agents with in vitro activity include rifampin, vancomycin, penicillin, ampicillin, chloramphenicol, imipenem, clindamycin, and clarithromycin. Penicillin and ampicillin should not be used alone.
3 In children, streptomycin dosage should not exceed 2 g/d.
4 Patients should be screened for hypersensitivity with small challenge dose of equine antitoxin before given full dose. Refer to package insert for explanation of scratch tests and intradermal tests used for sensitivity.

DOD = Department of Defense

Adapted from references 7 and 10 to 22.

infectious waste must be ensured. The ICP may consult with local waste management companies and local or state governmental medical waste programs for recommendations. The ICP will work in tandem with Occupational Health to ensure that hospital employees potentially exposed to infectious agents receive appropriate prophylaxis and surveillance for illness (see Table 20-4).

Mass Casualty Event

If a mass casualty event occurs, the facility will receive guidance from the local, state, and federal agencies. ICPs may be called upon to provide input for creation of educational messages for all hospital staff and patients and ongoing hospital-based surveillance for new and severely ill cases.

Special Considerations

Pre-Event Smallpox Vaccination of Healthcare Workers

In an effort to prepare the United States for a potential bioterrorism attack using the smallpox virus, the ACIP and the HICPAC have recommended identifying HCWs (Table 20-5) who can be vaccinated and trained to provide direct medical care for the first smallpox patients requiring hospitalization and to evaluate and manage patients who are suspected of having smallpox.[26] In addition, individuals administering the smallpox vaccine must be vaccinated. Previously vaccinated HCWs should be considered first to receive the vaccine to decrease the potential of adverse side effects (Table 20-6). The vaccinia (smallpox) vaccine is a live virus that does not cause smallpox; however, the vaccinia virus is shed from the vaccination site

TABLE 20-5. INFECTION CONTROL PROTOCOLS FOR CATEGORY A AGENTS

Agent	Anthrax	Plague	Smallpox	Tularemia	Botulinum	Hemorrhagic Fever Viruses
Isolation Precautions*	Standard *Cutaneous* Contact precautions if lesions are draining Use soap and water after removing gloves or touching surfaces. Waterless, alcohol-based hand hygiene products are not effective in removing *Bacillus anthracis*[8]	Droplet precautions for the first 48 hours of antimicrobial therapy and until clinical improvement has taken place.	Airborne and contact	Standard	Standard If flaccid paralysis is suspected to be from acute meningitis, droplet precautions (for *N. meningitidis* and *H. influenzae*) until diagnosis confirmed.	Airborne and VHF-specific barrier precautions, which includes N-95 masks or high-efficiency particulate respirator, double gloves, impermeable gowns, leg and shoe coverings, face shields, goggles for eye protection, and dedicated medical equipment (ie, stethoscopes, glucose monitors, point of care analyzers).[6]
Patient Placement	No restrictions	May cohort	Negative pressure isolation room required	No restrictions	No restrictions	Negative pressure isolation room required
Patient Transport	No restrictions	Not recommended. If necessary, patient should wear surgical mask.	Not recommended. If necessary, patient should wear surgical mask.	No restrictions	No restrictions	Not recommended. If necessary, patient should wear a surgical mask.
Discharge	No special discharge instruction needed	No special discharge instruction needed	Discharged when determined no longer infectious	No special discharge instruction needed	No special discharge instruction needed	Discharged when determined no longer infectious. Convalescing patients from filoviral/arenaviral infection should refrain from sexual activity for 3 months.[6]

TABLE 20-5. INFECTION CONTROL PROTOCOLS FOR CATEGORY A AGENTS (CONTINUED)

Agent	Anthrax	Plague	Smallpox	Tularemia	Botulinum	Hemorrhagic Fever Viruses
Cleaning, Disinfection of room and equipment	Disinfect surfaces using a 1:100 dilution of household bleach: ¼ cup to 1 gallon water	Disinfect surfaces using a 1:100 dilution of household bleach: ¼ cup to 1 gallon water	All bedding and clothing must be autoclaved or laundered in hot water and bleach. Environmental Protection Agency (EPA)-approved hospital disinfectants are effective for cleaning surfaces	Routine terminal cleaning of room with hospital-approved disinfectant	Routine terminal cleaning of room with hospital-approved disinfectant	Disinfect all surfaces using a US EPA-registered hospital disinfectant or a 1:100 dilution of household bleach. Discard dedicated equipment or disinfect equipment prior to leaving room. Soiled linen should be placed in leak-proof bags at the site of use and transported directly to the decontamination area. Linens may be decontaminated in a gravity displacement autoclave or incinerated. Linens may be laundered using a normal hot water cycle with bleach if standard precautions are followed and linens are placed directly into washing machine without sorting.
Postmortem Care	Cremation preferred. If autopsies are performed, all related instruments and materials should be autoclaved or incinerated	Aerosol generating procedures (ie, bone sawing) are not recommended. If necessary, must wear high-efficiency particulate air filtered masks and perform procedure in a negatively ventilated pressure room	Cremation preferred, and mortuary workers should be vaccinated	Aerosol-generating procedures should be avoided	Per routine	The corpse should be wrapped in sealed leak-proof material. Do not embalm. Cremation preferred or bury promptly in a sealed casket. Autopsy only by specially trained personnel using VHF-specific barrier precautions, HEPA-filtered respirators, and negative pressure rooms

*Standard precautions should be used for the care of all patients. All employees and other healthcare workers caring for patients and/or handling patient specimens must take measures to prevent exposure to blood and/or body fluids. The purpose of this practice is to establish procedures to minimize the risk of occupational infection by bloodborne and/or other infectious agents. Standard precautions should be applied to all patients regardless of diagnosis or presumed infection status. Standard precautions apply to all Category A, B, and C agents.

Adapted from references 1 to 6 and 10 to 22.

TABLE 20-6. PRE-EVENT SMALLPOX VACCINATION OF HEALTHCARE WORKERS

Selection of Healthcare Workers for Smallpox Vaccine

➤ Emergency department staff (includes physicians and nurses caring for children and adults)
➤ Intensive care unit staff (includes pediatricians and pediatric intensive care specialists)
➤ General medical unit staff, including internists, family physicians
➤ Medical subspecialists, including ID specialists
➤ Infection control professionals
➤ Respiratory therapists
➤ Radiology technicians
➤ Security personnel
➤ Housekeeping staff (eg, those involved in maintaining the healthcare environment and decreasing risk for fomite transmission).

Contraindications to Smallpox Vaccination in Pre-Event Setting

➤ History or presence of eczema or atopic dermatitis (V,H[1])
➤ Acute, chronic, or exfoliative skin conditions[†] (V,H)
➤ Immunosuppression[§] (V,H)
➤ Pregnancy (V,H)
➤ Breastfeeding (V)
➤ Children and adolescents <18 years (V)
➤ Vaccine component allergy (V)
➤ Known coronary disease including (V)
  ➤ Previous myocardial infarction or angina
  ➤ Congestive heart failure (V)
  ➤ Cardiomyopathy (V)
  ➤ Stroke or transient ischemic attack (V)
  ➤ Chest pain or shortness of breath with activity (V)
  ➤ Other heart conditions under the care of a physician (V)

In addition, the smallpox vaccine should NOT be given if the vaccinee has 3 or more of the following risk factors:

➤ Hypertension
➤ High blood cholesterol level
➤ Diabetes
➤ A first-degree relative (eg, mother, father, brother, sister) who had a heart condition before the age of 50
➤ Smokes cigarettes

Vaccine-Related Adverse Events

➤ Inadvertent inoculation (nonocular)
➤ Ocular vaccinia
➤ Pyogenic infection of vaccination site
➤ Eczema vaccinatum
➤ Generalized vaccinia
➤ Mycocarditis/pericarditis
➤ Postvaccinial encephalitis or encephalomyelitis
➤ Myocardial infarction

[1]V = Vaccinees, H = Household contacts (people with prolonged intimate contact with the potential vaccinee [eg, sexual contacts] and others who might have direct contact with the vaccination site).
[†]Conditions include burns, impetigo, *varicella zoster*, *herpes*, severe acne, or psoriasis.
[§]Conditions include human immunodeficiency virus, acquired immunodeficiency syndrome, leukemia, lymphoma, generalized malignancy, solid organ transplantation, cellular or humoral immunodeficiencies, or therapy with alkylating agents, antimetabolites, radiation, or high-dose corticosteroids.
Vaccination of children and adolescents aged <18 years not recommended in the pre-event smallpox vaccination program.

Adapted from references 26 to 28.

for 4 to 14 days after inoculation and until the scab separates from the skin. Vaccinia can be transmitted from an unhealed vaccination site to other people by close contact. It is important to caution the vaccinee about the following to prevent autoinoculation and infection of people within close contact: (1) keep the vaccination site covered with gauze and a semipermeable dressing; (2) do not touch, scratch, or rub the site; (3) avoid person-to-person contact with susceptible individuals; (4) avoid touching or rubbing the site to prevent transfer of vaccinia virus to the eye or surrounding skin; (5) dressings used to cover the site should be changed every 3 to 5 days and more frequently if exudate accumulates; (6) discard used gauze/semipermeable dressing in a sealed plastic bag; and (7) hand hygiene is required after contact with the vaccination site or any materials that have come into contact with the site.[26,28] Using correct hand hygiene prevents the majority of inadvertent inoculations and contact transmissions after changing dressings or having contact with the vaccination site. The vaccination site should be assessed by a trained clinician at day 6, 7, or 8 to verify a "take" or proper response to the vaccination.[28] Some individuals who receive the vaccinia vaccine may experience adverse reactions. Adverse reactions range from mild (fever, headache, fatigue, myalgia, chills, local skin reactions, nonspecific rashes, erythema multiforme, lymphadenopathy, and pain at the vaccination site) to severe (see Table 20-6).[27,28] Adverse events must be reported immediately to the Vaccine Adverse Event Reporting System (VAERS). Reports can be submitted through the internet at http://secure.vaers.org/ VaersDataEntryintro.htm.

In the event of a confirmed smallpox exposure, the benefits of vaccination to protect against smallpox disease outweigh the potential vaccine side effects. In the setting of a confirmed smallpox case or outbreak, close contacts of the case(s) and potentially the larger community would be eligible to receive the vaccine. People exposed to smallpox are generally protected from smallpox if vaccinated within 2 to 3 days of exposure; vaccination within 4 to 5 days following exposure may protect against a fatal outcome.[17]

INTERNET RESOURCES

Bioterrorism is a rapidly evolving field and requires access to current information. Additional information about bioterrorism and bioterrorism preparedness may be found using the internet resource list (Table 20-7); Table 20-7 is not all-inclusive and should serve as a general guide.

CONCLUSION

ICPs play a pivotal role in preparing facilities to meet the challenges of biological terrorism. ICPs must actively seek opportunities to develop relationships with all hospital departments to develop clear lines of communication that could be instantly accessed in the event of a bioterrorism threat. Additionally, working relationships should be pre-established with outside agencies, such as the local and state health departments; medical/nursing professional associations at the state, national, and international level; and nongovernmental disaster response organizations. ICPs should strive to remain current regarding bioterrorism issues by attending local and state bioterrorism seminars; reviewing the CDC's bioterrorism Web site at least weekly; and attending and participating in local, state, and national bioterrorism drills. Institutions that have developed a Hospital Response Plan, practiced tabletop drills and mock bioterrorism disaster drills, and provided education for their HCWs will be better prepared in the event of an actual bioterrorism attack.

REFERENCES

1. Centers for Disease Control and Prevention. Biological and chemical terrorism: strategic plan for preparedness and response. Recommendations of the CDC Strategic Planning Workgroup. *MMWR Morbid Mortal Wkly Rep*. 2000;49(RR-4):1-8.

2. Rotz LD, Khan AS, Lillibridge SR, Ostroff SM, Hughes JM. Public health assessment of potential biological terrorism agents. *Emerg Infect Dis*. 2002;8:225-230.

3. Centers for Disease Control and Prevention. (March 24, 2003). Public Health emergency preparedness and response. Available at http://www.bt.cdc.gov/ agent/anthrax/ lab-testing/index.asp. Accessed May 23, 2003.

4. The American Hospital Association. 2002. Chemical and bioterrorism preparedness checklist. Available at http://my.premierinc.com/all/safety/resources/disaster_re adiness/downloads/22_aha_prepardness_checklist.doc. Accessed May 5, 2003.

5. Evans G. Bioterrorism fears put ICPs front and center following WTC, Pentagon attacks. *Hosp Infect Control*. 2001;28:141-147.

6. The American Hospital Association, Office of Emergency Preparedness, US Department of Health and Human Services. (2000, August). Hospital preparedness for mass casualties: summary of an invitational forum. 1-35. Available at http://www.hospitalconnect.com/ahapolicyfo rum/rsources/content/disasterpreparedness.doc. Accessed on May 5, 2003.

TABLE 20-7. INTERNET RESOURCES

Local, State, Federal, and International Agencies

Centers for Disease Control and Prevention
http://www.cdc.gov

CDC Bioterrorism Preparedness and Response Program
http://www.bt.cdc.gov

New York City Department of Health
http://www.nyc.gov/html/doh/html/cd/wtc8.html

New York State Department of Health
http://www.health.state.ny.us

California Department of Health
http://www.dhs.cahwnet.gov/ps/dcdc/bt

State Public Health Departments
http://www.statepublichealth.org

Health Alert Network: Public Health Practice Program Office
http://www.phppo.cdc.gov/han/index.asp

World Health Organization
http://www.who.int/health_topics/bioterrorism/en

Academic and Other Educational Institutions

Johns Hopkins University Center for Civilian Biodefense Studies
http://www.hopkins-biodefense.org

Saint Louis University School of Public Health, Center for the Study of Bioterrorism and Emerging Infections
http://www.bioterrorism.slu.edu

Agency for Healthcare Research and Quality in cooperation with the University of Alabama School of Medicine
www.bioterrorism.uab.edu

Monterey Institute of International Studies: Center for Nonproliferation Studies
http://cns.miis.edu

Societies and Organizations

The Society for Healthcare Epidemiology of America, Inc.
http://www.shea-online.org/BTprep.html

Association for Professionals in Infection Control and Epidemiology
http://www.apic.org

Infectious Disease Society of America; Bioterrorism Information and Resources
http://www.idsociety.org/BT/ToC.htm

American Society for Microbiology
http://www.asmbiodefense.org

7. Henretig FM, Cieslak TJ. Bioterrorism and pediatric emergency medicine. *Clin Pediatr Emerg Med*. 2001;2:211-222.

8. Henning KJ, Brennan PJ, Hoegg C, O'Rourke E, Dyer BD, Grace TL. Health system preparedness for bioterrorism: bringing the tabletop to the hospital. *Infect Control Hosp Epidemiol*. In press.

9. Centers for Disease Control and Prevention. (December 13, 2001). CDC Plague information: public health emergency preparedness and response. Available at http://www.bt.cdc.gov/agent/plague/index.asp. Accessed May 23, 2003.

10. Centers for Disease Control and Prevention. (December 13, 2001). CDC Tularemia information: public health emergency preparedness and response. Available at http://www.bt.cdc.gov/agent/tularemia/index.asp. Accessed May 23, 2003.

11. Centers for Disease Control and Prevention. (May 13, 2003). CDC Botulism information: public health emergency preparedness and response. Available at http://www.bt.cdc.gov/Agent/Botulism?botulismlabprotocol.pdf. Accessed May 23, 2003.

12. Borio L, Inglesby T, Peters CJ, et al. Hemorrhagic fever viruses as biological weapons; medical and public health management. *JAMA*. 2002;287:2391-2405.

13. Inglesby TV, O'Toole T, Henderson DA, et al. Anthrax as a biological weapon, 2002; updated recommendations for management. *JAMA*. 2002;287:2236-2252.

14. Weber DJ, Sickbert-Bennett E, Gergen MF, Rutala WA. Efficacy of selected hand hygiene agents used to remove *Bacillus atrophaeus* (a surrogate of *Bacillus anthracis*) from contaminated hands. *JAMA*. 2003;289:1274-1277.

15. Inglesby TV, Dennis DT, Henderson DA, et al. Plague as a biological weapon; medical and public health management. *JAMA*. 2000;283:2281-2290.

16. Chanteau S, Rahalison L, Ralafiarisoa L, et al. Development and testing of a rapid diagnostic test for bubonic and pneumonic plague. *Lancet*. 2003;361:211-216.

17. Henderson DA, Inglesby TV, Bartlett JG, et al. Smallpox as a biological weapon; medical and public health management. *JAMA*. 1999;281:2127-2137.

18. Constantin CM, Martinelli AM, Bonney EA, Strickland OL. Smallpox: an update for nurses. *Biol Res Nurs*. 2003; 4:282-294.

19. Dennis DT, Inglesby TV, Henderson DA, et al. Tularemia as a biological weapon; medical and public health management. *JAMA*. 2001;285:2763-2773.

20. Arnon SS, Schechter R, Inglesby TV, et al. Botulinum toxin as a biological weapon; medical and public health management. *JAMA*. 2001;285:1059-1069.

21. Centers for Disease Control and Prevention. (September 19, 1998). Notice to readers: Management of patients with suspected viral hemorrhagic fever-United States. Available at http://www.cdc.gov/mmwr/preview/mmwrhtml/ 00038033.htm. Accessed on May 26, 2003.

22. Irvin CB, Nouhan PP, Rice K. Syndromic analysis of computerized emergency department patients' chief complaints: an opportunity for bioterrorism and influenza surveillance. *Ann Emerg Med*. 2003;41:447-452.

23. Pottinger JM, Herwaldt LA, Perl TM. Basics of surveillance, an overview. In: Herwaldt LA, Decker M, eds. *A Practical Handbook for Hospital Epidemiologists*. Thorofare, NJ: SLACK Incorporated; 1998: 59-78.

24. Draft framework for evaluating syndromic surveillance systems for bioterrorism preparedness. Available at www.cdc.gov/epo/dphsi/phs/syndromic.htm. Accessed on June 2, 2003.

25. Henning KJ. Syndromic surveillance. In: Smolinski MS, Hamburg MA, Lederberg J, eds. *Microbial Threats to Health: Emergence, Detection and Response*. Washington, DC: The National Academies Press; 2003:309-350.

26. Centers for Disease Control and Prevention. Recommendations for using smallpox vaccine in a pre-event vaccination program; supplemental recommendations of the Advisory Committee on Immunization Practices (ACIP) and the Healthcare Infection Control Practices Advisory Committee (HICPAC). *MMWR Morbid Mortal Wkly Rep*. 2003;52(RR-7):1-16.

27. Centers for Disease Control and Prevention. (March 31, 2003). Smallpox vaccine and heart problems. Available at http://www.bt.cdc.gov/agent/smallpox/vaccination/heart-problems.asp. Accessed June 2, 2003.

28. Centers for Disease Control and Prevention. Smallpox vaccination and adverse reactions; guidance for clinicians. *MMWR Morbid Mortal Wkly Rep*. 2003;52(RR-4):1-29.

CHAPTER TWENTY-ONE

EMPLOYEE HEALTH/OCCUPATIONAL MEDICINE

David K. Henderson, MD

INTRODUCTION

An institution's occupational medicine program represents one of three vital programs that provide occupational medical and safety support for its HCWs. The other 2 programs are the institution's biosafety program and its hospital epidemiology program. These 3 programs work in concert to ensure the health and safety of workers and patients in healthcare institutions. This chapter will review the intersection of these 3 programs in screening workers for IDs, in providing education to HCWs, in providing immunoprophylaxis, in ensuring an adequate infrastructure for the safe provision of care, and in participating in the management of employee exposures to infectious agents.

SEROLOGIC SCREENING AND IMMUNIZATION

Preplacement Examination

Prior to entry into the workplace, hospital personnel should be evaluated by the occupational medicine service to ensure fitness for duty. The most important aspect of this evaluation is the employee's medical history. From the perspective of the hospital epidemiologist, the most important aspect of the employee's medical history is his or her communicable disease history. An "entry-onto-duty" focused physical examination is performed by some occupational medical services; others require that the employee's personal physician provide results from a recent physical examination.

Laboratory Evaluation

Routine, unfocused laboratory testing is of limited value in prescreening potential employees. Screening should be limited to diseases presenting significant or unique risks to patients and other staff (eg, VZV serology in children's hospitals or oncology centers; rubella in obstetrical and gynecology settings). Some institutions that primarily provide care to children or immunocompromised patients screen all employees for varicella immunity, whereas others consider a history of chickenpox to be reliable evidence of immunity. Routine serologic screening of potential hepatitis B vaccine recipients is generally not cost-effective, unless the prevalence of infection is high enough in the population of HCWs being screened to avoid vaccination of enough employees to pay for the screening process. Routine screening for susceptibility to MMR is not advisable. Individuals who cannot document that they were adequately vaccinated or that they had physician-diagnosed infection may be given the MMR vaccine. If an institution wishes to ensure that all employees are immune to these childhood illnesses, immunity to these infections should be made a condition of employment. History alone is not adequate to determine rubella immunity; serological examination should be required.

Screening for Prior Tuberculosis Infection

The occupational medicine, hospital epidemiology, and institutional biosafety programs should work together to establish an effective ongoing tuberculosis prevention program, including a tuberculosis surveillance system. This scope of the program should be based on the history of transmission of tuberculosis in the institution and the prevalence of tuberculosis in the hospital's catchment. Each new employee should receive intradermal Mantoux skin testing, using the 2-step approach, during his or her initial evaluation, unless the employee has documentation of prior active tuberculosis, a previously positive skin test, and/or completion of therapy for infection. Use of "control" skin tests (eg, candida, mumps) is not advisable. Occupational medicine staff should evaluate skin tests using stringent, consistent criteria. Positive skin tests should be managed according to existing guidelines.[1]

PRE-EVENT IMMUNOPROPHYLAXIS

As noted above, immunizations against certain IDs are advisable for healthcare providers. Certainly, all HCWs whose jobs entail exposure to blood or blood-containing body fluids should be immunized against hepatitis B (Table 21-1). The occupational medicine service and the hospital epidemiology service should work together to ensure that an efficient program is in place to educate staff about the occupational risks for bloodborne pathogen infection and to provide hepatitis B immunization. Depending on the institution, immunization against MMR and varicella may be appropriate. If the risk for transmission of these childhood exanthems is present in your institution, or, conversely, if transmission of these infections may present life-threatening risks to immunosuppressed patients in your institution, you may wish to consider establishing ongoing immunization programs for your providers. For most institutions, the risks for spread of influenza A and B are substantial. For this reason, institutional occupational medicine service providers should offer voluntary influenza vaccination to all providers who have patient contact. The beneficial effects of influenza immunization include decreasing the spread of the virus in the institution, decreasing worker absenteeism during influenza epidemics, and decreasing healthcare costs.

INFECTIOUS DISEASE SURVEILLANCE FOR EMPLOYEES

The one ID for which active surveillance is almost uniformly recommended for healthcare employees is tuberculosis. A detailed description of an ongoing prevention and surveillance program for tuberculosis is beyond the scope of this chapter; however, in addition to ensuring that the program is tailored to the unique aspects of risk in their own environments, institutions should develop programs that address the variable risks for exposure of individuals in differing job categories.[1] At a minimum, HCWs who have prior negative Mantoux tests should be retested annually. Staff members who, based on their job categories, are at higher risk for occupational exposures to tuberculosis (eg, critical care physicians and nurses, pulmonologists, anesthesiologists, respiratory therapists) should be tested more frequently.

EDUCATION/ORIENTATION

Employee education is another area in which the biosafety, hospital epidemiology, and occupational medicine programs should work together. New employee orientation should contain basic information about infection control and prevention and should provide detailed resources for additional information. Educational efforts should focus on the routine use of standard/universal precautions and handwashing to decrease the risk of transmitting infection. Ongoing educational programs for staff should emphasize basic tenets of infection control, such as standard/universal precautions, optimal use of personal protective devices, handwashing, vaccine safety and efficacy, and HCW illnesses that require occupational medicine evaluation (eg, conjunctivitis, varicella, zoster, other childhood illnesses, jaundice, diarrhea).

OUTBREAK INVESTIGATION

The occurrence of clusters of infections caused by the same organism is another instance where cooperation and collaboration among the occupational medicine, hospital epidemiology, and biosafety programs are essential. Depending on the type of epidemic, the hospital epidemiology team will likely conduct the "shoe-leather" studies, identify individuals at risk, and refer them to the occupational medicine service. Occupational medicine will conduct careful interviews, provide postexposure treatment as appropriate, and (in collaboration with hospital epidemiology and biosafety) try to identify factors that are associated with a risk for transmission. During an outbreak, effective communication and daily interaction among these 3 groups is essential to effective interdiction.

Exposure Management and Postexposure Treatment

The occupational medicine program plays a key role in exposure management and postexposure treatment. Again, for effective postexposure management, the occupational medicine team needs to be aligned philosophically with both the institution's hospital epidemiology team, as well as with the institution's administration.

TABLE 21-1. IMMUNIZATIONS RECOMMENDED FOR HOSPITAL EMPLOYEES

Immunization	Indications	Dose	Contraindications
Diphtheria	In an outbreak or following documented exposures for employees who have not been immunized in the past 10 years or those who lack serological evidence of immunity	0.5 mL IM of Td vaccine (tetanus and diphtheria toxoids)	Known hypersensitivity to thimerosal or any component of the vaccine
Hepatitis A	Employees working in high-risk areas (eg, dietary, cafeteria, hepatitis ward) who do not have serologic evidence of previous Hepatitis A infection	1.0 mL IM at 0 and 6 to 12 months	Known hypersensitivity to any component of the vaccine
Hepatitis B	All employees at risk for occupational exposure to blood or body fluids	1.0 mL IM (deltoid) at 0, 1, and 6 months	Yeast sensitivity/allergy
Influenza	All hospital employees	0.5 mL IM annually	History of anaphylactic reaction to eggs or prior doses of flu vaccine
Measles*	Employees who have never had physician-diagnosed measles or laboratory evidence of immunity	0.5 mL SC of trivalent MMR vaccine	Pregnancy, history of anaphylactic reaction to eggs or neomycin, severe febrile illness, immunosuppression, recent receipt of IV immunoglobulin
Mumps*	Employees who have never had physician-diagnosed mumps, laboratory evidence of immunity, or proof of vaccination on or after their first birthday	As for measles (above)	As for measles (above)
Meningococcus	In institutional outbreak caused by organism of the A, C, Y, or W-135 strains, vaccination may be useful	0.5 mL of reconstituted vaccine	Safety in pregnancy uncertain; sensitivity to thimerosal or any other component of the vaccine
Pneumococcus	Employees older than 65 years of age or who have underlying cardiac, pulmonary, liver, renal, or immuno-compromising disease	0.5 mL SC or IM; booster dose	Safety in pregnancy undocumented

TABLE 21-1. IMMUNIZATIONS RECOMMENDED FOR HOSPITAL EMPLOYEES (CONTINUED)

Immunization	Indications	Dose	Contraindications
Rubella	Employees who have never received the live vaccine on or after their first birthday or who do not have serological proof of immunity	As for measles (above)	As for measles (above)
Tetanus	Employees who sustain tetanus-prone wounds, those who never completed the initial series, and those who have not received a booster dose within 10 years	Initial series: 0.5 mL IM of tetanus-diphtheria toxoid at 0, 1, and 6 to 12 months booster: 0.5 mL IM	History of neurological or hypersensitivity reaction following a previous dose; first trimester of pregnancy
Varicella	Employees with patient contact who have no history of chickenpox and negative varicella titer**	0.5 mL at 0 and 4 to 8 weeks	Hypersensitivity to vaccine, gelatin, neomycin; immunosuppression or immunodeficiency; active TB; febrile, illness; pregnancy

ICU = intensive care unit; IM = intramuscular; SC = subcutaneous; IV = intravenous; TB = tuberculosis
* HCWs who have never received measles vaccine and have no history of immunity to measles require 2 doses of MMR, separated by no less than 1 month.
** Current USPHS/CDC/Advisory Committee on Immunization practices recommendation.

Hepatitis A Virus

Hepatitis A virus (HAV) is not commonly transmitted in the hospital. Transmission occurs from individuals who are acutely infected (there is no carrier state in HAV infection). Instances in which HAV has been transmitted in healthcare institutions include transmission from neonates to staff members (because the disease is most often accompanied by few signs or symptoms in the very young), transmission from individuals incubating the disease who are hospitalized for other reasons, and rare instances of transfusion-transmitted infection.[2]

Transmission

HAV is transmitted primarily via the fecal-oral route. Peak infectivity for HAV occurs at the time when fecal excretion of HAV is greatest. Peak fecal excretion occurs during the incubation period (prior to the development of clinical signs and symptoms and jaundice, when it occurs). Whereas infants often shed the virus in their stools for weeks or months, most adult patients no longer shed virus by the time they develop signs and symptoms consistent with hepatitis.

Criteria for Exposure

Those employees at greatest risk for infection include:
➤ Hospital employees exposed to the stool or gastric contents of patients shedding HAV
➤ Patrons consuming food not cooked since being prepared by an individual shedding HAV
➤ Close or intimate contact with friends or family members shedding HAV in their stool

Postexposure Prophylaxis

Though the CDC does not recommend routine postexposure prophylaxis for HCWs exposed to patients infected with HAV, at the Clinical Center of the National Institutes of Health, we do provide postexposure prophylaxis with standard immune serum globulin (ISG) (0.02 mL/kg intramuscularly) for HCWs who meet the criteria for exposure outlined above. Depending on the timing of exposure, consider determining the exposed HCW's anti-HAV status prior to administering immunoglobulin. At a minimum, a baseline HAV serology should be drawn prior to treatment. If time permits serological testing, ISG need not be administered to individuals who have positive HAV serologies. Again, based on the clinical circumstance, one could also consider immunization with the HAV vaccine. Whereas the HAV vaccine is not routinely indicated for HCWs, its use may be prudent for employees who have a high likelihood of recurring exposure. If given within 2 weeks of exposure, ISG prevents disease or lessens the severity of clinical illness with approximately 80% to 90% efficacy. Occupational medicine providers should obtain follow-up for any exposed individual who develops clinical illness and should routinely follow up with all exposed personnel 2 to 3 months following the exposure event with anti-HAV serologies. If anti-HAV is positive, staff should evaluate for IgM anti-HAV to document recent infection.

Control Measures

HCWs known or suspected of having HAV infection should be relieved of patient care duties. If infection is confirmed, the HCW should not return to patient care duties until 7 days after clinical signs and symptoms have resolved. To prevent HAV transmission to others, HCWs should be instructed to use meticulous hygiene (ie, handwashing, use of gloves, no food preparation or food sharing).

Hepatitis B Virus

Prior to the development of the hepatitis B virus (HBV) vaccine, hepatitis B represented one of the most significant workplace risks for healthcare providers. As a result of exposures to HBV in the workplace, HCWs were at significantly increased risk for HBV infection when compared to the population at large.

Transmission

HBV is transmitted parenterally, with percutaneous exposure to infected blood the most important mode of occupational transmission. Mucous membrane exposure also may result in infection. HBV also can be transmitted sexually and perinatally. Both acutely and chronically infected individuals transmit infection, with those infected individuals who have "e" antigen (HBeAg) representing the largest risk for infection. The risk for transmission of HBV following a parenteral exposure to blood from an "e" antigen-positive patient is 27% to 43% per exposure; whereas the risk associated with exposure to blood from a hepatitis B surface antigen (HBsAg) positive, but HBeAg negative, individual is approximately 6% to 10%.[2]

Criteria for Exposure

Any worker who sustains a percutaneous, mucous membrane, or nonintact skin exposure to blood or body fluids that may contain blood from an HBsAg-positive patient (or a patient whose HBV serologies cannot be determined) should be considered exposed. Source patients with unknown serologies should be tested as soon as possible after the exposure.

Postexposure Prophylaxis

If a HCW who has not been immunized with the HBV vaccine sustains an occupational exposure to HBV, the worker should be given 0.06 mL/kg of hepatitis B immune globulin (HBIG) intramuscularly (IM). Ideally, this first dose should be administered within 24 hours of the exposure. The first dose of the HBV vaccine series should be administered at the same time, followed by additional doses 1 and 6 months later. Prior to treatment, a baseline anti-HBs level should be drawn. If positive, no additional treatment is indicated. For previously vaccinated HCWs, an anti-HBs level should be drawn and measured. Workers whose anti-HBs levels are ≥10 mIU/mL are protected. Although not routinely recommended by the CDC, we administer a booster dose of HBV vaccine to employees who are known to have had protective antibody levels but whose levels have fallen below 10 mIU/mL. Employees who have antibody levels below 10 mIU/mL and who were never demonstrated to have made an adequate vaccine response should be treated as if they had not responded (ie, they should be given both a single dose of HBIG and a vaccine booster). For employees who for some reason cannot be vaccinated, a second dose of HBIG should be administered 1 month following the first.[2,3]

Control Measures

Universal vaccination of HCWs against HBV should be the primary goal of the occupational medicine service. Vaccination of HCWs, which provides immunity in ≥93% of vaccinees, should mitigate the risk for HBV transmission from patients to providers. Whereas patient-to-provider transmission occurs far more frequently than does provider-to-patient transmission, the latter type of transmission does occur, particularly when the provider is HBeAg positive and conducts invasive procedures. More than 400 instances of iatrogenic HBV transmission have been reported in the literature. Current US Public Health Service guidelines recommend restricting the practices of HCWs who are HBeAg positive.[4]

Hepatitis C Virus

HCWs are at risk for hepatitis C virus (HCV) infection as a result of parenteral or mucous membrane exposures to blood from patients infected with HCV.[5] A significant proportion of individuals who develop productive HCV infection develop chronic infection and are at risk for serious sequelae, such as chronic active hepatitis, cirrhosis, hepatocellular carcinoma, and death.

Transmission

Occupational risk for HCV transmission is likely linked to the same routes of transmission as those for HBV. Occupational HCV infection has been most frequently associated with parenteral exposures. A few instances of mucous membrane transmission have been reported, and a risk for unapparent parenteral transmission (due to exposure of nonintact skin to blood of an HCV-infected individual) likely also occurs, albeit at a substantially lower rate than is the case for HBV. The risk for occupational infection associated with a single parenteral exposure has been estimated at approximately 2%.[5]

Criteria for Exposure

Occupational medicine staff should consider any HCW who has sustained a percutaneous, mucous membrane, or nonintact skin exposure to the blood or body fluid potentially containing blood from an HCV-infected patient as having been exposed. As is the case for HBV infection, in instances in which the source patient for an exposure is unknown, cannot be tested, or is known to have epidemiological risk factors associated with HCV infection, the worker also should be considered exposed.

Postexposure Management

All HCV-exposed individuals should be tested for aminotransferases (alanine and aspartate) as well as for HCV antibody with a sensitive and specific antibody test at baseline and again at least 15 weeks after exposure. The HCW also should be encouraged to seek prompt medical attention for any symptoms suggestive of systemic illness or acute hepatitis. Immune serum globulin should not be administered for occupational exposures to HCV. Neutralizing antibodies to HCV are highly strain specific and have not been shown to afford protection against reinfection. Additionally, even if antibody were protective, donors for current immune globulin preparations are screened for hepatitis C antibody and are eliminated from the donor pool if found to be anti-HCV positive. HCV infection also has been associated with the administration of HCV-contaminated intravenous immunoglobulin (IVIG) in 2 clusters. Some investigators have advocated using PCR technology to monitor exposed HCWs for HCV RNA and then using immunomodulators to treat the HCWs who become infected. Both "pre-emptive therapy" and "watchful waiting" strategies have been proposed as reasonable strategies for postexposure management.[5] As yet, data from studies of HCWs treated with these approaches are too preliminary to provide the basis for formal recommendation for an optimal management strategy.

Control Measures

Avoidance of exposures through the routine use of universal/standard precautions is the only effective preventive strategy currently available. Iatrogenic transmission of HCV from providers to their patients has been uncommon, particularly in the United States. The experience in the United Kingdom has been quite distinctive, in that HCV transmission from providers to patients seems to be occurring at higher rates than in the United States. Although the limited data available effectively preclude

identifying factors associated with risk for iatrogenic transmission, the fact that 2 gynecologists, 3 cardiac or thoracic surgeons, and an orthopedic surgeon are involved in reported cases suggest that risk factors for transmission are likely to be similar to those identified for HBV transmission. Due to several clusters of provider-to-patient transmission of HCV in the United Kingdom, U.K. public health authorities have issued practice restrictions for HCV-infected providers. In the United States, neither the US Public Health Service nor professional organizations have, at least as yet, recommended restricting the practices of HCV-infected providers.

Human Immunodeficiency Virus

The magnitude of risk from each exposure to HIV is approximately 0.3% per parenteral exposure.[6-8] Though this risk is substantially smaller than those for other bloodborne infections, the consequences of infection are life altering.[7,8]

Transmission

HIV is transmitted parenterally, sexually, and vertically (across the placenta, perinatally, or via breastfeeding). Occupational transmission has been reported after percutaneous, mucous membrane, and nonintact skin exposure to HIV-infected blood. HIV is present in much lower amounts in other blood cell-containing body fluids, including inflammatory exudates, amniotic fluid, saliva, and vaginal secretions. The risk of seroconversion following mucous membrane or nonintact skin exposure is too low to be estimated with precision.

Criteria for Exposure

Any HCW who has sustained a percutaneous, mucous membrane, or nonintact skin exposure to blood or body fluid potentially containing blood from an HIV-infected patient should be considered exposed. The risk for infection associated with any discrete exposure depends on a number of variables including inoculum size, exposure severity, and the stage of the source patient's illness (ie, circulating viral burden).

Postexposure Management and Postexposure Antiretroviral Prophylaxis

The efficacy of antiretroviral chemoprophylaxis for occupational HIV exposure will likely never be definitively established in a prospective clinical trial. Nonetheless, a variety of types of studies provide indirect evidence of the efficacy of postexposure prophylaxis.[7,8] Current US Public Health Service recommendations for post-exposure prophylaxis are included in Table 21-2,[3] and recommended antiretroviral regimens are detailed in Table 21-3.[3] The fact that treatment is immediately accessible should be widely publicized throughout the institution. All employees should be aware of the postexposure prophylaxis program and how it works. Occupational medicine staff mem-

TABLE 21-2. CENTERS FOR DISEASE CONTROL AND PREVENTION RECOMMENDATIONS FOR POSTEXPOSURE PROPHYLAXIS FOR PERCUTANEOUS, MUCOUS MEMBRANE, AND NONINTACT SKIN EXPOSURES TO HIV

Exposure Type	HIV-Positive, Class 1[a] — Asymptomatic HIV infection or known low viral load (eg, <1500)	HIV-Positive, Class 2[a] — Symptomatic HIV infection, AIDS, acute seroconversion, or known high viral load	HIV Status or Source Unknown	HIV-Negative
Less severe percutaneous exposure, (eg, solid needle, superficial injury)	Recommend basic PEP	Recommend expanded PEP	Generally, no PEP warranted; consider basic PEP[b] for source with HIV risk factors[c]	No PEP warranted
More severe percutaneous exposure (eg, large-bore hollow needle, deep puncture, visible blood on device, or needle used in patient's artery or vein)	Recommend expanded PEP	Recommend expanded PEP	Generally, no PEP warranted; consider basic PEP[b] for source with HIV risk factors[c]	No PEP warranted
Small volume mucous membrane/nonintact skin exposure (eg, few drops or brief contact)	Consider basic PEP[b]	Recommend basic PEP	Generally, no PEP warranted; consider basic PEP[b] for source with HIV risk factors[c]	No PEP warranted
Large volume mucous membrane/nonintact skin exposure (eg, major blood splash or prolonged contact)	Recommend basic PEP	Recommend expanded[d] PEP	Generally, no PEP warranted; consider basic PEP[b] for source with HIV risk factors[c]	No PEP warranted

[a] If drug resistance is a concern, obtain expert consultation. Initiation of PEP should not be delayed pending expert consultation, and, because expert consultation alone cannot substitute for face-to-face counseling, resources should be available to provide immediate evaluation and follow-up care.

[b] The designation "consider PEP" indicates that PEP is optional and should be based on an individualized decision between the exposed health-care worker and the treating clinician.

[c] If PEP is offered and taken, and the source is later determined to be HIV-negative, PEP should be discontinued.

[d] For a discussion of "basic" and "expanded" PEP, see Table 21-3.

Adapted from Centers for Disease Control and Prevention. Updated U.S. Public Health Service guidelines for the management of occupational exposures to HBV, HCV, and HIV and recommendations for postexposure prophylaxis. *MMWR.* 2001;50(RR-11):1-52.

TABLE 21-3. CURRENT US PUBLIC HEALTH SERVICE RECOMMENDATIONS FOR BASIC AND EXPANDED CHEMOPROPHYLAXIS REGIMENS FOR OCCUPATIONAL EXPOSURES TO HIV

HIV exposures with a recognized transmission risk	"Basic Regimen"	Zidovudine (ZDV) (GlaxoSmithKline Inc, Philadelphia, Pa) plus Lamivudine (3TC) (GlaxoSmithKline, Inc, Philadelphia, Pa)
	Alternative "Basic Regimen"	Stavudine (d4t) (Bristol-Myers Squibb, Inc, Princeton, NJ) plus Lamivudine d4t plus Didanosine (ddI)[b,c] (Bristol-Myers Squibb, Inc, Princeton, NJ)
HIV exposures for which the nature of the exposure suggests an elevated transmission risk[a]	A "Basic Regimen" plus one of the following agents	Indinavir[b] (Merck Inc, White House Station, NJ) Nelfinavir (Agouron Pharmaceuticals, La Jolla, Calif) Abacavir (GlaxoSmithKline Inc, Philadelphia, Pa) or Efavirenz (Bristol-Myers Squibb, Inc, Princeton, NJ)[b,d]

[a] Elevated risk is associated with "larger" volume of blood and/or blood containing a high titer of HIV.

[b] Agent(s) not advisable for use in pregnancy.

[c] New recommendations (due for publication in 2004) will likely include additional basic regimens, incorporating newly marketed antiretrovirals, such as Tenofovir (Gilead Sciences, Foster City, Calif), boosted protease inhibitors, and emtricitabine

[d] New recommendations (due for publication in 2004) will likely include additional agents and combinations for the "expanded" regimen that incorporate newly marketed antiretrovirals, such as Tenofovir, boosted protease inhibitors, Emtricitabine (Gilead Sciences, Foster City, Calif), and, perhaps, Fuzeon (Roche Laboratories, Nutley, NJ).

Adapted from Centers for Disease Control and Prevention. Updated U.S. Public Health Service guidelines for the management of occupational exposures to HBV, HCV, and HIV and recommendations for postexposure prophylaxis. *MMWR.* 2001;50(RR-11):1-52.

bers have to be very familiar with what constitutes an exposure and must make certain that they do not over-prescribe antiretrovirals. Prescribing physicians should carefully choose a regimen that can be taken by the HCW. Prescribing staff also need to be cognizant of the source-patient's therapy and viral burden (when this information is immediately available) and should use this information in developing an optimal regimen. If the prescriber is not familiar with the primary or alternative agents, he or she should get assistance from ID physicians who are used to prescribing antiretrovirals. To the extent that it is possible, prescribers should become familiar with the agents, their side effects, and the appropriate strategies to manage toxicity. Prescribing staff also should carefully monitor all HCWs who are taking antiretrovirals for the development of signs of toxicity as well as for adherence to the regimen.

The occupational medical service should also have ready access to (and frequently should seek the advice of) expert consultants. If no experts are immediately available, the CDC/University of California PEPline is available either by telephone at (888) 448-4911 or via the Internet at http://pepline.ucsf.edu/pepline.

Other Considerations

Several additional issues must be taken into consideration when considering postexposure chemoprophylaxis. Counseling and serologic testing of exposed personnel should be performed as soon as possible after exposure. These services should be available 24 hours per day. All personnel involved in postexposure evaluation and counseling, including emergency room workers, must be trained in and familiar with institutional protocols. Follow-up serologic testing should be performed at 6 weeks, 3 months, and 6 months after the exposure. Exposed workers should be instructed to return immediately for clinical evaluation if they develop signs or symptoms of either drug toxicity or of the acute retroviral infection (eg, fever, rash, lymphadenopathy). Occupational HIV exposure can cause severe psychological symptoms, including depression, anxiety, anger, fear, sleep disturbances, conversion symptoms, suicidal ideation, and psychosis. Postexposure counselors should be alert to these possibilities and be quick to refer the employee to specialists in crisis intervention and counseling, if necessary.

Provider-to-Patient Transmission

Transmission of HIV from HCW to patient occurs extremely uncommonly.[7,8] Current US Public Health Guidelines recommend that individual states construct guidelines that are equivalent to the published CDC guidelines of 1991.[4] Although individual state guidelines vary markedly, some include restricting the practices of HIV-infected providers who perform what CDC termed "exposure-prone" procedures. The CDC guidelines clearly recommend that HIV-infected HCWs who do not perform "exposure-prone invasive procedures" need not have their practices restricted.

Cytomegalovirus

Cytomegalovirus (CMV) is a member of the herpes virus family that may be transmitted from patients to hospital employees, but the risk for nosocomial transmission is so small that it has never been measured or estimated. Infants and immunosuppressed patients (eg, HIV-infected patients, bone marrow/stem cell and organ transplantation patients) serve as the largest reservoirs for CMV in the hospital.[9]

Transmission

CMV is transmitted by several routes: direct contact, sexual contact, congenitally, and by transfusion. HCWs most likely become infected by direct inoculation when their hands become contaminated with infected bodily fluid and they touch the mucous membranes in their mouths, noses, or eyes. CMV can be found in the blood, urine, saliva, respiratory secretions, tears, feces, breast milk, semen, and cervical secretions of infected patients.

Control Measures

If hospital personnel follow recommended handwashing and infection control practices, their risk of acquiring CMV is miniscule. Available data suggest that staff who work regularly with adult patients who are likely to shed CMV in large amounts (eg, end-stage HIV-infected patients, severely immunosuppressed, oncology, or transplant patients) are no more likely to contract CMV than employees who do not have patient contact. Data regarding the risk of CMV infection from working closely with pediatric patients, who also may shed virus, are contradic-

tory, but, to my knowledge, transmission has never been definitively established. Screening employees for evidence of previous CMV infection is neither practical nor cost effective and is not recommended. Because primary infection with CMV during pregnancy may be associated with fetal damage, some institutions allow CMV-naïve pregnant employees the opportunity to transfer to "lower risk" units if they wish, provided that staffing levels are adequate. Employees who have acute CMV-related illnesses do not need to be relieved of patient care duties. By following careful handwashing and routine infection control practices, they can prevent transmission of the virus.

Varicella-Zoster Virus

VZV is the etiologic agent of *varicella* (chickenpox) and of *H. zoster* (shingles). VZV is highly communicable and a well-recognized cause of nosocomial outbreaks among patients and employees. VZV infection is a particular problem for pediatric institutions and those institutions providing care for severely immunocompromised patients.[9]

Transmission

VZV is transmitted as a result of direct contact with respiratory secretions or vesicle fluid and via the airborne route, through inhalation of small particle aerosols produced by patients who have varicella and disseminated zoster infection. For patients who have classical dermatomal zoster, most authorities believe that transmission occurs only following direct contact with vesicular fluid containing the virus. The incubation period for primary infection is 11 to 20 days. Viral shedding occurs during late incubation (2 to 3 days prior to the eruption of cutaneous lesions). For this reason, patients who have varicella should be considered infectious from 48 hours (at a minimum) before lesion onset to the time the lesions crust over. Patients and employees who have dermatomal zoster should be considered infectious from 24 hours prior to the appearance of the first lesion to the time the lesions crust over.

Criteria for Exposure

Any household contact of a person who has a systemic infection with VZV (ie, either chickenpox or disseminated zoster) should be considered to be exposed. Any employee who worked either face-to-face, in the same room, or at an adjacent bed on a larger ward of a patient with a varicella or disseminated zoster patient should be considered potentially exposed. HCWs who have prolonged contact with the patient's clothing or bedding, as during changing of bed linens or a bed bath, may also be exposed to vesicular fluid containing the virus, and, therefore, should also be considered as potentially exposed.

Postexposure Prophylaxis

Varicella-zoster immune globulin is available for postexposure prophylaxis of exposed individuals who are at risk for serious sequelae of primary infection. If administered within 96 hours of exposure, VZIG (125 units/10 kg up to a total of 625 units) modifies and attenuates disease rather than prevents infection. If the exposed employee does not report a history of chickenpox, a sensitive serology should be obtained. Exposed employees who do not have measurable antibody should be considered candidates for VZIG or immunization with the VZV vaccine. All immunocompromised seronegative contacts, irrespective of age, and all exposed nonimmunocompromised susceptible pregnant women should receive VZIG. VZIG administration may prolong the incubation period for up to 28 days. Susceptible, exposed, hospitalized patients who cannot be discharged should be maintained in isolation for the full period.

Control Measures

Exposed employees should be placed on work restriction or furloughed from day 8 to day 21 postexposure (day 28 if VZIG is given). Work restrictions should include no direct patient contact, a requirement to work only with immune individuals, no attendance at group meetings, avoiding use of the cafeteria and other common areas, and entering and exiting the hospital by the shortest and safest route (ie, not through the lobby). For some hospitals, VZV outbreaks and potential outbreaks are frequent, costly, time-consuming, and labor-intensive. Each occupational medicine service should tailor its program to the specific needs of the hospital. Some settings (eg, pediatrics hospitals, oncology centers) prospectively determine each employee's VZV immune status. This approach will almost unquestionably be cost effective in such settings. Development of a systematic approach to a potential outbreak is the key to a successful investigation.[9] For postexposure management, VZIG is now more widely available. The VZV vaccine is also available; however, its role in postexposure management is not yet clear. Approximately 5% of adults are susceptible; however, there are substantial geographical variations in the endemic rate of primary infection. Because of the distinctive nature of the viral exanthem, the HCW's VZV history is reasonably reliable (approximately 98% sensitive). The VZV vaccine is efficacious in immunocompetent children, although breakthrough infection does occur (ie, in the setting of a household exposure). When breakthrough infection occurs, the disease is often attenuated. Vaccine efficacy in adults is less clear, although the vaccine is recommended by the US Public Health Service for use in susceptible HCWs.

Herpes Simplex Virus

Herpetic whitlow and other localized herpes simplex virus (HSV) infections occur after occupational exposure, but serious or disseminated HSV disease from occupational exposure is unlikely in immunocompetent employees. However, hospital employees can transmit HSV infections to high-risk patients with serious consequences.[9]

Transmission

Transmission of HSV occurs through direct contact with open lesions or body fluids from individuals shedding the virus.

Control Measures

Because parents with *Herpes labialis* can transmit the virus to infants, these parents should not kiss infants. Employees also should not work with infants or immunocompromised hosts during active *H. labialis* episodes. Similarly, employees with herpetic whitlow should not care for immunosuppressed patients until the lesion has healed. Although such employees probably do not pose a significant risk to patients if they wear gloves, the risk of transmission in this setting has not been well studied.

Influenza

Both community and nosocomial outbreaks of influenza are common and cause significant morbidity and mortality, especially among elderly and immunocompromised patients. Nosocomial influenza epidemics can be caused by both influenza A and influenza B strains. An often-underappreciated aspect of an influenza epidemic is HCW absenteeism, which, in an epidemic setting, can have dramatic implications for patient safety.

Transmission

Influenza is transmitted via small-particle aerosols. Viral shedding begins approximately 24 hours before onset of symptoms and can continue for up to 10 days. Young children may be infectious for even longer periods of time. Because one infected patient may transmit the infection to many others, nosocomial outbreaks can be explosive and can result in serious morbidity and mortality.

Control Measures

Prevention of influenza among hospital employees depends on the success of the institution's annual immunization campaign. Vaccine efficacy in HCWs has been definitively demonstrated in a placebo-controlled trial published by Wilde and colleagues in 1999.[10] Vaccination of high-risk patients prior to influenza season also is essential. In another study, HCW vaccination was associated with a substantial decrease in mortality among elderly, at-risk patients.[11] Early recognition of influenza combined with droplet isolation precautions for suspected or confirmed cases is critical in the prevention of nosocomial outbreaks. Once an outbreak occurs, all at-risk individuals should receive chemoprophylaxis (ie, with rimantadine, oseltamivir, or amantidine) as well as the influenza vaccine. Chemoprophylaxis should be administered for 14 days following immunization. HCWs who refuse vaccination should take rimantadine 100 mg/day or oseltamivir

75 mg/twice daily until the epidemic subsides. Employees who have suspected or confirmed influenza should not work until they are symptom-free and should not work for at least the first 5 to 7 days following the onset of symptoms.

Adenovirus (Epidemic Keratoconjunctivitis)

Adenovirus accounts for most highly contagious episodes of keratoconjunctivitis. Outbreaks of epidemic keratoconjunctivitis are common in hospitals, especially among personnel working in outpatient settings such as an ophthalmology clinic.

Transmission

Adenoviral keratoconjunctivitis is spread by direct contact with infected people and contaminated inanimate fomite reservoirs (eg, tonometry equipment, ophthalmologic solutions). The incubation period ranges from 4 to 24 days, and the illness lasts up to 4 weeks. The conjunctivitis often (but not always) is accompanied by upper respiratory tract symptoms and/or other systemic symptoms (eg, fever, diarrhea, myalgias).

Control Measures

Effective control measures include removing infected HCWs from direct patient care duties, emphasizing strict handwashing, and eliminating/disinfecting potential environmental reservoirs. Personnel should be educated to report to the occupational medicine service for evaluation whenever they develop conjunctivitis.

Parvovirus B19

Human parvovirus B19 causes erythema infectiosum (fifth disease) in children and an illness manifested by fever, rash, and arthropathy in adults. Most parvoviral infections are mild and self-limited (many cases are asymptomatic). People at high risk for serious disease include patients with chronic hemolytic anemia (who may develop aplastic crisis as a result of the infection); pregnant women, in whom parvovirus can cause *hydrops fetalis* and fetal demise; and immunodeficient patients, including those with HIV infection and hematologic malignancies, who may develop chronic anemia and persistent infection with the virus.

Transmission

Parvovirus B19 is found in blood and respiratory secretions from the fifth to the 15th days of the acute illness. Patients who have parvovirus detected in blood most often have systemic symptoms. Transmission occurs via direct person-to-person contact, fomites, or through inhalation of droplet nuclei carrying the virus.

Control Measures

Placing patients with known or suspected infection in droplet isolation precautions effectively prevents nosoco-

mial parvovirus transmission. Women in the first half of pregnancy should not work with patients known or suspected to be infected with parvovirus. An exposed pregnant employee should be tested for evidence of prior infection. A positive IgG titer at the time of exposure represents prior infection and immunity. Susceptible pregnant employees who are exposed should be referred to an obstetrician and followed for an IgM response (representing acute parvovirus B19 infection). Nonpregnant employees who are exposed should be observed for the development of symptoms. Employees who develop acute parvovirus B19 infection should not work until several days after symptoms resolve. No employee with suspected parvovirus B19 infection should work directly with patients at risk for serious sequelae from infection with this agent.

Respiratory Syncytial Virus, Parainfluenza, and Other Respiratory Viruses

Respiratory syncytial virus (RSV) is the most common cause of lower respiratory infection in infants and young children. RSV can cause severe and sometimes fatal illnesses, especially among infants who have cardiopulmonary disease or who are immunocompromised. During the winter, nosocomial outbreaks frequently occur in association with community outbreaks. Because completely protective antibody responses rarely develop after infection, virtually everyone is susceptible, and nosocomial RSV transmission is common. The other respiratory viruses also occur seasonally and may cause serious infection and even mortality in immunocompromised stem cell or bone marrow transplantation patients.

Transmission

Patients who have RSV infection expel large quantities of virus in secretions. RSV can survive on inanimate objects for hours. Thus, HCWs may contaminate their hands from contact with a fomite reservoir and then subsequently inoculate their own conjunctivae or nasal mucosa. Alternatively, close contact can result in transmission via large droplet nuclei that are produced when patients sneeze, cough, or talk. Patients who have parainfluenza or other respiratory virus infections usually transmit these infections though direct contact with infectious secretions.

Control Measures

Control measures include strict handwashing (whether or not gloves are worn) after contact with patients or potentially contaminated articles. HCWs also should wear masks and facial shields or eye-nose goggles (if available) for all contact with potentially RSV-infected patients. Because of the environmental risk for RSV transmission, they should wear gowns when soiling is likely. Masks alone do not completely prevent RSV transmission because they do not adequately protect the conjunctivae from viral inoculation. RSV-infected employees or those with symptoms of upper respiratory tract infection should not work with infants or young children. Cohorting patients and staff and limiting visitors (especially siblings and others with respiratory symptoms, especially during the winter months) also are important in preventing RSV transmission. For parainfluenza and other respiratory virus infections, hospital epidemiology and occupational medicine staff should pay meticulous attention to staff illness and/or minor respiratory symptoms. We recommend limiting infected individuals' personal effects in their rooms and in the institution while they are infected (to decrease the potential for inadvertent fomite spread). Finally, especially for severely immunocompromised transplant patients, the institution may limit visitors and try to keep the at-risk patients from congregating with large groups of patients or visitors.

Severe Acute Respiratory Syndrome

SARS burst onto the public health landscape in the late fall of 2002. In developed and developing countries, HCWs were at substantial risk for infection. In Toronto, for example, more than 50% of cases occurred in healthcare providers.[12] Because the virus causing this new syndrome has not previously been known to cause infection in humans, the entire population is presumed to be both immunologically naïve and susceptible.

Transmission

The coronavirus responsible for SARS is most commonly spread by direct contact, although substantial concern exists that certain infected patients (ie, "supershedders") may transmit the infection through the air via small droplet aerosols. The virus is also extremely stable in the environment (albeit easily disinfected). Thus, HCWs may become infected as a result of contamination from contact with a fomite reservoir, from direct patient care activities, and by exposure to supershedder-generated aerosols.

Control Measures

Control measures include meticulous attention to isolation and infection control policies, including strict handwashing after contact with patients or potentially contaminated articles. HCWs also should wear particulate respirators or powered, air-purifying respirators when in the room with an infected patient. Because of the environmental risk, special procedures should be developed for decontaminating items from the patients' rooms. In epidemic settings, cohorting patients and staff and excluding visitors are important in preventing SARS transmission.

Measles, Mumps, and Rubella

A resurgence of measles in the United States began in 1989 and has been associated with an increase in measles transmission in hospitals. Similarly, rubella outbreaks have increased in frequency and have often involved nosocomial transmission. Importantly, index cases in many nosocomial rubella outbreaks are employees, rather than patients. Because rubella can devastate the fetus during the first trimester of pregnancy, hospital outbreaks can have major medical and financial sequelae. Mumps incidence has increased since 1987, largely on college campuses, although hospital transmission also occurs.

Transmission

Measles, one of the most highly communicable of all IDs, is transmitted by aerosol. Measles can be transmitted from an index case to susceptibles by aerosol over extremely large distances, presumably because only a very small number of viral particles are needed to cause infection. Viral shedding begins 9 to 10 days after exposure and lasts for up to 10 days. Rubella also is highly communicable, but is spread by direct contact with infectious nasopharyngeal secretions. Infected individuals can shed virus for up to 1 week before they develop the rash. Asymptomatic people may both shed virus and transmit disease. Adults shed virus for approximately 4 days after rash onset, but infants with congenital rubella syndrome can shed virus for months. Mumps is spread by droplet nuclei and by direct contact with the saliva of infected people. Viral shedding may occur for up to 9 days before parotitis develops and for an equal period thereafter.

Control Measures

Employees can be protected from MMR by appropriate vaccination. Routine serologic screening of employees for immunity to these pathogens is not cost effective, and no increased risk is involved in giving MMR to immune individuals. Immunocompro-mised people who cannot receive live virus vaccines (with the exception of HIV-infected people, who are candidates for MMR) may be protected from severe measles infection if they receive immunoglobulin within 3 days after a documented exposure. Pregnant employees who are seronegative for rubella should not work with patients suspected of having rubella infection and should be relieved from patient care duties during rubella outbreaks. Due to theoretical risk of the rubella vaccine to the fetus, women of childbearing age should not receive the vaccine unless they are known not to be pregnant. Susceptible pregnant employees who are exposed to patients with rubella should be referred to their obstetrician for careful follow-up, including testing for anti-rubella IgM, which indicates acute infection. Employees with measles, rubella, or mumps infection should not care for patients until 7 days after the rash appears for measles, until 5 days after the rash appears for rubella, or until 9 days after the onset of parotitis for mumps. Susceptible personnel who are exposed to the above pathogens should be relieved from patient care duties from days 5 through 21 after exposure for measles, from days 7 through 21 after exposure for rubella, and from days 5 through 26 after exposure for mumps.

Meningococcal Meningitis and Meningococcemia

N. meningitidis transmission in the hospital setting is extremely uncommon, but the potentially devastating nature of meningococcal disease produces a great deal of concern and anxiety whenever a meningococcal infection is diagnosed.

Transmission

N. meningitidis is transmitted by direct contact with respiratory secretions or by direct contact with cultures of the organism. Risk from casual or brief contact with infected patients is minimal. Transmission within the hospital is rare. Patients are infectious for 24 to 48 hours after appropriate antibiotic therapy is initiated.

Criteria for Exposure

Only employees who have direct contact with infected respiratory secretions or laboratory employees who inadvertently handle *N. meningitidis* cultures without using appropriate protection (gowns and gloves for routine procedures and biologic safety cabinet for procedures that may aerosolize organisms) require chemoprophylaxis. HCWs who have only typical institutional exposures to patients who have meningococcal disease are not felt to be at risk for infection. Exposed staff who have sustained "intimate" exposure to respiratory secretions (eg, those performing "mouth-to-mouth" resuscitation) should be offered chemoprophylaxis. Chemoprophylaxis often is requested by many more employees than have been meaningfully exposed.

Postexposure Prophylaxis

Exposed HCWs can be treated with rifampin (600 mg orally twice daily for 2 days), ciprofloxacin (500 to 750 mg orally), ceftriaxone (250 mg IM or IV), or azithromycin (500 mg orally). Due to its ease of delivery, single-dose ciprofloxacin has replaced rifampin as the prophylactic therapy of choice at many institutions. However, ciprofloxacin should not be administered to children or pregnant women. Employees taking rifampin should be warned about red urine, stained contact lenses, and the adverse interaction with contraceptives resulting in lower, often ineffective levels. Laboratory employees who sustain percutaneous exposure to *N. meningitidis* require penicillin (rather than rifampin) prophylaxis. Susceptibility testing should be performed on all isolates to ensure effective chemoprophylaxis. Immunization of hospital personnel offers no further benefit after chemoprophylaxis for sporadic cases of meningococcal disease; however, in epidemics known to be caused by serotypes A, C, Y, or W-135, quadrivalent vaccine may be administered. More highly immunogenic conjugate vaccines are in efficacy trials;

serotype B vaccines derived from outer-membrane protein vesicles containing serotype B lipooligosaccharide are also in development.

Control Measures

Patients who have meningococcal disease should be placed on droplet isolation precautions (a negative pressure room is not required) for the first 24 to 48 hours of antibiotic therapy, despite the low risk of nosocomial transmission. The local health department should be notified to arrange prophylaxis of household and community contacts.

Methicillin-Resistant and Vancomycin-Resistant Staphylococcus aureus

MRSA infection and carriage have increased dramatically during the past decade. These isolates have become major endemic pathogens in many healthcare institutions. Although hospital employees do not appear to be at substantial risk for acquiring serious staphylococcal disease from patients, patients can develop infections after contact with employees who are MRSA carriers. Only a few strains of VRSA have been identified to date. Nonetheless, the specter of an epidemic of nosocomial VRSA infections is a frightening thought. Patients or staff infected with these isolates should be managed with extreme caution.

Transmission

S. aureus is transmitted primarily by direct contact. HCWs who are transient carriers can transmit MRSA among colonized and susceptible patients. Less commonly, HCWs who are chronically colonized or infected may transmit MRSA to patients. The anterior nares are the primary reservoir for MRSA, but the axilla, hands, and perineum also can be colonized.

Control Measures

During nosocomial outbreaks, cultures should be obtained of the hands and anterior nares of HCWs who are epidemiologically linked to infected patients, and MRSA-colonized employees should be treated. Mupirocin (1 cm length of ointment twice daily intranasally for 5 days) eliminates carriage in most employees, although resistance may emerge, and many recolonize over time. Employees who have skin conditions or upper respiratory infections and who are known MRSA carriers are at risk of becoming significant disseminators. Such individuals should receive appropriate medical care and should be managed on a case-by-case basis by occupational medicine staff.

Group A Streptococci

Whereas pharyngitis and skin infections are the most common manifestations of group A streptococcal infection, invasive disease is increasing in frequency.

Nosocomial group A streptococcal outbreaks have been linked to employees who were infected or colonized.

Transmission

Transmission occurs following direct contact with infected secretions, although airborne spread is also likely, as suggested in outbreaks associated with rectal, vaginal, and scalp carriers.

Control Measures

When a nosocomial case of group A streptococcal disease is identified, an investigation should be instituted to locate carriers. Only employees who are epidemiologically linked to cases should have cultures obtained. Pharyngeal, rectal, vaginal, and skin lesion cultures should be obtained. If culture-positive and epidemiologically linked to transmission, an employee should be removed from patient care until carriage is eliminated. Oral or intramuscular penicillin are the treatments of choice; erythromycin is an effective alternative.

Diphtheria

Although increasing in frequency in parts of the developing world (eg, parts of the former Soviet Union), diphtheria is extremely rare in the United States. Nonetheless, one recent study suggests that adult immunity to diphtheria is waning in the United States,[13] so the risk for nosocomial transmission, should a case be hospitalized, is clearly increasing. In one study, only 60.5% of Americans over the age of 6 had protective levels of diphtheria antibody; among people 70 years of age, only 30% had protective levels of antibody against diphtheria.[13]

Transmission

Transmission occurs following direct contact with infected secretions.

Control Measures

HCWs in the United States have generally been vaccinated with diphtheria toxoid and will likely have some immunological memory. Patients with classic diphtheria should be placed on strict isolation precautions. Patients who have skin/wound diphtheria should be placed on contact isolation precautions. Use of recommended barrier precautions in combination with universal/standard precautions should limit the risk for occupational acquisition.

Postexposure Management

No clear recommendations have been made for management of HCWs exposed to diphtheria; however, if one applies recommendations for "close contacts," one should boost with adult-dose Td vaccine (tetanus-diphtheria toxoids) if the individual has not been immunized within the past 5 years. In addition, exposed HCWs who are uncertain about diphtheria immunity should be given erythromycin, 1000 mg daily, orally, in 4 doses of 250 mg each, for 7 to 10 days. Benzathine penicillin 1.2 MU intramuscularly is an acceptable alternative.[14]

Pertussis

Pertussis is also reasonably uncommon in the United States; however, adult cases reported to CDC increased in the 1990s by approximately 4 fold. As is the case with diphtheria, adult immunity to pertussis is frequently inadequate. Recent studies of adults who have persistent cough for more than 2 weeks (both in the community and HCWs in particular) demonstrated that up to 15% of HCWs and 25% of adults in the community have pertussis as the most likely etiology for their coughs (based on serological evidence).

Transmission

Transmission occurs following direct contact with infected secretions.

Control Measures

Patients with pertussis should be placed on respiratory isolation (ie, routine use of gloves and mask) until 7 days after effective antibiotic therapy has been administered. Use of standard barrier precautions in combination with universal/standard precautions should limit the risk for occupational acquisition.

Postexposure Management

As was the case for diphtheria, no definitive recommendations have been made for management of HCWs sustaining occupational exposure to pertussis; however, if one applies recommendations for "close contacts," occupational medicine staff should administer azithromycin 500 mg orally, followed by 250 mg orally, once daily for 5 days. Clarithromycin is also effective. Both newer macrolides are better tolerated than erythromycin. Boosting HCWs with the acellular vaccine may ultimately present a reasonable alternative to antimicrobial chemoprophylaxis, although this vaccine is not yet approved for use in adults and its use in this setting should be considered experimental. In the United States, the acellular vaccine is only available in combination with other toxoids (eg, diphtheria, tetanus).

Tuberculosis

The national incidence of tuberculosis increased during the AIDS epidemic, but is once again on the decline, except in certain municipal areas. Nonetheless, because of its ability to spread insidiously, the disease remains as a major concern for occupational medicine practitioners. Reports of nosocomial transmission of MDR tuberculosis are even more alarming and require increased vigilance to protect hospital employees. As noted previously, institutions should develop comprehensive respiratory protection programs for their workers.

Transmission

M. tuberculosis is transmitted by droplet nuclei produced during expiratory efforts (coughing, sneezing, talking) of patients who have pulmonary or laryngeal tuberculosis.

Criteria for Exposure

Any close or even casual (ie, same ward or clinic) contact with an infectious (smear-positive) patient who is not appropriately isolated should be considered a potential exposure. Each exposure scenario should be evaluated individually, as some circumstances may present substantially lower levels of risk.

Control Measures

In the hierarchy of controls, administrative controls (ie, maintaining a high index of suspicion for the diagnosis of tuberculosis, developing and implementing policies and procedures that place patients in isolation until the diagnosis is excluded) are by far the most effective in protecting employees from work-related tuberculosis exposure and infection. Engineering controls (eg, appropriately constructed isolation rooms that have negative pressure air flow and more than 12 air changes an hour) are next in importance. In instances in which exposures occur, exposed employees should undergo Mantoux tuberculin skin testing at baseline and then 6 weeks after exposure. Skin test converters should be treated according to currently published US Public Health Service guidelines.[1] The occupational medicine program should use expert IDs consultant assistance to assist with the management of employees who convert their PPD after exposure to a patient with MDR tuberculosis. Because MDR-tuberculosis infection usually is rapidly fatal in HIV-positive people, employees infected with HIV who work in areas of high MDR-tuberculosis prevalence should be advised against working with high-risk patient populations (eg, AIDS and pulmonary patients).

CONCLUSION

HCWs regularly place themselves at risk for occupational infections as a result of caring for patients. As our understanding of the pathogenesis and epidemiology of these IDs has increased, we have been able to develop more effective strategies to protect the HCW from occupational infection. As additional information about these syndromes is gathered, guidelines and recommendations will continue to be modified. To maintain state-of-the-art protection strategies, personnel in hospital epidemiology programs, occupational medicine programs, and biosafety programs must keep abreast of the medical literature, paying special attention to modifications of US Public Health Service/CDC guidelines.

REFERENCES

1. Centers for Disease Control and Prevention. Guidelines for preventing the transmission of Mycobacterium tuberculosis in health-care facilities. *MMWR.* 1994;43(RR-13):1-132.

2. Beekmann SE, Henderson DK. Nosocomial viral hepatitis in healthcare workers. In: Mayhall CG, ed. *Hospital Epidemiology and Infection Control.* 3rd ed. Philadelphia, Pa: Lippincott, Williams and Wilkins; 2003;1337-1360.

3. Centers for Disease Control and Prevention. Updated U.S. Public Health Service guidelines for the management of occupational exposures to HBV, HCV, and HIV and Recommendations for Postexposure Prophylaxis. *MMWR.* 2001;50(RR-11):1-52.

4. Centers for Disease Control. Recommendations for preventing transmission of human immunodeficiency virus and hepatitis B virus to patients during exposure-prone invasive procedures. *MMWR.* 1991;40(RR-8):1-9.

5. Henderson DK. Managing occupational risks for hepatitis C transmission in the health care setting. *Clin Microbiol Rev.* 2003;16(3):546-568.

6. Henderson DK, Fahey BJ, Willy ME, Schmitt JM, Carey K, Koziol DE. Risk for occupational transmission of human immunodeficiency virus type 1 (HIV-1) associated with clinical exposures: a prospective evaluation. *Ann Intern Med.* 1990;113:740-746.

7. Henderson DK, Gerberding JL. Human immunodeficiency virus in the health-care setting. In: Mandell G, Dolin R, Bennett J, eds. *Principles and Practice of Infectious Diseases.* 6th ed. New York, NY: Churchill-Livingstone; 2003.

8. Henderson DK, Gerberding JL. Healthcare worker issues, including occupational and nonoccupational postexposure management. In: Dolin RMH, Saag MS, eds. *AIDS Therapy.* 2nd ed. New York, NY: Churchill Livingstone; 2002:327-346.

9. Henderson DK. Nosocomial herpes virus infections. In: Mandell G, Dolin R, Bennett J, eds. *Principles and Practice of Infectious Diseases.* 6th ed. New York, NY: Churchill-Livingstone; 2003.

10. Wilde JA, McMillan JA, Serwint J, Butta J, O'Riordan MA, Steinhoff MC. Effectiveness of influenza vaccine in health care professionals: a randomized trial. *JAMA.* 1999;281(10):908-913.

11. Carman WF, Elder AG, Wallace LA, et al. Effects of influenza vaccination of health-care workers on mortality of elderly people in long-term care: a randomised controlled trial. *Lancet.* 2000;355(9198):93-97.

12. Henderson DK. Hospital preparedness for emerging and highly contagious infectious diseases—getting ready for SARS or whatever comes next. In: Mandell GL, Dolin R, Bennett JE, eds. *Principles and Practice of Infectious Diseases.* 6th ed. New York, NY: Churchill-Livingstone; 2003.

13. McQuillan GM, Kruszon-Moran D, Deforest A, Chu SY, Wharton M. Serologic immunity to diphtheria and tetanus in the United States. *Ann Intern Med*. 2002;136(9):660-666.

14. Magdei M, Melnic A, Benes O, et al. Epidemiology and control of diphtheria in the Republic of Moldova, 1946-1996. *J Infect Dis*. 2000;181 Suppl 1:S47-S54.

SUGGESTED READING

Agah R, Cherry JD, Garakian AJ, Chapin M. Respiratory syncytial virus (RSV) infection rate in personnel caring for children with RSV infections. Routine isolation procedure vs routine procedure supplemented by use of masks and goggles. *Am J Dis Child*. 1987;141(6):695-697.

Atkinson WL, Markowitz LE, Adams NC, Seastrom GR. Transmission of measles in medical settings-United States, 1985-1989. *Am J Med*. 1991;91(3B):320S-324S.

American College of Occupational and Environmental Medicine. ACOEM guidelines for protecting health care workers against tuberculosis. *J Occup Environ Med*. 1998;40(9):765-767.

Baptiste R, Koziol D, Henderson DK. Nosocomial transmission of hepatitis A in an adult population. *Infect Control*. 1987;8(9):364-370.

Barnhart S, Sheppard L, Beaudet N, Stover B, Balmes J. Tuberculosis in health care settings and the estimated benefits of engineering controls and respiratory protection. *J Occup Environ Med*. 1997;39(9):849-854.

Bell LM, Naides SJ, Stoffman P, Hodinka RL, Plotkin SA. Human parvovirus B19 infection among hospital staff members after contact with infected patients. *N Engl J Med*. 1989;321(8):485-491.

Beltrami EM, Williams IT, Shapiro CN, Chamberland ME. Risk and management of blood-borne infections in health care workers. *Clin Microbiol Rev*. 2000;13(3):385-407.

Benenson AS, ed. *Control of Communicable Diseases in Man*. 16th ed. Washington, DC: American Public Health Association; 1995.

Diodati C. Mandatory vaccination of health care workers. *CMAJ*. 2002;166(3):301-302.

Dworsky ME, Welch K, Cassady G, Stagno S. Occupational risk for primary cytomegalovirus infection among pediatric health-care workers. *N Engl J Med*. 1983;309(16):950-953.

Gundlach DC. Protecting health care workers from the occupational risk of disease. *QRB Qual Rev Bull*. 1988;14(5):144-146.

Hallak KM, Schenk M, Neale AV. Evaluation of the two-step tuberculin skin test in health care workers at an inner-city medical center. *J Occup Environ Med*. 1999;41(5):393-396.

Jarvis WR, Bolyard EA, Bozzi CJ, et al. Respirators, recommendations, and regulations: the controversy surrounding protection of health care workers from tuberculosis. *Ann Intern Med*. 1995;122(2):142-146.

Joint Tuberculosis Committee of the British Thoracic Society. Control and prevention of tuberculosis in the United Kingdom: code of practice 2000. *Thorax*. 2000;55(11):887-901.

Larsen NM, Biddle CL, Sotir MJ, White N, Parrott P, Blumberg HM. Risk of tuberculin skin test conversion among health care workers: occupational versus community exposure and infection. *Clin Infect Dis*. 2002;35(7):796-801.

Lewy R. Organization and conduct of a hospital occupational health service. State of the art reviews. *Occup Med*. 1987;2:617-638.

Maunder R, Hunter J, Vincent L, et al. The immediate psychological and occupational impact of the 2003 SARS outbreak in a teaching hospital. *CMAJ*. 2003;168(10):1245-1251.

Moore RM Jr., Kaczmarek RG. Occupational hazards to health care workers: diverse, ill-defined, and not fully appreciated. *Am J Infect Control*. 1990;18(5):316-327.

Nardell EA. Issues facing TB control (4.1). Nosocomial tuberculosis transmission—problems of health care workers. *Scott Med J*. 2000;45(5 Suppl):34-37.

O'Reilly FW, Stevens AB. Sickness absence due to influenza. *Occup Med (Lond)*. 2002;52(5):265-269.

Omenn GS, Morris SL. Occupational hazards to health care workers: report of a conference. *Am J Ind Med*. 1984;6(2):129-137.

Polder JA, Tablan OC, Williams WW. Personnel health services. In: Bennett JV, Brachman PS, eds. *Hospital Infections*. 3rd ed. Boston, Ma: Little, Brown and Co; 1992:31-61.

Rehermann B. Interaction between the hepatitis C virus and the immune system. *Semin Liver Dis*. 2000;20(2):127-141.

Sepkowitz KA. Occupationally acquired infections in health care workers. Part I. *Ann Intern Med*. 1996;125(10):826-834.

Sepkowitz KA. Occupationally acquired infections in health care workers. Part II. *Ann Intern Med*. 1996;125(11):917-928.

Sobaszek A, Fantoni-Quinton S, Frimat P, Leroyer A, Laynat A, Edme JL. Prevalence of cytomegalovirus infection among health care workers in pediatric and immunosuppressed adult units. *J Occup Environ Med*. 2000;42(11):1109-1114.

Swinker M. Occupational infections in health care workers: prevention and intervention. *Am Fam Physician*. 1997;56(9):2291-2300, 2303-2306.

Takaki A, Wiese M, Maertens G, et al. Cellular immune responses persist and humoral responses decrease two decades after recovery from a single-source outbreak of hepatitis C. *Nat Med*. 2000;6(5):578-582.

Thomas DL, Factor SH, Kelen GD, Washington AS, Taylor E Jr., Quinn TC. Viral hepatitis in health care personnel at The Johns Hopkins Hospital. The seroprevalence of and risk factors for hepatitis B virus and hepatitis C virus infection. *Arch Intern Med*. 1993;153(14):1705-1712.

Valenti WM. Infection control and the pregnant health care worker. *Am J Infect Control*. 1986;14(1):20-27.

Weber DJ, Rutala WA. Risks and prevention of nosocomial transmission of rare zoonotic diseases. *Clin Infect Dis*. 2001;32(3):446-456.

Wharton M, Cochi SL, Hutcheson RH, Schaffner W. Mumps transmission in hospitals. *Arch Intern Med*. 1990; 150(1):47-49.

Zimmerman RK, Middleton DB, Smith NJ. Vaccines for persons at high risk due to medical conditions, occupation, environment, or lifestyle, 2003. *J Fam Pract*. 2003;52(1 Suppl):S22-S35.

CHAPTER TWENTY-TWO

TUBERCULOSIS INFECTION CONTROL IN HEALTHCARE SETTINGS

Henry M. Blumberg, MD

INTRODUCTION AND BRIEF HISTORICAL OVERVIEW

Tuberculosis is spread person to person by an airborne route. Interestingly, TB has been recognized and accepted by the medical community as a potential occupational hazard only for several decades.[1] The risk of transmission of *Mycobacterium tuberculosis* from patients with TB disease to other hospitalized patients and healthcare workers was established by the 1950s when, as noted by Myers et al, "a rapid decline of TB in the general population made the disease among physicians more conspicuous."[1-3] With the introduction of effective chemotherapy for TB in the 1950s and a progressive decline in the incidence of TB in the United States until the mid 1980s, the risk of occupational infection and clinical TB declined among healthcare workers. There were only scattered reports of hospital outbreaks in the 1960s, 1970s, and early 1980s.[4-7] With this decline, less and less attention was paid toward TB infection control measures in hospitals. Thus few healthcare facilities were prepared for the changing epidemiology of TB in the mid 1980s and early 1990s.

Between 1985 and 1992, there was a resurgence of TB in the United States with a 20% increase in the number of TB cases reported. This resurgence was fueled by the decay of the public health infrastructure (due to underfunding) and the HIV epidemic.[8-10] The surge of TB cases combined with neglect toward TB control activities and ineffective TB infection control measures led to a number of reports of nosocomial transmission of TB in the late 1980s and early 1990s.[11-21] A number of these explosive and devastating outbreaks involved transmission of MDR strains of *M. tuberculosis* to patients and HCWs that was associated with significant morbidity and mortality, especially among HIV-infected and other immunocompromised persons.

Several factors, which are outlined in Table 22-1, contributed to these outbreaks of TB in hospitals. Breaks in basic TB infection control strategies—such as delays in the suspicion and diagnosis of TB, delays in identification of drug resistance, and delays in initiation of appropriate therapy—postponed proper isolation and prolonged infectiousness of patients. Second, respiratory isolation often was inadequate. For example, airborne infection isolation rooms had positive rather than negative pressure, air recirculated from isolation rooms to other areas, doors to isolation rooms were left open, isolation precautions were discontinued too soon, and healthcare workers did not wear adequate respiratory protection.[22]

Implementation of effective TB infection control measures recommended in the CDC's *Guidelines for Preventing the Transmission of Mycobacterium tuberculosis in Health-Care Settings, 1994*[23] and the decreasing incidence of TB in the community since 1992 led to a dramatic decrease in the risk of nosocomial transmission of TB in healthcare settings in the United States.[9,24,25] The control of TB in healthcare settings contributed to enhanced TB control in the community, which was also facilitated by rebuilding of the public health infrastructure and the greatly expanded use of directly observed therapy. A hierarchy of TB infection control measures including administrative (the most important), engineering, and personal respiratory protection controls have reduced nosocomial transmission significantly and prevented transmission of TB in healthcare settings.[9] Despite the decreasing incidence of TB in the United States,[26] TB infection control remains an important responsibility of healthcare personnel.[27] Failure to be vigilant and recognize undiagnosed patients with TB can result in nosocomial transmission as highlighted by a recent report by the CDC of nosocomial transmission of TB at a hospital in Washington, DC.[28]

TABLE 22-1. FACTORS FACILITATING NOSOCOMIAL TRANSMISSION OF TUBERCULOSIS

1. Inefficient infection-control procedures
   A. Delayed suspicion and diagnosis
      ➤ Clustering of patients with unsuspected TB with susceptible immunocompromised patients
      ➤ Delayed recognition of TB in HIV-infected patients because of "atypical" presentation or low clinical suspicion leading to misdiagnosis (HIV+ or HIV-)
      ➤ Failure to recognize and isolate patients with active pulmonary disease
   B. Failure to recognize ongoing infectiousness of patients
2. Laboratory delays in identification and susceptibility testing of *M. tuberculosis* isolates
3. Inadequate respiratory isolation facilities and engineering controls
   A. Lack of airborne infection isolation rooms
   B. Recirculation of air from isolation rooms to other parts of the hospital
4. Delayed initiation of effective anti-TB therapy

Adapted from Sepkowitz KA. Tuberculosis and the healthcare worker: a historical perspective. *Ann Intern Med.* 1994;120:71-9.

This chapter is not intended to provide an exhaustive summary of TB infection control measures; the CDC's 1994 TB guidelines have discussed these measures in detail and it is anticipated that revised CDC TB infection control guidelines will be issued in 2005. Rather, the basic framework for developing a TB control program is emphasized, including how to assess the risk of TB in a healthcare delivery setting, how to prioritize control measures based on their effectiveness, and how to meet current regulatory requirements.

INSTITUTIONAL CONTROLS FOR THE PREVENTION OF NOSOCOMIAL TUBERCULOSIS

Nosocomial TB is driven by the occurrence of disease in the community served by the hospital or healthcare system[25] and the efficacy of TB infection control measures instituted by a healthcare institution. Rates of TB in the United States have decreased significantly over the past decade[26] but still vary widely by geographic area. Frequently, inner-city areas have the highest rates of TB.[29]

An effective TB infection control program requires early identification, airborne infection isolation, and effective treatment of persons who have active TB disease.[23] The importance of an effective TB infection control program is highlighted by the devastating outbreaks of TB, including MDR-TB that occurred in the late 1980s and early 1990s and were associated with high rates of mor-

bidity and mortality, especially among HIV and immunocompromised patients and healthcare workers.[11-22] The termination of these outbreaks and prevention of nosocomial transmission of TB followed implementation of effective TB control program.[9,24,25,30-32] Policies and procedures regarding TB infection control should be developed by all healthcare facilities, which reflect their risk and patient population served. All healthcare settings need a TB infection control program designed to detect TB disease early and to isolate and promptly refer or treat persons who have TB disease. The major goals of a TB infection control program are outlined in Table 22-2.

Assignment of Responsibility

The first step in establishing an effective TB infection control program is for an institution to assign responsibility to a specific person or persons and ensure they have the authority and support to implement such a program. The person or persons should have expertise or access to expertise in the areas of infection control and healthcare epidemiology, infectious diseases, public health, employee health, engineering, and clinical microbiology. Frequently this responsibility is given to an institution's Infection Control Committee. The group should develop written TB infection control policies that are based on the institution's risk assessment. Policies and procedures should be reviewed on at least an annual basis and updated as indicated. At large institutions located in urban areas that care for sizable numbers of patients with TB, it has been very useful to designate an individual (eg, one of the ICP) to serve as the coordinator of TB infection control activities.

TABLE 22-2. MAJOR GOALS IN THE CONTROL AND PREVENTION OF NOSOCOMIAL TUBERCULOSIS

1. Airborne infection isolation of patients as soon as TB is suspected, whether during emergency care or on admission to the institution.

2. Start empirical anti-TB therapy as soon as TB is suspected with an appropriate regimen including at least 2 drugs to which the organism is likely to be susceptible. (Generally, a 4-drug regimen of RIPE* will be employed.)

3. Comply with isolation procedures during the patient's hospitalization until laboratory and clinical evidence eliminates the possibility of TB or the risk of transmission.

4. Conduct laboratory studies as soon as possible to confirm or exclude the presence of TB and to identify multidrug-resistant strains of *M. TB.*

5. Enhance occupational health services to monitor for infection and disease in HCWs.

6. Discharge TB patients from acute care only when they are no longer infectious or when arrangements have been made for appropriate isolation from contact with susceptible individuals (eg, in a stable home or another stable location with no new persons exposed).

7. Cooperate closely with public health and other community agencies to provide resources that ensure the completion of therapy (eg, direct observation).

8. TB-related HCW education to support the above goals.

* R = rifampin, I = isoniazid, P = pyrazinamide, E = ethambutol

Adapted from Sepkowitz KA. Tuberculosis and the healthcare worker: a historical perspective. *Ann Intern Med.* 1994;120:71-9; and McGowan JE. Nosocomial tuberculosis: new progress in control and prevention. *Clin Infect Dis.* 1995;21:489-505.

Risk Assessment

Tuberculosis is not evenly distributed among the population; it is more common among foreign-born persons, inner-city residents, ethnic/racial minorities, the homeless, and indigent persons. Additionally, TB incidence can vary widely and is not evenly distributed in the United States by geographic areas. Even within a defined metropolitan area, TB case rates can vary widely.[29] Therefore, a "one size fits all approach" is not appropriate for TB infection control, and the measures implemented should reflect the risk of the institution.[25] All healthcare settings should conduct regular, periodic (at least annual) TB risk assessments regardless of whether patients with suspected or confirmed TB disease will receive care at their institution.

The TB risk assessment determines the risk of nosocomial transmission of *M. tuberculosis* in the healthcare setting by examining a numbers of factors, including community incidence of TB disease; number of patients with TB disease presenting for care at the healthcare facility, regardless of whether they receive care in the setting or are transferred to another healthcare setting; timeliness of the recognition, isolation, and evaluation of patients with suspected or confirmed TB; and evidence for transmission

of *M. tuberculosis* in the setting. Local or state public health departments can help infection control personnel obtain information about their community's TB profile. Other sources of information on TB cases include extended-care facilities, schools, homeless shelters, and prisons. Even if there are no reported cases of TB in a community, the infection control staff still should determine if patients with TB may have been admitted or treated in the facility. Good sources for this information are the microbiology laboratory's database, infection control records, and medical record databases containing discharge diagnoses, autopsy, and surgical pathology reports.[27]

The institutional risk of TB can be categorized (ie, by the size of the institution and the number of persons with active disease seen at the institution) into low risk, medium risk, or ongoing transmission categories. In general, a risk classification is determined for the entire setting although in certain circumstances such as a large healthcare organization that encompasses several sites, specific areas can be defined by geography, functional units, or location. Hospitals with ≥200 beds that provide care for <6 patients with TB per year are categorized as *low risk* while those which care for ≥6 patients with TB per year are considered *medium risk*. For inpatient settings with <200 beds, those that provide care to <3 TB patients in the past

---

TABLE 22-3. HIERARCHY OF TUBERCULOSIS INFECTION-CONTROL MEASURES

1. Administrative controls (most essential component)
   - Careful screening of patients, isolation, early diagnosis, and treatment
   - HCW-directed measures
   - Comprehensive TST program for HCWs
   - HCW education
2. Environmental controls
   - Airborne infection isolation (ie, negative pressure) rooms; a single pass ventilation system is preferred; use HEPA filtration if recirculation of air is necessary
   - UV germicidal irradiation (eg, in selected locations such as emergency room waiting areas)
3. Personal respiratory protection equipment (including use of N-95 respirator masks)

---

year are considered low risk and those with ≥3 TB cases in the past year are considered *medium risk*. Outpatient clinics, outreach, or home health settings that provide care to <3 patients with TB per year are considered low risk and those that provide care for ≥3 patients are considered *medium risk*. Tuberculosis clinics and outreach programs as well as other outpatient settings where care of persons with TB disease is provided should be classified as *medium risk*. Any institution, clinic, or setting with evidence of patient-to-patient or patient-to-HCW transmission of *M. tuberculosis* or evidence of ongoing nosocomial transmission of TB should be classified as *potential ongoing transmission* until appropriate infection control measures have been implemented and transmission has been demonstrated to have been stopped. *Potential ongoing transmission* should be a temporary classification only. When nosocomial transmission of TB is suspected, immediate investigation, active steps, and corrective steps should be implemented. This may include consultation with public health officials or experts in healthcare epidemiology and infection control. Evidence of potential nosocomial transmission of TB includes clusters of tuberculin skin test (TST) conversion in healthcare workers, increased rates of healthcare worker TST conversions, a healthcare worker with potentially infectious TB, unrecognized TB disease in patients or healthcare workers, or recognition of an identical strain of *M. tuberculosis* in patient or healthcare workers with TB disease.

Based on the finding of the risk assessment, the appropriate level of administrative, environmental, and respiratory protection policies to prevent occupational exposure to and nosocomial transmission of TB can be determined. The frequency of TST of healthcare workers is also based on the finding of the risk assessment and discussed in additional detail below.

HIERARCHY OF TUBERCULOSIS INFECTION CONTROL MEASURES

A "hierarchy of controls," which include administrative controls, engineering controls, and respiratory protection (Table 22-3), are recommended by CDC to prevent nosocomial transmission of TB.[23] Implementation of this hierarchy has been noted to be effective in terminating outbreaks and preventing nosocomial transmission of TB.[9] A TB infection control program should achieve the following goals: early identification of patients with TB disease, prompt airborne infection isolation (AII), and prompt diagnosis and effective treatment of persons with active disease (or rapid transfer of the patient to another facility that treats patients with TB if the admitting facility does not). The specific control measures can be prioritized based on their relative effectiveness in reducing risk of transmission and are discussed below.

Administrative Controls

Administrative controls are the most important TB infection control measures and consist of measures to reduce the risk of exposure to persons with infectious TB (see Table 22-3). A healthcare facility should implement administrative controls first because these controls most effectively reduce the risk of nosocomial transmission.[9,24] Early identification and AII are the keys to controlling and preventing nosocomial TB. As noted previously, nosocomial transmission of TB has occurred primarily because of the failure to recognize and isolate patients with infectious TB. Administrative controls include developing and implementing effective policies and protocols to assure that persons likely to have TB disease are identified rapidly, isolated properly, evaluated clinically, and treated appropriately. It requires that HCWs carefully evaluate patients upon their initial encounter and promptly isolate any patient who they suspect may have TB until laboratory and clinical evidence eliminates this diagnosis. Hospitals can implement an early identification and isolation protocol more efficiently by authorizing both nurses and physicians to isolate patients with suspected TB and by developing policies that allow staff to isolate automatically certain patients (eg, patients for whom TB is in the differential diagnosis or from whom specimens are ordered for acid-fast bacilli [AFB] smear or culture).[24] Many institutions have implemented policies that include mandatory respiratory isolation for certain types of patients in order to facilitate the success of administrative controls.[2,24,32] Moreover, because patients with HIV infection may present with "atypical" signs and symptoms, some facilities isolate all patients with HIV infection who have clinical symptoms suggestive of TB (eg, fever, cough, and/or an abnormal chest radiograph) until appropriate cultures are negative. For example, at Grady Memorial Hospital in Atlanta, which cares for large numbers of patients with TB including those who are HIV co-infected, the respiratory isolation policy requires that all patients admitted to the hospital with known TB, those with TB in the differential diagnosis or who have sputum or respiratory specimens for AFB ordered, and those who are HIV infected and have an abnormal chest x-ray be placed in AII until TB is "ruled out." Generally the diagnosis is excluded by obtaining 3 negative AFB smears of sputum or other respiratory specimens. AII precautions, policies, and procedures should be developed based on the local epidemiology of the disease in the community served by a particular facility.

The protocol for early identification of patients with TB and the definition of "suspect case" will determine the number of isolation rooms required. It should be anticipated that some patients who do not have TB will be isolated (ie, overisolation) to prevent nosocomial transmission. The degree of overisolation will depend on the institution's policy and the prevalence of TB in the community and patient population served by the institution. At our institution, the "rule out" ratio of patients isolated to patients found to have TB disease is about 9:1.[33,34] In a low prevalence Midwestern state (Iowa), a group of investigators predicted that as many as 93 patients would be isolated without TB for every case of TB diagnosed.[35] The expected "rule out" ratio is not well defined and likely varies by geographic area based on the prevalence of TB in the community and at the facility served. However, because there is little margin of error when detecting persons with TB disease in that a single person with undiagnosed TB can lead to an outbreak,[23,28] a high sensitivity is required and therefore some degree of overisolation is to

be expected. At large institutions, increased efficiency in the evaluation of patients who subsequently "rule out" for TB has been demonstrated by clustering AII rooms on a respiratory isolation ward.[33] This enhanced efficiency can provide significant cost savings to the institution and better use of AII rooms, which are often in limited supply.

Surveillance for Latent Tuberculosis Infection

Surveillance for latent TB infection in healthcare workers is a component of the administrative controls. The appropriate frequency of tuberculin skin testing of HCWs is determined by the risk assessment described above. Given the low positive predictive value of the TST when testing low risk and low prevalence populations for latent TB infection (LTBI),[9,36] frequent testing of HCWs in low-incidence and low-risk settings is not recommended because it will lead to false-positive results. In fact, testing of very low risk persons can result in the majority of positive tests being false positives. Institutions need to also recognize that false positive TSTs have occurred when institutions have switched brands of purified protein derivative (PPD) reagent, for example from Tubersol (Aventis Pasteur, Swiftwater, Pa) to Aplisol (Peradale Pharmaceuticals, Rochester, Mich).[37] All HCWs should undergo baseline tuberculin skin testing (with 2-step testing if not previously tested in the preceding year) at the time of employment.[23] Two-step baseline testing can help identify LTBI in new personnel who otherwise would be classified as recent conversions. This is especially true of institutions that have a large number of employees.[38]

It is not recommended that HCWs in low-risk settings (as determined by the risk assessment) undergo routine periodic follow-up testing; follow-up testing is recommended only if there is an exposure to a patient with active TB (ie, patient not initially isolated but later found to have laryngeal or pulmonary TB). HCWs working at medium-risk settings should undergo baseline and annual skin testing as well as testing after a TB exposure episode. Institutions with ongoing nosocomial transmission should carry out TST of at risk healthcare workers every 3 months until it is documented that transmission has been terminated. Surveillance for TST conversions is one way to assess the efficacy of an infection control program (eg, in medium-risk settings), a cluster of conversions may be the first indication of ongoing nosocomial transmission. In addition, this surveillance is a mechanism of demonstrating termination of transmission in situations where there has been ongoing nosocomial transmission.

When performing tuberculin skin testing of healthcare workers, the Mantoux method should be used. PPD is injected intradermally (0.1 mL [5 tuberculin units]) and the degree of induration is recorded in mm at 48 to 72 hours after placement.[36] HCWs with a positive TST (either at baseline or during follow-up testing) should have a chest radiograph performed to exclude active disease. If an abnormal chest x-ray is found, the HCW should be removed from the work setting until active disease is excluded. HCWs with a negative chest radiograph found to have LTBI who are at increased risk for progression to active disease (eg, recent conversion, underlying medical condition) should be strongly encouraged to take and complete therapy for LTBI. The infection control staff working closely with the Employee Health Clinic staff should consider a number of important issues when developing a program for tuberculin testing of healthcare workers. Institutions should assume responsibility for surveillance and mandate testing of all HCWs working at a particular institution (eg, all paid and unpaid staff, including students, agency nurses, residents, attending physicians, volunteers, and others) and not just employees. This is particularly important in an era of outsourcing when many HCWs may not be employees of the institution that they are working at. For institutions where routine follow-up testing is warranted (eg, medium risk), TST results should be recorded in the individual employee's health record and in an aggregate database of all TST results. TST conversion rates should be calculated for the facility as a whole and, if appropriate, for specific areas of the facility and for occupational groups. TST conversion rates should be calculated by dividing the number of PPD-test conversions among HCWs in each area or group (ie, the numerator) by the total number of previously PPD-negative HCWs tested in each area or group (ie, the denominator). In collaboration with Employee Health Clinic staff, infection control personnel should interpret TST conversion rates. If the number of workers in a particular area is small, the conversion rate may be high, although the actual risk may not be higher than in other areas. In contrast, statistical analysis may miss significant problems when the number of workers is small. If HCWs become TST positive (ie, have a TST conversion), the infection control staff should investigate to determine whether the likely source is in the facility or in the community. Of note, HCWs in some facilities are more likely to be exposed to TB in the community than in the hospital[39,40]; this may particularly be the case following implementation of effective TB infection control measures. One challenge of TST programs is to ensure that the staff reports to employee health for TST placement and for follow-up assessment. Some facilities have improved compliance by offering TST testing at the work site, thereby removing the time and distance barriers and increasing peer pressure. Others have tied TST to issuance of employee identification badges, which are required to work at the facility, and to the physician credentialing process.

For over 100 years, the TST had been the only diagnostic test available for LTBI and remains the primary test used for diagnosis of LTBI. Given the limitations of the TST,[9,36] the development of more effective diagnostic tests is desperately needed.[41] An alternative to TST is now available for the diagnosis of LTBI, including baseline and serial testing of healthcare workers. A whole blood γ-interferon release assay (IγRA) marketed under the trade name QuantiFERON-TB (Cellestis Inc, Valencia, Calif) has been approved by the FDA, and the CDC has published guidelines on the appropriate use of this test in selected populations.[42] The IγRA is based on the quantification of γ-interferon released from sensitized lymphocytes in whole blood incubated overnight with PPD from *M. tuberculosis* and control antigens. As a diagnostic test, the IγRA requires phlebotomy, can be accomplished after a single patient visit, assesses responses to multiple antigens simultaneously, and does not boost anamnestic immune responses.[42] Limitations of the IGRA include the need to draw blood and process it within 12 hours after collection and limited laboratory and clinical experience with the assay. Results of the QuantiFERON-TB and TST were moderately concordant.[43] Confirmation of a positive QFT result with TST is recommended before initiation of treatment for LTBI for low-risk patients but not for those at high risk. It is hoped in the future that improved diagnostic tests for LTBI will be developed that permit implementation of alternatives to the TST. Other blood-based diagnostic tests including Elispot and newer generation IγRA tests, which use TB specific antigens, are being investigated but these are not currently clinically available.[44,45]

Education

HCW education is a critical component of an effective TB infection control program.[2] HCWs should receive training and education on the variety of components of an effective TB infection control program and their responsibilities in implementing and carrying out the institution's infection control plan. HCWs need to appreciate the risk of occupational exposure to patients with TB as well as the measures (eg, hierarchy of controls) and policies adopted by the healthcare facility to prevent nosocomial transmission of TB. Tuberculosis education should be provided at the time of employment and then subsequently each year. Basic information should be provided to all HCWs and more in-depth education and training can be provided on a targeted basis to HCWs working in areas or settings where patients at risk or with TB may receive care. OSHA requires that US healthcare facilities provide annual training. A number of institutions have incorporated this TB-related education into their OSHA-mandated bloodborne pathogen training.

Long-Term Care Facilities

Many of the considerations for control of TB in hospitals described in this section apply to extended care facilities including the risk assessment recommendations. Elderly persons residing in a nursing home are at a higher risk of developing active TB than those elderly persons living at home in the community.[46,47] As in the hospital setting, effective TB control measures for extended care facilities include a high index of suspicion, prompt detection of active cases, isolating infectious cases, initiating appropriate therapy, identifying and evaluating contacts, and, when appropriate, conducting targeting testing and treatment of LTBI. Generally, LTCFs do not have airborne infection isolation rooms and therefore patients with suspected TB should be referred to acute care hospitals. Patients found to have TB should not be admitted or readmitted to a LTCF until they are determined to be noninfectious. All residents entering LTCFs should have a baseline TST performed (using 2-step testing) unless documented to be previously positive. Persons found to have a positive TST should have a chest radiograph performed and if negative, evaluated for treatment of LTBI.[36] Stead has published data indicating the value of treating LTBI in elderly residents of nursing homes as a means to preventing future outbreaks.[48]

Environmental Controls

The second level of controls are *environmental controls*, which reduce or eliminate *M. tuberculosis*-laden droplet nuclei in the air. These controls include local exhaust ventilation, general or central ventilation, air filtration with HEPA filters, and air disinfection with ultraviolet germicidal irradiation (UVGI).

Local Exhaust Ventilation

Local exhaust ventilation is a source control method used for capturing airborne contaminants including infectious droplet nuclei or other infectious particles before they are dispersed into the general environment. Local exhaust ventilation using a booth, hood, or tent can be an efficient engineering control technique because it captures a contaminant at its source. Local exhaust ventilation should be used for cough-inducing (eg, sputum induction booth) and aerosol-generating procedures. If local exhaust ventilation is not feasible, cough-inducing and aerosol-generating procedures (eg, bronchoscopy) should be preformed in a room that meets the requirements of an AII room.

General Ventilation

General ventilation includes mechanisms that dilute and remove contaminated air and control the direction of airflow to prevent an infectious source from contaminating the air in nearby areas. These mechanisms include maintaining negative pressure and circulating air to dilute and remove infectious droplet nuclei (eg, room air exchanges). Airflow should be from more clean areas to more contaminated (or less clean) areas[49,50]; thus, air should flow from corridors into AII rooms to prevent the spread of TB. AII rooms are used to house patients with suspected or confirmed TB being cared for at a healthcare facility. AII rooms should have negative pressure to prevent the escape of droplet nuclei, and the CDC recommends a minimum of 6 air exchanges per hour (and 12 air changes per hour if feasible) to decrease the concentration

of infectious particles. For newly constructed or renovated facilities, a minimum of 12 air exchanges per hour for AII rooms is recommended by the CDC.[23] A single pass ventilation system is the preferred choice for AII rooms; in such cases after air passes through the room or area, 100% of that air is exhausted to the outside. If this is not possible, HEPA filtration must be employed to filter air from an AII room that is recirculated into the general ventilation system. HEPA filtration must also be used when discharging air from local exhaust ventilation booths or enclosures (eg, sputum induction booths).

The number of AII rooms and the location of these rooms (eg, wards, emergency department, intensive care unit) should be determined based on results of the risk assessment. Grouping of AII rooms in one area (eg, respiratory isolation ward) may facilitate the care of patients with suspected or proven TB[33] and the installation and maintenance of optimal environmental controls. AII rooms should be checked regularly to ensure they are under negative pressure using smoke tubes or other devices. The CDC recommends that these rooms be checked before occupancy and daily while occupied by a patient with suspected or confirmed TB. When negative pressure is required, the CDC and AIA recommend the pressure differential should be >0.01 inch of water. Detailed recommendations for designing and operating ventilation systems have been published in recent years.[49-51] A maintenance plan that outlines the responsibility and authority for maintenance of the environmental controls and addresses staff training needs should be part of the written TB control plan. Standard operating procedures should include the notification of infection control personnel before performing maintenance on ventilation systems serving TB patient care areas.

Portable Air Filtration Units

Portable room-air recirculation units (which are often referred to as portable air filtration units or portable HEPA filters) have been shown to be effective in removing bioaerosols and aerosolized particles from room air[52] and therefore may be helpful in reducing airborne disease transmission. If portable devices are used, units with relatively high volumetric airflow rates that provide maximum flow through the HEPA filter are preferred. Placement of the units is important and should be selected to optimize the recirculation of AII room air through the HEPA filter. These portable units may be useful as an interim engineering control measure. These units enable hospitals to establish TB isolation rooms in outpatient departments and in patient-care areas when other TB isolation rooms are in use. In addition, facilities that do not have isolation rooms can use these units to convert general patient rooms to TB isolation rooms.[27] Effectiveness of these portable units is affected by the room's configuration, the furniture and persons in the room, and the placement of the HEPA filtration unit relative to the supply air vent and exhaust grilles. Portable air filtration units may also include ultraviolet germicidal irradiation as discussed below.

Ultraviolet Germicidal Irradiation

UVGI is an air cleaning technology that can be used in a room or corridor to irradiate the air in the upper portion of the room (upper air irradiation), installed in a duct to irradiate air passing through the duct (duct irradiation), or incorporated into room air-recirculation units. The CDC considers UVGI to be a supplementary measure for TB control and recommends that UVGI not be used as a substitute for negative pressure or HEPA filtration.[23] Others have advocated more vigorously for an expanded role of UVGI for TB infection control.[53] Air-cleaning technologies, such as UVGI and HEPA filtration, can be used to increase equivalent air changes per hour (ACH) in waiting areas and AII rooms. Studies suggest that a 30-W UV fixture provides the equivalent of 20 or more room air exchanges, depending on the air-mixing and flow patterns.[54,55] Air mixing, air velocity, relative humidity, UVGI intensity, and lamp configuration affect the efficacy of UVGI systems.

In upper-room air irradiation, UVGI lamps are suspended from the ceiling or mounted on the wall with a shield at the bottom of the lamp to direct the rays upward. As the air circulates, nonirradiated air moves from the lower to the upper part of the room, and irradiated air moves from the upper to the lower part of the room. For upper-air systems, airborne microorganisms in the lower, occupied areas of the room must move to the upper part of the room to be killed or inactivated by upper-air UVGI. For optimal efficacy of upper-air UVGI, relative humidity should be maintained at ≤60%, a level that is consistent with current recommendations for providing acceptable indoor air quality and minimizing environmental microbial contamination in indoor environments.[56] The most useful places to consider using UVGI include locations in high TB prevalence; areas that are difficult to control through ventilation measures alone such as waiting rooms, emergency rooms, corridors, and other central areas of a facility where patients with undiagnosed TB could contaminate the air including operating rooms; and adjacent corridors where procedures are performed on patients with TB disease. Details about the types of UVGI, their applications, and limitations can be found in the CDC guidelines and in other resources.[23,57]

UVGI-containing portable room air cleaners are another area where UVGI has been used in healthcare facilities. In portable room air-recirculation units containing UVGI, a fan moves a volume of room air across UVGI lamps to disinfect the air before it is recirculated back to the room. Some portable units contain both a HEPA filter (or other high-efficiency filter) as well as UVGI lamps. One study has reported that portable room air cleaners with UVGI lamps

are effective (>99%) in inactivating or killing airborne vegetative bacteria.[58] Potential uses of portable room air cleaners with UVGI include in AII rooms as a supplemental method of air cleaning, waiting rooms, emergency departments, corridors, central areas, or other large areas where individuals with undiagnosed TB could potentially contaminate the air.

There are a number of health and safety issues related to the use of UVGI. For example, short-term overexposure to UV radiation can cause erythema, photokeratitis, and conjunctivitis.[23,59,60] If UVGI is used (eg, in upper air UVGI systems), it is important that the UVGI fixtures be designed and installed to ensure that UVGI exposures to occupants are below current safe exposure levels. Health-hazard evaluations by CDC/National Institute for Occupational Safety and Health (NIOSH) have identified potential problems at some facilities using UVGI systems.[23] These include overexposure of HCWs to UVGI and inadequate maintenance, training, labeling, and use of PPE. It is believed that in most instances, properly designed, installed, and maintained UVGI fixtures provide protection from most, if not all, of the direct UVGI in the lower room.[53] When UVGI is used, it is important that these systems be monitored appropriately, as would be expected with other types of engineering controls, that responsible individuals maintain them, and that HCWs receive appropriate education about UVGI safety-related issues.[2]

Personal Respiratory Protection

Personal respiratory protection is the last step in the hierarchy of TB control measures. It is recommended that personal respiratory equipment (eg, N-95 respirators) be used when entering high risk areas where exposure to airborne *M. tuberculosis* may occur (eg, AII rooms, rooms where cough-producing or aerosol-producing procedures are performed, and bronchoscopy suites where procedures are performed on patients with suspected or proven TB). The most controversial area of TB infection control has involved personal respiratory protection because of federal mandates from the OSHA regarding fit testing and due to lack of data on the precise level of effectiveness of respiratory protection in protecting HCWs from *M. tuberculosis* transmission in healthcare settings has not been determined. Prior to 1996, OSHA had mandated the use of HEPA respirators in healthcare facilities. Two cost-effectiveness analyses performed at the University of Virginia and involving VA hospitals suggested that HEPA respirators would offer negligible additional efficacy at a great cost (eg, $7 million per case of TB prevented).[61,62] However, all federal agencies involved in this issue (NIOSH, OSHA, and the CDC) are in agreement that the minimal acceptable respiratory protection is a NIOSH-certified N-95 respirator.[63]

On October 17, 1997, OSHA published a proposed standard for occupational exposure to TB.[64] The Institute of Medicine of the National Academies of Sciences (IOM) was subsequently asked by the US Congress to evaluate the risk of TB among HCWs and the impact of the proposed OSHA TB standard. The IOM published a report in 2001 entitled, *Tuberculosis in the Workplace*.[9] The IOM report questioned the validity of the OSHA risk assessment that the standard was based on and noted that the risk of occupational exposure to TB and HCW risk of occupationally acquired infection had decreased significantly following implementation of CDC recommended TB infection control guidelines and decreasing incidence of TB in the community. The IOM report also concluded that CDC recommended guidelines[23] were effective in terminating outbreaks and preventing nosocomial infection of TB. A survey by CDC and the American Hospital Association has noted that most hospitals had implemented CDC recommended TB infection control guidelines by the mid 1990s.[65] In 2003, OSHA announced that it had decided to withdraw this proposal[66] because "it does not believe a standard would substantially reduce the occupational risk of TB infection."

Despite not issuing a separate TB standard, OSHA maintains regulatory control over TB in healthcare settings under the Code of Federal Regulations (CFR) Title 29, Part 1910.139 (29CFR1910.139) and compliance policy directive CPL 2.106 (*Enforcement Procedures and Scheduling for Occupational Exposure to Tuberculosis*).[67] On December 31, 2003, OSHA announced in the *Federal Register* that it was applying the General Industry Respiratory Protection Standard (1910.134) to respiratory protection against TB in healthcare settings.[68] The impact of this decision is that healthcare facilities are now required by OSHA to perform annual fit testing rather than just at the time of employment as had been the case previously.

Fit testing has been an extremely contentious issue. Observational studies have demonstrated that TB outbreaks were terminated prior to the availability or use of N-95 or HEPA respirators or use of fit testing.[25] Fit testing is time consuming and logistically difficult, and can be expensive at large institutions that may have thousands of healthcare workers. There is no definitive data of the benefit of fit testing and recent publications by NIOSH have demonstrated a variety of problems with fit testing. Coffey et al reported that when the most rigorous criterion of fit testing was used (the 1% pass/fail criterion recommended by the American National Standards Institute and required by OSHA), a substantial majority of tested individuals failed the fit test for 17 of 21 brands of N-95 respirators tested; thus most individuals could not be successfully fitted.[9,69] There are a number of different methodologies available for fit testing although in healthcare facilities, the qualitative fit method is most commonly

used. In an additional investigation, Coffey et al compared 5 methods for fit-testing N95 respirators using both qualitative and quantitative methods.[70] The authors found wide variation in results between these fit testing methods and that none of the 5 methods met criteria for determining whether a fit test adequately screened out poorly fitting respirators. They concluded that the accuracy of fit testing methods and the fitting characteristics of N-95 respirators need to be improved.

In a more recent investigation, Coffey and colleagues at NIOSH reported on the fitting characteristics of 18 different models of N-95 respirators using 4 different analytical methods used to measure the performance of N-95–respirators.[71] Coffey found that the most important characteristic in providing protection was the inherent fitting characteristics of the N-95 respirators. Only 3 of the 18 N-95 respirators had good fitting characteristics and met the expected level of protection without fit testing. Passing a fit test, however, did not guarantee the wearer an adequately fitting respirator. There was little additional benefit of fit testing for those models of respirators with good fitting characteristics. Poor fitting respirators with fit testing continued to be inferior to good fitting respirators without fit testing. Thus, those respirators with good fitting characteristics provided better protection out of the box without fit testing than did respirators with poor fitting characteristics after fit testing. These findings led the NIOSH authors to conclude that given the "current state of fit testing, it may be of more benefit to the user to wear a respirator model with good-fitting characteristics without fit testing than to wear a respirator model with poor-fitting characteristics after passing a fit-test."[71] In 1995, NIOSH published new certification regulations for particulate respirators.[72] Unfortunately, there is no provision requiring good fit characteristics as part of the certification process.

OSHA permits a HCW to reuse a N-95 respirator as long as it maintains its structural and functional integrity and the filter material is not damaged or soiled. Each facility should include in its TB control program policy a protocol that defines when a disposable respirator must be discarded (eg, if it becomes contaminated with blood or other body fluids). Healthcare facilities should strongly consider selecting a brand of N-95 respirator based on its fit characteristics (ie, whether it has good fitting characteristics) as outlined by Coffey et al.[71] In addition to selecting N-95 respirators, each healthcare facility needs a complete respiratory protection program. Components of the OSHA respiratory protection standard require that an institution:

➤ Assign responsibility for the program to a specific person or group

➤ Write procedures for all aspects of the program

➤ Screen all employees for medical conditions that prevent them from wearing respirators

➤ Train and educate employees about respiratory protocols (and TB infection control measures)

➤ Fit test the respirators on each employee (on an annual basis) and have employees check the fit each time they use a respirator

➤ Develop policies and procedures that describe how to inspect, maintain, and reuse respirators, and define when respirators are contaminated and must be discarded

➤ Evaluate the program periodically

Despite the limitations of fit testing,[9,69-71] it is currently required by OSHA on an annual basis. A qualitative fit testing method is generally used for fit testing disposable N-95 respirators at most healthcare facilities. This method involves exposing the employee to saccharin. Some individuals are not sensitive to saccharin's taste. In addition, some data suggest that saccharin may be a carcinogenic. It has been recommended that healthcare facilities should follow the manufacturer's instructions and recommendations for fit testing.[23] OSHA requires that healthcare facilities screen employees to determine whether they can wear respirators. Other than severe cardiac or pulmonary disease, few medical conditions should preclude the use of disposable respirators. Many facilities use a general questionnaire to screen employees for medical conditions and to determine whether an employee should be evaluated further. Personal respiratory protection (eg, N-95 respirator) should be used by persons entering rooms in which patients with suspected or confirmed infectious TB are being isolated (eg, airborne infection isolation rooms), persons present during cough-inducing or aerosol-generating procedures performed on patients with suspected or confirmed infectious TB, and persons in other settings where administrative and environmental controls are not likely to protect them from inhaling infectious airborne droplet nuclei. This includes emergency medical technicians and other persons who transport patients who might have infectious TB in ambulances or other vehicles and persons who provide urgent surgical or dental care to patients who might have infectious TB. In addition, laboratory workers conducting aerosol-producing procedures involving specimens that might contain *M. tuberculosis* should also use respiratory protection. Detailed recommendations about the environment (including use of a biosafety cabinet and other biosafety procedures) used for carrying out such procedures has been published by CDC and the National Institutes of Health.[73]

It is recommended that visitors to airborne infection isolation rooms or other areas where patients with suspected or confirmed infectious TB are present should wear a N-95 respirator. Visitors can be given N-95 respirators and instructed in their use but do not need to be fit tested.

As discussed above, OSHA's minimum requirement for respiratory protection is the N-95 respirator. However, particular situations may warrant more protective respirators. Modeling studies have suggested that the benefits of respiratory protection are directly proportional to the presence of the risk.[74] For example, personnel who perform extremely high-risk procedures, such as bronchoscopy on patients with known or suspected MDR TB, may need additional respiratory protection. One example of a more protective respirator is a powered air-purifying respirator. NIOSH has published a guide on respirators for TB that describes the type of respirators that are available.[72]

LABORATORY DIAGNOSIS

Laboratory tests (eg, AFB smear and culture) are necessary to confirm or exclude the diagnosis of TB and to identify resistant isolates of *M tuberculosis*.[75,76] If a clinical laboratory cannot perform the most rapid tests, the hospital may need to send specimens to a referral laboratory. This will become increasingly the case in low-incidence areas.[77] The healthcare facility must ensure that arrangements comply with the CDC's guidelines for transporting specimens and reporting results (eg, AFB smear results should be reported within 24 hours of specimen collection). The use of nucleic acid amplification tests may be useful when caring for HIV co-infected patients where recovery of nontuberculous mycobacteria may be common. Given the relatively low positive predictive value of a positive AFB smear of sputum from a HIV-infected person, nucleic acid amplification tests that identify whether *M. tuberculosis* is present can help facilitate care of patients. Reports have indicated a high sensitivity and specificity for the test for AFB smear-positive specimens.[78] Those patients who are AFB respiratory smear positive but found to not have TB based on nucleic acid amplification results could have isolation discontinued and therapy discontinued in an expeditious fashion rather than having to wait several weeks for results of a culture.

TREATMENT OF TUBERCULOSIS DISEASE AND LATENT TUBERCULOSIS INFECTION

Clinicians should start empirical therapy as soon as they suspect that the patient has TB disease. The current recommendation is to begin empirical therapy with a four-drug regimen (isoniazid, rifampin, pyrazinamide, and ethambutol).[76] Definitive therapy depends on sensitivity testing. The American Thoracic Society, the IDSA, and the CDC have published revised guidelines on the treatment of TB disease that provide detailed guidance.[76] Directly observed therapy is an important component of therapy and has been demonstrated to improve completion rates and outcome.[79]

Treatment of LTBI has been demonstrated to be effective in reducing the risk of progression to active disease and is recommended for those individuals at increased risk of progression, including healthcare workers. Recommendations for the treatment of LTBI have been published and updated[36,80] (Table 22-4). It should be noted that short course (2-month) LTBI therapy with rifampin plus pyrazinamide is no longer recommended for the treatment of LTBI because of reports of increased severe hepatoxicity and deaths associated with this regimen.[80] However, the use of rifampin and pyrazinamide remain an important component of a multidrug regimen in the treatment of TB disease.[76]

Despite the benefits of therapy for the treatment of LTBI, HCWs have historically had poor rates of initiation and completion of LTBI therapy with the majority of healthcare workers not initiating or completing therapy.[81-83] However, in the context of a comprehensive TB infection control program[84] and programs that have focused efforts on delivering LTBI therapy to HCWs,[85] much higher rates of initiation and completion have been reported. For example, investigators in St. Louis reported that 98% of HCWs with LTBI initiated isoniazid therapy and 82% completed therapy at Barnes-Jewish Hospital. The authors of this study attributed their high initiation and completion rates to active follow-up, consisting of physician counseling and monthly phone consultations by nurses at the institution's Occupational Health Department along with free services and medication. Foreign-born HCWs who had received BCG were less likely to complete therapy in the St. Louis study and the authors recommend addressing cultural barriers that may lead to refusing therapy and nonadherence with therapy.

Improved infection control measures and decreasing incidence of TB over the past decade have led to a significant reduction in HCW risk.[9] Following the establishment of effective TB control measures in hospitals, for many HCWs, community factors pose a greater risk for TB infection than occupational exposure.[39,40] At many institutions, a large proportion of HCWs are foreign born and may be found to have LTBI at the time of employment, presumably due in large part to infection acquired in their home countries, which may have a high incidence of disease. Thus in part, surveillance for LTBI among HCWs is part of a public health strategy for treating those with LTBI who may be at increased risk for progression (eg, immigrants to the United States within the past 5 years).

Discharge Planning and Collaboration With Public Health

Healthcare facilities and local and state public health officials have responsibilities to work closely with each other to further TB control in the community and state. Public health officials can provide important data to healthcare facilities regarding incidence of TB in the community, which is needed for the institution's risk assessment. It is important for healthcare facilities to establish contact with local public health authorities and report TB cases to them. All US states require that TB cases be reported and often the physician caring for the patient is responsible for this. Frequently infection control departments have assumed this responsibility for their facility to ensure the reporting occurs in a timely fashion. Healthcare facilities and public health officials need to also work closely with regards to discharge planning in order to ensure a seamless transition of care from an inpatient setting to an outpatient clinic (eg, TB Clinic at the patient's local health department) and to help ensure that patients are not lost to follow-up after discharge. A written policy or critical pathway management of TB patient discharges that provides guidance as to what constitutes an appropriate transfer (for programs that do not provide care to patients with proven or suspected TB but refer to other sites) or discharge (for sites that do provide care) should be established and included as part of a TB infection control program.[25] For example these measures may include ensuring that patients be discharged on an appropriate anti-TB regimen, patients have arrangements to ensure close follow-up after discharge (eg, patient is contacted in the hospital by the public health outreach worker who will provide directly observed therapy following hospital discharge, and patients meet appropriate criteria for discharge (eg, be medically ready for discharge and have a stable home or other stable location if potentially infectious).[2]

Summary

Much progress has been made over the past decade in greatly reducing the risk of occupational exposure to TB and occupationally acquired infection due to *M. tuberculosis*. The CDC recommended guidelines (ie, hierarchy of controls) have been shown to be effective in preventing terminating outbreaks and in preventing nosocomial transmission of TB.[9,23] The improved safety for healthcare workers (and patients) has been due to a combination of improved infection control measures implemented in hospitals and a decrease in the incidence of TB in the com-

TABLE 22-4. ABBREVIATED GUIDELINES FOR THE TREATMENT OF LATENT TUBERCULOSIS INFECTION

Drug	Interval and Duration	Comments*
Isoniazid	Daily for 9 months**+	**Preferred regimen.** In HIV-infected persons, isoniazid may be administered concurrently with nucleoside reverse transcriptase inhibitors (NRT Is), protease inhibitors, or non-nucleoside reverse transcriptase inhibitors (NNRT Is).
	Twice weekly for 9 months**+	Directly observed therapy (DOT must be used with twice-weekly dosing).
Isoniazid	Daily for 6 months**	Not indicated for HIV-infected persons, those with fibrotic lesions on chest radiographs, or children.
	Twice weekly for 6 months**	DOT must be used with twice-weekly dosing.
Rifampin++	Daily for 4 months	Used for persons who are contacts of patients with isoniazid-resistant, rifampin-susceptible TB.
		In HIV-infected persons, most protease inhibitors or delavirdine should not be administered concurrently with rifampin. Rifabutin with appropriate dose adjustments can be used with protease inhibitors (saquinavir should be augmented with ritonavir) and NNRT Is (except delavirdine). Clinicians should consult Web-based updates for the latest specific recommendations.

* Interactions with HIV-related drugs are updated frequently and are available at http://www/aidsinfo.nih.gov/guidelines.
+ Recommended regimen for persons aged <18 years
** Recommended regimen for pregnant women
++ The substitution of rifapentine for rifampin is not recommended because rifapentine's safety and effectiveness have not been established for patients with LTBI

Adapted from Centers for Disease Control and Prevention. Update: adverse event data and revised American Thoracic Society/CDC recommendations against the use of rifampin and pyrazinamide for treatment of latent tuberculosis infection-United States, 2003. *MMWR.* 2003;52:735-739.

munity. The annual risk of TST conversion among HCWs has been reported at some institutions to be in the range of 2 to 4 per 1000 person years worked, even in high prevalence areas in the United States.[40,86] Recommendations made in this chapter focus on TB infection control for the United States (and would be applicable to other industrialized countries). The WHO has published guidelines for limited resource areas.[87] More detailed guidelines for TB infection control have been published by the CDC[23] and it is anticipated that revised CDC TB infection control guidelines will be published in 2005. Despite progress made, a number of controversial areas remain, including mandates regarding respiratory protection and fit testing and the appropriate role of UVGI. It is essential that guidelines and regulatory requirements be evidenced based as much as possible and that research continue into unresolved

scientific issues. Finally, HCWs must remain vigilant. Even in a decreasing era of TB, failure to consider the diagnosis and take appropriate infection control measures can lead to nosocomial transmission of TB in healthcare facilities.[28]

REFERENCES

1. Sepkowitz KA. Tuberculosis and the healthcare worker: a historical perspective. *Ann Intern Med.* 1994;120:71-79.

2. Blumberg HM. Tuberculosis infection control. In: Reichman LB, Hershield E, eds. *Tuberculosis: A Comprehensive International Approach.* 2nd ed. New York: Marcel-Dekker, Inc.; 2000;609-644.

3. Myers JA, Diehl HS, Boynton RE, Horns HL. Tuberculosis in physicians. *JAMA.* 1955;158:1-8.

4. Lincoln EM. Epidemic of tuberculosis. *Adv Tuberc Res.* 1965;14:157-201.

5. Alpert ME, Levison ME. An epidemic of tuberculosis in medical school. *N Engl J Med.* 1965;332:92-98.

6. Ehrenkranz NJ, Kirklighter JL. Tuberculosis outbreak in a general hospital: evidence for airborne spread of infection. *Ann Intern Med.* 1972;77:377-382.

7. Catanzaro A. Nosocomial tuberculosis. *Am Rev Respir Dis.* 1982;125:559-562.

8. Menzies D, Fanning A, Yuan L, Fitzgerald M. Tuberculosis among healthcare workers. *N Engl J Med.* 1995;332:92-98.

9. Institute of Medicine (IOM). Committee on regulating occupational exposure to tuberculosis. In: MJ Field, ed. *Tuberculosis in the Workplace.* Washington, DC: National Academy Press; 2001.

10. Snider DE Jr, Roper WL. The new tuberculosis. *N Engl J Med.* 1992;326:703-705.

11. Jarvis WR. Nosocomial transmission of multidrug-resistant *Mycobacterium tuberculosis. Res Microbiol.* 1993; 144:117-122.

12. Fischl MA, Uttamchandani RB, Caikos G, et al. An outbreak of tuberculosis caused by multidrug-resistant tubercle bacilli among patients with HIV infection. *Ann Intern Med.* 1992;117:177-183.

13. Beck-Sague C, Dooley SW, Hutton MD, et al. Hospital outbreak of multidrug-resistant *Mycobacterium tuberculosis* infections: factors in transmission to staff and HIV-infected patients. *JAMA.* 1992;268:1280-1286.

14. Edlin BR, Tokars JI, Grieco MH, et al. An outbreak of multidrug-resistant tuberculosis among hospitalized patients with the acquired immunodeficiency syndrome. *N Engl J Med.* 1992;326:1514-1521.

15. Dooley SW, Villarino ME, Lawrence M, et al. Nosocomial transmission of tuberculosis in a hospital unit for HIV-infected patients. *JAMA.* 1992;267:2632-2634.

16. Zaza S, Blumberg HM, Beck-Sague C, et al. Nosocomial transmission of *Mycobacterium tuberculosis*: role of healthcare workers in outbreak propagation. *J Infect Dis.* 1995;172:1542-1549.

17. Aita J, Barrera L, Reniero A, et al. Hospital transmission of multidrug-resistant *Mycobacterium tuberculosis* in Rosario, Argentina. *Medicina.* 1996;56:48-50.

18. Jereb JA, Klevens RM, Privett TD, et al. Tuberculosis in healthcare workers at a hospital with an outbreak of multidrug-resistant *Mycobacterium tuberculosis. Arch Intern Med.* 1995;24(155):854-859.

19. Coronado VG, Beck-Sague CM, Hutton MD, et al. Transmission of multidrug-resistant *Mycobacterium tuberculosis* among persons with human immunodeficiency virus infection in an urban hospital: epidemiologic and restriction fragment length polymorphism analysis. *J Infect Dis.* 1993;168:1052-1055.

20. Pearson ML, Jereb JA, Frieden TR, et al. Nosocomial transmission of multidrug-resistant *Mycobacterium tuberculosis*. A risk to patients and healthcare workers. *Ann Intern Med.* 1992;117:191-196.

21. Ikeda RM, Birkhead GS, DiFerdinando GT Jr, et al. Nosocomial tuberculosis: an outbreak of a strain resistant to seven drugs. *Infect Control Hosp Epidemiol.* 1995;16:152-159.

22. Jarvis WR. Nosocomial transmission of multidrug-resistant *Mycobacterium tuberculosis. Am J Infect Control.* 1995;23:146-151.

23. Centers for Disease Control and Prevention. Guidelines for preventing the transmission of *Mycobacterium tuberculosis* in health-care settings, 1994. *MMWR.* 1994;43(RR-13):1-132.

24. Blumberg HM, Watkins DL, Berschling JD, et al. Preventing the nosocomial transmission of tuberculosis. *Ann Intern Med.* 1995;122:658-663.

25. McGowan JE. Nosocomial tuberculosis: new progress in control and prevention. *Clin Infect Dis.* 1995;21:489-505.

26. Centers for Disease Control and Prevention. Trends in tuberculosis—United States, 1998-2003. *MMWR.* 2004;53:209-214.

27. Pugliese G, Tapper ML. Tuberculosis control in healthcare. *Infect Control Hosp Epidemiol.* 1996;17:819-827.

28. Centers for Disease Control and Prevention. Tuberculosis outbreak in a community hospital—District of Columbia, 2002. *MMWR.* 2004;53:214-216.

29. Sotir, MJ, Parrott P, Metchock B, et al. Tuberculosis in the inner city: impact of a continuing epidemic in the 1990's. *Clin Infect Dis.* 1999;29:1138-1144.

30. Wenger PN, Otten J, Breeden A, Orfas D, Beck-Sague CM, Jarvis WR. Control of nosocomial transmission of multidrug-resistant *Mycobacterium tuberculosis* among healthcare workers and HIV-infected patients. *Lancet.* 1995;345:235-240.

31. Maloney SA, Pearson ML, Gordon MT, del Castillo R, Boyle JF, Jarvis WR. Efficacy of control measures in preventing nosocomial transmission of multidrug-resistant tuberculosis to patients and healthcare workers. *Ann Intern Med.* 1995;122:90-95.

32. Fazal BA, Telzak EE, Blum S, et al. Impact of a coordinated tuberculosis team in an inner-city hospital in New York City. *Infect Control Hosp Epidemiol.* 1995;16:340-343.

33. Egan KB, MK Leonard, N White, HM Blumberg. An Investigation of a Dedicated Respiratory Isolation Unit in Ruling Out Patients for Tuberculosis. In: 2002 Southern Regional Meetings of the American Federation for Medical Research. New Orleans, Louisiana: February 2002.

34. Black CL, Parrott, PL, White N, Ray SM, Blumberg HM. Increased efficiency in the evaluation of patients after the implementation of a dedicated respiratory isolation unit. In: 4th Decennial International Conference on Nosocomial and Healthcare-Associated Infections. CDC: Atlanta, GA, March 2000.

35. Scott B, Schmid M, Nettleman M. Early identification of and isolation of inpatients at high risk for tuberculosis. *Arch Intern Med.* 1994;154:326-330.

36. American Thoracic Society, Centers for Disease Control and Prevention. Targeted tuberculin testing and treatment of latent tuberculosis infection. *Am J Resp Crit Care Med*. 2000;161:S221-S247.

37. Blumberg HM, White N, Parrott P, Gordon W, Hunter M, Ray S. False-positive tuberculin skin test results among healthcare workers. *JAMA*. 2000;283:2793.

38. Horowitz HW, Luciano BB, Kadel JR, Wormser RP. Tuberculin skin test conversions in hospital employees vaccinated with bacille Calmette-Guérin: recent *Mycobacterium tuberculosis* infection or booster effect? *Infect Control Hosp Epidemiol*. 1995;23:181-187.

39. Bailey TC, Fraser VJ, Spitznagel EL, Dunagan WC. Risk factors for a positive tuberculin skin test among employees of an urban, midwestern teaching hospital. *Ann Intern Med*. 1995;122:580-585.

40. Larsen NM, Biddle CL, Sotir MJ, White N, Parrott P, Blumberg HM. Risk of tuberculin skin test conversion among healthcare workers: occupational versus community exposure and infection. *Clin Infect Dis*. 2002;35:796-801.

41. Institute of Medicine. *Ending Neglect: The Elimination of Tuberculosis in the United States*. Washington, DC: National Academy Press; 2000.

42. Centers for Disease Control and Prevention. Guidelines for using the QuantiFERON®-TB test for diagnosing latent *Mycobacterium tuberculosis* infection. *MMWR Morb Mortal Wkly Rep*. 2002;51:1-5.

43. Mazurek GH, LoBue PA, Daley CL, et al. Comparison of a whole-blood interferon gamma assay with tuberculin skin testing for detecting latent *Mycobacterium tuberculosis* infection. *JAMA*. 2001;286:1740-1747.

44. Ewer K, Deeks J, Alvarez L, et al. Comparison of T-cell-based assay with tuberculin skin test for diagnosis of *Mycobacterium tuberculosis* infection in a school tuberculosis outbreak. *Lancet*. 2003;361:1168-1173.

45. Brock I, Weldingh K, Lillebaek T, Follmann F, Andersen P. Comparison of a new specific blood test and the skin test in tuberculosis contacts. *Am J Respir Crit Care Med*. In press.

46. Centers for Disease Control and Prevention. Prevention and control of tuberculosis in facilities providing long-term care to the elderly: recommendations of the Advisory Council for the Elimination of Tuberculosis. *MMWR*. 1990;39(RR-10).

47. Ijaz K, Dillaha JA, Yang Z, Cave MD, Bates JH. Unrecognized tuberculosis in a nursing home causing death with spread of tuberculosis to the community. *J Am Geriatr Soc*. 2002;50:1213-1218.

48. Stead WW. Tuberculosis among elderly persons, as observed among nursing home residents. *Int J Tuberc Lung Dis*. 1998;2(Suppl 1):S64-70.

49. American Society of Heating RaA-CE. Healthcare facilities. *1999 ASHRAE Handbook: HVAC Applications*. Atlanta, Ga: ASHRAE; 1999: 7.1-7.13.

50. American Institute of Architects. *Guidelines for Design and Construction of Hospital and Healthcare Facilities*. Washington, DC: American Institute of Architects; 2001.

51. American Conference of Governmental Industrial Hygienists. *Industrial Ventilation: A Manual of Recommended Practice*. 24th ed. Cincinnati, Ohio: ACGIH; 2001.

52. Rutala WA, Jones SM, Worthington JM et al. Efficacy of portable filtration units in reducing aerosolized particles in the size range of *Mycobacterium tuberculosis*. *Infect Control Hosp Epidemiol*. 1995;16:391-98.

53. Nardell EA. Environmental infection control of tuberculosis. *Seminars in Respiratory Infections*. 2004;4:307-319.

54. Nardell EA. Interrupting transmission from patients with unsuspected tuberculosis: a unique role for upper-room ultraviolet air disinfection. *Am J Infect Control*. 1995; 23:156-164.

55. Nardell EA. Fans, filters, or rays? Pros and cons of the current environmental tuberculosis control technologies. *Infect Control Hosp Epidemiol*. 1993;14:681-685.

56. American National Standards Institute, American Society of Heating RaA-CE. *Standard 55—Thermal Environmental Conditions for Human Occupancy*. Atlanta, Ga: ASHRAE; 1992.

57. First M, Nardell E, Chaaission W, et al. Guidelines for the application of upper-room ultraviolet germicidal irradiation for preventing transmission of airborne contagion-Part II: design and operations guidance. *ASHRAE Trans*. 1999;105:877-887.

58. Green CF, Scarpino PV. The use of ultraviolet germicidal irradiation (UVGI) in disinfection of airborne bacteria. *Environ Eng Policy*. 2003;3:101-107.

59. Brubacher J, Hoffman RS. Hazards of ultraviolet lighting used for tuberculosis control. *Chest*. 1996;109:582-583.

60. Talbot EA, Jensen P, Moffat HJ et al. Occupational risk from ultraviolet germicidal irradiation (UVGI) lamps. *International J Tuberculosis Lung Dis*. 2002;6:738-741.

61. Adal KA, Anglim AM, Palumbo CL, Titus MG, Coyner BJ, Farr BM. The use of high-efficiency particulate air-filter respirators to protect hospital workers from tuberculosis. A cost-effectiveness analysis. *N Engl J Med*. 1994;331:169-173.

62. Nettleman MD, Fredrickson M, Good NL, Hunter SA. Tuberculosis control strategies: the cost of particulate respirators. *Ann Intern Med*. 1994;121:37-40.

63. Jarvis WR, Bolyard EA, Bozzi CJ, et al. Respirators, recommendations, and regulations: the controversy surrounding protection of healthcare workers from tuberculosis. *Ann Intern Med*. 1995;122:142-146.

64. Department of Labor, Occupational Safety and Health Administration. Occupational exposure to tuberculosis: proposed rule. *Federal Register*. 1997;62:54159-54308.

65. Managan LP, Bennett CL, Tablan N, et al. Nosocomial tuberculosis prevention measures among two groups of U.S. hospitals, 1992 to 1996. *Chest*. 2000;117:380-384.

66. Department of Labor, Occupational Safety and Health Administration (OSHA). Occupational exposure to tuberculosis; proposed rule; termination of rulemaking respiratory protection for *M. tuberculosis*; final rule; revocation. *Federal Register.* 2003;68:75767-75775.

67. US Department of Labor. Tuberculosis: OSHA standards. Available at: http://www.osha.gov/SLTC/tuberculosis/standards.html. Accessed May 14, 2004.

68. Department of Labor, Occupational Safety and Health Administration (OSHA). Respiratory protection for *M. tuberculosis*. 29 CFR Part 1910 [Docket No. H-371]. *Federal Register.* 2003;68:75776-75780.

69. Coffey CC, Campbell DL, Zhuang Z. Simulated workplace performance of N95 respirators. *Am Ind Hyg Assoc J.* 1999;60(5):618-24.

70. Coffey CC, Lawrence RB, Zhuang Z et al. Comparison of five methods for fit-testing N-95 filtering-facepiece respirators. *Appl Occup Environ Hyg.* 2002;17:723-730.

71. Coffey CC, Lawrence RB, Campbell DL, Zhuang Z, Calvert CA, Jensen PA. Fitting characteristics of eighteen N-95 filtering-facepiece respirators. *J Occup Environ Hyg.* 2004;1:262-271.

72. National Institute for Occupational Safety and Health (NIOSH). Respiratory protective devices; final rules and notice. *Federal Register.* 1995;60(110):30336-30398.

73. Department of Health and Human Services, Centers for Disease Control and Prevention and National Institutes of Health, Richmond JY, McKinney RW, eds. *Biosafety in Microbiological and Biomedical Laboratories.* 4th ed. Washington, DC: US Government Printing Office: Washington; 1999.

74. Fennelly K, Nardell E. The relative efficacy of respirators and room ventilation in preventing occupational tuberculosis. *Infect Control Hosp Epidemiol.* 1998;19:754-759.

75. American Thoracic Society and Centers for Disease Control and Prevention. Diagnostic standards and classification of tuberculosis in adults and children. *Am J Respir Crit Care Med.* 2000;161:1376-1395.

76. Blumberg HM, Burman WJ, Chaisson RE, et al; American Thoracic Society, Centers for Disease Control and Prevention and the Infectious Diseases Society. Treatment of tuberculosis. *Am J Respir Crit Care Med.* 2003;167:603-662.

77. Advisory Council for the Elimination of Tuberculosis (ACET). Tuberculosis elimination revisited: obstacles, opportunities, and a renewed commitment. *MMWR Recomm Rep.* 1999;48(RR-9):1-13.

78. Centers for Disease Control and Prevention. Notice to readers: update: nucleic acid amplification tests for tuberculosis. *MMWR.* 2000;49:593-602.

79. Chaulk CP, Kazandjian VA. Directly observed therapy for treatment completion of pulmonary tuberculosis: consensus statement of the public health tuberculosis guidelines panel. *JAMA.* 1998; 279:943-948.

80. Centers for Disease Control and Prevention. Update: adverse event data and revised American Thoracic Society/CDC recommendations against the use of rifampin and pyrazinamide for treatment of latent tuberculosis infection—United States, 2003. *MMWR Morb Mortal Wkly Rep.* 2003;52:735-739.

81. Barrett-Connor E. The epidemiology of tuberculosis in physicians. *JAMA.* 1979;241:33-38.

82. Fraser VJ, Kilo CM, Bailey TC, Medoff G, Dunagan WC. Screening of physicians for tuberculosis. *Infect Control Hosp Epidemiol.* 1994;15:95-100.

83. Gieseler PJ, Nelson KE, Crispen RG. Tuberculosis in physicians: compliance with preventive measures. *Am Rev Respir Dis.* 1987;135:3-9.

84. Camins BC, Bock N, Watkins DL, Blumberg HM. Acceptance of isoniazid therapy by healthcare workers after tuberculin skin test conversion. *JAMA.* 1996; 275:1013-1015.

85. Shukla SJ, Warren DK, Woeltje KF, Gruber CA, Fraser VJ. Factors associated with the treatment of latent tuberculosis infection among health-care workers at a midwestern teaching hospital. *Chest.* 2002;122:1609-1614.

86. Wilson JCE, Blumberg HM. Low risk of house staff tuberculin skin test conversion at an inner-city hospital in a high endemic area. In: *Annual Meeting of the Infectious Diseases Society of America.* Chicago, Ill: Infectious Diseases Society of America; 2002.

87. World Health Organization. *Guidelines for the prevention of tuberculosis in healthcare facilities in resource-limited settings.* Geneva: World Health Organization; 1999.

CHAPTER TWENTY-THREE

INFECTION CONTROL IN LONG-TERM CARE FACILITIES

Lindsay E. Nicolle, MD and Richard A. Garibaldi, MD

BACKGROUND

Many individuals in developed countries reside for extended periods in LTCFs. While different types of institutions provide a wide variety of services to diverse groups of patients, the majority of residents in these facilities are elderly people who reside in nursing homes. Approximately 43% of Americans who became 65 years old in 1990 will reside in a nursing home for some time before they die.[1] Infection control programs are necessary in these facilities to limit morbidity and mortality from infections and to achieve optimal use of resources.

Infections are common in LTCFs. Reported rates of infection in nursing homes have varied from 1.8 to 9.4 per 1000 resident-days (Table 23-1). The prevalence of infection has varied from 1.6% to 14%.[2] This wide variation in reported rates reflects differences in patient populations, definitions of infection, and surveillance methods used.

The most common endemic infections in nursing homes affect the urinary tract, upper and lower respiratory tracts, gastrointestinal tract, conjunctiva, and skin (eg, decubitus ulcers, cellulitis, and vascular ulcers). SSIs, the second most common cause of nosocomial infections in acute-care facilities, are uncommon. Outbreaks of infections occur frequently.[2] The most common etiologic agents of outbreaks are listed in Table 23-2.

Residents of LTCFs have numerous comorbidities and impaired functional status; between 10% and 30% of these patients die each year. Consequently, the morbidity and mortality that is specifically attributable to infections rather than due to the underlying disease may be difficult to assess. Morbidity may include further functional impairment or a need for transfer to an acute-care facility. Pneumonia, with a reported case-fatality ratio of 6% to 23%, is the only infection that contributes substantially to mortality. The case fatality ratio for bacteremias is also quite high, ranging from 10% to 25%; however, bacteremia is uncommon in LTCFs.[2]

At present, little is known about the costs of infections in LTCFs. Some factors that may contribute to increased costs include evaluation by nursing and medical staff, laboratory and radiologic tests, antimicrobial therapy, intensified nursing care, infection control efforts, and transfer of residents to acute-care facilities.

REASONS FOR INCREASED RISK OF INFECTION IN LONG-TERM CARE FACILITY RESIDENTS

Changes in body systems that occur with aging increase the risk of infection (Table 23-3). The specific contributions of aging-associated alterations in immune function are not clear. However, nonimmune aging-associated changes that enhance the patient's susceptibility to infection occur in virtually all body systems.

The institutionalized elderly have numerous comorbidities that substantially increase their risk of infection. For instance, urologic abnormalities, such as prostatic hypertrophy, are associated with urinary tract infections. Chronic obstructive lung disease and congestive heart failure increase a patient's risk of developing pneumonia. Diabetes or vascular insufficiency may lead to more frequent and severe skin infections. Functional impairment, including decreased mobility and incontinence (usually secondary to comorbidities), further increases the risk that a patient will develop an infection.

Therapeutic interventions may also increase the risk of infection for individual patients. Approximately 5% to 10%

TABLE 23-1. REPORTED INCIDENCE AND PREVALENCE OF COMMON INFECTIONS IN NURSING HOMES

	Incidence Per 1000 Days	Percent Prevalence
All infections	1.8 to 9.4	1.6 to 13.9
Urinary infections		
Symptomatic	0.19 to 2.2	2.6 to 3.5
Asymptomatic	1.1	15 to 50
Respiratory tract		
Lower (pneumonia, bronchitis)	0.3 to 4.7	0.3 to 5.8
Sinusitis/otitis	0.003 to 2.3	1.5
Skin/soft tissue	0.14 to 1.1	5.6 to 8.4
Infected pressure ulcers	0.1 to 0.3	2.6 to 24
Cellulitis/cutaneous abscesses	0.19 to 0.23	7.2 to 8.7
Conjunctivitis	0.17 to 1.0	5 to 13
Candida infections	0.28	33 to 47
Bacteremia	0.2 to 0.36	—
Gastrointestinal infections	0 to 2.5	0.5 to 1.3

TABLE 23-2. ETIOLOGIC AGENTS IDENTIFIED AS CAUSES OF LONG-TERM CARE FACILITY OUTBREAKS

	Viral	Bacterial	Other
Respiratory	Common cold viruses	*S. pneumoniae*	
	Influenza	*H. influenzae*	
	Respiratory syncytial virus	*M. tuberculosis*	
	Parainfluenza[1,3]	*Bordetella pertussis* (rare)	
	Coronavirus	Group A streptococcus	
Gastrointestinal	Rotavirus	*Salmonella* spp	*Giardia lamblia*
	Norwalk-like viruses	*E. coli* 0157:H7	
	Astroviruses (rare)	*Shigella* spp	
		C. difficile	
		S. aureus (food poisoning)	
		C. perfringens (food poisoning)	
		Bacillus cereus (food poisoning)	
		Aeromonas hydrophilia (rare)	
		Campylobacter jejuni (rare)	
Skin infections		Group A streptococcus	Scabies
		S. aureus	

of residents in nursing homes will have long-term indwelling urinary catheters, and these patients always will be bacteriuric.[2] The increasing use of other invasive procedures, such as hemodialysis and chronic respirators with tracheostomy, puts patients in LTCFs at risk for bloodstream and pulmonary infections. Percutaneous feeding tubes lead to infections at the stoma site. Medications such as antidepressants, with atropine-like side effects, will dry oral secretions and increase the frequency of pharyngeal colonization. In addition, these drugs inhibit bladder contraction and impede urine flow, which may predispose patients to urinary tract infections.

In institutions, high-risk patients are clustered together in distinct geographic units, dining facilities, recreational activities, and physical or occupational therapy. This clustering may facilitate transmission of pathogens from one resident to another. Organisms may be transmitted through the air (eg, tuberculosis, influenza), on the hands of staff or patients (eg, *S. aureus* or uropathogens), and by contaminated items (eg, food).

TABLE 23-3. FACTORS THAT MAY PROMOTE INFECTION IN LONG-TERM CARE FACILITY RESIDENTS

Factor	Aging-Associated Changes
Skin	Epidermal thinning, decreased elasticity, subcutaneous tissue, vascularity, and wound healing
Respiratory tract	Decreased cough reflex, elastic tissue, mucociliary transport, IgA
Gastrointestinal tract	Decreased gastric acidity and motility
Genitourinary tract	Decreased estrogen effect on mucosa, decreased prostatic secretions, increased prostatic size
Immune system	Thymic involution, decreased antibody production, decreased T cells, decreased mitogen stimulation, decreased fever response, decreased interleukin-2, and increased autoantibodies
Chronic illness	Diabetes, congestive heart failure, vascular insufficiency, chronic obstructive pulmonary disease, neurologic impairment, dementia
Nutritional impairment	Decreased cell-mediated immunity and wound healing
Functional impairment	Immobility, incontinence, impaired mental status, poor hygiene
Invasive devices	Indwelling urinary catheter, tracheostomy, feeding tube gastrostomy, central intravenous catheter
Institutionalization	Increased person-to-person contact

SPECIAL CONSIDERATIONS FOR INFECTION CONTROL PROGRAMS IN LONG-TERM CARE FACILITIES

There are fundamental differences between LTCFs and acute-care facilities.[3] In some cases, these differences require epidemiologists to approach infection control differently in each setting.

Resources

In LTCFs, the resources and expertise available for establishing and operating infection control programs are limited. Specific problems include the following:

➤ In many facilities, individuals responsible for the infection control program are part-time workers. They have numerous other responsibilities that limit the time available for infection control and reduce its priority.

➤ Some facilities have limited access to personnel with expertise in IDs, microbiology, and infection control practices to assist in dealing with infections.

➤ Some facilities have minimal or no employee health programs. They may have limited resources to educate staff to prevent infections, conduct immuniza-

tion programs, screen for tuberculosis, or manage HCWs who may be ill with an infection.

➤ The medical literature provides limited evidence to support the effectiveness of specific practices to limit the transmission of infections in LTCFs.

Personnel

Compared to staff in acute-care facilities, staff in LTCFs often have less training in infection control and other patient care practices. Furthermore, staff turnover in LTCFs is higher than that in acute-care facilities, making it difficult to train personnel adequately in infection control practices.

Patient-Related Issues

The clinical approach to the diagnosis and management of patients in LTCFs differs from that practiced in the community or in acute-care facilities. The reasons for this include the following:

➤ The ability to communicate may be impaired for many patients in LTCFs.

➤ Access to radiologic and laboratory facilities may be limited, and specimens or patients may need to be transferred off site for testing.

➤ Clinical criteria to diagnose infections have been developed for younger populations with fewer co-morbidities. Most LTCF residents have chronic symptoms that may make it difficult to identify and evaluate acute changes in clinical status that represent a new infection.

➤ IDs in the elderly patient may have nonclassical presentations. For instance, impaired elderly patients who have infections may present with acute confusion rather than prominent localizing findings. Compared to younger patients, the elderly have a relatively blunted temperature response; therefore, a higher proportion of infected patients may be afebrile.

➤ Certain microbiologic specimens have limited diagnostic use in this population. For example, gram-negative organisms frequently colonize the oropharynx of elderly patients who are in institutions.[2] Sputum specimens obtained from these patients may be contaminated by the colonizing organisms. In addition, 30% to 50% of noncatheterized elderly residents of nursing homes are bacteriuric; in these patients, a positive urine culture has a low positive predictive value for diagnosing symptomatic urinary infection.[4]

➤ In general, the use of standard clinical diagnostic tests has not been evaluated for patients in LTCFs. The optimal use of laboratory tests for management of infection in this population and the appropriate empiric approach to treatment are not well established.

DEVELOPING AN INFECTION CONTROL PROGRAM IN THE LONG-TERM CARE FACILITY

Infection control programs should be developed to serve the specific needs of a given institution and its patient population. The basic components of such a program include administration, personnel, surveillance for infections, policies, and education.[3]

Administration

An effective reporting structure must be defined. It is essential that the infection control program has a close working association with the medical director, administrator, or nursing supervisor for the LTCF. Responsibility and authority should be defined clearly and the structure developed to ensure an efficient and effective infection control program.

Personnel

The size and complexity of the institution will determine the number of individuals needed to work on infection control. At least one individual must have responsibility for the infection control program. If an individual is responsible for other programs in the institution in addition to infection control, his or her specific commitment to infection control must be defined clearly.

Personnel with responsibility for infection control must have a good understanding of the basic principles of microbiology, IDs, epidemiology, program management, and patient and staff education.

Individuals with expertise in areas such as outbreak investigation, IDs, antimicrobial use, and microbiology should be identified and consulted when needed.

Surveillance for Infections

Surveillance to identify infected patients and outbreaks of infections is an essential component of the infection control program.[3] Standard definitions, appropriate for LTCFs, should be used to identify infections at each site. Some recommended definitions have been published.[5]

Infection control personnel should use case-finding methods that are appropriate for the available resources and characteristics of the institution. Methods may include walking rounds, nursing-generated reports, chart reviews, and laboratory or medication record reviews. When an infection control program is initially being developed for a facility, prevalence surveys may be useful. Generally, incidence surveys are more useful for ongoing programs.

Infection control personnel should analyze data, review findings, and report results to the administration and to their infection control committee at least quarterly. Incidence rates generally should be reported as the number of infections per 1000 resident days.

The surveillance program should enable infection control personnel to identify outbreaks of influenza, gastrointestinal illness, scabies, and other common problems in a timely manner so that appropriate control measures can be implemented.

Policies

Policies regarding the identification and control of infections must be developed, reviewed, updated, and monitored to document adherence. Some specific issues to be addressed by institutional policies include the following:

➤ Handwashing

➤ Standard precautions and additional isolation practices

➤ Environmental cleaning, laundry, and waste disposal

➤ Food preparation, holding, and transport

➤ Preadmission screening of residents for infections (eg, tuberculosis)

➤ Immunization policies (eg, influenza, *S. pneumoniae*)

➤ Management of patients with infections, especially those who may require special infection control precautions

➤ Identification and management of residents with antimicrobial-resistant organisms

➤ Outbreak identification, investigation, and control

➤ Review of antimicrobial use[6,7]

➤ Employee health issues including tuberculosis screening, immunizations, and work restriction when employees have potentially transmissible infections

Education

Ongoing education of staff, residents, and visitors is an important component of the infection control program. All individuals working in the facility, including medical staff, should know risk factors for infection and methods for minimizing each resident's risk of infection. These programs should be developed with input from the groups of employees for which they are targeted.

SPECIAL INFECTION PROBLEMS

Influenza

Influenza outbreaks occur frequently in LTCFs[8] and may be disruptive because many patients and staff members become ill within a short time. Outbreaks have been associated with substantial patient mortality. Each facility should develop a specific plan for managing influenza that includes the following:

➤ Yearly immunization programs for patients and staff

➤ Clinical and epidemiologic definitions of influenza

➤ Surveillance for possible outbreaks

➤ Criteria defining when and from whom diagnostic specimens should be collected

➤ Response to outbreaks, including when to place restrictions on residents or visitors

➤ Notification of local authorities

➤ Recommendations for prophylactic and therapeutic use of antiviral medications (eg, agent, dose, patient exclusions, triggers for initiating prophylaxis, and criteria for deciding which patients will receive prophylaxis)

Gastrointestinal Illness, Including Clostridium difficile

Outbreaks of gastrointestinal illness are common in LTCFs.[9] Sporadic episodes of diarrhea may be caused by infectious bacteria or viruses or by noninfectious condi-

tions including medications or diet.[10] Specific components in a program to control diarrheal illness should include the following:

➤ Clinical definitions to identify individual cases and outbreaks of diarrheal disease

➤ Criteria that define when specimens and laboratory tests should be obtained

➤ A description of infection control practices, including isolation precautions required for patients with suspected infectious diarrheal illness

➤ A protocol for the use of oral rehydration therapy

➤ Protocols for antimicrobial therapy of infected patients and staff (eg, metronidazole for moderate-to-severe *C. difficile* colitis)[10]

➤ Staff education programs

Clusters of patients with diarrhea may be caused by foodborne pathogens, including those associated with toxins (eg, *Bacillus cereus*, *S. aureus*), as well as bacterial, viral, or parasitic infections. Management of such clusters should include the following:

➤ Epidemiologic investigation that includes the number of cases; number of people at risk; and the characterization of cases by time, place, and person

➤ Identification of the source of infection (eg, food item, person, utensil)

➤ Elimination or treatment of the source

➤ Staff education to limit transmission and to prevent future outbreaks

➤ Appropriate management of infected residents and personnel

Scabies

To manage scabies effectively, personnel in LTCFs must understand the disease and follow a systematic approach to identifying and treating affected patients.[11] Issues that must be addressed include clinical and microscopic diagnostic criteria; treatment for infected patients (5% permethrin or 1% lindane); management of exposed patients, staff, and household contacts; handling of contaminated bedding and clothing; and follow-up of treated subjects.

Group A Streptococcal Skin Infections

LTCFs should define how they will identify individual cases and outbreaks of streptococcal disease.[12] They also must define which infection control precautions should be instituted when streptococcal infections are identified.

For severe outbreaks, or in instances when initial control measures are not effective, infection control personnel should have criteria for performing a culture survey to identify colonized patients and staff or for undertaking mass treatment of residents.[12]

Tuberculosis

The most important strategy for preventing spread of tuberculosis is early identification and treatment of possibly infectious patients.[13] LTCFs need to monitor skin-test conversion among residents and staff, identify and evaluate patients with pulmonary symptoms consistent with tuberculosis, isolate patients with potential or proven pulmonary tuberculosis, trace exposed patients and staff, and initiate prophylactic isoniazid therapy.

Bloodborne Pathogens

Policies must be developed for the management of patients with potential bloodborne infections, including hepatitis B, hepatitis C, and HIV infection. These policies should describe the practice of standard precautions, include guidelines for the use of gloves and other barriers during patient care, and discuss methods to limit needlestick exposures and other percutaneous injuries.

Multiply-Resistant Organisms

Some patients in nursing homes are at increased risk of colonization or infection with antimicrobial-resistant organisms.[2] Institutional programs should define multiply-resistant organisms, provide guidelines for the management of patients who are colonized or infected with resistant organisms, and review and restrict antimicrobial use when appropriate. Certain patients may require isolation precautions; however, standard infection control precautions, such as appropriate handwashing, environmental cleaning, and wound care, usually will be sufficient.[14,15]

LTCFs should develop policies regarding transferring patients with resistant organisms to other institutions or accepting such patients from other institutions. In general, a resistant organism should not preclude transferring or accepting a patient. However, the institution that transfers the patient should always notify the accepting institution before the patient is transferred so that the staff of the latter facility can be prepared.[15]

REFERENCES

1. Kemper P, Murtaugh C. Lifetime use of nursing home care. *N Engl J Med.* 1991;324:595-600.

2. Nicolle LE, Strausbaugh LJ, Garibaldi RA. Infections and antibiotic resistance in nursing home. *Clin Micro Reviews.* 1996;9:1-17.

3. Smith PW, Rusnak PG. Infection prevention and control in the long-term care facility. *Infect Control Hosp Epidemiol.* 1997;18:831-849.

4. Nicolle LE, SHEA Long Term Care Committee. Urinary tract infections in long term care facilities. *Infect Control Hosp Epidemiol.* 2001;22:167-175.

5. McGeer A, Campbell B, Emori TG, et al. Definitions of infection for surveillance in long-term care facilities. *Am J Infect Control.* 1991;19:1-7.

6. Nicolle LE, Bentley D, Garibaldi R, Neuhaus E, Smith P, SHEA Long Term Care Committee. Antimicrobial use in long-term care facilities. *Infect Control Hosp Epidemiol.* 2000;21:537-545.

7. Loeb M, Bentley DW, Bradley S, et al. Development of minimum criteria for the initiation of antibiotics in residents of long term care facilities: results of a consensus conference. *Infect Control Hosp Epidemiol.* 2001;22:120-124.

8. Bradley SF, SHEA Long Term Care Committee. Prevention of influenza in long term care facilities. *Infect Control Hosp Epidemiol.* 1999;20:629-637.

9. Bennett RG. Diarrhea among residents of long-term care facilities. *Infect Control Hosp Epidemiol.* 1993;14:397-404.

10. Simor AE, Bradley SF, Strausbaugh LJ, Crossley K, Nicolle LE, SHEA Long Term Care Committee. *Clostridium difficile* in long term care facilities for the elderly. *Infect Control Hosp Epidemiol.* In press.

11. Segelau J. Scabies in long-term care facilities. *Infect Control Hosp Epidemiol.* 1992;13:421-425.

12. Schwartz B, Ussery XT. Group A streptococcal outbreaks in nursing homes. *Infect Control Hosp Epidemiol.* 1992;13:742-747.

13. Centers for Disease Control. Prevention and control of tuberculosis in facilities providing long-term care to the elderly. *MMWR.* 1990;39(No. RR-10):7-13.

14. Boyce JM, Jackson MM, Pugliese G, et al. Methicillin-resistant *Staphylococcus aureus* (MRSA): a briefing for acute care hospitals and nursing facilities. *Infect Control Hosp Epidemiol.* 1994;15:105-115.

15. Strausbaugh LJ, Crossley KB, Nurse BA, Thrupp LD, SHEA Long Term Care Committee. Antimicrobial resistance in long-term care facilities. *Infect Control Hosp Epidemiol.* 1995;17:120-129.

SUGGESTED READING

Smith PW, ed. *Infection Control in Long-Term Care Facilities.* 2nd ed. Albany, NY: Delmar Publishers, Inc; 1994.

Strausbaugh LJ, Joseph C. Epidemiology and prevention of infections in long-term care facilities. In: Mayhall G, ed. *Hospital Epidemiology and Infection Control.* Philadelphia, Pa: Lippincott, Williams & Wilkins, 1999;1461-1482.

CHAPTER TWENTY-FOUR

INFECTION CONTROL
IN THE OUTPATIENT SETTING

Deborah M. Nihill, RN, MS, CIC; Loreen A. Herwaldt, MD; Shanon Smith, MD; Cheryl D. Carter, RN, BSN; and Tammy Lundstrom, MD

INTRODUCTION

Healthcare delivery is undergoing dramatic changes. Innovative medical technologies have allowed HCWs to perform many diagnostic and therapeutic procedures in the outpatient setting. Consequently, the proportion of medical care that is provided in the outpatient setting is increasing rapidly. For example, 80% to 90% of all cancer care is delivered in the outpatient setting and more than half of all hospital-based operations are done in ambulatory surgery centers.[1] From 1992 to 2001, patient visits to hospital outpatient departments increased from 56.6 million to 83.7 million visits. This represents a 48% increase, although the population in the United States increased by only 12% during the same time period. Office-based physician practices account for 80% of ambulatory healthcare delivered by nonfederal physicians, with 880.5 million patient visits in 2001.[2,3]

Given these statistics, hospital epidemiologists and ICPs must develop programs that address infection control issues across the entire spectrum of care and not focus exclusively on the inpatient setting. In addition to the clinical and monetary incentives to address infection control issues in the outpatient setting, the CDC recommends and the OSHA mandates that HCWs in the outpatient setting incorporate the Bloodborne Pathogen Standard[4] and tuberculosis guidelines into their practices.[5] Moreover, the JCAHO requires that within a particular healthcare organization the infection control policies and procedures that are applied in the inpatient setting and in the outpatient setting are consistent in intent and application.[6]

HCWs and infection control personnel traditionally have considered the risk of infection to be low in the ambulatory-care setting. However, few investigators have systematically evaluated the rates of infection in outpatient populations. Investigators who have attempted to conduct surveillance in outpatient populations have often encountered substantial problems that have precluded instituting such programs into the routine practice of infection control. These include lack of resources, lack of education and training, lack of administrative support, and lack of time (multiple duties), and lack of computerized data sources.

To date, experts in infection control and agencies such as the CDC have not recommended specific surveillance systems in ambulatory care. However, essential elements of infection control programs in the outpatient setting have been developed and defined.[7-11] It has been noted that risk for transmission of nosocomial infections in ambulatory care settings is more likely to occur in 1 of 2 manners: congregation of patients in waiting rooms or other common areas, and in association with invasive procedures.[12] Despite the dearth of data and guidelines, the infection control staff must develop programs that address the special needs of the ambulatory-care setting because this is where most medical care will be given in the 21st century.

For the purposes of this chapter, we will define outpatient or ambulatory care as any medical services provided to patients who are not admitted to inpatient hospital units. Infection control in the outpatient or ambulatory setting is a very broad topic because the scope of medical services provided outside of the traditional inpatient setting and the types of facilities providing these services have expanded exponentially. Even conventional hospitals that specialize in hospital-based care have numerous areas in which persons other than inpatients are waiting, visiting, or undergoing treatment. Although most hospitals have an infection control program, planning and provision of resources for expansion beyond inpatient units is often inadequate. Numerous outpatient facilities have sprung up that are independent of hospitals, including ambulatory treatment centers, urgent-care centers, outpatient surgical centers, and radiology and imaging clinics. Third-party payers have encouraged this development and now demand that a large proportion of medical care be given in the outpatient setting. Challenges for infection control in outpatient and ambulatory care settings include determining which infections to conduct surveillance, to whom the data will be reported, and who will be responsible for implementing the changes.[13]

This chapter will discuss general principles of infection control in the outpatient setting, as well as specific considerations for some specific areas. However, we will not discuss specific infection control issues for ambulatory surgery centers, home healthcare, or dental offices. Readers who need information on those topics are referred to recent reviews.[14-18]

COMMON PROBLEMS ENCOUNTERED

Persons who conduct infection control efforts in any outpatient setting will encounter problems that either do not occur in the inpatient setting or are exaggerated in the outpatient setting compared with the inpatient setting. We will discuss some of these problems briefly.

The population of persons in the outpatient setting often is very difficult to define. For example, exposures to communicable diseases such as SARS, measles, or tuberculosis can occur in clinic waiting areas, hospital registration areas, or in other large open areas in which many people congregate. Infection control personnel may have difficulty identifying what patients, family members, and staff members were in the area at a particular time. Similarly, infection control personnel may have difficulty determining the rate of device-related infections in outpatients because patients who acquire these infections may be treated elsewhere and because the denominator (ie, the number of persons with devices) is very difficult to determine.

Most surveillance methodologies were developed for use in the inpatient setting and are of limited use in the outpatient setting. The surveillance methods that have been tested in the outpatient setting often are labor-intensive and lack sensitivity and specificity. Clinic schedules often are very busy and leave little time for formal educational programs. Moreover, unlike hospital-based programs, freestanding facilities might not have on-site continuing education programs.

Staff in some outpatient facilities turn over rapidly, and these changes make it difficult to achieve and maintain an adequate level of infection control knowledge among staff members. Telephone calls and registration usually are handled by persons with the least medical knowledge.

Thus, patients who have contagious diseases might not be identified and triaged appropriately.

Personnel in clinics often care for many patients and do many procedures during a day. Given current budget constraints, the number of staff members and the amount of equipment often are limited. Thus, the staff might cut corners to meet the demands of the schedule. For example, HCWs might not wash their hands when appropriate or they might not clean, disinfect, or sterilize equipment properly.

Many outpatient medical facilities were not designed with infection control input, and thus are not adequately laid out with infection control principals in mind. For example, most outpatient facilities do not have negative-air-pressure rooms, and the air often is recirculated without filtration. In addition, outpatient facilities might have only one entrance and one waiting area, making these clinics ideal places in which airborne pathogens, such as *Mycobacterium tuberculosis*, VZV, or SARS coronavirus can spread. Moreover, many outpatient facilities have inadequate space to allow the staff to maintain separate clean and dirty areas, and storage is often a challenge.

EXPOSURES TO BLOODBORNE PATHOGENS

The OSHA Bloodborne Pathogen Standard specifies that all healthcare institutions, including outpatient facilities, must implement policies and procedures to protect HCWs from exposures to bloodborne pathogens.[4] Infection control personnel must ensure that the inpatient and outpatient facilities within their institution implement the same general policies and procedures (ie, a single standard of practice) to prevent exposures (see Chapter 28 for additional information on implementing a bloodborne pathogen program). However, some of the specific policies might be different in the 2 settings because the staffs provide different services in each setting.

HCWs in the ambulatory setting are at risk for exposure to blood and body fluids.[19-24] Staff members in emergency departments may be at the highest risk because they frequently provide acute care for persons who have traumatic injuries or are critically ill.[19,20] Despite their exposure to blood and body fluids, HCWs in the outpatient setting often do not comply with precautions designed to protect them from bloodborne pathogens.[22-24]

Devices with engineered safety features are required by OSHA and federal legislation in inpatient as well as outpatient settings.[25,26] ICPs face challenges engaging frontline outpatient staff members in the selection of particular devices. Educational programs related to the safe use of these devices are problematic because sites of care may be widely scattered, requiring a traveling road show for effective education.

In addition to HCWs, patients are also at risk for acquiring HBV, HCV, and HIV through medical care provided in the outpatient setting.[27-38] Contaminated multidose vials, equipment that was cleaned and disinfected improperly, and reuse of needles have been associated with transmission of these pathogens, both in isolated cases and in outbreaks.[27-40] In addition, lax infection control injection procedures have also been noted during employee vaccination programs.[41] These findings underscore the need for appropriate staff training and monitoring of infection control practices in these settings.

HAND HYGIENE

The CDC *Guideline for Hand Hygiene in Healthcare Settings* are applicable to the inpatient as well as the outpatient setting.[42] Studies of hand hygiene compliance in the outpatient setting have found adherence ranging from 31% to 74%.[42-45] As in the inpatient setting, improvements are needed, and attention should be paid to installing waterless hand hygiene agents appropriately in outpatient settings. See Chapter 19 for additional information on hand hygiene.

RESPIRATORY INFECTIONS IN THE OUTPATIENT SETTING

Several outbreaks have illustrated that bacterial and viral pathogens can be transmitted within outpatient facilities by airborne or droplet spread. Particular characteristics of the outpatient setting, such as the following, might enhance the likelihood that these pathogens will be transmitted:

➤ Many people congregate in waiting rooms
➤ Many contagious patients come to outpatient facilities for evaluation and treatment, particularly during endemic or epidemic periods for viral infections
➤ Outpatient facilities frequently have inadequate triage systems
➤ The number of air exchanges in the building often is low, and the air often is recirculated

Increased attention has been focused on transmission of respiratory pathogens in the outpatient setting with the emergence of SARS and avian influenza. The likelihood of transmission of respiratory pathogens in the outpatient setting can be reduced through the use of "respiratory etiquette" protocols,[46] which include:

➤ Post visual alerts at the entrance to outpatient facilities instructing those reporting for care to report respiratory symptoms
➤ Cover nose/mouth when coughing or sneezing
➤ Use tissues to contain respiratory secretions and dispose of them in the nearest waste receptacle after use
➤ Perform hand hygiene after contact with respiratory secretions and contaminated objects/materials
➤ Provide tissues and no-touch receptacles for used tissue disposal
➤ Provide conveniently located hand washing agents (either waterless or soap/towels if sink available)
➤ Offer masks to persons who are coughing
➤ Triage coughing individuals out of common waiting area as soon as possible

TUBERCULOSIS IN THE AMBULATORY SETTING

Several outbreaks demonstrate that HCWs[47-51] and patients[52-55] can become infected when exposed to outpatients who have undiagnosed tuberculosis or to patients with known tuberculosis when the isolation precautions are not optimal. HCWs have transmitted *M. tuberculosis* to patients infrequently.

The most important element of a tuberculosis control program is early identification and isolation of patients with suspected or confirmed infectious tuberculosis, which includes respiratory etiquette protocols. Triage personnel and staff members who perform the initial evaluation in ambulatory-care facilities must be educated about how and when to institute respiratory etiquette protocols based on patient symptoms and risk factors.[56] Unfortunately, in many settings "tuberculosis is often unsuspected, and isolation measures are often not used."[57]

If staff members in outpatient departments or facilities perform special procedures such as sputum induction, bronchoscopy, aerosolized pentamidine treatments, or pulmonary function testing, the units must have adequate facilities (ie, booths or other enclosures meeting ventilation requirements for tuberculosis isolation) to prevent airborne spread of *M. tuberculosis*. However, a survey conducted by the CDC in 1992 revealed that patients with tuberculosis often were treated in emergency departments, but few emergency departments were equipped appropriately to care for patients with suspected tuberculosis.[58]

Infection control personnel should help the staff in the ambulatory-care areas of their healthcare center develop comprehensive protocols for identifying and treating patients with respiratory signs and symptoms. As part of this process, infection control personnel should help create screening tools that staff can use to identify such patients.

MEASLES AND RUBELLA

The incidence of measles and rubella in the United States has decreased substantially since appropriate vaccines were introduced. However, both continue to be transmitted within healthcare facilities and in the outpatient setting.[59-70]

Several infection control precautions can prevent measles and rubella transmission in medical settings: proper ventilation, infection control policies stipulating that all staff members must be immune,[67] appropriate immunization protocols for patients, and prompt triage of patients who have febrile exanthems. However, proper ventilation may be difficult to achieve in many outpatient settings because buildings are built to be energy efficient, which often means the buildings are airtight, and the ventilation systems recirculate air.[62] In addition, because the incidence of measles and rubella is low, few HCWs recognize these illnesses. Consequently, patients with measles may be misdiagnosed and may not be isolated appropriately.[61]

Appropriate triage begins with the telephone conversation during which clinic appointments are scheduled. The scheduler should ask the caller for the patient's chief complaint. If the patient has a fever and a rash or respiratory symptoms, the appointment should be scheduled at the end of the day or during times of the day when few patients are present.[63] Patients who must come to the clinic when other patients are present should wear a mask, enter through a separate entrance, and go directly to an examination room. If a patient arrives unannounced at a clinic or emergency department, the staff at the registration desk should ask whether the patient has fever and a rash or respiratory symptoms. If the answer to this question is yes, the patient should put on a mask and go to an examining room (preferably one with negative air pressure) immediately.

EPIDEMIC KERATOCONJUNCTIVITIS

Adenovirus, particularly type 8, has caused numerous outbreaks of keratoconjunctivitis in ophthalmology clin-

ics.[71-83] However, basic infection control precautions could prevent spread of this virus among patients and staff in those clinics. The infection control staff should ensure that its ophthalmology clinic and emergency departments have developed the following appropriate policies and procedures[45,76,84]:

➤ HCWs should wear gloves for possible contact with the conjunctiva.

➤ Equipment, including tonometers, should be cleaned and disinfected according to recommendations by the CDC,[79] the American Academy of Ophthalmology,[84] or the manufacturers. (Note that the methods for cleaning and disinfecting tonometers vary with the type of tonometer. Moreover, tonometers must be rinsed appropriately and thoroughly to prevent chemical keratitis).[85]

➤ If a nosocomial outbreak is identified, all open ophthalmic solutions should be discarded, and the equipment and environment should be cleaned and disinfected thoroughly.

➤ During an outbreak, unit doses of ophthalmic solutions should be used.

➤ During outbreaks, patients with conjunctivitis should be examined in a separate room with designated equipment, supplies, and ophthalmic solutions.

➤ During an outbreak, elective procedures such as tonometry should be postponed.

➤ HCWs who work in any outpatient area and who have adenovirus conjunctivitis should not work until the inflammation has resolved, which may take 14 or more days.

OTHER TRANSMISSIBLE AGENTS

Bordetella pertussis outbreaks in the community have spread to outpatient settings within hospitals.[86,87] VZV, influenza virus, and parvovirus B19 all have been transmitted in the inpatient setting, and many exposures to VZV occur in clinics and physicians' offices. However, we did not find published descriptions of outbreaks in the ambulatory setting caused by VZV, influenza virus, or parvovirus B19. Outbreaks may in fact occur, but they might not be recognized, or persons who investigate them might not report them. The general infection control precautions recommended to prevent spread of respiratory pathogens will help prevent spread of these etiologic agents. Vaccines currently are available for all of these agents except for parvovirus B19.

INFECTION CONTROL ISSUES RELATED TO DEVICES

Infections Related to Bronchoscopic and Gastrointestinal Endoscopic Procedures Done in the Outpatient Setting

Eleven million endoscopic procedures are performed in the United States each year, many of which are done in the outpatient setting. Many inpatient HCFs have bronchoscopy or gastrointestinal endoscopy suites that serve both inpatients and outpatients. Private physicians and physicians in freestanding clinics also do endoscopy in their offices. Moreover, the number and type of procedures performed and the number of patients undergoing these procedures continue to increase.

Given the nature of the procedures and the limitations of surveillance systems, infections associated with endoscopic procedures are very difficult to identify unless they occur in clusters. Despite these limitations, numerous investigators have reported outbreaks of infection related to endoscopic procedures.[88-109] Most outbreaks could have been prevented if the endoscopy staff had followed basic infection control procedures.

Flexible fiberoptic endoscopes have allowed physicians to do procedures that are not possible with rigid endoscopes. However, flexible endoscopes present problems not encountered with rigid endoscopes. The most important problem is that flexible endoscopes are very difficult to clean and disinfect because they have several long, narrow internal channels and because they cannot be steam sterilized. Consequently, endoscopes must be reprocessed by persons who understand the internal structure of the devices and who take the time necessary to clean and disinfect these devices meticulously. Although professional societies have published guidelines for reprocessing endoscopes,[88,110-112] the protocols used for those procedures have not been standardized,[113,114] and different endoscopes must be reprocessed by different methods. Moreover, because endoscopes are very expensive, endoscopy staff may try to save money by using a small number of endoscopes to evaluate and treat a large number of patients. The staff may not be able to process the equipment properly in the time allowed between patients.[115]

This topic has been well reviewed in articles by Spach et al,[89] Ayliffe,[90] and Weber and Rutala.[91] Factors that have allowed flexible endoscopes to transmit pathogenic organisms have included the following:

➤ Failure to clean and disinfect the blind channel in endoscopes used to examine the biliary tree[94]
➤ Failure to disinfect endoscopes and accessory equipment (eg, suction-collection bottles, rubber connection tubing) properly between procedures[92,97-99]
➤ Failure to sterilize biopsy forceps[93,98]
➤ Failure to dry endoscopes completely before storage[95]
➤ Failure to wash endoscopes before disinfecting them[107]
➤ Use of contaminated water[95]
➤ Use of tap water to rinse endoscopes[96,104]
➤ Use of unfiltered tap water in automatic endoscope washers[116]
➤ Improper maintenance with subsequent contamination of automatic endoscope washers[108]
➤ Use of inadequate disinfectants[99]
➤ Use of contaminated suction valves[102]
➤ Use of endoscopes with internal defects that prevent adequate cleaning and disinfection[105]

Despite numerous reports of outbreaks, endoscopy suites often do not reprocess endoscopes properly. Several studies conducted in different countries document that staff in many endoscopy suites continue to make the same errors that have caused the outbreaks listed above.[114,115,117-121]

The policies and procedures needed in an endoscopy suite for infection control, cleaning, and disinfection are not more complicated or substantially different from those needed in other healthcare settings. However, the procedures must be followed precisely because endoscopes are such complex semicritical instruments that they are difficult to clean even when the staff reprocess these devices conscientiously.[122] Staff members might be intimidated by the complexity of the cleaning and disinfection process. To overcome these barriers, the infection control staff should read the published recommendations for cleaning and disinfecting endoscopes[88,110-112] and should understand the basic principles of disinfection and sterilization.[123] Infection control staff also should spend time in the endoscopy suite to learn from the staff and to identify potential infection control problems. Together, staff from both programs should review the policies and procedures to ensure that they are consistent with current recommendations and guidelines and that they are consistent in intent and application throughout the HCF.

Infection control personnel should be aware that new ion plasma, vaporized hydrogen peroxide, and 100% ethylene oxide sterilizers do not reliably kill organisms in narrow lumens when serum and salt are present.[124,125] Thus, these methods may not be adequate for processing flexible endoscopes, especially if they have not been cleaned scrupulously. Infection control personnel should discuss with staff in the endoscopy suite the limitations of these technologies and, at present, probably should discourage their use in this setting.

Endoscopy clinics that are not a part of a larger medical center may not have direct access to infection control personnel or to training in infection control. Regardless of the endoscopy suite's location, staff members must be trained to clean and disinfect endoscopes meticulously. The endoscopy staff also should understand basic principles of infection control, including methods for preventing transmission of routine bacterial pathogens to patients and to staff, methods for preventing spread of bloodborne pathogens, and methods for cleaning and disinfection. One person should be responsible to ensure that staff members are educated properly, that they always comply with the specified procedures, and that all equipment is handled and maintained properly.

Disposable Devices

With the increased pressure for cost containment, HCWs and administrators are questioning why many devices marketed for single use cannot be reprocessed and reused. This issue is not unique to the outpatient setting, but, in this setting, the pressure to reuse single-use items might be greater, or the infection control oversight might be substantially less than in the inpatient setting. Examples of single-use items that often are reused in the outpatient setting include syringes, plastic vaginal specula, mouthpieces for pulmonary function machines, cardiac catheters, and oral airways. An ambulatory HCF that chooses to reprocess single-use devices must develop a comprehensive quality-assurance program to ensure that the products are cleaned, disinfected, or sterilized adequately and that the items retain their integrity and function.[126] Institutions that reprocess those devices, not the manufacturers, assume the liability. Thus, infection control personnel would be wise to identify which single-use products are being reused and to ensure that the devices are reprocessed and tested for function and integrity appropriately. Readers interested in a more in-depth discussion of this topic should read the recent review by Greene.[127]

Flash Sterilization of Surgical Equipment

Steam sterilization of patient-care items for immediate use, or "flash sterilization," was designed to process items that had become contaminated during a sterile procedure but were essential for that procedure. The time required for flash sterilization is very short. Thus, all of the parameters (eg, time, temperature) must be met precisely. The persons doing flash sterilization must keep meticulous records to document that these parameters have been met. In addition, flash sterilization will not work if the device is contaminated with organic matter or if air is

trapped in or around the device. The efficacy of flash sterilization also will be impaired if either the sterilizer or the flash pack are not working properly. Moreover, because the devices are used immediately (ie, before the results of biological indicators are known), personnel in ambulatory surgery centers that use flash sterilization must record which devices were used for specific patients, so that patients can be followed if the load was not processed properly.

Many institutions have expanded the use of flash sterilization well beyond its intended and approved uses. Some of the changes are reasonable, but some jeopardize the efficacy of sterilization. Infection control professionals whose outpatient facilities use flash sterilization should read two pertinent publications by the Association for the Advancement of Medical Instrumentation (AAMI).[128,129] Infection control professionals should then assess whether their institution is using this process properly.

OTHER INFECTION CONTROL ISSUES

Multidose Vials

Multidose vials are used frequently in the inpatient and outpatient setting because they may be more convenient and cheaper than single-dose vials. However, studies in the literature indicate that up to 27% of used multidose vials are contaminated with bacterial pathogens.[130-132]

Although the actual risk of infection associated with multidose vials remains unknown, the risk of infection appears to be low if multidose vials are used properly. However, the staff in a busy outpatient clinic might not adhere to appropriate infection control precautions. Indeed, numerous outbreaks in such clinics attest to the fact that multidose vials can be an important reservoir or vehicle for bacterial and viral pathogens.[30,32,133-138]

Antimicrobial Resistant Pathogens

Antimicrobial resistance is increasing among many pathogenic gram positive, gram negative, viral, and fungal pathogens. Examples include VRE,[139-141] MRSA, glycopeptide-intermediate *S. aureus* (GISA), and VRSA.[139-147] Many of these organisms are spread on the hands of personnel and by contaminated patient-care equipment or environmental surfaces. Consequently, the organisms could be spread in both the inpatient and outpatient settings. Infection control personnel, therefore, must work across the spectrum of healthcare settings (ie, inpatient units, central surgical suites, ambulatory surgical centers, endoscopy suites, hospital-based and freestanding ambulatory clinics, LTCFs, and home care) if they want to control the spread of these organisms effectively. Efforts to control antimicrobial resistant organisms in the outpatient setting will cross disciplines, departments, and organizations. Hence, these efforts may be very difficult to coordinate. General infection control measures such as containment of patients' secretions/excretions, proper hand hygiene, and appropriate environmental cleaning can impact cross-transmission of these important pathogens. Specific recommendations have been made for VRE,[139,140] MRSA,[140] and VRSA.[147] Updated CDC and Prevention Isolation guidelines are expected to be released in 2004 and are expected to further address resistant pathogens.

Medical Waste

Like hospitals, HCFs and agencies that operate in the ambulatory setting produce infectious wastes. However, these institutions may not have an expert in waste management on their staff, and they may not have ready access to appropriate processing (eg, autoclaves) and disposal facilities (eg, incinerators). In addition, because these facilities often operate for profit, the staff might feel pressured to take shortcuts.

An in-depth discussion of medical waste is beyond the scope of this chapter. Readers who must develop waste-management programs for outpatient facilities should read several excellent reviews of this topic.[123,148,149] We will review a few of the basic principles, most of which were discussed by Morrison in his review of the topic.[148]

The control plan must meet city, county, state, and federal regulations. Healthcare organizations must comply with all regulatory requirements; penalties can be imposed for noncompliance.

Infection control personnel should help other staff to do the following:

➤ Define which items are noninfectious waste and which are infectious

➤ Develop protocols and procedures for separating infectious waste from noninfectious waste; labeling the infectious waste properly; and transporting, storing, and disposing of infectious waste safely

➤ Develop contingency plans for managing waste spills and inadvertent exposures of visitors or HCWs

➤ Develop programs to teach staff to handle infectious waste

Infection control personnel also could help staff identify ways to minimize infectious waste. Examples include the following:

➤ Stop discarding noninfectious waste, such as wrappers and newspapers, in infectious waste containers

➤ Substitute products that do not require special modes of disposal (eg, needleless intravenous systems) for those that must be discarded in the infectious waste (eg, needles)

INFECTION CONTROL IN SPECIAL SETTINGS

Dialysis Centers

Background

Dialysis centers can be associated with hospitals (on-site or at a distance), or they can be freestanding. In the former case, the infection control staff should ensure that the policies and procedures in the unit are consistent with those in the hospital. The freestanding dialysis units resemble other freestanding medical facilities in that they usually are for-profit organizations, and they rarely have trained infection control staff.

Bloodborne Pathogens

The primary infection control issue in dialysis centers is transmission of bloodborne pathogens, such as HBV, HCV, and HIV. To date, transmission of HBV has been the most common problem. Use of good infection control precautions and the hepatitis B vaccine have decreased the risk of transmission substantially in this setting. Staff members should always use standard precautions when they handle blood and other specimens, such as peritoneal fluid, which can contain high levels of HBsAg and HBV.[150]

In this section, we will review some basic infection control precautions for dialysis units by summarizing the main points from an excellent chapter by Favero et al.[150] Infection control personnel who need detailed information should read that chapter and several other articles.[150-153]

Infection control precautions designed to prevent transmission of hepatitis B in dialysis centers include the following[150]:

➤ Patients and staff members should be screened for HBsAg and anti-HBsAg when they enter the unit.

➤ Dialysis centers should survey susceptible patients and HCWs routinely for HBsAg and anti-HBsAg to determine whether transmission of HBV has occurred in the unit.

➤ Patients who are HBsAg carriers should undergo dialysis in a separate room designated only for use by such patients. If this is impossible, patients who are HBsAg carriers should be dialyzed on dedicated machines in an area that is separated from the area in which HBV-seronegative patients are dialyzed.

➤ Medications in multidose vials should not be shared among patients.

➤ Staff members should not care for patients who carry HBsAg and for seronegative patients during the same shift.

➤ Ideally, the same hemodialysis equipment should not be used for both HBsAg-seropositive and HBsAg-seronegative patients. However, when this is not possible, the machines should be disinfected using conventional protocols, and the external surfaces should be cleaned or disinfected using soap and water or a detergent germicide.

➤ HBsAg-positive patients should not participate in dialyzer reuse programs.

➤ Centers that do peritoneal dialysis should separate HBsAg-positive patients from those who are HBsAg-negative and should observe precautions similar to those used for hemodialysis patients because peritoneal fluid can transmit HBV to susceptible persons.

Hepatitis D virus (HDV) has been transmitted in dialysis centers. Therefore, patients who are infected with HDV should be dialyzed on dedicated machines in an area that is separated from all other dialysis patients, especially those who are HBsAg-positive.[150] If there is evidence that HDV has been transmitted within the unit, patients should be screened for delta antigen and antibody to delta antigen.

HCV has caused outbreaks in dialysis centers.[154] However, there is no consensus on using specific precautions for patients who have antibody to HCV or for those who are infected with HIV.[150,154,155] General procedures that are recommended include:

➤ The staff should use precautions that limit exposure to blood and body fluids.[154]

➤ The staff always should clean and disinfect all instruments and environmental surfaces that are touched routinely.[154]

➤ Articles should not be shared among patients.[154]

➤ The center should measure liver enzymes for all patients to determine whether any patients have evidence of non-A and non-B hepatitis, including HCV.[150]

➤ If liver enzymes from several patients increase during a short time period, staff should identify the etiology of each patient's hepatitis, so that the staff can determine whether an outbreak exists.[150]

➤ Hemodialysis centers could conduct serological surveys of their patient and staff populations to determine the baseline prevalence of hepatitis C in their center and to determine whether the prevalence has changed over time.[150]

If transmission of bloodborne pathogens occurs in a dialysis unit, staff must determine how the organism was transmitted and what infection control procedures have been violated. To facilitate such investigations, Favero et al have recommended that dialysis centers maintain detailed records on the following[150]:

➤ The lot number of all blood and blood products used

➤ All mishaps such as blood leaks or spills, and dialysis machine malfunctions

➤ The location, name, or number of the dialysis machine used for each dialysis session

➤ The names of staff members who connect and disconnect the patient to and from a machine

➤ Results of serologic tests for hepatitis

➤ All accidental needle punctures and similar accidents sustained by staff members and patients

Staphylococcus aureus

Patients on dialysis have high rates of *S. aureus* nasal carriage (up to 81%).[156] *S. aureus* also is a leading cause of infections in patients on dialysis. Moreover, the risk of *S. aureus* infection is significantly higher for dialysis patients who carry this organism in their nares than for patients who do not carry it.[156,157]

Most dialysis patients are infected by the *S. aureus* strains that they carry in their nares.[158,159] Thus, the most effective preventive strategies involve decolonization of the nares. Several investigators have documented that prophylactic use of rifampin or mupirocin can prevent *S. aureus* infections in dialysis patients.[156-161] However, mupirocin resistance can develop rapidly.

Approximately 10% to 20% of *S. aureus* infections in patients on continuous ambulatory peritoneal dialysis (CAPD) occur in noncarriers or are caused by strains other than those carried by the patients. Thus, HCWs in dialysis units, family members, and home healthcare staff must practice basic infection control precautions to prevent spread of *S. aureus* to dialysis patients.[162,163] Of note, dialysis center patient was the source of the first VRSA infection in the world.[145]

Outbreaks in Dialysis Centers

Numerous outbreaks have occurred in dialysis centers.[31,32,136,154,164-168] Most of the outbreaks were caused by major deficiencies in basic infection control practices. The primary errors were inadequate or improper disinfection processes, poor compliance with precautions to prevent spread of bloodborne pathogens, and allowing HBsAg-positive and HBsAg-negative patients to share multidose vials of medications. Bacterial pathogens other than *S. aureus* that have been reported to cause outbreaks in dialysis patients include coagulase-negative staphylococci,[169] gram-negative bacilli (*Enterobacter cloacae, P. aeruginosa,* and *E. coli* from contaminated dialysis machine valves),[170] and *Pasturella multocida.*[171]

In 1999, the CDC initiated a voluntary national system to monitor and prevent infections in outpatient dialysis centers. Results identified a vascular access infection rate of 3.2 per 100 patient-months overall.[172] However, rates varied significantly by type of vascular access: rates were lowest for natural arteriovenous fistulas and highest for noncuffed catheters (0.56 versus 11.98),[172] confirming a finding that had been previously reported.[173] Infection control professionals armed with this knowledge can impact infection rates through education of physicians and dialysis staff regarding access selection, where appropriate.

INFECTION CONTROL IN PHYSICAL THERAPY

Physical therapy facilities can be located in hospitals, in clinics, or can be freestanding. Many of these facilities provide services to outpatients. Physical therapy facilities have not been documented to be the source of outbreaks except in the case of infections associated with hydrotherapy. However, the absence of data is no cause to be sanguine because all the elements necessary for transmission of pathogens exist in physical therapy centers. In addition, few investigators have looked rigorously for evidence of transmission in this setting.

The APIC has published the only recommendations for infection control in physical therapy.[174] However, these recommendations provide limited guidance because little information is available regarding appropriate infection control precautions specific for this setting.[175,176] The following text outlines a few basic infection control principles for physical therapy centers that are summarized from an excellent review written by Linnemann.[175]

Infection control professionals who advise physical therapy units should ensure that the staff implement the following recommendations:

➤ All mats, table tops, and equipment handles should be covered with impervious materials, so that these items can be cleaned frequently.

➤ Cleaning supplies should be stored where they are readily accessible, so that staff can clean the equipment whenever necessary, not just at the scheduled times.

➤ Handwashing sinks or alcohol-based hand rubs should be located such that therapists can wash or disinfect their hands easily after each patient or between patients if they are helping more than one patient at a time.

➤ Physical therapists should be educated regarding standard precautions and the mechanisms by which organisms are transmitted.

➤ Physical therapists should understand that they could transmit infectious agents as they move from patient to patient and should know what precautions are necessary to prevent spread of pathogens.

➤ Therapists should wear gloves and gowns when they could contaminate their hands or clothing.

➤ Patients who have active infections caused by transmissible organisms or who are infected or colonized with resistant organisms should not use the facility. If such patients are allowed to use the facility, the staff must use appropriate precautions to prevent spread of these organisms.

OCCUPATIONAL SAFETY AND HEALTH ADMINISTRATION INSPECTIONS

A full discussion of OSHA inspections in the ambulatory setting is beyond the scope of this chapter. However, infection control personnel must understand that OSHA's regulations also apply to facilities that provide care to outpatients. Persons who must ensure that their outpatient facility complies with OSHA's regulations must understand the Bloodborne Pathogen Standard[4] and the CDC tuberculosis recommendations.[5] For additional information on OSHA inspections, see Chapter 28.

Outpatient facilities associated with hospitals might be at greater risk of an OSHA inspection than are physicians' offices. However, OSHA does inspect offices operated by doctors of medicine and osteopathy.[177,178] Most inspections result from complaints filed by employees. Common violations in physicians' offices "involve personal protective equipment such as gloves and gowns, employee information and training requirements, records of training sessions, storage of those records, development of an exposure control plan, and procedures for laundering of personal protective equipment."[178] It is important to remember that outpatient settings are not exempt from requirements for implementation of sharps safety devices.

CONCLUSION

By now, you probably are overwhelmed completely and are wondering where to begin. Obviously, one person or one program cannot assess all of the areas that we have discussed in this chapter. Thus, we would recommend that infection control staff members assess their own institutions to determine the following:

➤ What type of outpatient facilities are present in your medical center (eg, only hospital-based clinics, units that provide services to both inpatients and outpatients, only freestanding clinics, or a mixture of on-site and off-site clinics owned by the medical center)?

➤ What types of patients are seen in the outpatient facilities (eg, young children, immunocompromised patients, healthy preoperative patients)?

➤ What types of procedures are performed in the outpatient facilities?

➤ Which procedures are performed most commonly?

➤ What types of infectious diseases are diagnosed and treated in the outpatient facilities?

➤ What resources are available for infection control?

➤ Do the administration and the clinicians support the infection control program?

Once you have identified the primary characteristics of your facility, you should review the policies and procedures in the major areas and conduct walking rounds to answer the following questions:

➤ Does the area have policies, procedures, and engineering controls to prevent transmission of bloodborne pathogens?

➤ Does the area have appropriate screening, triage, isolation protocols, and engineering controls to prevent the spread of airborne agents?

➤ Does the area have appropriate screening, triage, and isolation for patients who may be infected or colonized with other infectious agents?

➤ Does the area have appropriate exposure management plans for bloodborne pathogens, measles virus, *M. tuberculosis*, VZV, *B. pertussis*, lice, and scabies?

➤ Does the staff understand and practice principles of asepsis, including those required to use multidose vials safely?

➤ Does the staff understand and practice appropriate cleaning, disinfection, and sterilization?

➤ Are the policies and procedures in this area consistent in content and intent with those from other areas in the medical center?

➤ Does the area have educational programs to teach staff precautions for respiratory pathogens, bloodborne pathogens, and other infectious agents? Do they document these programs adequately?

Once you have answered these questions, you should set priorities. We would suggest that all outpatient facilities should focus first on the following preventive measures:

➤ Ensure that the staff complies with the tuberculosis recommendations and Bloodborne Pathogen Standards published by the CDC and OSHA, respectively.

➤ Implement "respiratory etiquette" protocols to prevent unnecessary patient and employee exposures.

➤ Ensure that the staff and patients have been vaccinated appropriately.

➤ Ensure that the staff practices good aseptic technique when handling multidose vials and that protocols and practices for cleaning, disinfection, and sterilization are appropriate.

Once they have addressed these priorities, infection control personnel then can address other issues, including whether or not to develop surveillance for surgical site infections after ambulatory surgery. For example, infection control personnel might be able to work with home-healthcare agencies to identify infections that are associated with inpatient medical care or with treatments given in hospital-based clinics or ambulatory-surgery centers.

Infection control personnel who begin to address infection control needs in the ambulatory setting have not only a huge task to accomplish but also an enormous opportunity. Infection control personnel who take on this challenge will help to improve the patient and health care professional safety as well as the quality of care provided, and will help their institutions survive in this extraordinarily competitive environment. In addition, those intrepid persons will help shape the course of healthcare over the next decade.

REFERENCES

1. Lamkin L. Outpatient oncology settings: a variety of services. *Seminars in Oncology Nursing*. 1994;10:227,229-235.

2. Hing E, Middleton K. *National Hospital Ambulatory Medical Care Survey: 2001 Outpatient Department Summary. Advance data from vital and health statistics; no 338*. Hyattsville, Maryland: National Center for Health Statistics; 2003.

3. Cherry D, Burt CW, Woodwell DA. *National Hospital Ambulatory Medical Care Survey: 2001 Summary. Advance data from vital and health statistics; no 337*. Hyattsville, Maryland: National Center for Health Statistics; 2003.

4. Department of Labor, Occupational Safety and Health Administration. 29 CFR Part 1920.1030, Occupational exposure to bloodborne pathogens, final rule. *Federal Register*. December 6, 1991;56:64,004-64,182.

5. Centers for Disease Control and Prevention. Guidelines for preventing the transmission of *Mycobacterium tuberculosis* in health care facilities, 1994. *MMWR*. 1994;43:1-133.

6. Joint Commission on Accreditation of Healthcare Organizations. Leadership standard. In: *Comprehensive Accreditation Manual for Hospitals: The Official Handbook*. Oakbrook Terrace, Ill: JCAHO; 1996:LD-1-LD-52.

7. Herwaldt LA, Smith SD, Carter CD. Infection control in the outpatient setting. *Infect Control Hosp Epidemiol*. 1998;19:41-74.

8. Friedman C, Barnette M, Buck AS, et al. Requirements for infrastructure and essential activities of infection control and epidemiology in out-of-hospital settings: a consensus panel report. Association for Professionals in Infection Control and Epidemiology and Society for Healthcare Epidemiology of America. *Infect Control Hosp Epidemiol*. 1999;20:695-705.

9. Nguyen GT, Proctor SE, Sinkowitz-Cochran RL, Garrett DO, Jarvis WI. Status of infection surveillance and control programs in the United States, 1992-1996. Association for Professionals in Infection Control and Epidemiology, Inc. *Am J Infect Control*. 2000;28:392-400.

10. Friedman C. Infection control outside the hospital: developing a continuum of care. *Qual Lett Healthc Lead*. 2000;12:12-13.

11. Health Canada. Nosocomial and Occupational Infections Section. Development of a resource model for infection prevention and control programs in acute, long term, and home care settings: conference proceedings of the infection prevention and control alliance. *Am J Infect Control*. 2004;32:2-6.

12. Nafziger DA, Lundstrom T, Chandra S, Massanari RM. Infection control in ambulatory care. *Infect Dis Clin North Am*. 1997;11(2):279-296

13 Jarvis WR. Infection control and changing health-care delivery systems. *Emerg Infect Dis*. 2001;7(2):170-173.

14. Meier PA. Infection control issues in same-day surgery. In: Wenzel RP, ed. *Prevention and Control of Nosocomial Infections*. 3rd ed. Philadelphia, Pa: Williams & Wilkins; 1997:262-282.

15. Wade BH. Outpatient/out of hospital care issues. In: Wenzel RP, ed. *Prevention and Control of Nosocomial Infections*. 3rd ed. Philadelphia, Pa: Williams & Wilkins; 1997:243-259.

16. Smith PW, Roccaforte JS. Epidemiology and prevention of infections in home health care. In: Mayhall CG, ed. *Hospital Epidemiology and Infection Control*. Philadelphia, Pa: Williams & Wilkins; 1996:1171-1176.

17. Molinari JA. Dental office. In: Olmsted RN, ed. *APIC Infection Control and Applied Epidemiology: Principles and Practice, Part I Section C, Practice Settings*. St Louis, Mo: Mosby-Year Book, Inc; 1996:88-1-88-20.

18. Centers for Disease Control and Prevention. Guidelines for infection control in dental health-care settings 2003. *MMWR*. 2003;52:1-76.

19. Kelen GD, Hansen KN, Green GB, Tang N, Ganguli C. Determinants of emergency department procedure- and condition—specific universal (barrier) precaution requirements for optimal provider protection. *Ann Emerg Med*. 1995;25:743-750.

20. Kelen GD, Green GB, Purcell RH, et al. Hepatitis B and hepatitis C in emergency department patients. *N Engl J Med*. 1992;326:1399-1404.

21. Sivapalasingam S, Malak SF, Sullivan JF, Lorch J, Sepkowitz KA. High prevalence of hepatitis C infection among patients receiving hemodialysis at an urban dialysis center. *Infect Control Hosp Epidemiol*. 2002;23:319-324.

22. Kelen GD, Green GB, Hexter DA, et al. Substantial improvement in compliance with universal precautions in an emergency department following institution of policy. *Arch Intern Med*. 1991;151:2051-2056.

23. Thurn J, Willenbring K, Crossley K. Needlestick injuries and needle disposal in Minnesota physicians' offices. *Am J Med*. 1989;86:575-579.

24. Miller KE, Krol RA, Losh DP. Universal precautions in the family physician's office. *J Fam Pract*. 1992;35:163-168.

25. OSHA Compliance Document. Occupational exposure to bloodborne pathogens; needlesticks and other sharp injuries; Final rule. 29 C.F.R. Part 1910 (January 18, 2001)

26. Federal Needlestick Safety and Prevention Act Pub. L. 106-430 (2000).

27. Kent GP, Brondum J, Keenlyside RA, LaFazia LM, Scott HD. A large outbreak of acupuncture-associated hepatitis B. *Am J Epidemiol*. 1988;127:591-598.

28. Stryker WS, Gunn RA, Francis DP. Outbreak of hepatitis B associated with acupuncture. *J Fam Pract*. 1986;22:155-158.

29. Canter J, Mackey K, Good LS, et al. An outbreak of hepatitis B associated with jet injections in a weight reduction clinic. *Arch Intern Med*. 1990;150:1923-1927.

30. Alter MJ, Ahtone J, Maynard JE. Hepatitis B virus transmission associated with a multiple-dose vial in a hemodialysis unit. *Ann Intern Med*. 1983;99:330-333.

31. Danzig LE, Tormey MP, Sinha SD, et al. Common source transmission of hepatitis B virus infection in a hemodialysis unit. *Infect Control Hosp Epidemiol*. 1995;16(suppl):P19. Abstract.

32. Rosenberg J, Gilliss DL, Moyer L, Vugia D. A double outbreak of hepatitis B in a dialysis center. *Infect Control Hosp Epidemiol*. 1995;16(suppl):P19. Abstract.

33. Hlady WG, Hopkins RS, Ogilby TE, Allen ST. Patient-to-patient transmission of hepatitis B in a dermatology practice. *Am J Public Health*. 1993;83:1689-1693.

34. Drescher J, Wagner D, Haverich A, et al. Nosocomial hepatitis B virus infections in cardiac transplant recipients transmitted during transvenous endomyocardial biopsy. *J Hosp Infect*. 1994;26:81-92.

35. Reingold AL, Kane MA, Murphy BL, Checko P, Francis DP, Maynard JE. Transmission of hepatitis B by an oral surgeon. *J Infect Dis*. 1982;145:262-268.

36. Ciesielski C, Marianos D, Ou CY, et al. Transmission of human immunodeficiency virus in a dental practice. *Ann Intern Med*. 1992;116:798-805.

37. Velandia M, Fridkin SK, Cardenas V, et al. Transmission of HIV in dialysis centre. *Lancet*. 1995;345:1417-1422.

38. Chant K, Lowe D, Rubin G, et al. Patient-to-patient transmission of HIV in private surgical consulting rooms. *Lancet*. 1993;342:1548-1549. Letter.

39. Centers for Disease Control and Prevention. Transmission of hepatitis B and C viruses in outpatient settings—New York, Oklahoma, and Nebraska, 2000-2002. *MMWR*. 2003; 52:901-906.

40. Katzenstein TL, Jorgensen LB, Permin H, et al. Nosocomial HIV-transmission in an outpatient clinic detected by epidemiologic and phylogenetic analyses. *AIDS*. 1999;13:1779-1781.

41. Centers for Disease Control and Prevention. Improper infection—control practices during employee vaccination programs—District of Columbia and Pennsylvania, 1993. *MMWR*. 1993;42:969-971.

42. Centers for Disease Control and Prevention. Guideline for hand hygiene in health-care settings. *MMWR*. 2002; 51(RR-16):1-56.

43. Cohen HA, Kitai E, Levy I, Ben-Amitai D. Handwashing patterns in two dermatology clinics. *Dermatology*. 2002;205(4):358-361.

44. Cohen HA, Matalon A, Amir J, Paret G, Barzilai A. Handwashing patterns in primary pediatric community clinics. *Infection*. 1998;26:45-47.

45. Aizman A, Stein JD, Stenson SM. A survey of patterns of physician hygiene in ophthalmology clinic patients encounters. *Eye Contact Lens*. 2003;29:221-222.

46. Centers for Disease Control and Prevention. Public health guidance document for community-level preparedness and response to severe acute respiratory syndrome (SARS) Available at www.cdc.gov. Accessed January 8, 2003.

47. Haley CE, McDonald RC, Rossi L, Jones WD, Haley RW, Luby JP. Tuberculosis epidemic among hospital personnel. *Infect Control Hosp Epidemiol*. 1989;10:204-210.

48. Centers for Disease Control. *Mycobacterium tuberculosis* transmission in a health clinic—Florida, 1988. *MMWR*. 1989;38:256-258,263-264.

49. Griffith DE, Hardeman JL, Zhang Y, Wallace RJ, Mazurek GH. Tuberculosis outbreak among HCW in a community hospital. *Am J Respir Crit Care Med*. 1995;152:808-811.

50. Sokolove PE, Mackey D, Wiles J, Lewis RJ. Exposure of emergency department personnel to tuberculosis: PPD testing during an epidemic in the community. *Ann Emerg Med*. 1994;24:418-421.

51. Calder RA, Duclos P, Wilder MH, Pryor VL, Scheel WJ. *Mycobacterium tuberculosis* transmission in a health clinic. *Bulletin of the International Union Against Tuberculosis and Lung Disease*. 1991;66:103-106.

52. Fischl MA, Uttamchandani RB, Daikos GL, et al. An outbreak of tuberculosis caused by multiple-drug-resistant tubercle bacilli among patients with HIV infection. *Ann Intern Med*. 1992;117:177-183.

53. Couldwell DL, Dore GJ, Harkness JL, et al. Nosocomial outbreak of tuberculosis in an outpatient HIV treatment room. *AIDS*. 1996;10:521-525.

54. Moore M, the Investigative Team. Evaluation of transmission of tuberculosis in a pediatric setting—Pennsylvania. Presented at the 46th Annual Epidemic Intelligence Service Conference; April 14-18, 1997; Atlanta, Ga; p 53.

55. Agerton TB, Valway S, Gore B, Poszik C, Onorato I. Transmission of multidrug-resistant tuberculosis via bronchoscopy. Presented at the 46th Annual Epidemic Intelligence Service Conference; April 14-18, 1997; Atlanta, Ga.

56. Sepkowitz KA. AIDS, tuberculosis, and the health care worker. *Clin Infect Dis*. 1995;20:232-242.

57. Moran GJ, McCabe F, Morgan MT, Talan DA. Delayed recognition and infection control for tuberculosis patients in the emergency department. *Ann Emerg Med*. 1995;26:290-295.

58. Moran GJ, Fuchs MA, Jarvis WR, Talan DA. Tuberculosis infection-control practices in United States emergency departments. *Ann Emerg Med*. 1995;26:283-289.

59. Davis RM, Orenstein WA, Frank JA, et al. Transmission of measles in medical settings: 1980 through 1984. *JAMA*. 1986;255:1295-1298.

60. Istre GR, McKee PA, West GR, et al. Measles spread in medical settings: an important focus of disease transmission? *Pediatrics*. 1987;79:356-358.

61. Centers for Disease Control. Measles—Washington, 1990. *MMWR*. 1990;39:473-476.

62. Bloch AB, Orenstein WA, Ewing WM, et al. Measles outbreak in a pediatric practice: airborne transmission in an office setting. *Pediatrics*. 1985;75:676-683.

63. Centers for Disease Control. Measles—Hawaii. *MMWR*. 1984;33:702,707-711.

64. Miranda AC, Falcao JM, Dias JA. Measles transmission in health facilities during outbreaks. *Int J Epidemiol*. 1994;23:843-848.

65. Centers for Disease Control and Prevention. Measles among children of migrant workers—Florida. *MMWR*. 1983;32:471-472,477-478.

66. Remington PL, Hall WN, Davis IH, Herald A, Gunn RA. Airborne transmission of measles in a physician's office. *JAMA*. 1985;253:1574-1577.

67. Krause PJ, Gross PA, Barrett TL, et al. Quality standard for assurance of measles immunity among health care workers. *Clin Infect Dis*. 1994;18:431-436.

68. Gladstone JL, Millian SJ. Rubella exposure in an obstetric clinic. *Obstet Gynecol*. 1981;57:182-186.

69. Fliegel PE, Weinstein WM. Rubella outbreak in a prenatal clinic: management and prevention. *Am J Infect Control*. 1982;10:29-33.

70. Centers for Disease Control and Prevention. Exposure of patients to rubella by medical personnel—California. *MMWR*. 1978;27:123.

71. Pellitteri OJ, Fried JJ. Epidemic keratoconjunctivitis report of a small office outbreak. *Am J Ophthalmol*. 1950;33:1596-1599.

72. Thygeson P. Office and dispensary transmissions of epidemic keratoconjunctivitis. *Am J Ophthalmol*. 1957;3:98-101.

73. Dawson C, Darrell R. Infections due to adenovirus type 8 in the United States, I: an outbreak of epidemic keratoconjunctivitis originating in a physician's office. *N Engl J Med*. 1963;68:1031-1034.

74. D'Angelo LJ, Hierholzer JC, Holman RC, Smith JD. Epidemic keratoconjunctivitis caused by adenovirus type 8: epidemiologic and laboratory aspects of a large outbreak. *Am J Epidemiol*. 1981;113:44-49.

75. Keenlyside RA, Hierholzer JC, D'Angelo LJ. Keratoconjunctivitis associated with adenovirus type 37: an extended outbreak in an ophthalmologist's office. *J Infect Dis*. 1983;147:191-198.

76. Buehler JW, Finton RJ, Goodman RA, et al. Epidemic keratoconjunctivitis: report of an outbreak in an ophthalmology practice and recommendations for prevention. *Infect Control*. 1984;5:390-394.

77. Craven ER, Butler SL, McCulley JP, Luby JP. Applanation tonometer tip sterilization for adenovirus type 8. *Ophthalmology*. 1987;94:1538-1540.

78. Koo D, Bouvier B, Wesley M, Courtright P, Reingold A. Epidemic keratoconjunctivitis in a university medical center ophthalmology clinic: need for re-evaluation of the design and disinfection of instruments. *Infect Control Hosp Epidemiol*. 1989;10:547-552.

79. Centers for Disease Control and Prevention. Epidemic keratoconjunctivitis in an ophthalmology clinic—California. *MMWR*. 1990;39:598-601.

80. Warren D, Nelson KE, Farrar JA, et al. A large outbreak of epidemic keratoconjunctivitis: problems in controlling nosocomial spread. *J Infect Dis*. 1989;160:938-943.

81. Colon LE. Keratoconjunctivitis due to adenovirus type 8: report on a large outbreak. *Annals of Ophthalmology*. 1991;23:63-65.

82. Jernigan JA, Lowry BS, Hayden FG, et al. Adenovirus type 8 epidemic keratoconjunctivitis in an eye clinic: risk factors and control. *J Infect Dis*. 1993;167:1307-1313.

83. Smith D, Gottsch J, Froggatt J, Dwyer D, Karanfil L, Groves C. Performance improvement process to control epidemic keratoconjunctivitis transmission. *Infect Control Hosp Epidemiol*. 1996;17(suppl):P36. Abstract.

84. American Academy of Ophthalmology. Updated recommendations for Ophthalmic Practice in Relation to the Human Immunodeficiency Virus and Other Infectious Agents. San Francisco, Calif: AAO; 1992.

85. Dailey JR, Parnes RE, Aminlari A. Glutaraldehyde keratopathy. *Am J Ophthal*. 1993;115:256-258.

86. Christie CDC, Marx ML, Marchant CD, Reising SF. The 1993 epidemic of pertussis in Cincinnati. Resurgence of disease in a highly immunized population of children. *N Engl J Med*. 1994;331:16-21.

87. Hardy IRB, Strebel PM, Wharton M, Orenstein WA. The 1993 pertussis epidemic in Cincinnati. *N Engl J Med*. 1994;331:1455-1455.

88. Members of the American Society for Gastrointestinal Endoscopy Ad Hoc Committee on Disinfection. Position statement. Reprocessing of flexible gastrointestinal endoscopes. *Gastrointest Endosc*. 1996;43:540-546.

89. Spach DH, Silverstein FE, Stamm WE. Transmission of infection by gastrointestinal endoscopy and bronchoscopy. *Ann Intern Med*. 1993;118:117-128.

90. Ayliffe GA. Nosocomial infections associated with endoscopy. In: Mayhall CG, ed. *Hospital Epidemiology and Infection Control*. Philadelphia, Pa: Williams & Wilkins; 1996:680-693.

91. Weber DJ, Rutala WA. Nosocomial infections associated with respiratory therapy. In: Mayhall CG, ed. *Hospital Epidemiology and Infection Control*. Philadelphia, Pa: Williams & Wilkins; 1996:748-758.

92. Beecham JH III, Cohen ML, Parkin WE. Salmonella typhimurium: transmission by fiberoptic upper gastrointestinal endoscopy. *JAMA*. 1979;241:1013-1015.

93. Dwyer DM, Klein EG, Istre GR, Robinson MG, Neumann DA, McCoy GA. Salmonella newport infections transmitted by fiberoptic colonoscopy. *Gastrointest Endosc*. 1987;33:84-87.

94. Struelens MJ, Rost F, Deplano A, et al. *Pseudomonas aeruginosa* and Enterobacteriaceae bacteremia after biliary endoscopy: an outbreak investigation using DNA macrorestriction analysis. *Am J Med*. 1993;95:489-498.

95. Classen DC, Jacobson JA, Burke JP, Jacobson JT, Evans RS. Serious pseudomonas infections associated with endoscopic retrograde cholangiopancreatography. *Am J Med*. 1988;84:590-596.

96. Low DE, Micflikier AB, Kennedy JK, Stiver HG. Infectious complications of endoscopic retrograde cholangiopancreatography: a prospective assessment. *Arch Intern Med*. 1980;140:1076-1077.

97. Earnshaw JJ, Clark AW, Thom BT. Outbreak of *Pseudomonas aeruginosa* following endoscopic retrograde cholangiopancreatography. *J Hosp Infect*. 1985;6:95-97.

98. Langenberg W, Rauws EAJ, Oudbier JH, Tytgat GNJ. Patient-to-patient transmission of *Campylobacter pylori* infection by fiberoptic gastroduodenoscopy and biopsy. *J Infect Dis*. 1990;161:507-511.

99. Akamatsu T, Tabata K, Hironga M, Kawakami H, Uyeda M. Transmission of *Helicobacter pylori* infection via flexible fiberoptic endoscopy. *Am J Infect Control*. 1996;24:396-401.

100. Birnie GG, Quigley EM, Clements GB, Follet EAC, Watkinson G. Endoscopic transmission of hepatitis B virus. *Gut*. 1983;24:171-174.

101. Singh S, Singh N, Kochhar R, Mehta SK, Talwar P. Contamination of an endoscope due to *Trichosporon beigelli*. *J Hosp Infect*. 1989;14:49-53.

102. Wheeler PW, Lancaster D, Kaiser AB. Bronchopulmonary cross-colonization and infection related to mycobacterial contamination of suction valves of bronchoscopes. *J Infect Dis*. 1989;159:954-985.

103. Wang H-C, Liaw Y-S, Yang P-C, Kuo S-H, Luh K-T. A pseudoepidemic of *Mycobacterium chelonae* infection caused by contamination of a fiberoptic bronchoscope suction channel. *Eur Respir J*. 1995;8:1259-1262.

104. Nye K, Shadha DK, Hodgkin P, Bradley C, Hancox J, Wise R. *Mycobacterium chelonei* isolation from broncho-alveolar lavage fluid and its practical implications. *J Hosp Infect*. 1990;16:257-261.

105. Pappas SA, Schaaff DM, DiCostanzo MB, King FW Jr, Sharp JT. Contamination of flexible fiberoptic bronchoscopes. *Am Rev Respir Dis*. 1983;127:391-392. Letter.

106. Steere AC, Corrales J, von Graevenitz A. A cluster of Mycobacterium gordonae isolates from bronchoscopy specimens. *Am Rev Respir Dis*. 1979;120:214-416.

107. Kolmos HJ, Lerche A, Kristoffersen K, Rosdahl VT. Pseudo-outbreak of *Pseudomonas aeruginosa* in HIV-infected patients undergoing fiberoptic bronchoscopy. *Scand J Infect Dis*. 1994;26:653-657.

108. Umphrey J, Raad I, Tarrand J, Hill LA. Bronchoscopes as a contamination source of *Pseudomonas putida*. *Infect Control Hosp Epidemiol*. 1996;17(suppl):P42. Abstract.

109. Hoffmann KK, Weber DJ, Rutala WA. Pseudo-outbreak of Rhodotorula rubra in patients undergoing fiberoptic bronchoscopy. *Am J Infect Control*. 1989;17:99. Abstract.

110. American Society for Gastrointestinal Endoscopy. Infection control during gastrointestinal endoscopy: guidelines for clinical application. *Gastrointest Endosc*. 1988;34(suppl):37S-40S.

111. Rutala WA. APIC guideline for selection and use of disinfectants. *Am J Infect Control*. 1996;24:313-342.

112. Nelson DB, Jarvis WR, Rutala WA, et al; Society for Healthcare Epidemiology of America. Multi-society guideline for reprocessing flexible gastrointestinal endoscopes. *Infect Control Hosp Epidemiol*. 2003;24:532-537.

113. Muscarella LF. Advantages and limitations of automatic flexible endoscope reprocessors. *Am J Infect Control*. 1996;24:304-309.

114. Reynolds CD, Rhinehart E, Dreyer P, Goldmann DA. Variability in reprocessing policies and procedures for flexible fiberoptic endoscopes in Massachusetts hospitals. *Am J Infect Control*. 1992;20:283-290.

115. Foss D, Monagan D. A national survey of physicians' and nurses' attitudes toward endoscope cleaning and the potential for cross-infection. *Gastroenterology Nursing*. 1992;15:59-65.

116. Reeves DS, Brown NM. Mycobacterial contamination of fibreoptic bronchoscopes. *J Hosp Infect*. 1995;30(suppl):531-536.

117. Van Gossum A, Loriers M, Serruys E, Cremer M. Methods of disinfecting endoscopic material: results of an international survey. *Endoscopy*. 1989;21:247-250.

118. Kaczmarek RG, Moore RM, McCrohan J, et al. Multi-state investigation of the actual disinfection/sterilization of endoscopes in health care facilities. *Am J Med*. 1992;92:257-261.

119. Axon ATR, Cockel R, Banks J, Deverill CEA, Newmann C. Disinfection in upper-digestive-tract endoscopy in Britain. *Lancet*. 1981;1:1093-1094.

120. Rutala WA, Clontz EP, Weber DJ, Hoffmann KK. Disinfection practices for endoscopes and other semicritical items. *Infect Control Hosp Epidemiol*. 1991;12:282-288.

121. Gorse GJ, Messner RL. Infection control practices in gastrointestinal endoscopy in the United States: a national survey. *Infect Control Hosp Epidemiol*. 1991;12:289-296.

122. Favero MS. Strategies for disinfection and sterilization of endoscopes: the gap between basic principles and actual practice. *Infect Control Hosp Epidemiol*. 1991;12:279-281.

123. Rutala WA. Disinfection, sterilization, and waste disposal. In: Wenzel RP, ed. *Prevention and Control of Nosocomial Infections*. 3rd ed. Philadelphia, Pa: Williams & Wilkins; 1997:539-593.

124. Alfa MJ, DeGagne P, Olson N, Puchalski T. Comparison of ion plasma, vaporized hydrogen peroxide, and 100% ethylene oxide sterilizers to the 12/88 ethylene oxide gas sterilizer. *Infect Control Hosp Epidemiol*. 1996;17:92-100.

125. Rutala WA, Weber DJ. Low-temperature sterilization technologies: do we need to redefine "sterilization"? *Infect Control Hosp Epidemiol*. 1996;17:87-91.

126. Food and Drug Administration. Compliance policy guide 7124.16. 9/24/87. Available from FDA Kansas City Regional Office.

127. Greene VW. Reuse of disposable devices. In: Mayhall CG, ed. *Hospital Epidemiology and Infection Control*. Philadelphia, Pa: Williams & Wilkins; 1996:946-954.

128. Association for the Advancement of Medical Instrumentation. *AAMI—good hospital practice: flash sterilization-steam sterilization of patient care items for immediate use (ST37)*. Arlington, Va: AAMI Steam Sterilization Hospital Practices Working Group, AAMI Sterilization Standards Committee; 1996.

129. Association for the Advancement of Medical Instrumentation. *AAMI—good hospital practice: guidelines for the selection and use of reusable rigid sterilization container systems (ST33)*. Arlington, Va: AAMI Steam Sterilization Hospital Practices Working Group of the Thermal Sterilization Subcommittee, AAMI Sterilization Standards Committee; 1996.

130. Longfield R, Longfield J, Smith LP, Hyams KC, Strohmer ME. Multidose medication vial sterility: an in-use study and a review of the literature. *Infect Control*. 1984;5:165-169.

131. Melnyk PS, Shevchuk YM, Conly JM, Richardson CJ. Contamination study of multiple-dose vials. *Ann Pharmacother*. 1993;27:274-277.

132. Mattner F, Gastmeier P. Bacterial contamination of multiple-dose vials: a prevalence study. *Am J Infect Control*. 2004;32:12-16.

133. Borghans JGA, Stanford JL. Mycobacterium chelonei in abscesses after injection of diphtheria-pertussis-tetanus-polio vaccine. *Am Rev Respir Dis*. 1973;107:1-8.

134. Kothari T, Reyes MP, Brooks N, Brown WJ, Lerner AM. Pseudomonas cepacia septic arthritis due to intra-articular injections of methylprednisolone. *Can Med Assoc J*. 1977;116:1230,1232. Letter.

135. Greaves WL, Hinman AR, Facklam RR, Allman KC, Barrett CL, Stetler HC. Streptococcal abscesses following diphtheria-tetanus toxoid-pertussis vaccination. *Pediatr Infect Dis J*. 1982;1:388-390.

136. Kantor RJ, Carson LA, Graham DR, Petersen NJ, Favero MS. Outbreak of pyrogenic reactions at a dialysis center: association with infusion of heparinized saline solution. *Am J Med*. 1983;74:449-456.

137. Stetler HC, Garbe PL, Dwyer DM, et al. Outbreaks of group A streptococcal abscesses following diphtheria-tetanus toxoid-pertussis vaccination. *Pediatrics*. 1985;75:299-303.

138. Nakashima AK, McCarthy MA, Martone MJ, Anderson RL. Epidemic septic arthritis caused by *Serratia marcescens* and associated with a benzalkonium chloride antiseptic. *J Clin Microbiol*. 1987;25:1014-1018.

139. Hospital Infection Control Practices Advisory Committee, Centers for Disease Control and Prevention. Recommendations for preventing the spread of vancomycin resistance. *Infect Control Hosp Epidemiol*. 1995;16:105-113.

140. Muto CA, Jernigan JA, Ostrowsky BE, Richet HM, Jarvis WR, Boyce JM, Farr BM. SHEA guideline for preventing nosocomial transmission of multidrug-resistant strains of *Staphylococcus aureus* and Enterococcus. *Infect Control Hosp Epidemiol*. 2003;24:362-386.

141. Frieden TR, Munsiff SS, Low DE, et al. Emergence of vancomycin-resistant enterococci in New York City. *Lancet*. 1993;342:76

142. Centers for Disease Control and Prevention. Update: *Staphylococcus aureus* reduced susceptibility of *Staphylococcus aureus* to vancomycin—United States, 1997. *MMWR*. 1997;46:813.

143. Sieradzki K, Roberts RB, Haber SW. The development of vancomycin resistance in a patient with methicillin-resistant *Staphylococcus aureus* infection. *N Engl J Med*. 1999;340:517.

144. Fridkin SK, Hageman J, McDougal LK, et al. Vancomycin-Intermediate *Staphylococcus aureus* Epidemiology Study Group. Epidemiological and microbiological characterization of infections caused by *Staphylococcus aureus* with reduced susceptibility to vancomycin, United States, 1997-2001. *Clin Infect Dis*. 2003;36:429-439.

145. Chang S, Sievert D, Hageman J, et al. Infection with vancomycin-resistant *Staphylococcus aureus* containing the vanA resistance gene. *N Engl J Med*. 2003;348:14.

146. Centers for Disease Control and Prevention Public Health Dispatch: vancomycin-resistant *Staphylococcus aureus*—Pennsylvania, 2002. *MMWR*. 2002;51

147. Centers for Disease Control and Prevention. Preventing the spread of vancomycin resistance-report from the Hospital Infection Control Practices Advisory Committee. *Federal Register*. May 17, 1994.

148. Morrison AJ Jr. Infection control in the outpatient setting. In: Wenzel RP, ed. *Prevention and Control of Nosocomial Infections*. 2nd ed. Philadelphia, Pa: Williams & Wilkins; 1993:89-92.

149. Reinhardt PA, Gordon JG, Alvarado CJ. Medical waste management. In: Mayhall CG, ed. *Hospital Epidemiology and Infection Control*. Philadelphia, Pa: Williams & Wilkins; 1996:1099-1108.

150. Favero MS, Alter MJ, Bland LE. Nosocomial infections associated with hemodialysis. In: Mayhall CG, ed. *Hospital Epidemiology and Infection Control*. Philadelphia, Pa: Williams & Wilkins; 1996:693-714..

151. Alter MJ, Favero MS, Moyer LA, Bland LA. National surveillance of dialysis-associated diseases in the United States, 1989. *Transactions American Society for Artificial Internal Organs*. 1991;37:97-109.

152. Band JD. Nosocomial infections associated with peritoneal dialysis. In: Mayhall CG, ed. *Hospital Epidemiology and Infection Control*. Philadelphia, Pa: Williams & Wilkins; 1996:714-725.

153. Garcia-Houchins S. Dialysis. In: Olmsted RN, ed. APIC *Infection Control and Applied Epidemiology: Principles and Practice, Part I Section C, Practice Settings*. St. Louis, Mo: Mosby-Year Book, Inc; 1996:89-1-89-15.

154. Niu MT, Alter JM, Kristensen C, Margolis HS. Outbreak of hemodialysis-associated non-A, non-B hepatitis and correlation with antibody to hepatitis C virus. *Am J Kidney Dis*. 1992;19:345-352.

155. Delarocque-Astagneau E, Baffoy N, Thiers V, et al. Outbreak of hepatitis C virus infection in a hemodialysis unit: potential transmission by the hemodialysis machine? *Infect Control Hosp Epidemiol*. 2002;23:328-334.

156. Yu VL, Goetz A, Wagener M, Smith PB, et al. *Staphylococcus aureus* nasal carriage and infection in patients on hemodialysis: efficacy of antibiotic prophylaxis. *N Engl J Med*. 1986;315:91-96.

157. Luzar MA, Coles GA, Faller B, et al. *Staphylococcus aureus* nasal carriage and infection in patients on continuous ambulatory peritoneal dialysis. *N Engl J Med*. 1990;322:505-509.

158. Ena J, Boelaert JR, Boyken L, Van Landuyt HW, Godard CA, Herwaldt LA. Epidemiology of *Staphylococcus aureus* infections in patients on hemodialysis. *Infect Control Hosp Epidemiol*. 1994;15:78-81.

159. Pignatari A, Pfaller M, Hollis R, Sesso R, Leme I, Herwaldt L. *Staphylococcus aureus* colonization and infection in patients on continuous ambulatory peritoneal dialysis. *J Clin Microbiol*. 1990;28:1898-1902.

160. Boelaert JR, Van Landuyt HW, Godard CA, et al. Nasal mupirocin ointment decreases the incidence of *Staphylococcus aureus* bacteremias in haemodialysis patients. *Nephrol Dial Transplant*. 1993;8:235-239.

161. The Mupirocin Study Group. Nasal mupirocin prevents *Staphylococcus aureus* exit-site infection during peritoneal dialysis. *J Am Soc Nephrol*. 1996;7:2403-2408.

162. Dryden MS, McCann M, Phillips I. Housewife peritonitis: conjugal transfer of a pathogen. *J Hosp Infect*. 1991;17:69-70. Letter.

163. Herwaldt LA, Boyken LD, Coffman S. Epidemiology of *S. aureus* nasal carriage in patients on continuous ambulatory peritoneal dialysis who were in a multicenter trial of mupirocin. Presented at the 36th Interscience Conference on Antimicrobial Agents and Chemotherapy; September 15-18, 1996; New Orleans, La. Abstract.

164. Gordon SM, Drachman J, Bland LA, Reid MH, Favero M, Jarvis WR. Epidemic hypotension in a dialysis center caused by sodium azide. *Kidney Int*. 1990;37:110-115.

165. Longfield RN, Wortham WG, Fletcher LL, Nauscheutz WF. Clustered bacteremias in a hemodialysis unit: cross-contamination of blood tubing from ultrafiltrate waste. *Infect Control Hosp Epidemiol*. 1992;13:160-164.

166. Flaherty JP, Garcia-Houchins S, Chudy R, Arnow PM. An outbreak of gram-negative bacteremia traced to contaminated O-rings and reprocessed dialyzers. *Ann Intern Med.* 1993;119:1072-1078.

167. Beck-Sague CM, Jarvis WR, Bland LA, Arduino MJ, Aguero SM, Verosic G. Outbreak of gram-negative bacteremia and pyrogenic reactions in a hemodialysis center. *Am J Nephrol.* 1990;10:397-403.

168. Hopkins DP, Cicirello H, Dievendorf G, Kondracki S, Morse D. An outbreak of culture-negative peritonitis in dialysis patients-New York. Presented at the 46th Annual Epidemic Intelligence Service Conference; April 14-18, 1997; Atlanta, Ga.

169. Spare MK, Tebbs SE, Lang S, et al. Genotypic and phenotypic properties of coagulase-negative staphylococci causing dialysis catheter-related sepsis. *J Hosp Infect.* 2003; 54:272-278.

170. Wang SA, Levine RB, Carson LA, et al. An outbreak of gram-negative bacteremia in hemodialysis patients traced to hemodialysis machine waste drain ports. *Infect Control Hosp Epidemiol.* 1999;20:746-751.

171. Kitching AR, Macdonald A, Hatfield PJ. Pasturella multocida infection in continuous ambulatory peritoneal dialysis. *NZ Med J.* 1996;23:59.

172. Tokars JI, Miller ER, Stein G. New national surveillance system for hemodialysis-associated infections: initial results. *Am J Infect Control.* 2002;30:288-295.

173. Stevenson KB, Adcox MJ, Mallea MC, Narasimhan N, Wagnild JP. Standardized surveillance of hemodialysis vascular access infections: 18-month experience at an outpatient, multifacility hemodialysis center. *Infect Control Hosp Epidemiol.* 2000;21:200-203.

174. Temple RS. Physical medicine and rehabilitation/occupational therapy/speech. In: Olmsted RN, ed. *APIC Infection Control and Applied Epidemiology: Principles and Practice, Part I Section D, Support Services and Facilities Management.* St Louis, Mo: Mosby-Year Book, Inc; 1996:114-1-114-5.

175. Linnemann CC. Nosocomial infections associated with physical therapy, including hydrotherapy. In: Mayhall CG, ed. *Hospital Epidemiology and Infection Control.* Philadelphia, Pa: Williams & Wilkins; 1996:725-730.

176. Goodman RA, Solomon SL. Transmission of infectious diseases in outpatient health care settings. *JAMA.* 1991;265:2377-2381.

177. Zuber TJ, Geddie JE. Occupational safety and health administration regulations for the physician's office. *J Fam Pract.* 1993;36:540-550.

178. Favero MS, Sadovsky R. Office infection control, OSHA, and you. *Patient Care.* 1993;27:117-121.

OTHER RESOURCES

American Society of Gastrointestinal Endoscopy (ASGE) and the Society of Gastroenterology Nurses and Associates. Reprocessing of Flexible Gastrointestinal Endoscopes. A white paper publication, December 1995. This document may be accessed through the ASGE home page http://www.asge.org. Select position papers, then select this title. Original copies may be obtained by writing to ASGE or by calling 508-526-8330.

American Academy of Ophthalmology's Updated Recommendations for Ophthalmic Practice in Relation to the Human Immunodeficiency Virus and Other Infectious Agents may be obtained from that society at 655 Beach St, San Francisco, CA 94109; telephone, 415- 561-8500; fax, 415-561-8533; web site, http://www.eyenet.org.

Centers for Disease Control. (CDC). Guidelines for preventing the transmission of tuberculosis in health-care settings, with special focus on HIV-related issues. *MMWR.* 1990;39

Core Curriculum On Tuberculosis. *What the Clinician Should Know.* 3rd ed. CDC, National Center for Prevention Services, Division of Tuberculosis Elimination, US Department of Health and Human Services, Atlanta Ga; 1994.

Department of Labor, OSHA. Occupational exposure to tuberculosis. *Federal Register.* 1997;62(201).

Diosegy AJ, MC Lord. What physicians need to know about OSHA: how to avoid tough new penalties. *North Carolina Medical Journal.* 1993;54:251-254.

ECRI Special Report. Reuse of Single-Use Medical Devices. 1997, ECRI 5200 Butler Pike, Plymouth Meeting, Pa 19462; telephone 610-825-6000; fax, 610-834-1275; e-mail ecri@hslc.org.

Heroux DL. Ambulatory care. In: Olmsted RN, ed. APIC *Infection Control and Applied Epidemiology: Principles and Practice, Part I Section C, Practice Settings.* St. Louis, Mo: Mosby-Year Book, Inc; 1996:83-1-83-15.

Heroux D, Garris J, Nahan J, Vivolo P. Ambulatory Care Infection Control Manual. © 1993, Group Health Cooperative, Group Health Cooperative of Puget Sound, 1809 Seventh Ave, Suite 1003, Seattle, Wash 98101. Publishing coordination and production by Laing Communications Inc., Redmond, Washington.

The Reuse of Single-Use Medical Devices. 1996, Canadian Healthcare Association, CHA Press, 17 York St, Suite 100, Ottawa, Ontario K1N 9J6, Canada.

CHAPTER TWENTY-FIVE

INFECTION CONTROL AND PATIENT SAFETY

Darren R. Linkin, MD and PJ Brennan, MD

INTRODUCTION

There is currently a strong, growing interest in patient safety in the United States. Fortunately for hospital epidemiologists, the practice of infection control is already a patient safety effort utilizing surveillance for adverse events and interventions to prevent harm to patients in the future. In this chapter, we will discuss the history and importance of patient safety, terms and techniques unique to the field, and the role of infection control.

SPACE SHUTTLE DISASTERS: THE IMPORTANCE OF SYSTEM ERRORS

The crash of the Challenger space shuttle in 1986 resulted in an investigation that found significant problems with how the National Aeronautics and Space Administration (NASA) managed significant safety threats in the space shuttle program. In particular, it was found that problems with the "O" rings that led to the crash had been known by NASA for years preceding the disaster.[1]

On February 1, 2003, the Columbia became the second space shuttle to be destroyed in flight, killing all on board. This is one of a number of prominent disasters that highlight the complex nature of the problems that affect safety. An investigation found that a falling foam chunk from another part of the shuttle damaged the left wing, allowing superheated air into the damaged wing, eventually leading to destruction of the shuttle. Similar foam debris was known to fall from the space shuttle on multiple earlier flights, but the problem was never adequately addressed. During the flight, engineers repeatedly asked for photos of the shuttle to be taken to assess for damage after the foam debris was spotted on video from the take-off. Due to lack of communication and a culture (shared attitude and behavior) of downplaying potential risks, NASA management did not allow the photographs to be taken.

Errors in management and politics also predated the Columbia's last flight. The NASA safety program personnel reported to managers running the program being assessed, creating a lack of independence in those evaluating and reporting on safety issues. There was a lack of strategic planning in NASA and the executive branch of the government. The space shuttle was originally designed as part of a broader (American) space station plan that was rejected; a huge amount of money and effort were funneled into a space shuttle program that had little reason to exist. The budget approved by Congress, however, was insufficient to allow for a robust safety program. In summary, the Columbia disaster was primarily the result of multiple pre-existing errors in the system for how the space shuttle program was run by NASA and the government.[2]

INTRODUCTION TO PATIENT SAFETY

While the field of safety has been an active source of investigation and planning in nonmedical fields starting in the 1960s, it was only in the past few years that the issue has gained national attention in the medical industry. In 1999, the Institute of Medicine (IOM) released, "To err is human," which estimated that 44,000 to 98,000 inpatients die each year from medical errors. Even the lower estimate would make medical errors the eighth leading cause of death in the United States, ahead of motor vehicle accidents and breast cancer. The cost of adverse events due to medical errors is estimated to be between $17 and $29 billion per year; the lower estimate is 2% of the United States' annual healthcare expenditures.[3] Clearly, medical errors lead to substantial mortality and cost. The well-publicized IOM report brought a renewed focus on patient safety, as well as an outpouring of studies and reviews addressing the topic. However, the response of the healthcare industry to introduce patient safety practices has been slow, leading to external pressures on healthcare organizations to examine and improve the safety of patients. Regulation has come in the form of patient safety requirements for healthcare organizations from the JCAHO.[4] Businesses have also joined in the fray: the Leapfrog Group[5] is a consortium of large businesses that purchase healthcare for their employees. The consortium recommends that its patients be cared for in hospitals that have taken particular patient safety measures, such as using computer physician order entry.

Compared with the delivery of healthcare, other industries have a far better safety record. For instance, fatalities with airline flights occur in 0.43 cases per million opportunities and baggage mishandling in approximately 1 per 100. The accuracy of inpatient medication delivery and adequate use of postmyocardial infarction medication are compromised in greater than 1 opportunity in 10. These differences were noted in the IOM report.[3] The report suggested that significant improvements in patient safety were needed and would require large changes in the paradigm of how safety is addressed in healthcare organizations.

Patient safety is more than the use of computer physician order entry or other interventions to prevent errors. It is a fundamental change in the way errors and adverse events are viewed. Previously, individuals have been singled out as the cause of an adverse event, leading to an organizational culture that emphasized blame and silence by HCWs when errors or adverse events are made. In the newer paradigm for patient safety, it is assumed that most workers are trying to do good work within the constraints of their job and that problems with the system are often the cause of adverse events. Optimally, a nonpunitive culture should emphasize reporting of problems, and improvements in the design of systems will be used to prevent adverse events in patients.[6]

PATIENT SAFETY TERMINOLOGY

To further understand errors and their consequences, a basic understanding of terms used in the safety field is necessary. Definitions and examples for these terms are given in Table 25-1.

While errors may lead to adverse events, each can occur without the other. The failure to give appropriate preoperative antibiotics is an error that does not invariably lead to a postoperative surgical site infection (an adverse event). This error is then a near miss. Conversely, SSI can occur even in the absence of errors. But, if infection is due to an error, it is a preventable adverse event.

POSTSURGICAL WOUND OUTBREAK: A MEDICAL ADVERSE EVENT

An example of an adverse event relating to infection control was published by the Agency for Healthcare Research and Quality (AHRQ) in its online morbidity and mortality forum.[8] The case vignette describes an increase in postoperative sternal wound infections. An investigation by the infection control team determined that the outbreak was occurring in patients operated on by one surgeon and his team. When observed during surgery, this team used "sloppy" technique, including having loose hair and jewelry while performing surgery. While contamination of surgical wounds by the operating room personnel was not proven in this case, studies have suggested that bacteria shed from surgical personnel—including from skin and hair[9,10]—is common and has led to outbreaks of postoperative infections.[11,12] While the operating room staff committed active errors (not properly covering hair and removing jewelry), these were likely related to errors in the system. For instance, the culture and leadership (individual surgeon and surgical chief) of the operating room permitted sloppy personal surgical attire. Other potential system errors may have included lack of sleep and rest by surgical team members, a rushed schedule that compromised safe practices to facilitate patient turnover, lack of access to properly fitting head coverings, and inadequate training of the operating room staff in infection control procedures.

LATENT SYSTEM ERRORS

In both examples given above, an individual did not act in error alone. Instead, there were multiple active errors due to several latent errors in the system. For instance, in the Columbia disaster, there were many faulty decisions made before and during the flight. However, these decisions were made in a system of poor communication (between engineers and managers) and a culture that downplayed risks instead of actively exploring potential problems. The investigation concluded that the disaster was primarily the result of NASA's "culture," not the act of

TABLE 25-1. SAFETY TERMINOLOGY[3,7]

Term	Definition	Example
Error	The failure of a planned action to be competed as intended (ie, error of execution) or the use of a wrong plan to achieve an aim (ie, error of planning)	Execution: right medication administered to the wrong patient by a nurse Planning: wrong medication ordered by a physician
Active error	Errors by individuals at the "front-line" of a complex process	Nurse administers a toxic dose of an aminoglycoside (that was incorrectly ordered and dispensed)
Slip	Errors of implementation (ie, failing to do a semiautomatic low-level behavior)	Failure to order contact isolation for an inpatient with a new culture growing VRE
Mistake	Errors of higher functioning during non-stereotypic behaviors	A physician makes the wrong diagnosis although the right diagnosis was evident
Latent error	System errors that lead to adverse events when combined with other factors	Chronic understaffing of nursing, which may increase the risk of subsequent active errors by overworked nurses
Adverse event	An unexpected negative outcome of a process; in the case of healthcare, the processes are medical interventions	Postoperative pneumonia in an otherwise healthy patient
Preventable adverse event	The subset of adverse events caused by errors	Postoperative wound infection after failure to use appropriate preoperative antibiotic prophylaxis
Sentinel event	A serious and unexpected adverse event	Death from postoperative pneumonia in an otherwise healthy patient
Near miss	An error that does not result in a preventable adverse event but could if the error were repeated in the future	Use of inadequately sterilized surgical instruments does not lead to a subsequent infection in the patient

any one individual.[2] In the case of the outbreak of sternal wound infections, bacteria shed from the hair of multiple individuals likely caused the wound contamination. These errors could only occur because of latent errors in training, leadership, group culture, or patient scheduling.

Adverse events are usually preceded by an active error by an individual. However, these errors are typically the result of latent errors that both increased the risk of the active error (eg, understaffing) and allowed the error(s) to progress to adverse events (eg, lack of engineering or procedural safety checks). Thus, system errors are thought to account for most adverse events.[6]

Multiple errors usually need to occur together in order for major adverse events to occur. James Reason's "Swiss cheese" model analogizes the multiple errors that precede an adverse event to holes in slices of Swiss cheese lined up like dominoes. The layers of cheese represent multiple barriers and safeguards to prevent adverse events from taking place. The holes in the cheese are active and latent errors. A hole in any one slice does not lead to an adverse event. Only when the holes in multiple layers momentar-

ily line up (multiple active and latent errors occurring together) do adverse events happen.[13]

TECHNIQUES FOR DETECTING AND INVESTIGATING ADVERSE EVENTS

Because sentinel events are severe adverse events, they are worthy of investigation in order to prevent further injuries or deaths. Two techniques used to investigate past and potential future adverse events are root cause analysis (RCA) and failure modes and effects analysis (FMEA), respectively. Infection control programs have traditionally used surveillance to benchmark infection rates against past rates at a single institution or from other medical centers, such as those available through the NNIS program at the CDC.[14] After a discussion of RCAs and FMEAs, we will contrast them with benchmarking and describe how the 3 approaches are complementary. While full instruction on how to perform an RCA and a FMEA is beyond the scope of this chapter, we will provide a conceptual overview of the techniques illustrated with theoretical examples that may be encountered in infection control.

Root Cause Analysis

An RCA is used to investigate a sentinel event in order to determine and correct its causes, preventing or decreasing the likelihood that the event will recur. RCAs start with a flow diagram of events that led to the adverse event. Next, a separate cause-and-effect diagram is made. Starting with the adverse event, the RCA team traces sequential causes of the event backward, elaborating the "roots" of the tree to determine underlying root causes of the event. Causal statements are then constructed to describe how a root cause(s) led to the adverse event(s), emphasizing latent system errors. Finally, recommendations are made for how to correct the root causes to prevent the adverse event from recurring. It is important for the investigators to both review the medical record as well as interview people involved in the process or event under study.[15]

An investigation of an unexpected death from a post-surgical wound infection could be performed using an RCA. The flow of events is first mapped, starting with the need for surgery, through details of the infection control practices and preoperative antibiotics used, and concluding with postoperative diagnosis and management of the infection up through the time of death. A causal diagram would elaborate the root cause of the infectious death, which may include death from infection, *caused by* (1) wound contamination, *caused by* lack of hospital guidelines for surgical attire for covering all head and face hair and (another branch) *caused by* (2) preoperative antibiotics starting after the skin incision, *caused by* scheduling not allowing for time for antibiotics preoperatively. Causal statements and recommendations may include the following: "Death from wound infection was caused by lack of adequate procedures for protection from wound contamination and proper timing of preoperative antibiotics. Recommendation will be for a surgical checklist prior to skin incision that includes checking for proper surgical attire by entire surgical team and completion of preoperative antibiotics prior to skin incision."

Failure Mode Effects Analysis

In general terms, an FMEA is a systematic method of identifying and preventing product, equipment, and process problems before they occur. Each way a system can fail is called a *failure mode*. Each failure mode has a potential *effect* (adverse event). As with RCAs, the first step is creating a flow chart of the system. Next, the FMEA

team brainstorms failure modes for each step and their potential effect. As with RCAs, people involved with the process under study should be interviewed (and/or included on the team). The *severity* of the effect, risk of *occurrence*, and ease of *detection* are then assessed on a scale (eg, of 1 to 10 where 10 is the worst). Each effect is then assigned a *risk priority number* (RPN), which is the product of the 3 scores (severity x occurrence x detection). In our example, the RPN (or *criticality*) of the effect will be on a scale from 1 to 1000. The potential effects of a system are then ranked from highest to lowest RPN score. The effects with the highest RPN—and all effects with an absolutely high RPN—are targeted for corrective action. After the intervention(s), the RPN of the effects are recalculated and referred to as the *resulting RPN*. Corrective actions should continue until the RPN or resulting RPN for all potential effects is at an acceptable level. An acceptable RPN level is not a number set in stone. The team performing the FMEA has to decide what an acceptable level of risk is in the system it is evaluating.

An example of an FMEA is the evaluation of a hospital's system for sterilizing surgical instruments. There are many steps in the process including cleaning, sterilization, and the evaluation of sterilization using biological tests (determining if the sterilizer properly killed a standard test sample of bacteria). Failing to list all sterilized instruments in a log may be a common occurrence (occurrence score: 7) but it is easily detected (detection score: 2) and does not lead to a severe effect (severity score: 2) giving a low RPN of 28 (7 x 2 x 2). Failing to exchange the ethylene oxide (ETO) canister in the ETO sterilizer during a sterilizer run may be an uncommon occurrence (occurrence score: 3) but may be difficult to detect without an automatic alarm system (detection score: 8) and operating with nonsterile instruments is likely to have a severe effect (severity score: 8) leading to a relatively higher RPN of 192 (3 x 8 x 8). An FMEA of this system would target the latter step first for corrective action.

Contrasting Root Cause Analysis, Failure Mode Effects Analysis, and Benchmarking

The advantages and disadvantages for using these 3 investigative techniques are listed in Table 25-2. Surveillance with benchmarking detects trends in infection rates even without an unexpected death or disability (ie, without a sentinel event). RCAs can uncover system errors that may not be explored in an outbreak case-control study that focuses on patient-level risk factors. Because it can be triggered by a single sentinel event, an RCA investigation can also be initiated sooner, before a benchmarking-based system would have detected the new problem. Finally, an FMEA investigates the potential for adverse events that have not yet occurred, preventing patient harm before it happens. Thus, the 3 techniques are complementary.

TABLE 25-2. COMPARING INVESTIGATION TECHNIQUES

	Advantages	Disadvantages
Surveillance, benchmarking (and outbreak investigation)	➤ Detects trends in adverse events that are not sentinel events ➤ Detects patient-level risk factors ➤ Quantitative results	➤ Need multiple events to trigger an investigation, with harm to those patients ➤ May not detect system-level errors ➤ Time- and cost-consuming
RCA	➤ Can initiate after 1 sentinel event ➤ Detects system errors	➤ Need to wait until sentinel event occurs, harming at least one patient ➤ Qualitative results may be susceptible to hindsight bias ➤ May not detect patient-level risk factors ➤ Time- and cost-consuming
FMEA	➤ Can initiate prior to an adverse or sentinel event ➤ Detects system errors	➤ Risk of potential events may not be anticipated until errors occur ➤ Qualitative results may be susceptible to hindsight bias ➤ May not detect patient-level risk factors ➤ Time- and cost-consuming

Healthcare-associated infections have traditionally been tracked using surveillance with benchmarking, then investigated with retrospective cohort or case-control studies. An outcome is (at least in part) typically attributed to or "caused" by a risk factor if the probability of finding the observed association between risk factor by chance alone is less than 0.05 (ie, a p-value of less than 0.05). This quantitative approach can be contrasted with the qualitative techniques of RCA and FMEA, which base decisions on the consensus of an investigative team. However, determining actual "causality" is based on the sum of the available evidence using Hill's classic criteria[16] and is not typically established by a single study. Furthermore, the results of any investigation need to be interpreted in the context of the study methods. While epidemiologists may be more comfortable with the results of a quantitative study, both qualitative and quantitative techniques have a useful role in investigating healthcare-related infections.

INFECTION CONTROL AND PATIENT SAFETY

Infection control is already working toward improving patient safety by focusing on the prevention of healthcare-associated infections. The 2004 JCAHO National Patient Safety Goals that will be required of hospitals include an infection control goal.[4] Reviewers have emphasized the role of infection control as a critical component of patient safety.[17,18] The following infection control activities promote patient safety by decreasing the risk of healthcare-associated infections:

1. Surveillance for healthcare-associated infections with feedback of infection rates to clinicians
2. Investigating and controlling outbreaks
3. Ensuring proper sterilization or disinfection of equipment for procedures and surgeries
4. Vaccination of vulnerable patients against preventable IDs
5. Evaluating and improving infection control practices that protect patients
   a. Hand hygiene
   b. Proper placement and care of invasive devices (eg, central venous catheters)
   c. Contact isolation of patients with IDs that are spread by HCWs
   d. Proper adherence to environmental infection control procedures by operating room staff (eg, completely covering head and face hair)
   e. Preoperative antibiotic prophylaxis when indicated
   f. Judicious use of antimicrobials

JCAHO REGULATIONS ADDRESSING INFECTION CONTROL

The JCAHO is the major source of accreditation at the intersection of patient safety and infection control. JCAHO published 6 National Patient Safety Goals that became effective on January 1, 2003. For 2004, a seventh goal has been added.[4] The seventh goal directly addresses issues in infection control: "*Reduce the risk of healthcare-acquired infections.*" There are 2 requirements to this goal:

1. "*Comply with current CDC hand hygiene guidelines.*" Category I recommendations in the hand hygiene guidelines are required by JCAHO, while Category II recommendations are "suggested." Compliance by the hospital will be assessed by interviews and observations of hospital staff. If there is more than a "sporadic" miss in compliance by staff, the hospital will be scored as noncompliant. The CDC hand hygiene recommendations are detailed in the "Hand Hygiene" chapter of this book.

2. "*Manage as sentinel events all identified cases of unanticipated death or major permanent loss of function associated with a healthcare-acquired infection.*" In their regulations, JCAHO specifies that all sentinel events must be evaluated with an RCA. The JCAHO emphasizes that this requirement is not new; it simply clarifies that an unanticipated death or loss of function should be reported even if it is due to a healthcare-associated infection. Whether a death is "unanticipated" depends on the patient's condition on admission. The death of an otherwise healthy adult admitted for an elective procedure would be unanticipated. If the patient was not likely to survive the hospitalization due to his or her baseline and admitting medical conditions, then his or her death would not be a sentinel event. Importantly, the JCAHO emphasizes that this requirement should not increase the surveillance already being performed (by infection control practitioners and other hospital personnel). Thus, a hospital's current sentinel event reporting system should clearly include events due to healthcare-associated infections. Another potential source of surveillance for these types of sentinel events is for infection control practitioners to report whether infections discovered through surveillance activities are related to subsequent patient deaths.

INFORMATION TECHNOLOGY AND SENTINEL EVENT REPORTING

The role of technology in improving the quality and safety of patient care in general has emphasized in recent reviews and reports publications.[6,19] One example is electronic reporting of adverse events by HCWs to the hospitals. The University of Pennsylvania Health System uses a computer-based system to collect spontaneous reports of adverse events. This system provides several advantages over alternative mediums (eg, paper based). Access to a hospital intranet-based program can be readily accessible at computer workstations. The information is quickly transmitted to administrators (including hospital epidemiologists) who can respond to the events. The reports can also be transmitted directly into a database. Thus, single sentinel events as well as trends in adverse events can be communicated efficiently, allowing for rapid response by the hospital administration and infection control team.

GETTING STARTED: PATIENT SAFETY AND INFECTION CONTROL AT YOUR HEALTHCARE INSTITUTION

➤ By performing surveillance for healthcare-associated infections, investigating outbreaks, and promoting good infection control practices, you are already contributing to patient safety.

➤ Ensure that a mechanism for reporting and investigating healthcare-associated infection sentinel events is in place at your hospital. This mechanism can take many forms, including passive surveillance by HCWs through a hotline, paper form, or computer-based form, or active surveillance by the infection control team or other hospital-based personnel. Other administrators may primarily run a sentinel event reporting, but input from infection control will be vital. The infection control team should also become familiar with RCA and FMEA techniques and may be called upon by the hospital to lead or at least participate on teams performing these investigations.

➤ Work toward establishing a nonpunitive culture with regard to medical errors. HCWs do not report to work with the intent of making mistakes. However, they routinely perform complex tasks under less than ideal conditions (eg, with inadequate training or as part of an understaffed department). Active errors by HCWs that led to adverse events were likely caused by (or allowed to happen by) system errors in how care is delivered. While active errors should be evaluated and corrected with improvements in systems, including retraining of the staff, they should not result in punitive action against the HCW. Only in such a nonpunitive culture will errors and adverse events be reported, allowing for investigation and system corrections to protect future patients.[6]

Conversely, there are blameworthy behaviors that merit action by healthcare organizations (personal communications James Bagian). The behaviors include errors by HCWs that occur while impaired (by alcohol or other drugs), while working outside the scope of their responsibility, from reckless behavior, or from intentionally harmful behavior. A nonpunitive environment does not mean that people are not responsible for their actions, but that staff members who committed errors will be encouraged to report mistakes and slips rather than hide them for fear of reprisal and that they will be valued for their reporting.

OTHER RESOURCES FOR FMEA AND RCA

➤ *Using failure mode and effects analysis to improve patient safety.*[20] This review article summarizes the history and methodology of FMEA using simple language and concepts.

➤ http://www.patientsafety.gov.[21] This Veterans Administration site has explanations and instructions for performing RCAs and FMEAs, as well as links to other resources. They describe a trademarked FMEA methodology referred to as a Healthcare FMEA.

➤ *Making healthcare safer: a critical analysis of patient safety practices (Chapter 5: Root Cause Analysis).*[22] This chapter—part of a report on patient safety from the AHRQ—describes the RCA process, then critically evaluates the evidence supporting its use as a tool to investigate medical sentinel events and improve patient safety. The report is available online (accessed on November 5, 2003, at http://www.ahcpr.gov/clinic/ptsafety/).

REFERENCES

1. Selected congressional hearings and report from the Challenger space shuttle accident: main page. GPO Access, 2003. Available at: http://www.gpoaccess.gov/challenger. Accessed October 22, 2003.

2. Report. Columbia accident investigation board, 2003. Available at: http://www.nasa.gov/ columbia/home. Accessed October 22, 2003.

3. Kohn LT, Corrigan JM, Donaldson MS. *To Err is Human: Building a Safer Health System.* Washington, DC: Committee on Quality Health Care in America, Institute of Medicine; 1999. Report No.: 0309068371.

4. National Patient Safety Goals. Joint Commission on Accreditation of Healthcare Organizations, 2003. Available at: http://www.jcaho.org/ accredited+organizations/ patient+safety/04+npsg/index.htm. Accessed October 20, 2003.

5. The Leapfrog Group for patient safety: rewarding higher standards, 2003. Available at: http://www.leapfroggroup. org/index.html. Accessed October 24, 2003.

6. *Crossing the Quality Chasm: A New Health System for the 21st Century.* Washington, DC: Committee on Quality Health Care in America, Institute of Medicine; 2001.

7. Reason J. *Human Error.* Cambridge, UK: Cambridge University Press; 1990.

8. Web M&M. Agency for Healthcare Research and Quality, 2003. Available at: http://www. webmm.ahrq.gov. Accessed October 30, 2003.

9. Bitkover CY, Marcusson E, Ransjo U. Spread of coagulase-negative staphylococci during cardiac operations in a modern operating room. *Ann Thorac Surg.* 2000; 69(4):1110-1115.

10. Hubble MJ, Weale AE, Perez JV, Bowker KE, MacGowan AP, Bannister GC. Clothing in laminar-flow operating theatres. *J Hosp Infect.* 1996;32(1):1-7.

11. Mastro TD, Farley TA, Elliott JA, et al. An outbreak of surgical-wound infections due to group A *streptococcus* carried on the scalp. *N Engl J Med.* 1990;323(14):968-972.

12. Dineen P, Drusin L. Epidemics of postoperative wound infections associated with hair carriers. *Lancet.* 1973; 2(7839):1157-1159.

13. Reason J. Human error: models and management. *BMJ.* 2000;320(7237):768-770.

14. National Nosocomial Infections Surveillance (NNIS) System Report, data summary from January 1992 to June 2002, issued August 2002. *Am J Infect Control.* 2002;30(8):458-475.

15. Vincent C. Understanding and responding to adverse events. *N Engl J Med.* 2003;348(11):1051-1056.

16. Hill AB. The environment and disease: association or causation? *Proc R Soc Med.* 1965;58:295-300.

17. Burke JP. Patient safety: infection control-a problem for patient safety. *N Engl J Med.* 2003;348(7):651-656.

18. Gerberding JL. Hospital-onset infections: a patient safety issue. *Ann Intern Med*. 2002;137(8):665-670.

19. Bates DW, Gawande AA. Improving safety with information technology. *N Engl J Med*. 2003;348(25):2526-2534.

20. Spath PL. Using failure mode and effects analysis to improve patient safety. *AORN J*. 2003;78(1):16-37; quiz 41-44.

21. VA National Center for Patient Safety, 2003. (Accessed October 29, 2003, at http://www.patientsafety.gov.)

22. Making health care safer: a critical analysis of patient safety practices. *Evid Rep Technol Assess* (Summ). 2001(43):i-x, 1-668.

ADMINISTRATIVE ISSUES

CHAPTER TWENTY-SIX

THE INFECTION CONTROL COMMITTEE

Virginia R. Roth, MD, FRCPC and Mark Loeb, MD, MSc, FRCPC

INTRODUCTION

The infection control committee plays an important role in ensuring patient safety through the prevention and control of infections in a HCF. Members of the committee should hold a leadership position within the hospital in order to serve as opinion leaders and to effect change when necessary. This committee is a mechanism for the infection control program to report activities including statistics, outbreaks, and proactive control measures. The infection control committee also drafts and disseminates policies and procedures on infection surveillance, prevention, control, and education. Because its responsibilities reach virtually all hospital departments, the infection control committee can serve as a liaison between departments responsible for patient care and supportive departments such as pharmacy, housekeeping, and maintenance. The committee should report to the facility's medical board or medical advisory committee and/or senior management.

Infection control committees vary in that some serve single HCFs (hospitals or LTCFs), while others are regional committees. As a general rule, the former are smaller committees (eg, membership from 8 to 12 members) while the latter are much larger because representation from various hospitals, public health, and/or LTCFs is required (eg, membership 15 to 25 members). Regardless of size, most infection control committees function in a reporting capacity. That is, a typical meeting will not involve a working group brainstorming over policy. Rather, the results of subcommittees formed to address specific issues (eg, policies on staff vaccination) will be presented and discussed. The outcome of such deliberations may be the approval of the policy or a request for the subcommittee to revise a policy for discussion at the next meeting.

MEMBERSHIP

The infection control committee should be multidisciplinary, with, at a minimum, representation from senior facility management, the physician group, and nursing. In addition, consideration should be given to representation from critical care, surgery, medicine, the microbiology laboratory, pharmacy, occupational health, the central processing department, housekeeping, and the local public health department. When establishing an infection control committee in your HCF, it is important to take an inventory of patient care activity, particularly where infection control challenges are likely to occur. For example, if your hospital has a large hematology/oncology department, then inviting a representative of this department might be wise. Representatives from hospital departments may be nominated by the departments and preferably should be in a position to make decisions.

The committee may be most effective if the chair is a physician leader and if both the chair and members are appointed or approved by the medical board. The chair may be the hospital epidemiologist. It is important to note that all members of the committee need not be present at all meetings, particularly if the committee is very large. Members from certain groups (eg, emergency services) may have ad-hoc status; if their presence is required, they are notified before the meeting.

FUNCTIONS

The functions of the infection control committee should include:

➤ Formulating and recommending policy on all matters pertaining to infection control.

➤ Serving in an advisory capacity to the medical and senior administration of the facility.

➤ Reviewing infection control surveillance data and developing an appropriate action plan.

➤ Reviewing outbreak situations and developing outbreak control measures.

➤ Approving infection control-related policy and procedures.

➤ Approving the annual goals and objectives of the infection control program.

The infection control committee is responsible for making final recommendations to the medical board with respect to policy. The actual deliberations about the specific details of policy do not necessarily occur during the committee meetings. Often, it is more efficient to have smaller working groups iron out a draft of the policy. This is circulated to committee members well in advance of the next meeting, where committee members voice their approval or concern about the policy. Policies may range from isolation precautions for multiresistant bacteria to skin-testing of hospital employees for tuberculosis.

Agenda items to be discussed at the infection control committee meeting may include the need to change policy in response to information gathered during the day-to-day work of ICP (eg, lack of adherence to guidelines for maximal sterile precautions when inserting central venous catheters) or in response to concerns of administrators (eg, lack of standardization of active surveillance for multiresistant organisms among different hospital sites in a health system). The committee recommendations on policy are then sent to the medical board for approval. The committee, therefore, serves as an advisory role for senior clinicians and administrators. Generally speaking, the recommendations of a good infection control committee are adhered to and usually are not challenged by hospital administration. Senior hospital administrators place a high value on the expertise of the infection control committee.

Surveillance data collected by the infection control program are regularly reviewed at committee meetings. Quarterly surveillance reports may be attached as an appendix to the agenda for an upcoming meeting or may be distributed at the meeting. It is important that the data are thoroughly discussed and interpreted. For example, an increase in the incidence of MRSA in July may be due to lack of adherence to infection control precautions among new housestaff and may signal the need for a more intensive educational effort targeted at this group.

Reviewing the handling of outbreaks is another important function of the infection control committee. During an outbreak, the outbreak management team is responsible for the investigation, including the implementation of appropriate infection control measures. This almost certainly will involve some but not all members of the infec-

tion control committee. The committee itself may not be charged with making "real time" decisions about outbreaks (although provisions should be made for calling an emergency meeting if needed) but definitely should review how the outbreak was handled as part of a quality improvement process. The committee is charged with providing a strategy for managing outbreaks, such as notification procedures and possibly the establishment of a formal outbreak team. This is particularly important when planning for serious threats such as bioterrorism and pandemic influenza.

In addition to approving infection control procedures and policies, it is important that the committee review the annual goals and objectives of the infection control program. Regular meetings should be held (eg, monthly). The infection control committee must also ensure that all appropriate facilities are available to the hospital personnel to maintain good infection control practices. The committee might, for example, have to advocate on behalf of the infection control team for more resources, such as hiring additional staff or updating computer software. The committee can coordinate the development of infection control rules and practices. It is important that the committee maintain a strong liaison with occupational health because often there is substantial overlap in content between these areas. Having the occupational health physician on the infection control committee is a good way to ensure effective communication.

Whether establishing a new infection control committee or taking over as chair of an existing committee, it is important to either establish or review the mission statement of the committee. The mission statement should summarize the overall goals of the committee.

RESPONSIBILITIES OF THE CHAIR

Ideally, the chair should have a strong background in infection control or infectious diseases in order to provide leadership and direction to members. The chair's responsibilities should be specified in writing and should include the following:

➤ Ensuring the plans and actions decided upon by the committee are implemented.

➤ Reviewing the membership list annually to ensure adequate representation from appropriate departments.

➤ Replacing members with poor attendance or who are unable to fulfill their mandate.

➤ Representing the committee as spokesperson.

➤ Appointing special subcommittees or task forces as required.

It is important that the chair have respect from committee members and the hospital administration generally. This will help ensure that the policies and recommendations of the committee are acted upon promptly. An ideal chair should be someone who is a good facilitator and who is able to convince others of the importance of new policies or practices, without being overly dogmatic or rigid. Usually, there are many items on the agenda during an infection control committee meeting. The chair must have the ability to facilitate important deliberation but at the same time move the agenda forward. The chair needs to have good delegation ability and must be capable of assigning tasks to subcommittees. The chair should also reserve the right to call an emergency infection control committee meeting at his or her discretion.

The chair of the committee is usually the official spokesperson for the committee. It is usually the chair who will sit on the medical board and may be called upon to defend or explain the committee's recommendations on certain issues. This may also include communications with the media, particularly likely if the chair is the HCF's hospital epidemiologist.

The chair should review the make up of the committee on an annual basis. New committee members may need to be added to the committee. For example, if the hospital undergoes extensive renovation, it may be reasonable to have a representative from the facility planning group on the committee. Individuals who do not contribute (by not attending meetings or by changing roles in the facility) should be replaced.

It is important that the chair of the committee have good administrative support. An administrative assistant needs to organize the meetings, distribute the minutes, and compile reports for distribution. Because these are legal documents, complete and accurate minutes of committee meetings must be maintained and distributed to committee members, the medical board, and department heads. The chair is also responsible for setting the agenda for each infection control committee meeting and making sure this is distributed to committee members well in advance of the meeting.

RESPONSIBILITIES OF THE MEMBERS

The responsibilities and office terms of the members should be specified in writing. Responsibilities should include the following:
➤ Participate in regular meetings.
➤ Work with other members on current infection control issues.
➤ Identify a delegate to attend in his or her absence.

➤ Report on committee activities and decisions to those whom they represent and initiate any necessary action.
➤ Bring forward concerns from their represented population.

It is important that members of the committee be carefully selected. When it is possible to choose between members to represent a particular department, for example, it is important to consider time commitments of the potential members. For example, it might not always be advantageous to select the chair of a department because he or she likely has substantial administrative or clinical commitments. Often, such an individual will have limited time for attending meetings, let alone participating on subcommittees. It is important to select people who have a track record of working collaboratively with others. An individual who is dogmatic and inflexible or who tends to dominate group discussions may be a liability because open discussion and a free exchange of information are essential. Members should delegate others to attend in their place when they cannot attend the meeting. It is important that members have good communication skills, as they will be responsible for communicating committee policies to other members of their department. Members of the committee should also be well respected by their peers and be approachable, so that concerns can be brought through the member to the committee.

REPORTING

Minutes should be kept of each committee meeting. Timely reporting of any actions and decisions to the medical board, senior management, and other relevant committees (eg, quality improvement committee) should be ensured. Reporting to outside agencies, such as the local public health department, also may be necessary to comply with reportable disease requirements.

SUGGESTED READING

Boyce JM. Hospital epidemiology in smaller hospitals. *Infect Control Hosp Epidemiol.* 1995;16:600-606.

Friedman C, Barnette M, Buck AS, et al. Requirements for infrastructure and essential activities of infection control and epidemiology in out-of-hospital settings: a consensus panel report. Association for Professionals in Infection Control and Epidemiology and Society for Healthcare Epidemiology of America. *Infect Control Hosp Epidemiol.* 1999;20:695-705.

Girouard S, Levine G, Goodrich K, et al. Infection control programs at children's hospitals: a description of structures and processes. *Am J Infect Control.* 2001;29:145-151.

Haley RW. The "hospital epidemiologist" in U.S. hospitals, 1976-1977: a description of the head of the infection surveillance and control program. Report from the SENIC project. *Infect Control*. 1980;1:21-32.

Scheckler WE, Brimhall D, Buck AS, et al. Requirements for infrastructure and essential activities of infection control and epidemiology in hospitals: a consensus panel report. Society for Healthcare Epidemiology of America. *Infect Control Hosp Epidemiol*. 1998;19:114-124.

CHAPTER TWENTY-SEVEN

DEVELOPING INFECTION CONTROL POLICIES AND GUIDELINES

Young S. Kim, MD; PJ Brennan, MD; and Elias Abrutyn, MD

INTRODUCTION

Practice guidelines, critical pathways, best practices, and policies are terms referring to documents that describe parameters within which clinical practice should occur in a healthcare organization. Typically, the hospital epidemiologist has had the important responsibility of creating infection control guidelines at the institutional level.

The Institute of Medicine defines practice guidelines as "systematically developed statements to assist practitioner and patient decisions about appropriate healthcare for specific clinical circumstances."[1] The preferred term, "practice guideline," implies a nonbinding document that allows the practitioner to exercise clinical judgment for individual cases; thus, we will use this term throughout this discussion. In contrast, "policy" suggests a binding regulation that excludes clinical judgment and thus carries undesirable overtones.

Guidelines have become commonplace in clinical practice in recent years, and there are now numerous available sources.[2-5] Hospitals, federal agencies, insurers, and physician organizations have developed clinical guidelines to satisfy a variety of agendas.[6-8] Interestingly, a physician's age and the type of practice and source of the guideline affect physicians' knowledge of guidelines and confidence in their content. Physicians often judge guidelines developed or supported by professional organizations as more credible than those provided by insurers.[9] In one view, the challenge for the hospital epidemiologist is not identifying topics or writing the guidelines, but rather developing statements that are credible, that are accepted by the practitioners in the institution, and that can be widely and effectively carried out after the writing is finished.

RATIONALE

In general, the goal of guidelines is to reduce variations in practice to achieve a desired outcome.[9] The benefits of practice guidelines include medical education, identification of a standard of care, increased compliance with recommended practices, and improved clinical results.[10] The creation of practice guidelines helps the hospital epidemiologist establish performance standards, comply with regulatory requirements, meet accreditation requirements, and improve the quality of care.

CREATION OF INSTITUTIONAL PERFORMANCE STANDARDS

Many industries establish standards for workers to increase performance consistency to enhance quality and reduce cost. Once established, standards also permit measurement of productivity and outcomes. The infection control policy manual and departmental infection control guidelines are examples of such standards. The hospital epidemiologist or infection control professional should write the manual and revise it periodically. With input from the hospital epidemiologist, each department should write and implement department-specific guidelines.

COMPLIANCE WITH REGULATORY REQUIREMENTS

Laws, local ordinances, regulations, and standards of municipal, county, state, and federal authorities influence activities in healthcare institutions so the hospital epi-

---

TABLE 27-1. METHODS FOR PRACTICE GUIDELINE DEVELOPMENT

➤ Informal consensus: the opinion of experts
➤ Formal consensus development: National Institutes of Health Consensus Statement Model
➤ Evidence-based: grounded in scientific evidence
➤ Explicit guideline development: uses scientific evidence and analytic methods to assess the benefits, harms, costs, and probability of various outcomes

---

demiologist may need to develop guidelines to help clinicians comply with extramural regulations. Such examples include institutional guidelines on the reporting of communicable diseases, consent requirements for HIV antibody testing, policies governing professional activities of HCWs with bloodborne diseases, reporting of communicable diseases to emergency services personnel under the Ryan White Act, and procurement of cadaveric organs for transplantation.

MEETING ACCREDITATION REQUIREMENTS

The JCAHO currently requires that hospitals have written infection control policies and documentation of procedures needed to conduct the organization's mission effectively.[11] The infection control officer should ensure the existence of these documents. Important examples of the required documentation include a defined program for nosocomial infection surveillance, prevention, and control; departmental infection control guidelines; and the institutional statement of the infection control officer's authority.

ACHIEVING QUALITY IMPROVEMENT

It has become increasingly important to care for patients using prescribed regimens to achieve improved clinical outcomes in an efficient manner. Practice guidelines and clinical pathways have become important tools to achieve these goals. Because many physicians view guidelines developed by insurers for this purpose with skepticism,[9] practice guidelines established by the hospital epidemiologist (with appropriate colleagues) are preferred and can play a critical role in shaping the institution's standards of care.

DEVELOPING PRACTICE GUIDELINES

Woolf[7] has described the approaches that the hospital epidemiologist can use to develop practice guidelines (Table 27-1). Each approach has strengths and weaknesses. The consensus approach has the advantage of speed, but its validity may be questioned. Evidence-based guidelines have emerged as the gold standard and have scientific rigor, but use of this approach may be limited when valid data for a particular topic are lacking. Explicit guideline development combines elements of several approaches to specify the benefits and costs of interventions. These analyses may exceed institutional capabilities. Table 27-2 outlines the process often used to develop practice guidelines. An evidence-based approach predominates, but the process may also include elements of consensus development. As additional approaches, we would add adapting published guidelines for local use or accepting established guidelines formally as the standard for the institution.

SELECTING A TOPIC FOR GUIDELINE DEVELOPMENT

To ensure a successful outcome, the hospital epidemiologist must choose appropriate and pertinent topics. Clinicians may suggest topics and advise the hospital epidemiologist on specialty and subspecialty concerns. Those who recently have joined the hospital staff can provide new insights into seemingly intractable problems. Some topics will be dictated by regulations (eg, local law, federal mandate, or a JCAHO Type I citation). In discretionary areas, the hospital epidemiologist should choose topics carefully. Above all else, the hospital epidemiologist must focus on improving the quality of care. Local infection control data should be used to identify areas of need. Infection rates that exceed benchmarks are good targets

TABLE 27-2. PROCESS OF GUIDELINE DEVELOPMENT

➤ Guideline planning
  ➣ Determine the purpose of the guideline
  ➣ Gather established guidelines
  ➣ Gather prior local guidelines
  ➣ Review/collect relevant infection control data
  ➣ Identify any deficiencies in practice
➤ Guideline development
  ➣ Identify key institutional personnel
  ➣ Gain concurrence on key points
  ➣ Finalize document
  ➣ Approval of key committees, departments, and hospital administration
➤ Guideline implementation
  ➣ Dissemination to key departments
  ➣ Education program for hospital staff, if needed
  ➣ Review/collect relevant infection control data after implementation
  ➣ Reassessment of guideline

for improvement through guideline development or revision. Infection rates exceeding published rates or rates from similar hospitals provide a powerful tool for the epidemiologist to help the hospital staff understand the problem and the need for change. For example, our rates of central venous catheter-related bloodstream infections were higher than those published by the NNIS System at the CDC. We examined who, how, where, and what type of catheters were inserted. We found that supplies for central venous catheters were in disparate locations, making it burdensome to assemble the proper sterile barrier supplies. In addition, the central venous catheter insertion and maintenance were suboptimal. We then formed a multidisciplinary committee to develop a new practice guideline using a published reference.[5,12] The guideline standardized the insertion procedure, care of central venous catheters, and ultimately helped reduce bloodstream infection rates.

TACKLING LARGER ISSUES

Developing guidelines and ensuring compliance with infection control practices for insertion and care of central venous, urinary catheters, or others may seem daunting, but improved practices in these important areas will have a greater effect on quality of care than minor, more easily achieved objectives. Your organization will measure your credibility by your recognition of critical issues for practice guideline development. Poor choice of topics and very limited or minor problems may erode your credibility. We list possible topics for practice guidelines in Table 27-3.

ANSWERING THE IMPORTANT QUESTIONS AND CHOOSING THE PARTICIPANTS

Writing guidelines is made easier and the guideline made more relevant by first answering the following questions. First, what is the impetus for the guideline and what are the desired goals? Second, who benefits from the guideline? Third, what parties will execute the new guideline? If the impetus is a widely recognized problem and improvement will benefit patients and staff, there may be a groundswell of support. If the impetus for action is unclear or the benefits of the guideline uncertain, you should reconsider your choice of topics because you may have difficulty finding support for such an undertaking. The answers to these questions will also help the hospital epidemiologist identify those who should participate in the process of properly defining the problem and the process to be used for guideline development.

Resistance to change is often encountered in clinical practice, but some changes are more difficult to promote than others. Mandates of regulatory agencies, such as the Bloodborne Pathogens Standard of the Occupational Safety and Health Administration, are among the most difficult policies to translate into hospital practice. People at various levels of an organization may oppose mandates. HCWs may find mandates burdensome; administrators find them costly; and patients may feel isolated by them. Although the infection control officers may have little enthusiasm for such mandates, they must bring the hospital into compliance. The hospital epidemiologist may have to convince administrators to implement these

TABLE 27-3. SUGGESTED TOPICS FOR PRACTICE GUIDELINE DEVELOPMENT

➤ Isolation precautions
➤ Triage and isolation of patients suspected of having tuberculosis
➤ Blood culture techniques
➤ Operating room traffic control
➤ Perioperative antimicrobial prophylaxis
➤ Outpatient surgery procedures
➤ Postoperative wound care
➤ Antimicrobial therapy
➤ Central venous catheter insertion practices
➤ Management of bladder catheters
➤ Management of ventilatory support equipment
➤ Maintenance of sterilizers and sterilization of critical devices
➤ Regulatory requirements
➤ Respirator training program
➤ Infection control precautions during hospital construction
➤ Notification of emergency medical personnel following exposure to transmissible diseases
➤ Bioterrorism

measures so that citations and fines can be avoided. Hospital epidemiologists can learn from the federal mandate process and can facilitate institutional acceptance of practice guidelines by bearing in mind our third question, "Who executes the policy change?" Although federal mandates allow for a period of public comment and debate, the scale of a national rule-making process may leave some clinicians feeling that the rule is an arbitrary dictum distant from the reality of clinical practice. It is critically important to understand that, at the institutional level, intramural and extramural guideline pronouncements may flounder unless key individuals in all affected departments "buy in" to the process even if the guidelines are based on sound infection control principles. The hospital epidemiologist can achieve "buy in" by actively engaging local opinion leaders in the development process. Participants in the process become resources who bring important viewpoints to the discussion and who bring credibility to the guidelines taken back to their constituents. This committee process may be more time-consuming, but the benefits far outweigh the burdens. As a general rule, the staff in key departments will accept, understand, and cooperate with guidelines that are developed with the input of their staff. Important personnel from hospital administration can be integral committee members to provide institutional support for the guideline and assist in its proper execution.

The next step is to establish a timeline for guideline development. Open-ended processes punctuated by monthly meetings may drag on and lose momentum. Meetings at shorter intervals (every 2 weeks) allow participants sufficient time to complete the work between meetings and to build momentum and enthusiasm for the

objectives. Defining the start and the end is helpful in gaining full cooperation. Assigning tasks for guideline development to important or critical committee members can help distribute the workload, and sharing the responsibility helps ensure a sense of ownership of the final document.

THE CONTENT

Choosing Benchmarks

A guideline should have a clear objective and should be written in plain, forthright language. Overreaching content and ambiguous language make a guideline unfocused and create confusion for its readers. The approach to developing the content of the guideline (see Table 27-1) will vary by institution, the topic chosen, the scientific evidence, and local experts. Guidelines should cite pertinent literature because clinicians may respond with skepticism to guidelines lacking supportive data, and guidelines should include institutional experience, if appropriate. The inclusion of the consensus of local or national expert panels is often very powerful.

The necessary elements for guidelines are described below.

➤ *Introduction*. This section provides the rationale and background for the document and sets out the objectives for creating the guideline and the factors leading to its development. The introduction may contain a glossary of key terms used subsequently.

➤ *Scope*. This section defines the circumstances and individuals to whom the guideline may apply.

➤ *Process.* This section describes the method of guideline development (eg, consensus, evidence-based).

➤ *Responsibility.* This section identifies the individuals who will ensure compliance and enforce the policy.

➤ *Implementation.* This section should contain an unambiguous, step-by-step description of the process and a list of equipment essential to the process. Accompanying diagrams may clarify procedures.

➤ *Appendices.* Some guidelines may overlap areas in which separate or complementary guidelines already exist. Take care not to contradict these preexisting documents (eg, nursing practice manuals). If you cross-reference these documents or include them as appendices to the guideline, you may avoid confusion.

➤ *Relevant References.* A list of all of the relevant references used to develop the guideline should be provided.

➤ *Conclusion.* At the end of the guideline, you should list the address, e-mail address, and the telephone number of people who can answer questions or clarify the content. When the appropriate hospital authority, usually the hospital epidemiologist, signs and dates the guideline, the document is complete. Remember to review guidelines periodically and keep a history of the revisions to ensure that they still are current. Document the review process, and enter the documentation in the infection control committee minutes.

IMPLEMENTATION

Memos, Movies, and More Work

Once the guideline has been written, the real work begins. Nothing is more frustrating than having months of work on a guideline lie dormant and unnoticed in a policy manual. The first step in implementing the written document is the administrative approval. Stepwise approval—starting with the hospital infection control committee and moving upward to medical staff committees, the medical staff, and, ultimately, hospital administration—is necessary before implementation can occur. Your presence at committee meetings may be required to answer questions to ensure smooth passage. You may need to advocate actively to facilitate acceptance.

If the guideline is to live after it is approved, the institution must educate its personnel. Memos announcing the new guideline are generally not effective; staff members seldom read or remember them. Traditional lectures

are not an efficient means to realize new guidelines given the time limitations of the hospital work environment. In-service educational programs are essential for all staff members who fall within the scope and responsibility of the guideline. Nursing staff educators skilled at professional development are ideal people to work with and conduct in-service programs for nurses. Educating physicians is more difficult, because they often practice autonomously. Presentations at department or division conferences or meetings are often the best venue for providing effective physician education. Demonstrating new procedures, either in person or by videocassette, may also work. Strategically placed posters, presentations, and periodic reiterations for the house staff may be needed to reinforce the changes. Undoubtedly, the most critical element is the support of hospital and departmental leaders. For example, if an intensive care unit director makes reduction of infection rates a priority, it is more likely that new practices guidelines will be introduced into practice.

MEASURING THE OUTCOME

The coin of the realm in healthcare is performance improvement. To determine the effectiveness of new guidelines, institutions must measure outcomes of interest and determine the effect of the guideline. The outcome of interest may be bloodstream infection rates, as in the example of a central venous catheter insertion guideline. To determine whether the practice guideline improves rates, the hospital epidemiologist will need to measure guideline compliance. For example, the epidemiologist could directly observe practice. If the guideline introduced a new product, the epidemiologist could assess how often HCWs use the product.

CONCLUSION

Practice guidelines will increase in importance as clinical outcomes become increasingly emphasized. Currently, many physicians remain unfamiliar with the content of guidelines, although they are aware of their existence.[6] Healthcare epidemiologists will be challenged to write clear, credible guidelines that are grounded in science and to bring them into practice through persistent and creative peer education.

ACKNOWLEDGMENT

Drs. Young and Abrutyn wish to acknowledge that this work was supported in part by a grant from the Tenet Healthcare Foundation.

REFERENCES

1. Field MJ, Lohr KN, eds. *Clinical Practice Guidelines: Directions for a New Program.* Washington, DC: National Academy Press; 1990.

2. *Clinical Practice Guidelines Directory, 1999.* 1st ed. Chicago, Ill: American Medical Association; 1999.

3. American College of Physicians Web Site, Current ACP Guidelines. Available at: http://www.acponline.org/sci-policy/guidelines/recent.htm. Accessed September 20, 2003.

4. Green E, Katz J, eds. *Clinical Practice Guidelines for the Adult Patient.* St. Louis, Mo: Mosby; 1994.

5. Abrutyn E, Goldmann DA, Scheckler WE, eds. *Infection Control Reference Service: The Experts' Guide to the Guidelines.* 2nd ed. Philadelphia, Pa: WB Saunders; 2001.

6. Woolf SH. Practice guidelines: a new reality in medicine, 1: recent developments. *Arch Intern Med.* 1990;150:1811-1818.

7. Woolf SH. Practice guidelines: a new reality in medicine, 2: methods of developing guidelines. *Arch Intern Med.* 1992;152:946-952.

8. Audet AM, Greenfield S, Field M. Medical practice guidelines: current activities and future directions. *Ann Intern Med.* 1990;113:709-714.

9. Tunis SR, Hayward RS, Wilson MC, et al. Internists' attitudes about clinical practice guidelines. *Ann Intern Med.* 1994;120:956-963.

10. Woolf SH. Practice guidelines: a new reality in medicine, 3: impact on patient care. *Arch Intern Med.* 1993; 153:2646-2655.

11. Joint Commission on Accreditation of Healthcare Organizations. Surveillance, prevention, and control of infections. *Comprehensive Accreditation Manual for Hospitals. The Official Handbook.* Oakbrook Terrace, Ill: JCAHO; 1996:IC1-IC25.

12. Guidelines for the prevention of intravascular catheter-related infections. *MMWR.* 2002;51:RR-10.

CHAPTER TWENTY-EIGHT

The Occupational Safety and Health Administration's Regulatory Role

Judene Bartley, MS, MPH, CIC; Gina Pugliese, RN, MS; and Tammy Lundstrom, MD

Introduction— OSHA Standards

OSHA is the federal agency that is authorized to conduct workplace inspections to determine whether employers are complying with the agency's safety and health standards. The General Duty Clause of the Occupational Safety and Health Act of 1970 requires that employers provide every worker with a safe and healthful workplace. OSHA may adopt a specific standard or regulation, such as the Bloodborne Pathogens standard, on which it bases all its inspections and enforcement actions. When a specific standard does not exist to apply to a perceived "hazard," such as protection against occupational exposure to *Mycobacterium tuberculosis*, OSHA must rely on the General Duty Clause for the authority to inspect the workplace and assess compliance with recognized "guidelines or standards of care," such as the CDC Guidelines. OSHA can issue citations under that clause if its compliance safety and health officers (CSHO) can demonstrate that the employer failed to keep the workplace free of a recognized hazard that was causing or was likely to cause death or serious physical harm and that a feasible and useful method of abatement existed. OSHA also expects facilities to be in compliance with all standards that may apply to the worksite, such as its standards for respiratory protection (29 CFR 1910.134; 29 CFR 1910.139); record keeping (29 CFR 1910.20); which requires CSHO access to employee exposure and medical records; and 29 CFR 1904, which requires a log and summary of occupational injuries and illnesses, called the OSHA 300 log; and hazard notification (29 CFR 1910.145); which requires that warnings be posted as needed.

OSHA withdrew its proposed *M. tuberculosis* (TB) standard in May 2003.[1] However, even without a formal standard, OSHA still has the authority to inspect worksites for occupational risks to TB under the General Duty Clause and continues to assess compliance with the CDC's TB Guidelines using a specific compliance directive issued in 1996 (CPL 2.106) to assist its CSHOs in interpreting CDC TB guidelines.[2,3]

Although there is no formal TB standard, OSHA has 2 respiratory protection standards that may apply in healthcare organizations. The first Respiratory Protection Standard (29.CFR 1910.134) issued October 5, 1998, applies to general industry, construction, shipyard, longshoring, and marine terminal workplaces for all exposures except TB. This standard may apply, for example, in the laboratory or plant operations for exposure to chemical fumes and may require specialized respirators. The second Respiratory Protection Standard (29 CFR 1910.139) is solely for protection from TB and addresses respirator selection, use, fit testing, and fit checking. This standard specifically addresses the use of N-95 respirators, requires an initial fit test and check, but does not require annual fit testing in lieu of a medical assessment based on specific criteria. All OSHA standards are easily located and downloaded from OSHA's Web site.[4] Additional information can be found in Chapter 22.

Understanding OSHA Through the Bloodborne Pathogen Standard

Of all the standards, the Bloodborne Pathogen Standard has had the greatest impact on worker protection in the healthcare setting and so will be used as the model to explain OSHA's processes and requirements.

OSHA first published its *Occupational Exposure to Bloodborne Pathogens Standard* in the December 6, 1991, *Federal Register*. When OSHA publishes a standard, it also publishes a compliance directive to assist the CSHO in interpreting the intent of the standard and to establish uniform inspection procedures. The compliance directive assists employers in determining the requirements for compliance with a standard and thus is valuable for developing specific procedures. The compliance directive for the Bloodborne Pathogen Standard was first issued in February 1992 and has undergone numerous revisions. The most recent revision was issued in November 2001 and reflects the requirements for the use of sharps safety devices outlined in the January 2001 revised Bloodborne Pathogen Standard.[5,6] These changes were mandated by the Needlestick Safety and Prevention Act signed into law on November 2000.[7] In developing worker protection programs, it is essential to review the federal OSHA standards, as well as state OSHA requirements and state laws, where applicable.

Bloodborne Pathogen Standard—Elements

Elements of a basic program to meet the requirements of the Bloodborne Pathogens Standard:

➤ A written exposure control plan that is accessible, includes a list of all job categories having occupational exposure to blood or other potentially infectious materials (OPIM), outlines a schedule for implementing all provisions of the standard, and states a procedure for reporting and investigating exposure incidents.

➤ Protocols that mandate that HCWs practice universal precautions (now included in standard precautions), describe how to implement work practice and engineering controls, and describe housekeeping schedules for cleaning and decontamination of equipment and disposal of regulated wastes.

➤ A program to provide personal protective equipment.

➤ A hepatitis B vaccination program.

➤ A postexposure evaluation and follow-up program that considers the latest CDC recommendations.

➤ A comprehensive hazard communication program that includes specific labels for regulated waste and for containers used to store or transport blood or OPIM, material safety data sheets, and programs to train employees.

➤ A recordkeeping system that is well maintained, is accessible to OSHA and employees, and includes records of training programs and employees' medical records.

If an institution has HIV or HBV research laboratories or production facilities, OSHA specifies additional requirements.

Current Focus

Federal Needlestick Safety and Prevention Act

On November 6, 2000, President Clinton signed into law the Needlestick Safety and Prevention Act.[6] This law authorized OSHA to revise the Bloodborne Pathogen Standard to require the use of devices with engineered sharps injury protection and a log with details of sharps-related injuries. Among the revisions, the Act specified that the definition of an engineering control be expanded to include safety devices and that safety device use be mandated.

OSHA's Revised Bloodborne Pathogen Standard

As mandated by the Needlestick Stick Safety and Prevention Act, OSHA issued its revision to the Bloodborne Pathogen Standard on January 18, 2001 in the Federal Register, with an effective date of April 18, 2001. The new requirements included the following:

➤ An expanded definition of an engineering control to include devices with engineered sharps injury protection and needleless systems.

➤ Exposure control plans that reflect changes in technology that reduce exposure to bloodborne pathogens and document the consideration, at least annually, of devices to minimize occupational exposure.

➤ Input solicited from nonmanagerial (ie, frontline) workers for identification, evaluation, and selection of devices and other controls. This process must be documented in the exposure control plan.

➤ A sharps injury log of percutaneous injuries with information on the type and brand of device involved, the department where the incident occurred, and an explanation of how the injury occurred.

State-Level OSHA Plans

Twenty-three states have state-approved OSHA plans. These state-level plans must incorporate regulations that are "at least as effective" (ie, at least as strict) as those set forth by OSHA at the federal level. As with all revisions in federal OSHA standards, the 23 states with state-approved OSHA plans were permitted an additional 6 months from the federal implementation date to review/revise their state OSHA regulations to include, at a minimum, the new federal OSHA requirements, but they may adopt stricter requirements. States with state-approved OSHA plans include Arkansas, Arizona, California, Connecticut, Hawaii, Iowa, Indiana, Kentucky, Maryland, Michigan, Minnesota, Nevada, North Carolina, New Mexico, New York, Oregon, South Carolina, Tennessee, Utah, Virginia, Vermont, Washington, and Wyoming. In Connecticut and New York, state programs cover public employees, and OSHA covers private employees.

State Laws

A number of states passed laws that mandated the use of sharps injury prevention devices. California was the first state to enact a law in September 1998 that mandated the state OSHA program revise its Bloodborne Pathogen Standard to require employers to implement sharps injury prevention technology, including needleless systems when applicable for IV access and needles with engineered sharps injury protection. The law also requires employers to record all exposure incidents, including the type and brand of the device involved in the injury, and to maintain a sharps injury log.

By December 2001, a total of 21 states had passed needle safety legislation; the bulk of the bills are patterned after California's. Many of these state laws have requirements similar to those in the revised OSHA standard as mandated by the new Federal Needlestick Safety and Prevention Act. If a state needle safety law has requirements that are more stringent than what the federal law requires, then the additional state requirements must be followed. For instance, some states require HCFs to report needlestick injury data to a state agency. States with specific needlestick and sharps safety prevention laws include Arkansas, Alabama, California, Connecticut, Georgia, Iowa, Maine, Maryland, Massachusetts, Minnesota, Missouri, New Hampshire, New Jersey, New York, Ohio, Oklahoma, Pennsylvania, Rhode Island, Tennessee, Texas, and West Virginia.

Bloodborne Pathogen Standard—Implementation Strategies

OSHA is currently citing healthcare organizations for lack of safety devices. OSHA may be flexible in issuing citations in some situations if there is evidence of safety devices already being used in some clinical applications and a written plan with a realistic timeline that outlines the process for completion of the selection, evaluation, and adoption of safety devices in all areas where sharps are used. The bloodborne exposure control plan should be revised to reflect the process that will be used to accomplish these goals.

Involvement of Frontline Workers

OSHA wants to ensure that management does not select devices without input from nonmanagerial workers—those responsible for direct patient care or potentially exposed to injuries from contaminated sharps. Input may be obtained from these frontline workers in any manner appropriate to the circumstances of the workplace. This input will be needed for identifying devices to consider, performing some type of assessment or evaluation of the devices, and selecting devices for implementation. Such input may be formal or informal; OSHA has explained that it does not prescribe any specific procedures for obtaining worker input. Frontline worker

involvement in the evaluation and selection of safety devices can help promote acceptance of these devices when they are implemented. Although it may not be feasible to involve every worker who will use a device in the selection and evaluation of every device, a representative sample of workers should always be included.

Device Evaluation

The evaluation process can be formal or informal. A formal evaluation might include a pilot study on a particular unit, with written evaluation forms completed by each worker. An informal evaluation might include bringing sample devices to the department or setting for a representative sample of frontline workers to evaluate them and provide informal feedback.

Nor are there exact formulas for the number of workers needed to evaluate a device, the number of devices to be evaluated, or the length of time an evaluation should be conducted. What is important is having a mechanism in place to solicit input from workers on an ongoing basis regarding their needs and preferences for safety devices. This input will be combined with data from exposure incidents and the sharps injury log and employee feedback, and will guide future decisions on selection and implementation of safety devices. In some cases, it may be necessary to replace the device that was originally selected with a more suitable device. This determination can only be made by the individual facility or work site based on its own data and experiences.

The final selection will be based on the preferences of the workers as they perform their duties and procedures using the safety devices. Preferences may vary for a single device, depending on the department and workers evaluating the device. The preferences are influenced by a number of factors—for example, prior experience with safety devices, type of clinical procedures being performed, noise or lighting in the clinical setting, or even the size of the worker's hands.

Other factors that might be considered in the final selection include characteristics listed in Table 28-1.

Sharps Injury Log

OSHA intends the sharps injury log to be used as a tool for identifying high-risk areas and providing information that may be helpful in evaluating devices. The confidential sharps injury log must include, at a minimum, the following information:

➤ Type and brand of the device causing the injury (if known)

➤ Department or work areas where incident occurred

➤ Description of the events surrounding the injury, including, for example

  ➤ Procedure being performed

  ➤ Body part affected

  ➤ Objects or substances involved in exposure

TABLE 28-1. SAFETY CHARACTERISTICS

Suitability for a range of uses across
  patient populations and procedures
Single- or 2-handed use
Extent of change in technique required
Undefeatable safety feature
Permanent coverage of the sharp
Patient safety
Breadth of product line

Active versus passive
Positioning of hands behind sharp
Indication of activation
Packaging
Interference with procedure
Right- or left-handed use
Studies in the literature on efficacy

OSHA explains that the sharps injury log may be kept in any format, such as electronic or paper. Employers may also use existing mechanisms for data collection, such as incident reports, provided that the necessary data are collected. The information from this sharps injury log can be used to guide the selection and evaluation of safety devices. The data from the sharps log are only one source of information for assessing the effectiveness of engineering controls. Employee interviews and informal feedback are other examples of input that should be considered. Trends in the data may be helpful in making a general assessment of the effectiveness of the sharps injury prevention program; however, calculation of rates of injury by device or brand is often inaccurate and misleading for a number of reasons: (1) Injuries are significantly underreported (up to 70% in some studies), which can influence the rates, and (2) individual facilities usually do not have enough data to calculate rates that are statistically significant and could not have occurred by chance, so in many cases, it is impossible to compare the relative ability of devices to reduce needlestick injuries.[8]

Conventional Needles and Exceptions

Conventional needles may still be needed. Safety devices are only required in situations where the needle may become contaminated. It is important to document those situations where conventional needles and devices may still be appropriate.

OSHA allows exceptions to the use of safer sharps technology when (1) there is no safety device commercially available to perform the specific procedure, (2) if employee safety is compromised by use of the safety device during a specific procedure, or (3) if patient safety is compromised by use of the safety device during a specific procedure. Exceptions allowed in a facility should be carefully researched and documented.

OSHA INSPECTIONS

OSHA lists its inspection priorities as imminent danger situations, catastrophes and fatal accidents, employee complaints, programmed inspections, and follow-up inspections. Rather than scheduled inspections, employee complaints have triggered nearly all healthcare inspections related to the Bloodborne Pathogen Standard. If an employee believes he or she is in imminent danger from a hazard or thinks there is a violation of an OSHA standard that may result in physical harm to workers, the employee may ask for an inspection. OSHA will withhold the employee's name from the employer if the employee so requests. OSHA will inform the employee of any actions taken and also will hold an informal review with an employee of any decision not to inspect.

Inspection Process

An inspection consists of 3 parts: an opening conference with the employer, a tour of the facility, and a closing conference.

The Opening Conference

At the opening conference, the CSHO first will explain the reasons for the inspection, the scope of the inspection, and any applicable OSHA standards. Although a complaint regarding the Bloodborne Pathogens Standard may have triggered the visit, OSHA almost certainly will conduct a complete survey, including hazardous chemicals, radiation safety, hazard communication, and so on. In some cases, the inspection may be terminated at this point if the CSHO finds that an exemption is appropriate, as in cases where an OSHA-funded consultation program is in progress. If an employee's complaint triggered the inspection, the CSHO will give a copy of the complaint to the employer. The CSHO will ask the employer to designate an employee representative. An employee representative (selected by the bargaining unit [union], employee members of the safety committee, or the employees) is entitled to attend the opening conference and to accompany the CSHO during the inspection.

Facility Tour

Healthcare epidemiologists and infection control professionals should accompany the CSHO during the tour to answer technical or clinical questions that may arise. They should be aware that in their interactions with the CSHO, it is likely they will be viewed by the CSHO as a representative of management, not as independent professionals. Infection control personnel may help to avert a citation simply by clarifying the hospital's protocols.

During the inspection, the CSHO will review policies, procedures, and training records; survey engineering controls; and observe employee practices. The CSHO will interview employees privately about their safety and work practices and likely their input into selecting safer devices to prevent needlestick injuries. The CSHO will review records of work-related injuries, illnesses, and fatalities and will check the OSHA 300 log, in which should be recorded all workplace injuries, including needlestick injuries, TB (Mantoux) skin-test conversions, cases of TB in employees, etc. During the tour, the CSHO will point out to the employer any unsafe working conditions and may take photographs or measurements to document the problem. The CSHO may specify corrective actions and may allow the hospital to correct the problems at this point. However, OSHA still may cite and fine the hospital for these deficiencies.

Closing Conference

At the closing conference, the CSHO will meet with the representatives of the employer and employees to discuss the problems and needs. The CSHO will provide an OSHA document that explains the employer's rights and responsibilities following the inspection. The CSHO will discuss all apparent violations, but will not indicate the proposed penalties at this time; the OSHA area director reviews the report and determines citations and proposes penalties. A facility spokesperson should explain to the CSHO how the employer has attempted to comply with the standards and should provide any information that can help OSHA to determine how much time may be needed to abate an apparent violation.

After the Inspection

Citations and Penalties

The area director will send citations and notices of proposed penalties to the hospital by certified mail. The hospital must post these citations on or near the areas where the alleged violations occurred. Penalties vary according to the seriousness of the violation. The area director may propose substantial fines, up to $70,000, for willful or repeated violations of a standard. Both the hospital and the employees have the right to appeal. Employees may request an informal review if OSHA decides not to issue a citation and may contest the time allowed for the hospital to eliminate the hazardous conditions.

Appeals

If the facility decides to contest a citation, an abatement period, or a proposed penalty, it must submit a written "Notice of Contest" to the area director within 15 working days from the time of the citation. The area director will forward the objection to the Occupational Safety and Health Review Commission (OSHRC), which operates independently of OSHA and which will assign the case to an administrative law judge. If the hospital fails to file a "Notice of Contest" within 15 days, the citation and proposed penalty will become a final order of the OSHRC that cannot be appealed.

An organization should not be afraid to contest citations. Challenging citations judged to be unfair or incorrect can lead to substantial reductions in fines at minimum. This is simply the process used by OSHA, and the local area offices expect further communication. Sometimes, it is possible to discuss issues informally with the area director of OSHA or meet face to face with additional documentation to support the reason for disagreement. The citation may be removed, or penalty fines may be reduced considerably.

TIPS FOR PREPARING FOR OSHA

Accountability

The healthcare epidemiologist and the administration must understand that the employer is responsible for compliance; employees have no responsibility whatsoever. It is the employer who controls the workplace, and the employer must use that control to ensure that employees comply. Therefore, the hospital administration must understand, promulgate, and enforce the regulations. The infection control department, the safety committee, and the occupational/employee health unit will bear much of the responsibility for developing and implementing the exposure control plan and the TB protection program. If there are employees who repeatedly fail to comply with regulations, OSHA will listen to efforts taken to educate and retrain such individuals, but documentation of training and communication records are essential to avoid citations.

Multidisciplinary Teams

Each institution will have its own best approach to managing these processes and responsibilities. A multidisciplinary group supports a proactive approach to an otherwise purely regulatory function. Many facilities have a subcommittee involving representatives from committees or functions such as infection control, safety, occupational health, risk management, and administrators to provide proactive direction, improve interdepartmental communications, and implement new policies and procedures. During an actual inspection, members of the group communicate with facility representatives accompanying the compliance officer and provide additional information when needed. After the inspection, members implement proposed corrective measures and help to prepare responses to any citations.

Mock Inspections

The healthcare epidemiologist must understand the key elements of the standards. The epidemiologist (and/or the multidisciplinary team) may want to conduct periodic surveys or mock OSHA inspections of healthcare departments to ensure compliance, check documentation, and identify problem areas. A comprehensive checklist based on the bloodborne pathogen rule may help the epidemiologist to evaluate each of the areas subject to inspection.[9] The infection control department should maintain records of these inspections.

Exposure Management

The management of employee exposures to blood, OPIM, and TB will vary according to each institution's plan, but infection control, employee health, and occupational medicine should work together to establish a post-exposure prophylaxis protocol. Infection control personnel should develop policies for handling prehospital exposures of nonemployed emergency medical personnel, visitors, students, and nonemployee physicians and their personnel. Administration, risk management, and the legal department should review these policies.

Education and Training

In larger institutions, the infection control department will not be able to assume the entire burden of initial employee training and the required annual updates. One widely used approach is termed "train the trainer." OSHA coordinators are designated in each department and are responsible for implementing regulations and teaching personnel about the standards that apply to their departments. If individuals at the departmental level are interested, their staff members are more likely to understand the regulations and to comply.

Videotapes made by the infection control department or online Web training may be helpful. Use of such resources, including computerized self-training modules, must include site-specific information, and a knowledgeable individual must be available to answer questions at the time the employee is participating in the training session.[10] Training sessions must be conducted during working hours, on the employer's time, and must cover topics specific to the employer's workplace, including details of the protection plan, names of people whom the employee must contact after an exposure, and method of medical follow-up.

OSHA's Consultation Service

OSHA has a free consultation service whereby a representative may be invited to evaluate your facility. The format is the same as for an OSHA inspection. They will inspect the facility for hazards, evaluate your safety and health program, conduct a conference to report their findings to management, provide a written report of recommendations and agreements, assist in implementing recommendations, including training, and conduct a follow-up inspection to determine whether the facility corrected the problems appropriately. If the facility receives a comprehensive consultation visit, corrects all specified hazards, and institutes the core elements of an effective safety and health program, the facility may be exempt from general schedule enforcement inspections for 1 year. However, if an employee files a complaint or if a fatality or catastrophe occurs within the year, OSHA may inspect the facility. The exemption provision applies only to states under the federal OSHA program, but some states that have their own enforcement plans have adopted similar provisions. Facilities cannot be fined under this program, and consultants do not report violations to the OSHA enforcement staff. However, OSHA requires that the facility correct all identified hazards. Consultation visits do not guarantee that the facility will pass a federal or state OSHA inspection. This process provides an opportunity to have OSHA answer questions and to clarify their regulations. OSHA provides multiple resources to assist in understanding and complying with its inspection process.[11]

Healthcare epidemiologists should seek to develop a cordial working relationship with their regional or state OSHA. By understanding the occupational health paradigm, finding common ground, and promoting dialogue, HCFs can change a "regulatory burden" into a proactive safety program that affects the overall safety culture of an organization.

REFERENCES

1. Department Of Labor (DOL) Final Rule Stage. Occupational Safety and Health Administration (OSHA) Occupational Exposure to Tuberculosis CFR Citation: 29 CFR 1910.1035. *Federal Register*. 2003;68(101):30588-30589.

2. Enforcement Policy and Procedures for Occupational Exposure to Tuberculosis. OSHA Directive CPL 2.106. Washington, DC: Occupational Safety and Health Administration; February 9, 1996.

3. Centers for Disease Control and Prevention. Guidelines for preventing the transmission of *Mycobacterium tuberculosis* in health-care facilities, 1994. *MMWR*. 1994; 43(RR-13).

4. OSHA standards and regulations: Available at: http://www.osha.gov/html/a-z-index.html. Accessed August 2, 2004.

5. *Enforcement Policy and Procedures for Occupational Exposure to Bloodborne Pathogens.* OSHA Directive CPL 2-2.69. Washington, DC: Occupational Safety and Health Administration; 2001.

6. US Department of Labor, Occupational Health and Safety Administration. Occupational exposure to bloodborne pathogens: needlesticks and other sharps injuries; final rule 29 CFR Part 1910. *Federal Register.* 2001;66:5318-5325.

7. Needlestick Safety and Prevention Act Law 106 430 Nov 6, 2000. 106th Congress of the United States of America. Available at: http://.thomas.loc.gov/. Accessed August 2, 2004.

8. Pugliese G, Germanson TP, Bartley J, et al. Evaluating sharps safety devices: meeting OSHA's intent. *Infect Control Hosp Epidemiol.* 2001;22(7):456-459.

9. OSHA Bloodborne Pathogen Program Assessment Tool. Available at: Premier Safety Institute: http://www.premier-inc.com/all/safety/resources/needlestick/downloads.htm. Accessed August 2, 2004.

10. Pugliese G. Preventing Occupational Sharps-Related Injuries-OSHA Compliance, APIC CEU Educational Website Module. Available at: www.apic.org. Accessed May, 2001.

11. OSHA Compliance resources on consultation service: Available at: http://www.osha.gov/dcsp/compliance_assistance/index.html. Accessed August 2, 2004.

CHAPTER TWENTY-NINE

PREPARING FOR AND SURVIVING A JOINT COMMISSION ON ACCREDITATION OF HEALTHCARE ORGANIZATIONS INSPECTION

Mary D. Nettleman, MD, MS

GETTING STARTED

The best advice is to start early and work continuously to prepare for JCAHO accreditation or re-accreditation. Most standards require that compliance be documented for at least 1 year prior to the survey. Although scheduled, formal evaluations by JCAHO are still the mainstay of accreditation, the organization will soon be putting increased emphasis on unannounced visits, interim data reporting, and continuous quality improvement.

The *Comprehensive Accreditation Manual for Hospitals*, published annually by JCAHO, is an ideal place to begin.[1] The accreditation manual contains standards that hospitals are expected to meet, as well as scoring guidelines and rules for accreditation. Many of these rules were based on recommendations from scientific societies including the SHEA.[2] All sections that apply to the epidemiologist should be read. In some institutions, the epidemiologist's responsibilities are confined to infection control. In other institutions, the responsibilities have been broadened. It is helpful to go over each standard individually and consider how compliance will be documented. One caution is that standards for infection control are not limited to the section labeled "Surveillance, Prevention, and Control of Infection." Sections on privacy, information management, waived testing, and others may apply to infection control activities.

JCAHO provides consultants, publishes newsletters, and holds frequent conferences. Conferences are helpful, and the speakers often have insight into changes planned for the future. For the novice, these events are a valuable introduction to the standards and to the survey process. Many hospitals avail themselves of JCAHO consultants prior to their scheduled survey.

It is especially useful to contact facilities that have been reviewed by the same survey team members (physician, nurse, and administrator) that will review your hospital. Information about the points emphasized by the team can be helpful. Of course, the team is permitted to evaluate compliance with any and all standards. Practically, however, it is impossible to cover every standard in detail in every care setting. Some surveyors are especially irritated if meetings are late. Some may prefer that the schedule be arranged in a certain way. Others may have personal preferences for their environment (room temperature, amount of walking, etc) or pet peeves that can be avoided. The epidemiologist should read the evaluation and recommendations from the last JCAHO visit. Surveyors will not hesitate to concentrate on areas that caused problems in the past.

DEMONSTRATING COMPLIANCE WITH SPECIFIC STANDARDS

Details of how to establish a quality improvement program are beyond the scope of this chapter. There should be evidence that the leadership is willing to spend time and money on quality improvement, as well as to provide direction and support for the program. Infection control should be part of the hospital performance improvement plan. Committee minutes should reflect discussion, conclusions, actions, and results of actions. There should be evidence that projects have improved the quality of care and patient outcome. Under no circumstances should minutes be altered after the committee has approved them. Falsification of data is considered grounds to deny accreditation. Interim reports to JCAHO should be based on credible data that can be produced when requested.

It is required that an individual who is qualified by virtue of education, training, certification, licensure, or experience manage the infection control program. For hospital epidemiologists, training in IDs and active membership in SHEA would fulfill this requirement. For infection control practitioners, certification by the Certification Board of Infection Control is an example of appropriate qualification. Some other qualifications also would fulfill the requirement.

Other specific standards can be found in the manual.[1] These include the existence of an effective surveillance program, effective reporting mechanisms, evidence of successful interventions, management systems for staff (including staff education and employee health), evidence of support for the infection control program, and attention to transmission of diseases from staff to patients. The JCAHO will expect that infection control efforts extend throughout the organization. The answer to the question "who is responsible for infection control?" is "everyone."[3]

The JCAHO "ORYX" system was designed to integrate data into the accreditation process, focusing on the outcome of care. As part of a pilot phase, selected hospitals have transmitted data to JCAHO where the results are compiled and compared to national standards. Examples of existing core measures that may be chosen include myocardial infarction, community-acquired pneumonia, pregnancy, and heart failure. SSIs, intensive care, pediatric asthma, and pain management will soon be added. The ORYX system will soon be standardized and required of all hospitals. JCAHO is currently using data generated from the ORYX system in its review process.

COMMON PITFALLS IN INFECTION CONTROL

Infection control is based on surveillance and action. The JCAHO will review surveillance data and will expect to see interventions that have reduced nosocomial infections. Interventions should address both control of outbreaks and prevention of infections. Merely having an infection control committee and surveillance data will not suffice. It is important to document success in improving care.

A common problem is for the infection control team to passively respond to questions put by the JCAHO surveyor. Surveyors don't know ahead of time what types of projects a specific hospital has initiated. Don't allow the surveyor to overlook your best projects. Bring your best projects to the attention of the surveyor. Modesty has no place during a survey. Tell the surveyor that your hospital is especially proud of these projects, and tell him or her why.

The infection control team should be prepared to answer questions about why the problem was selected, who was involved in designing the intervention, and the current status of the problem. Infection control issues that are high volume (affect a large number of patients or occur frequently), high risk, or problem prone (complicated invasive procedures or vulnerable populations) are considered to have high priority by the JCAHO.

Another pitfall is that an otherwise excellent infection control team may not produce excellent documentation. If a successful intervention cannot be found in any minutes or publications or written presentations, it is invisible to surveyors.

It is important to realize that the JCAHO will require the hospital to follow its own policies. Many hospitals have been cited for failing to follow their own policies, yet many continue to make policies that are impractical to implement. The infection control committee should have significant input into all policies regarding nosocomial infections.

Surveyors may find a nurse, physician, or house staff member and ask him or her how to clean up a blood spill or dispose of infectious waste. Surveyors might ask HCWs when they last were tested for tuberculosis. They might ask a physician what he or she would do if the needle disposal box were too full to use. Surveyors may also talk with patients to ensure that educational goals have been met.

Policies are required to address tuberculosis exposure, bloodborne pathogens, isolation guidelines, employee health, medical waste disposal, and surveillance/reporting activities for patients and staff. Policies should be made with the input of multiple disciplines and should be updated annually.

Common problems that JCAHO finds with infection control programs include using nonstandard definitions of nosocomial infections, failing to trend data to identify outbreaks or the outcome of interventions, insufficient time is allotted to infection control activities, or lack of a written description of the infection control program.[3] The last point is often overlooked: it is important to write down the description of the infection control program and to update it annually. The program description should demonstrate a coordinated approach across the organization.

Some key questions come up frequently.[3] These include asking how hospital staff are involved in infection control. The answer should highlight the fact that staff involvement begins at the time of hire with in-services and vaccination. Staff should be involved at all levels of the program, including identifying infections, providing input on control of infections, and participating in interventions.

MOCK SITE VISITS

In between triennial surveys, many hospitals have found it useful to stage mock site visits. A multidisciplinary team usually is chosen to review each clinical area and to score compliance with JCAHO standards. Some hospitals hire outside agencies (including JCAHO-based mock surveyors) to perform the mock site visit. The purpose of the review is to identify problem areas and to give HCWs an opportunity to improve their presentation skills. Continuous Survey Readiness (CSR) is a program whereby hospitals in a region subscribe and receive a dedicated JCAHO expert, consultation, updates, and conferences.

OTHER SETTINGS

The JCAHO surveys a variety of healthcare institutions including hospitals, independent clinics, LTCFs, assisted living facilities, clinical laboratories, and student health programs. Special standards may exist for these facilities. Please contact the JCAHO (www.jcaho.org) for information.

TIPS FOR SURVIVING THE SURVEY

All surveyors bring with them their own experiences and personalities. Surveyors often spend a lot of time away from home and frequently endure stressful, even hostile, situations. Courtesy and hospitality will create a good working environment. Most surveyors appreciate time at the end of the day to summarize their work and begin written reports. Schedules are usually tight, so meetings and tours should begin on time. Staff should be prompt. Committee minutes and policies should be organized and accessed easily. Presentations should be concise and given by knowledgeable individuals. Whenever possible, data should be shown in graphic form.

THE SURVEY SCHEDULE

Healthcare organizations are surveyed about every 3 years. The usual survey team consists of a physician, a nurse, and an administrator, who review all areas of the hospital. The JCAHO also conducts unannounced, 1-day surveys on a small number of randomly chosen hospitals. Random surveys evaluate infection control activities as well as other standards. The JCAHO will also conduct an unannounced survey when it becomes aware of potentially serious patient care or safety issues. The JCAHO usual-

ly give the organizations 24 to 48 hours advance notice of an unscheduled survey. Recently, the JCAHO has begun requiring a Periodic Performance Review (see below). This requires organizations to evaluate compliance with all standards through an electronic extranet tool provided 15 months after their on-site survey.

SURVEY OUTCOME

Every standard will be scored, and the score translated to a grid. Significant deficiencies will result in Type I or Type II recommendations. Depending on the type of deficiency, the organization will be given a time frame in which to remediate the problem and prove subsequent compliance through a written report or during a second visit.

Accreditation decisions are made public. The decisions are (1) Accreditation with full standards compliance; (2) accreditation with requirements for improvement; (3) conditional accreditation (marginal performance); (4) preliminary denial of accreditation; or (5) denial of accreditation. Of the hospitals surveyed in 2001, 12% received accreditation with full standards compliance, 87% received accreditation with requirements for improvement, and 1% received conditional accreditation.

PUBLICITY

Results of JCAHO surveys are available to the public. Detailed descriptions of compliance with standards are available on the Internet or by request. Results are compared to national averages. At the current time, the JCAHO does not publicize nosocomial infection rates.

THE FUTURE

As discussed, the JCAHO has adopted a program it calls "Shared Visions—New Pathways." This process will require submission of a mid-cycle self-evaluation, the "Periodic Performance Review," and a plan for remediation of any deficiencies. Data on ORYX core measures and other information will be transmitted to JCAHO electronically and used to direct on-site visits. The goal is to focus on critical areas of patient care and reduce paperwork through consolidation of standards. Detailed scores would no longer be available to the public, but alternate performance data may be released. Surveyors will be required to pass an examination to demonstrate competence before being allowed to go on site visits. Beginning in January 2006, JCAHO plans to conduct all regular accreditation surveys on an unannounced basis.

For 2003, JCAHO announced an additional National Patient Safety Goal: "Reduce the risk of health care acquired infections." This has 2 specific components: (1) "Comply with current CDC hand hygiene guidelines," and (2) "Manage as sentinel events all identified cases of unanticipated death or major permanent loss of function associated with a health care-acquired infection." For the hand hygiene compliance, all Category I recommendations will be required to be implemented; see Chapter 19 for details on hand hygiene and the CDC recommendations. Chapter 26 has additional information on sentinel events and root cause analysis.

SUMMARY

The JCAHO has recognized the importance of infection control. Its regulations have meant that hospitals could not eliminate infection control programs for budget reasons. More recently, the JCAHO has emphasized the importance of broad support for infection control throughout the institution. With some foresight and planning, hospital epidemiologists should be able to achieve full accreditation for their infection control programs. Continued emphasis on good infection control practices, including hand hygiene, will be especially important once the JCAHO begins to routinely conduct unannounced surveys.

REFERENCES

1. Joint Commission on Accreditation of Healthcare Organizations. *Comprehensive accreditation manual for hospitals. The official handbook*. Chicago, Ill: JCAHO; 2002.
2. Scheckler WE, Brimhall D, Buck AS, et al. Requirements for infrastructure and essential activities of infection control and epidemiology in hospitals: a consensus panel report. Society for Healthcare Epidemiology of America. *Am J Infect Control*. 1998;26:47-60.
3. *Infection Control: Meeting Joint Commission Standards*. Chicago, Ill: Joint Commission on Accreditation of Healthcare Organizations; 1998.

CHAPTER THIRTY

PRODUCT EVALUATION

Lynn Slonim Fine, PhD, MPH, CIC and William M. Valenti, MD

INTRODUCTION

The current healthcare environment is dominated by managed care and capitated reimbursement, which have reduced the financial resources available to HCFs substantially. More than ever, clinicians and administrators must spend healthcare dollars wisely, without sacrificing the quality of care or safety. In addition, nosocomial infections increase the cost of healthcare substantially, and the cost of these infections is not reimbursed under capitated programs. Thus, hospitals now have tremendous incentive to lower nosocomial infection rates. In theory, one way to reduce the incidence of nosocomial infections is to use devices that have a lower risk of infection than other products. Over the past few years, manufacturers have released a staggering number of products purported to decrease infections. These products usually cost more than the standard products. Administrators and staff in HCFs must evaluate such devices and other products that may affect infection rates to determine whether they are efficacious and thus worth the added cost. For example, in compliance with CDC Guidelines for Hand Hygiene, hospitals are purchasing wall-mounted dispensers of alcohol hand gel. While this is initially a large expenditure, the presence of the hand gel should increase compliance with hand hygiene practices and decrease the rate of nosocomial infections, ultimately saving money.

TRANSMISSION OF NOSOCOMIAL PATHOGENS

The infection control literature provides evidence that most pathogens acquired in HCFs are transmitted by people and medical devices. The inanimate environment (eg, walls, floors, countertops, food, and water) plays a minor role in transmission of pathogens. The inanimate environment should be cleaned and maintained routinely as part of the HCF's overall maintenance plan as much as to control infection. Infection control activities designed to decrease infections should focus more on the role of people, invasive procedures, and medical devices such as catheters, endoscopes, and surgical equipment. Thus, when evaluating a product, HCWs should consider the various modes by which pathogens are transmitted (eg, common vehicle, droplets, airborne) to determine whether the device might facilitate or decrease transmission of important nosocomial pathogens.

The infection control literature documents numerous outbreaks and pseudo-outbreaks attributed to problems with disinfection and sterilization of equipment and invasive devices. Table 30-1 describes several outbreaks that demonstrate ways in which medical devices can become contaminated. Some outbreaks have occurred because the equipment was designed poorly or because the instructions for cleaning and disinfection were inadequate.

HCWs who evaluate the performance of invasive medical devices and equipment for purchasing should consider the following:

➤ Look for design flaws that could make the device hard to clean and disinfect.

➤ Determine whether the instructions for cleaning and disinfection meet current standards.

➤ Determine whether the HCF can clean and disinfect the device adequately (ie, the facility has the equipment needed to reprocess the device; the staff have been, or will be, trained to reprocess the device; and the staff have adequate time to reprocess the device properly).

➤ Review the literature to see whether similar devices have caused outbreaks at other institutions and

TABLE 30-1. EXAMPLES OF OUTBREAKS CAUSED BY CONTAMINATED EQUIPMENT

Author	Problem	Equipment	Error	Resolution
Srinivasan et al[1]	Recovery of *P. aeruginosa* from BAL specimens	Olympus bronchoscope	Contaminated via loose biopsy-port cap	Manufacturer recall of instruments
Kressel et al[2]	Pseudo-outbreak of *Mycobacterium chelonei* and *Methylobacterium mesophilicum*	Endoscope/ bronchoscope	Contaminated automated washers	Hospital purchased new instruments and paracetic acid sterilization system
Lemaitre et al[3]	Patients colonized or infected with *Sphingomonas paucimobilis*	Reusable nickel-plated temperature probes in ventilator circuits	The manufacturer's recommendation to wipe the probe with alcohol before reuse was inadequate	The probes were replaced with a more expensive probe that could be cleaned manually and gas sterilized
Bennett et al[4]	Pseudo-outbreak of *Mycobacterium xenopi*	Bronchoscopes, endoscopes, brushes	Contaminated tap water	Installation of submicron filter on water supply
Agerton et al[5]	Transmission of multidrug-resistant *Mycobacterium tuberculosis*	Bronchoscope	Inadequate cleaning and disinfection of bronchoscope	Strict adherence to cleaning/disinfection policies
Rudnick et al[6]	Gram-negative bacteremia in open heart surgery patients	Pressure-monitoring equipment	Pressure monitoring equipment that was left uncovered overnight in the operating room became contaminated when housekeepers sprayed disinfectant on the floor	Pressure-monitoring equipment was assembled just before procedures, and housekeepers stopped spraying disinfectant solutions while cleaning
Livernese et al[7]	Colonization/ infection with VRE	Electric thermometers	Contaminated rectal thermometer probes	Isolation of colonized/infected patients and removal of electronic thermometers
Brooks et al[8]	*Clostridium difficile*-associated diarrhea	Electric thermometers	Contaminated rectal thermometer handles	Replaced electronic thermometers with disposable thermometers
Flaherty et al[9]	Gram-negative bacteremia in hemodialysis patients	Hemoflow F-80 dialyzers	Contaminated O-rings	Changed procedure to require that O-rings be removed and immersed in disinfectant

TABLE 30-2. CATEGORIES FOR VALUE ANALYSIS

Category 1

This product is strongly recommended for all hospitals and strongly supported by well-designed experimental or epidemiological studies.

Category 2

This product is strongly recommended for all hospitals and viewed as effective by experts in the field, based on a strong rationale and suggestive evidence, even though definitive studies have not been done.

Category 3

This product is suggested for implementation in many hospitals and is supported by suggestive clinical or epidemiologic studies, a strong theoretical rationale, or definitive studies. This product is applicable to some, but not all, hospitals.

Category 4

The role of this product has not been defined because the evidence is insufficient or consensus has not been reached.

Category 5

This product is unnecessary: recommendations that HCFs use this product conflict with current data and the opinions of most experts in infection control.

Adapted from Garner J, the Hospital Infection Control Practices Advisory Committee. Guideline for isolation precautions in hospitals, part II: recommendations for isolation precautions in hospitals. *Infect Control Hosp Epidemiol.* 1996;17:60-80.

what factors (eg, design flaw, improper use, improper disinfection) caused the outbreaks.

Other equipment-related outbreaks have occurred because staff did not know how to clean and disinfect the equipment, took short cuts to save time or money, or did not maintain the device properly. In this era of cost containment, the staff may be tempted to save time and money by changing disinfection and sterilization protocols and procedures. These outbreaks emphasize that the basic, time-honored principles of infection control, such as proper reprocessing of reusable patient-care devices, regular maintenance of equipment, and effective staff education, are as important (or perhaps more important) as purchasing expensive, high-tech devices touted to lower infection rates.

A STANDARDIZED METHOD FOR ANALYZING PRODUCTS

The CDC has published guidelines for isolation precautions in hospitals.[10] This document provides a framework that the product assessment team (described below) can apply when evaluating products and equipment (Table 30-2). The isolation guidelines rank procedures according to whether scientific data support their use. Each new prod-

uct or device does not need to be assessed with this rigor. However, the similar hierarchical ranking may help the team evaluate whether specific products and equipment could benefit the institution in general and the overall infection control effort in particular. This approach allows the HCF to determine whether published data apply to their situation, and it allows personnel to use their common sense and experience when definitive scientific data are not available (categories 2 and 3). In addition to ranking products on the basis of published data, members of the product assessment team must assess a product's priority for implementation in that institution.

Healthcare providers may have difficulty evaluating whether products and equipment will be cost effective in their facilities. The task is especially difficult if the manufacturers do not provide peer-reviewed publications to support their claims, but only provide advertisements, promotional materials, or anecdotal information (eg, testimonials). We recommend that the HCF form a multidisciplinary team that will do the following:

➤ Define priorities based on the facility's rates of infections, rates of sharps injuries, or other pertinent data.

➤ Develop criteria regarding product design and performance.

➤ Assess published data regarding the product or similar products.

➤ Gather information regarding the experiences of similar facilities.

➤ Review Health Device Alerts distributed by the U.S. Food and Drug Administration and ECRI (formerly the Emergency Care Research Institute), an independent nonprofit health services research agency.

➤ Plan a trial period for the product in the appropriate clinical settings to determine whether the product functions well.

➤ Assess the results of the trial period.

➤ Analyze the cost benefit or cost effectiveness in their institution.

The multidisciplinary team should include members from the purchasing and stores departments, central sterile supply, the infection control program, and at least one representative of the staff who will use the product. In some situations, representatives from the facility's administration and from the finance department should also participate. Infection control personnel can help the team by assessing the product's effect on important parameters such as the rates of infections and sharps injuries. The person who represents the primary users should assess whether the product is likely to meet their needs and to be accepted.

After the multidisciplinary team has identified products or equipment that meet the predefined criteria, the members should decide whether these items must be tested before the institution purchases them. Chiarello states that HCWs are likely to reject new devices, despite infection control or safety advantages, if the staff members do not like to use them.[11] The team should assess the results of the trial period, including cost, staff satisfaction, adverse reactions, rates of infection, rates of injuries, the frequency of malfunction, the ease of cleaning and disinfection, and other appropriate information, before deciding whether or not to recommend the product.

In this era of managed care, the cost and the cost effectiveness of a product have become increasingly important. The assessment of the cost effectiveness is easy if the same product is cheaper when obtained from a different supplier or if an equivalent product, which is made by another company, is cheaper. In these situations, the multidisciplinary team could discuss the substitution, inform the primary users of the minor change, and work with the purchasing and stores departments to ensure a seamless transition.

The multidisciplinary team may need to analyze more thoroughly some products or equipment, particularly those that are more expensive than the products currently used in the facility. Cost-effectiveness analysis (CEA) is a method that many HCFs have used for this purpose.[12] CEA allows the team to determine a ratio of the incremental costs for devices to the expected change in outcomes. This method forces the members to consider the cost of the product, the change in outcome that the product should produce, and the scientific principles of disease transmission before the team determines whether a product should be purchased. Furthermore, CEA can help the multidisciplinary team convince the administration that a more expensive product should be purchased because the expected outcome would be improved significantly or because the complication rate would be decreased significantly and, thus, the overall cost to the institution would be decreased.

Laufer and Chiarello used CEA to evaluate 3 devices designed to prevent needlesticks.[12] They used the following formula to estimate the cost of preventing a needlestick injury with each of the devices:

$$\frac{\text{Incremental costs of devices}}{\text{(Injuries without devices)} - \text{(Injuries with devices)}}$$

The cost to prevent a needlestick injury varied substantially with the device evaluated. The authors estimated the cost of preventing one needlestick injury to be $984 if protective injection equipment was used, $1,574 if an intravenous system with recessed needles was used, or $1,877 if a needleless intravenous system was used. To date, no one has determined whether such devices, which cost more money than most systems currently in use, will be cost effective if used long term.

EXAMPLES

In the following paragraphs, several products that are purported to reduce the risk of infection in HCFs will be addressed. Each intervention will have a category adapted from the CDC's isolation guidelines assigned to it. In addition, Table 30-3 gives examples of products that the manufacturers claim will reduce infection rates and the classification that we assigned to the devices. However, a caveat is necessary. The literature in this field changes rapidly. Therefore, infection control personnel who must purchase products should not rely on this assessment, but also should review current literature prior to making their decision.

PROTECTING HEALTHCARE WORKERS FROM BLOODBORNE PATHOGENS

Hepatitis B vaccine reduces the risk of hepatitis B infection in HCWs exposed to blood and body fluids. Therefore, hepatitis B vaccine is a Category 1 intervention (see Table 30-2). In the era of HIV infections, equipment

TABLE 30-3. ASSESSMENT OF DEVICES PURPORTED TO DECREASE THE RISK OF INFECTION

Device	Supporting Evidence	Category[10]
Needleless device	Strongly recommended and supported by literature	1
Antibiotic-coated (minocycline and rifampin) intravenous catheters	Strongly recommended and supported by literature	1
Silver-coated intravenous catheters	Strongly recommended and supported by literature	1
Antibiotic-coated urinary catheters	Not available	3,4
Copper-based paint or other anti-bacterial paint	Not available	5

that reduces the risk of needlesticks is worth the extra expense because these injuries are a primary mode by which this virus is transmitted to HCWs. The OSHA's new Compliance Directive for the 1991 Bloodborne Pathogens Standard, issued in November 1999, calls for the use of safety needles and needleless IV devices (see Chapter 28 on OSHA). The NIOSH also published an alert, "Preventing Needlestick Injuries in Health Care Settings," in November 1999. This alert recommended that employers eliminate the use of needles when safe and effective alternatives are available, implement the use of devices with safety features, and evaluate use to determine which are most effective and acceptable.

Once these guidelines were published, hospitals referred to their Value Analysis committee for guidance in selecting needleless products to introduce into their institutions. Characteristics of safety or needleless devices should include the following: the safety feature is an integral part of the device and the device should work passively (ie, it requires no activation by the user). If user activation is necessary, the safety feature should be engaged with a single-handed technique, allowing workers' hands to remain behind the exposed sharp. In addition, it must be easy to determine whether the safety feature has been activated, and the safety feature should remain protective through disposal. The device must obviously be easy to use, safe, and effective in patient care. Many companies market devices designed to prevent needlesticks. The manufacturers claim that their products reduce the risk of sharps injuries and, therefore, reduce the risk of infection with HIV and other bloodborne pathogens. Devices that prevent needlestick injuries are essential for all HCFs in which needles are used.

Studies indicate that needlestick prevention systems, such as needleless intravenous access systems, decrease needlestick accidents.[13,14] Interestingly, studies examining safety needle use have also found that HCWs may not use these devices or may use them incorrectly, thereby increasing the risk of injury.[15] These devices have been shown to decrease needlestick injuries when used properly, and their use would be a Category 1 intervention (see Table 30-2). It is critical that HCWs are properly educated on how to use the devices to facilitate their implementation. Input from HCWs before deciding on a product is also essential to expedite the introduction of a new technology.

All HCFs must strive to maximize the HCW's safety by minimizing the risk of exposure to infectious material. The multidisciplinary team should know the epidemiology of needlestick injuries in their hospital, so that the team can develop a program that will be efficacious. Thus, the team must know what group of workers is experiencing needlesticks; how, where, and when needlestick injuries occur; and what devices and procedures are associated most frequently with these accidents. They should evaluate any available data on several different devices that might lower the rate of the most common injuries or the rates of injuries having the highest risk of transmitting bloodborne pathogens in their hospital. The team should know the incidence of infection with bloodborne pathogens in their patient population and should identify the areas in the facility that treat these patients most frequently. The team should use these data to determine which needlestick-prevention devices to introduce into their hospital.

PROTECTING PATIENTS, HEALTHCARE WORKERS, AND VISITORS FROM PATHOGENS IN THE ENVIRONMENT

Manufacturers often claim that their products will reduce the risk of infection from organisms found in the environment. Occasionally, some of these claims find their way into credible publications, only to confuse individuals who are assessing the value of these products for their hospitals. A report on the bactericidal effects of copper-based paints illustrates this point.[16] The author showed that copper-based paints kill bacteria and then concluded that "such paints could be used to render surfaces self-disinfecting in strategic locations where environmental causation of nosocomial infections is suspected."[16] This conclusion conflicts with current infection control thought on the role of the environment in infection transmission. In an accompanying editorial, Rutala and Weber wisely point out that walls always harbor bacteria, but they never have been linked by scientific data to nosocomial infection.[17] At best, self-disinfecting paint would be a Category 4 intervention. We think that self-disinfecting paint is more likely to be a Category 5 intervention: use of this product is unnecessary and is in conflict with current infection control thought.

Companies that produce disinfectants may try to capitalize on HCWs' fears of HIV infection by claiming that their products kill HIV on contact. However, most agents that are used to clean floors, countertops, and other surfaces readily kill HIV. In addition, HIV is inactivated rapidly by several products that are inexpensive and readily available, including 10% chlorine bleach, 50% ethanol, 35% isopropyl alcohol, hydrogen peroxide, and soap and water.[18] Thus, an expensive new product is not needed to clean areas contaminated by blood because existing products are cheaper and do the job adequately. Thus, a new product designed specifically for this purpose would be in Category 5. Rather than buying an expensive new product, personnel from the infection control program and from the housekeeping department should educate HCWs how to manage blood spills and should develop policies and procedures that clearly specify when and how to clean the environment and how to manage blood spills and other emergencies.

PREVENTING TRANSMISSION OF *MYCOBACTERIUM TUBERCULOSIS*

In some instances, the multidisciplinary team must consider the big picture when evaluating the infection-associated risks and benefits of particular products. For example, when developing their tuberculosis control program, HCFs must consider the nature of the individual facility, the frequency with which tuberculosis patients are seen in the facility, and tuberculin (PPD) conversion rates of employees. Institutions also must comply with the guidelines from regulatory or advisory agencies, such as OSHA and the CDC (see Chapter 22).

Data in the literature indicate that UV lights kill *M. tuberculosis*. However, most experts do not think that

UV light alone is adequate, and the CDC's guidelines state that UV lights cannot substitute for proper air handling units, but could be used as an adjunctive measure.[19] Thus, UV light would be a Category 4 strategy, because a consensus has not been reached.

CONCLUSION

In many cases, the purchaser cannot choose a product solely on the manufacturer's claims or on the cost. We recommend that HCFs develop a multidisciplinary team to evaluate products carefully. The team would review the literature, benchmark experience from other hospitals, and review the manufacturer's materials to determine whether the product could perform as required, has an equal or lower risk of infection compared with the current product, and would be cost effective. Products that meet these criteria should be tested by the staff who will use them to ensure that the products will be accepted and used properly after they are introduced into general use.

Infection control personnel may find the process of evaluating products to be quite complex and time consuming. However, we feel that this task will assume greater importance as managed care increases its presence in healthcare delivery and as new, emerging infectious diseases are identified (eg, sudden acute respiratory syndrome) or anticipated (eg, smallpox). Infection control personnel must ensure that the risk of infections does not increase as HCFs drastically reduce the cost of care. Many infection control programs already are being asked whether their hospitals can cut costs by substituting one product for another or one procedure for another. Other, less fortunate infection control programs have discovered that changes had been made only when an investigation of increased infection rates identified the substitution of a cheaper product. Infection control personnel who help their institutions to assess products carefully will enable these HCFs to survive the current financial crisis without sacrificing the quality of care or employee safety.

REFERENCES

1. Srinivasan A, Wolfenden L, Song X, et al. An outbreak of *Pseudomonas aeruginosa* infections associated with flexible bronchoscopes. *N Engl J Med*. 2003;348:221-227.

2. Kressel AB, Kidd F. Pseudo-outbreak of *Mycobacterium chelonei* and *Methylobacterium mesophilicum* caused by contamination of an automated endoscopy washer. *Infect Control Hosp Epidemiol*. 2001;22:414-418.

3. Lemaitre D, Elaichouni A, Hundhausen M, et al. Tracheal colonization with *Sphingomonas paucimobilis* in mechanically ventilated neonates due to contaminated ventilator temperature probes. *J Hosp Infect*. 1996;32:199-206.

4. Bennett SN, Peterson DE, Johnson DR, et al. Bronchoscopy-associated *Mycobacterium xenopi* pseudoinfections. *Am J Respir Crit Care Med.* 1994;150: 245-250.

5. Agerton T, Valway S, Gore B, et al. Transmission of a highly drug-resistant strain (strain W1) of *Mycobacterium tuberculosis*: community outbreak and nosocomial transmission via a contaminated bronchoscope. *JAMA.* 1997;278:1073-1077.

6. Rudnick JR, Beck-Sague CM, Anderson R, et al. Gram-negative bacteremia in open-heart-surgery patients traced to probable tap-water contamination of pressure-monitoring equipment. *Infect Control Hosp Epidemiol.* 1996; 17:281-285.

7. Livernese LL, Dias S, Samel C, et al. Hospital-acquired infection with vancomycin-resistant *Enterococcus faecium* transmitted by electronic thermometers. *Ann Intern Med.* 1992;117:112-116.

8. Brooks SE, Veal RO, Kramer M, Dore E, Schupf N, Adachi. Reduction in the incidence of *Clostridium-difficile*-associated diarrhea in an acute care hospital and a skilled nursing facility following replacement of electronic thermometers with single-use disposables. *Infect Control Hosp Epidemiol.* 1992;13:98-103.

9. Flaherty J, Garcia-Houchins S, Chudy R, Arnow P. An outbreak of gram negative bacteremia traced to contaminated O-rings in reprocessed dialyzers. *Ann Intern Med.* 1993;119:1072-1078.

10. Garner J, the Hospital Infection Control Practices Advisory Committee. Guideline for isolation precautions in hospitals, part II: recommendations for isolation precautions in hospitals. *Infect Control Hosp Epidemiol.* 1996;17:60-80.

11. Chiarello LA. Selection of needle stick prevention devices: a conceptual framework for approaching product evaluation. *Am J Infect Control.* 1995;23:386-395.

12. Laufer FN, Chiarello LA. Application of cost-effectiveness methodology to the consideration of needle stick prevention technology. *Am J Infect Control.* 1994;22:75-82.

13. Lawrence LW, Delclos GL, Felknor SA, et al. The effectiveness of a needleless intravenous connection system: an assessment by injury rate and user satisfaction. *Infect Control Hosp Epidemiol.* 1997;18:175-182.

14. Yassi A, McGill ML, Khokhar JB. Efficacy and cost-effectiveness of a needleless intravenous access system. *Am J Infect Control.* 1995;23:57-64.

15. L'Ecuyer PB, Schwab EO, Iademarco E, Barr N, Aton EA, Fraser VJ. Randomized prospective study of the impact of three needleless intravenous systems on needlestick injury rates. *Infect Control Hosp Epidemiol.* 1996;17:803-808.

16. Cooney TE. Bactericidal activity of copper and noncopper paints. *Infect Control Hosp Epidemiol.* 1995;16:444-446.

17. Rutala WA, Weber DJ. Environmental interventions to control nosocomial infections. *Infect Control Hosp Epidemiol.* 1995;16:442-443.

18. Centers for Disease Control and Prevention. Recommendations for preventing transmission of HTLV III/LAV in the workplace. *MMWR.* 1985;34:682-686.

19. Valenti WM. Tuberculosis in the HIV era: everything old is new again. *Am J Infect Control.* 1992;20:35-36.

SUGGESTED READING

Centers for Disease Control and Prevention. Evaluation of safety devices for preventing percutaneous injuries among health-care workers during phlebotomy procedures-Minneapolis-St. Paul, New York City, and San Francisco, 1993-1995. *MMMR.* 1997;46(2):21-29.

Occupational Safety and Health Administration (OSHA) Subject Page for Needle Sticks (http://www.osha-slc.gov/needlesticks/index.html).

National Institute for Occupational Safety and Health (NIOSH) Alert: Preventing Needlestick Injuries in Health Care Settings (http://www.cdc.gov/niosh/2000-108.html).

US Food and Drug Administration Center for Devices and Radiological Health (http://www.fda.gov/cdrh/index.html).

ECRI (formerly the Emergency Care Research Institute) (http://www.ecri.org/).

Centers for Disease Control and Prevention Emerging Infectious Diseases (http://www.cdc.gov/ncidod/eid/index.htm).

CHAPTER THIRTY-ONE

INFECTION CONTROL ISSUES IN CONSTRUCTION AND RENOVATION

Sherry A. David, RN, BS, CIC; Jose A. Fernandez, RA; and Loreen A. Herwaldt, MD

INTRODUCTION

Hospital construction and renovation projects pose many challenges to infection control personnel, in part because these projects can increase the risk of nosocomial infections. In addition, resources important to good infection control practices may be disrupted or may not be available during the projects. Finally, infection control personnel must assess whether the plans comply with infection control guidelines and regulations established by their city, county, and state, by regulatory and accrediting agencies, and by the federal government. To successfully meet these challenges, infection control personnel must collaborate with engineers, nurse managers, administrators, architects, and physicians before, during, and after the construction projects.

During, maintenance, renovation, and construction, bacterial or fungal microorganisms in the dust and dirt can contaminate air handling or water systems, which can transmit these organisms to susceptible persons. Seemingly benign activities or changes in the healthcare environment can increase the risk of infection for susceptible patients. For example, to install a phone line, telecommunication staff may remove dust-covered ceiling tiles. When maintenance workers replace carpet, they may expose fine debris filtered through the carpet over many years. Activities such as cutting into walls may disturb mold growing in areas where the plumbing or the windows leaked. When plumbers cap off of a water line to convert an exam room into an office, they create a dead end, which could encourage growth of *Legionella* spp in the water system. Moreover, the air handling or water systems may be shut down for periods to allow modifications or additions. During the time these systems are nonfunctional, routine infection control measures, such as handwashing, may be difficult to maintain. Reinstituting these sys-

tems also may increase the risk of infections such as Legionnaires' disease. Furthermore, routine clinical practice and traffic patterns may need to be substantially modified during construction projects to ensure that basic infection control precautions are maintained.

Current patient populations in hospitals, clinics, and care centers are sicker than those in the past. The numbers of elderly patients, immunocompromised patients, and patients with significant underlying illnesses have increased and these patients are at increased risk of acquiring infections associated with maintenance, renovation, and construction. Thus, infection control staff, especially infection control practitioner (ICP), have a tremendous opportunity and responsibility to protect patients, visitors, and staff members during such projects. This chapter will identify the potential risks involved in maintenance, renovation, and construction activities and provide practical solutions to decrease these risks. Although not specifically discussed in this chapter, excavation and demolition projects near patient-care areas create similar infection control issues. Infection control personnel who must deal with these projects should read the article by Streifel et al.[1]

ROLE OF THE INFECTION CONTROL TEAM

The primary goal of the infection control team during maintenance, renovation, or construction in HCFs is to protect susceptible patients, visitors, and healthcare workers (HCW) from acquiring infections. The APIC published a State-of-the Art Report: *The Role of Infection Control During Construction in Healthcare Facilities*, 1999,[2] which is an excellent resource. This report suggests that the role of the infection control team is to provide infection control expertise throughout a project (ie, from the design phase until the area is ready to use). Thus, infection control personnel should participate in construction projects from the inception so that they can identify potential infection control problems created by the project and can design solutions prospectively. In addition, infection control personnel should understand the purpose of the project, so they can assess whether or not the design will facilitate good infection control practice.

The infection control team must collaborate with the architects, engineers, and maintenance staff to develop comprehensive maintenance, renovation, and construction policies that define the procedures necessary to maintain a safe environment. An Infection Control Risk Assessment (ICRA) is an essential part of these policies.[2,3] The ICRA helps the infection control personnel and other members of a multidisciplinary planning team determine the infectious risks associated with each project. By forcing the team to identify the patient population at risk and the magnitude of the project, the ICRA helps the team identify important preventive strategies such as what type of barriers are necessary, whether workers need to wear protective attire and use special entrances and exits, and whether particle counts are necessary.

A caveat is necessary. During construction projects, infection control personnel will be asked to judge the value of many designs or products. Often, infection control personnel will be asked to determine how much space is necessary for a certain function, which products (eg, vinyl versus carpet) should be used, and what air handling requirements must be met, and any of a number of other questions. The persons asking the questions may genuinely want to know the answers, or they may have hidden agendas that they hope the hospital epidemiology program will endorse. In addition, the epidemiology staff members may find themselves mediating between opposing sides, including department directors who want vast amounts of space and the latest innovations, and administrators who want to limit the costs. To avoid costly mistakes and political landmines, infection control personnel must ask many questions to determine what the real issues are; how the product, equipment, room, or clinic will be used; what possible solutions are available; what the budgetary limitations are; and what infection control principles or external regulations apply. In addition, infection control personnel may need to review the medical literature, governmental codes, guidelines from architectural and engineering societies and accrediting agencies, and product descriptions, to determine which of the products or designs is within the project's budget and also balances the infection control requirements with patient and employee safety and satisfaction.

As healthcare budgets shrink, the expertise of infection control personnel will become more important during construction and renovation projects. Simultaneously, infection control personnel will feel increasing pressure to choose the cheapest products or design. Despite the pressures, infection control personnel must remember their primary goals and recommend the products or design that will achieve these goals most effectively. The appropriate products or designs may be more expensive initially; but, in the long run, they probably will be less costly, as they may prevent outbreaks, or they may last longer and require less maintenance.

Infection control personnel often are the only clinical personnel who work on all construction and renovation projects. Thus, they may have to be the watchdogs for the entire project to make sure that the design and the construction meets the appropriate standards.

Many of the above comments are based on common sense. However, our experience and the medical literature testify that common sense answers often are not chosen during construction projects.[4-34] Table 31-1 lists design and construction errors that we have encountered in our practice of infection control.

RISKS ASSOCIATED WITH MAINTENANCE, RENOVATION, AND CONSTRUCTION IN HEALTHCARE FACILITIES

Persons at Risk of Acquiring Infections Related to Maintenance, Renovation, and Construction

In a healthcare setting, special precautions are needed to protect susceptible or immunocompromised patients from acquiring infections related to maintenance, renovation, or construction. The persons who are most susceptible to these infections have immunologic disorders (eg, infection with human immunodeficiency virus, or congenital immune deficiency syndromes) or are on immunosuppressive therapy (eg, radiation, chemotherapy, steroids, anti-organ rejection drugs, anti-TNF antibodies). Severely neutropenic patients (absolute neutrophil count of ≤500 cells/mL) such as those who have undergone allogeneic or autologous hematopoietic stem cell transplants (HSCT) or patients with leukemia who are receiving intensive chemotherapy are at highest risk of these infections.[35] However, patients with underlying diseases such as chronic obstructive pulmonary disease, cancer, cardiac failure, or diabetes are also at increased risk compared with healthy persons.[1]

TABLE 31-1. DESIGN AND CONSTRUCTION ERROR

➤ Air intakes placed too close to exhausts or other mistakes in the placement of air intakes
➤ Incorrect number of air exchanges
➤ Air-handling system functions only during the week or on particular days of the week
➤ Air vents not reopened after the construction is finished
➤ No negative-air-pressure rooms built in a large, new inpatient building
➤ Carpet placed where vinyl should be used
➤ Wet-vacuum system in the operating suite pulls water up 1 floor into a holding tank rather than down 1 floor
➤ Aerators on faucets
➤ Sinks located in inaccessible places
➤ Patient rooms or treatment rooms do not have sinks in which healthcare workers can wash their hands
➤ Room or elevator doors too narrow to allow beds and equipment to be moved in and out of rooms or elevators

Organisms Causing Infections Related to Maintenance, Renovation, and Construction

The two most common microorganisms causing healthcare-associated outbreaks during construction-type activities are *Legionella* spp[5-8] and *Aspergillus* spp.[6-32]

Legionella

Legionella spp are ubiquitous aquatic microorganisms that can be isolated in 20% to 40% of fresh water environments and from soil and dust. There are 42 species of *Legionella* and 54 serogroups. *Legionella pneumophila*, serogroup 1, causes 90% of the 10,000 to 20,000 cases of Legionnaires' disease (Legionellosis) annually.[3] Cooling towers, potable water systems, and heating and air-conditioning systems can be contaminated with *Legionella* spp. These organisms can be transmitted via aerosols, which are inhaled, or by potable water, which is injested. During construction, *Legionella* can be introduced directly into the water when pipes are disrupted and become contaminated with soil. If a water system is already contaminated, organisms in the biofilm can be released into the water by changes in water pressure (eg, when a plumbing system is repressurized). *Legionella* can multiply rapidly in stagnant water. Therefore, pipes that have not been used for a considerable period of time should be flushed for more than 5 minutes before the water is used.[37]

In general, *Legionella* outbreaks have been related to contaminated water. However, one outbreak was associated with the installation of a lawn sprinkler system. Investigators postulated that *L. pneumophila* was aerosolized during excavation and inhaled by susceptible people who acquire Legionnaires' disease.

Aspergillus

Fungi are ubiquitous in both indoor and outdoor environments. There are approximately 900 fungal species[38] but *A. fumigatus* and *A. flavus* are the species that cause invasive disease most frequently. *Aspergillus* spp. can be found anywhere in a hospital; however, during construction activities, dust, dirt, and debris that harbor these organisms can be released into the air in quantities that can be harmful to susceptible patients. In general, healthy persons are not susceptible to infections caused by *Aspergillus* but immunocompromised patients may become severely ill and may die from these infections.

Additional Construction Related Health Risks

There are other problems with fungi and mold that can occur during maintenance and renovation of HCFs. Fungi may be growing behind walls, above false ceilings, or in any area that may have had water leaks or high humidity. Mold grows quickly and can contaminate water-soaked building materials within 48 hours. Species such as *Penicillium*,[39] *Fusarium*, *Trichoderma*, *Memnomiella*, and *Stachybotrys chartarum* can produce potent mycotoxins that are harmful to persons who inhale them or touch them with bare skin. Mold-related illness can range from mild allergic rhinitis symptoms—with symptoms such as runny nose, sneezing, and itchy eyes—to hypersensitivity pneumonitis, an allergic reaction to mold that becomes worse with repeated exposures and can cause permanent lung damage. Toxins produced by molds can cause a severe illness called organic dust toxic syndrome, which can start after exposure to a single heavy dose of allergen. The signs and symptoms are abrupt onset of fever, flu-like symptoms, and respiratory difficulty within hours of exposure.

If employees discover discoloration or a musty odor in an area that is undergoing maintenance or is being renovated, the area needs to be assessed and mold remediation must be done before the project is finished. The workers should tape a tight barrier of plastic around the affected area and report it immediately to the project manager. Only persons trained in mold remediation should clean the area. If the area is small, trained maintenance or housekeeping staff who are wearing goggles without venting holes, N95 respirators, and gloves can clean the area with a mild detergent. Large areas of mold may need to be addressed by a professional mold remediation contractor who uses protective attire and engineering controls such as barriers and HEPA-filtered negative airflow machines. Infection control policies should define when these special precautions are needed.[40]

OVERVIEW OF GUIDELINES, STANDARDS, AND REGULATIONS GOVERNING MAINTENANCE, RENOVATION, AND CONSTRUCTION IN HEALTHCARE FACILITIES

A number of agencies have produced important resources for infection control personnel who are helping with maintenance, renovation, and construction projects. The most important of documents are provided by the following organizations:

➤ American Institute of Architects (AIA), www.aia.org
➤ APIC, www.apic.org
➤ American Society for Healthcare Engineers of the American Hospital Association (ASHE), www.ashe.org
➤ American Society of Heating, Refrigeration, and Air-Conditioning Engineers (ASHRAE), www.ashrae.org
➤ CDC, www.cdc.gov
➤ JCAHO, www.jcaho.org
➤ OSHA, www.osha.gov

American Institute of Architects Guidelines for Design and Construction of Healthcare Facilities

The American Institute of Architects with assistance from the US Department of Health and Human Services developed a book entitled *Guidelines for Design and Construction of Healthcare Facilities*, 2nd edition, 2001.

Some states have adopted these guidelines as their codes, while others have specific codes and use the AIA Guidelines in conjunction with them. Infection control teams should obtain a copy of the AIA Guidelines and their state's regulations and make sure that their facility complies with both.[3]

The AIA Guidelines indicate that HCFs must incorporate infection control considerations into every project. For example, the Guidelines recommend appropriate locations and requirements for: clean and soiled workrooms, storage facilities for clean linen, handwashing stations, housekeeping rooms, patient toilet rooms, airborne infection isolation (AII) rooms, and protective environment rooms (Table 31-2). The AIA *Guidelines* mandate in Chapter 5 that a multidisciplinary team complete an ICRA for each project.

Guideline for Environmental Infection Control in Health-Care Facilities, 2003

The CDC and the HICPAC recently published the *Guideline for Environmental Infection Control in Health-Care Facilities*, 2003,[41] an extensive document that describes "environmental infection control strategies and engineering controls" to help prevent transmission of infectious agents.

Construction issues are interspersed throughout the document, but most of the recommendations regarding construction are in *Recommendation—Air, Section II, Construction, Renovation, Remediation, Repair, and Demolition* (Table 31-3).

Joint Commission on Accreditation for Healthcare Organizations

The Joint Commission evaluates and accredits nearly 17,000 healthcare organizations and programs in the United States. The JCAHO cites the AIA Guidelines in their Management of the Environment of Care (EC) Standard[42] and recommends that healthcare organizations follow the guidelines when planning to renovate existing space or construct new facilities. Surveyors will assess whether HCFs comply with the Environment of Care Standards, the AIA guidelines, and the CDC's recommendations for protecting patients, visitors, and HCWs during maintenance, renovation, and construction projects (see Table 31-2).

INFECTION CONTROL RISK ASSESSMENT

Team Development

Whether the project involves remodeling an existing area or building a new one, the staff members must do an

TABLE 31-2. GUIDELINES, RECOMMENDATIONS, AND STANDARDS

Source	Key Points	Summary/Information
AIA Guidelines: Chapter 7 General Hospital	1. Infection control risk assessment (ICRA)	1. Mandated in Chapter 5
	2. Toilet rooms	2. Patient access without entering a hallway (7.2.A5) Staff toilets (7.2.B6)
	3. Handwashing stations	3. Required in all patient bathrooms & in all patient bedrooms (7.2.A4) Convenient access at nurse stations (7.2.B1), medication station, nourishment station (7.2.B4)
	4. Emergency Service	4. At least 1 airborne infection isolation (AII) room (7.9.C7)
	5. Finishes	5. Floor materials shall be cleanable; OR and C-section floors will be monolithic and joint free (7.28.B4 & 7.28.B5); walls shall be washable (7.28.B6); ceilings in semi-restricted area shall be smooth, able to be scrubbed with chemicals, nonabsorptive, and without revices (7.28.B8); no carpets in protective isolation rooms and monolithic floors (7.28.B9)
	6. Sputum induction; glutaraldehyde use	6. Same as AII rooms (7.31.D23); negative air flow with 15 air changes per hour unless recirculating hood designed for glutaraldehyde is used (7.31.D25)
	7. Ventilation requirements	7. Table 7.2 lists all the special requirements needed for room ventilation
	8. Clean and soiled workrooms	8. Separate from each other (7.2.B11. & 7.2.B12.)
	9. Clean linen	9. Designated area or closed cart; can be in clean workroom (7.2.B14.)
	10. Housekeeping rooms	10. One per each nursing unit/floor (7.2.B22.)
	11. Airborne infection isolation room(s)	11. Determined for each facility based on the ICRA and the patient population (7.2.C - 7.2.C7.)
	12. Protective Environment Rooms	12. Must have handwashing station in the room; walls, floors, and ceilings must be sealed to prevent leakage; permanent device to monitor air flow (7.2.D-7.2.D7.)
CDC Guidelines for Environmental Infection Control in Health-Care Facilities: Recommendations- Air Section II	1. ICRA	1. Convene a multidisciplinary team including infection control to coordinate the project
	2. Education	2. Educate the construction team about dispersal of fungal spores
	3. Mandatory adherence agreements	3. Written into the contract
	4. Infection control surveillance	4. Review microbiologic data and other means of surveillance for fungal infections
	5. Control measures	5. Define the scope of activity; determine barrier/infection control practice needs; relocate patient/staff; conduct measures to prevent contamination through HVAC systems; create negative air pressure in work zone and monitor barriers
	6. Monitor the construction environment	6. Infection control professional should make rounds
	7. Conduct an epidemiologic investigation in cases of health-care acquired *Aspergillus* infections or other fungal disease	7. Use airborne particle sampling to evaluate barrier integrity; conduct an environmental assessment as indicated; perform corrective measures to eliminate fungal contamination
CDC Guidelines: Recommendations- Water Section VII Cooling Towers & Evaporative Condensers	1. Planning construction of new healthcare facilities	1. Locate cooling towers so that drift is directed away from air-intake system; design to minimize the volume of aerosol drift
CDC Guidelines: Recommendations- Environmental Services	1. Construction activities	1. Develop strategies for pest control

TABLE 31-2. GUIDELINES, RECOMMENDATIONS, AND STANDARDS (CONTINUED)

Source	Key Points	Summary/Information
JCAHO 2004 Standard: EC.7.10 *The hospital plans for managing utilities*	➤ Promote a safe, controlled environment of care ➤ Reduce the potential for hospital-acquired illness ➤ Assess and minimize risks of utility failure ➤ Ensure operational reliability of utility systems	➤ Develop a process for designing, installing and maintaining appropriate utility systems—eg, domestic water, cooling towers, and ventilation systems including pressure relationships, air exchange rates, air filtration efficiencies ➤ Control of elements used in healthcare: biological agents, gases, fumes, dust
JCAHO 2004 Standard: EC.8.30 *The organization manages the design and building of the environment when it is renovated, altered, or newly created*	➤ This Standard refers to the AIA Guidelines, state and county regulations and codes or standards that provide equivalent design criteria; ICRA ➤ Identify hazards that could compromise patient care	➤ Follow AIA Guidelines for Design and Construction of Hospital and Healthcare Facilities and local rules and regulations ➤ Development of an ICRA to address the effect of construction activities on air quality, infection prevention and control, utility requirements, noise, vibration and emergency procedures

ICRA before the project begins. A multidisciplinary team that includes persons with expertise in infection control, risk management, facility design, construction, ventilation, and safety (Figure 31-1) should do the ICRA to ensure that the project meets all the standards and codes.[3] Infection control personnel should help complete the ICRA and should participate in projects from their inception so that they can identify infection control issues early and they can make suggestions prospectively, not after the design is complete.

Notification of Team Members

Infection control personnel should be notified of all major and/or high-risk projects so that they can determine which precautions are needed. However, infection control personnel must be available to consult on any project.[2] Maintenance personnel can do minor maintenance and renovation projects that have low risk for patients without direct input from the infection control team if infection control personnel previously developed clear policies and procedures describing how to manage the infection control risks created by these projects and if they educated the maintenance personnel who will do these activities.

Each facility needs a mechanism whereby infection control personnel are notified that the planning phase of a project will begin soon. In small hospitals, the person responsible for renovation and construction could simply call the ICP and invite him or her to the first meeting or could notify the ICP and other persons who should be on the team at a meeting of another committee such as the

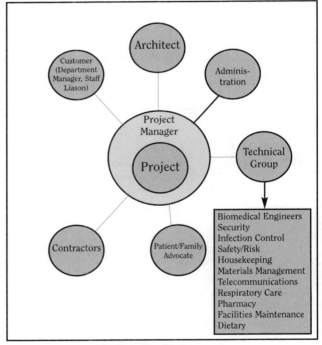

Figure 31-1. Infection control risk assessment.

Environment of Care, Risk or Safety. Large hospitals, which have many projects underway at the same time, should develop a more formal process for notifying infection control personnel and other ICRA team members to ensure that they can participate. To facilitate planning, some HCFs have regularly scheduled meetings at which new projects are discussed and updates are provided on current projects.

Infection Control Risk Assessment Matrix for Construction and Renovation

The multidisciplinary team must address the following key points when they are doing the ICRAs[2,9]:

➤ The team must assess the type of patients (ie, risk factors) treated in the affected area and the services that are provided there. In particular, the team should ask whether the area/facility cares for patients who are highly susceptible to fungal or *Legionella* infections.

➤ The team should assess whether essential services, such as power, medical gas, water, sewer, and fire protection, might be disrupted and should develop a contingency plan to provide these services if 1 or more are affected by the project.

➤ The team should evaluate areas that are above, below, and adjacent to the affected area and determine whether any phase of the project will affect these areas adversely. The team must develop a plan to minimize problems and infection risks on the other units.

➤ The team must determine whether the patients on the affected or nearby units need to be relocated during the project to protect them from possible infectious risks or to provide an environment conducive to healing (eg, to limit noise).

➤ The team must decide what types of barriers are necessary to decrease the risk of infection and should assign responsibility for inspecting the barriers and the cleanliness of both the work area and the area immediately adjacent. The barriers and detailed descriptions of other infection control measures should be included in the project specifications so that the costs of these measures can be included in the cost of the project.

➤ The team must discuss how the ventilation system will be affected by the project and must determine what measures should be taken to protect the ventilation system and to maintain good quality air in the surrounding areas. For example, the team should determine whether the supply and return ducts need to be sealed. They should also ensure that the ventilation system around the affected area is balanced and that appropriate pressure relationships are maintained. On the basis of the types of patients in adjacent areas, the team should decide whether to obtain particle counts before and during the project.

These questions are formalized in the ICRA Matrix (see Table 31-3). The matrix is a tool that can help infection control personnel and other members of the multidisci-

plinary team systematically identify the infection precautions needed for the project. The first task in the matrix is to identify the "type of construction project activity." There are 4 types (A to D) that range from noninvasive procedures or simple inspection to major demolition and construction projects. Next the team must identify the areas affected by the project and thereby determine how susceptible the patients in these areas are to construction-related infections (ie, determine the patients' level of risk). Subsequently, (step 3), the team uses the information about the project type and the patients' risk group to determine the class of precautions necessary for the project. The matrix specifies the precautions necessary for each classification. The matrix then requires the team to answer 11 questions about the project that will help them identify prospectively most important infection control issues.

Infection control personnel need to understand that the matrix is only a guide. The team must assess each project individually and must flexibly apply the principles in the matrix. Not all projects fit exactly into the parameters listed in the matrix. Thus, infection control personnel and the team must use their best judgment when their project falls between classifications.

Infection control personnel should educate unit staff, architects, engineers, maintenance personnel, and construction workers about infection risks associated with construction and about appropriate methods for minimizing these risks. Education is a continual process, because different hospital staff members will be involved in each project and because many people involved with maintenance, renovation, and construction are contract workers. Infection control personnel could develop a brochure, which discusses basic infection control issues in construction projects, and a checklist, which itemizes infection control essentials, to answer particular questions and prevent problems that occur frequently (eg, number and location of sinks, type of ceiling tiles, type of floor, and wall coverings).

HCFs should include the infection control requirements in the written contract, so the contractors know what they are expected to do. If the construction team consistently ignores infection control policies, the hospital should levy a fine or the contractors should not be allowed to do other projects in the hospital.

Infection Control Risk Assessment Construction Permit

The ICP or another ICRA team member should fill out the Infection Control Construction Permit during the design phase of the project. The Permit identifies the project's location, start and end date, project manager, the type of construction activity, the patient risk group, the Class selected for the particular project, and the necessary

TABLE 31-3. INFECTION CONTROL RISK ASSESSMENT: MATRIX OF PRECAUTIONS FOR CONSTRUCTION AND RENOVATION

Step One: Using the following table, identify the Type of Construction Project Activity (Type A-D)

TYPE A	*Inspection and noninvasive activities.*
	Includes, but is not limited to:
	➤ Removing ceiling tiles for visual inspection limited to 1 tile per 50 square feet
	➤ Painting (but not sanding)
	➤ Working on wallcoverings, electrical trim work, minor plumbing, and activities that do not generate dust or require cutting into walls or access to ceilings other than for visual inspection
TYPE B	*Small scale, short duration activities that create minimal dust*
	Includes, but is not limited to:
	➤ Installing telephone and computer cabling
	➤ Accessing chase spaces
	➤ Cutting into walls or ceilings where dust migration can be controlled
TYPE C	*Work that generates a moderate to high level of dust or requires demolition or removal of any fixed building components or assemblies*
	Includes, but is not limited to:
	➤ Sanding walls for painting or wall covering
	➤ Removing floorcoverings, ceiling tiles and casework
	➤ Constructing new walls
	➤ Working on ducts or electrical wiring above ceilings (minor)
	➤ Moving or placing cables (major)
	➤ Any activity that cannot be completed within a single workshift
TYPE D	*Major demolition and construction projects*
	Includes, but is not limited to:
	➤ Activities that require consecutive work shifts
	➤ Activities that require heavy demolition or removal of a complete cabling system
	➤ New construction

Step Two: Using the following table, identify the Patient Risk Groups that will be affected. If more than 1 risk group will be affected, select the higher risk group:

Low Risk	Medium Risk	High Risk	Highest Risk
➤ Office areas	➤ Cardiology	➤ Cardiac Care Unit	➤ Any area caring for immunocompromised patients
	➤ Echocardiography	➤ Emergency Room	➤ Burn Unit
	➤ Endoscopy	➤ Labor & Delivery	➤ Cardiac Cath Lab
	➤ Nuclear Medicine	➤ Laboratories (specimen)	➤ Central Sterile Supply
	➤ Physical Therapy	➤ Newborn Nursery	➤ Intensive Care Units
	➤ Radiology/MRI	➤ Outpatient Surgery	➤ Medical Unit
	➤ Respiratory Therapy	➤ Pediatrics	➤ Negative pressure isolation rooms
	➤ Other patient care areas not identified in *High Risk* or *Highest Risk* categories	➤ Pharmacy	➤ Oncology
		➤ Post Anesthesia Care Unit	➤ Operating rooms including C-section rooms
		➤ Surgical Units	

TABLE 31-3. INFECTION CONTROL RISK ASSESSMENT: MATRIX OF PRECAUTIONS FOR CONSTRUCTION AND RENOVATION (CONTINUED)

Step Three: Match the Patient Risk Group (Low, Medium, High, Highest) with the planned Construction Project Type (A, B, C, D) on the following matrix, to find the Class of Precautions (I, II, III or IV) or level of infection control activities required.

Class I-IV Precautions are delineated on the following page.

IC MATRIX - CLASS OF PRECAUTIONS: CONSTRUCTION PROJECT BY PATIENT RISK

| Patient Risk Group | Construction Project Type | | | |
	TYPE A	TYPE B	TYPE C	TYPE D
LOW Risk Group	I	II	II	III/IV
MEDIUM Risk Group	I	II	III	IV
HIGH Risk Group	I	II	III/IV	IV
HIGHEST Risk Group	II	III/IV	III/IV	IV

Note: Infection Control approval will be required when the Construction Activity and Risk Level indicate that Class III or Class IV control procedures are necessary.

DESCRIPTION OF REQUIRED INFECTION CONTROL PRECAUTIONS BY CLASS

	During Construction Project	Upon Completion of Project
CLASS I	1. Use methods that minimize dust. 2. Immediately replace a ceiling tile displaced for visual inspection.	1. Clean work area when task is completed.
CLASS II	1. Prevent dust from dispersing into air. 2. Use mist (water) on work surfaces to control dust while cutting. 3. Seal unused doors with duct tape. 4. Block off and seal air vents. 5. Place dust mat at entrance and exit of work area 6. Remove or isolate HVAC system in work areas. 7. Contain construction waste in tightly covered containers before transport.	1. Wipe work surfaces with disinfectant. 2. Wet mop and/or vacuum area with HEPA filtered vacuum before leaving. 3. Re-integrate HVAC system.
CLASS III	1. Isolate HVAC system in area where work is being done to prevent contamination. 2. Complete all critical barriers ie, sheetrock, plywood, plastic, to seal work area from nonwork area or use control cube method before construction begins. 3. Maintain negative air pressure within work site; use HEPA-equipped air filtration units. 4. Contain construction waste in tightly covered containers before transport. Cover transport receptacles or carts.	1. Do not remove barriers from work area until completed project is inspected by the owner's Safety Department and Infection Control Department and thoroughly cleaned by the owner's Environmental Services Department. 2. Remove barrier materials carefully to minimize spreading dirt and debris created by construction. 3. Vacuum work area with HEPA-filtered vacuums. 4. Wet mop area with disinfectant. Do not sweep. 5. Reintegrate HVAC system.

TABLE 31-3. INFECTION CONTROL RISK ASSESSMENT: MATRIX OF PRECAUTIONS FOR CONSTRUCTION AND RENOVATION (CONTINUED)

CLASS IV

1. Isolate HVAC system in area where work is being done to prevent contamination of duct system.

2. Complete all critical barriers ie, sheetrock, plywood, plastic, to seal area from non-work area or implement control cube method before construction begins.
3. Maintain negative air pressure within work site; use HEPA-equipped air filtration units.
4. Seal holes, pipes, conduits, and punctures.

5. Construct anteroom. All personnel must use anteroom so they can be vacuumed using a HEPA vacuum cleaner before leaving work site or they can wear cloth or paper coveralls that are removed each time they leave the work site.
6. All personnel entering work site are required to wear shoe covers and change them each time they exit the work area.
7. Contain construction waste before transport in tightly covered containers. Cover transport receptacles or carts.

1. Do not remove barriers from work area until completed project is inspected by the owner's Safety Department and Infection Control Department and thoroughly cleaned by the owner's Environmental Services Department.
2. Remove barrier material carefully to minimize spreading dirt and debris created by construction.

3. Vacuum work area with HEPA-filtered vacuums.

4. Wet mop area with disinfectant. Do not sweep.

5. Re-integrate HVAC system.

Step 4. Identify the areas surrounding the project area, assessing potential impact

Unit Below	Unit Above	Lateral	Lateral	Behind	Front
Risk Group	Risk Group	Risk Group	Risk Group	Risk Group	Risk Group

Step 5. Identify specific site of activity eg, patient rooms, medication room, etc.

_____

Step 6. Identify issues related to: ventilation, plumbing, electrical systems (ie, Are outages likely to occur during the project?).

_____

TABLE 31-3. INFECTION CONTROL RISK ASSESSMENT: MATRIX OF PRECAUTIONS FOR CONSTRUCTION AND RENOVATION (CONTINUED)

Step 7. Identify necessary containment measures based on the classification of the project. What types of barriers (eg, solids wall barriers) are needed? Is HEPA filtration required?

_____

(Note: Renovation/construction area shall be isolated from the occupied areas during construction and shall be at negative pressure with respect to surrounding areas).

Step 8. Consider potential risk of water damage. Is there a risk due to compromising structural integrity (eg, wall, ceiling, roof) ?

_____

Step 9. Work hours: Can or will the work be done during nonpatient care hours?

_____

Step 10. Do plans allow for adequate number of isolation/negative airflow rooms?

_____

Step 11. Do the plans allow for the required number & type of handwashing sinks?

_____

Step 12. Does the infection control staff agree with the minimum number of sinks for this project? (Verify against AIA Guidelines for types and area).

_____

Step 13. Does the infection control staff agree with the plans relative to clean and soiled utility rooms?

_____

Step 14. Plan to discuss the following containment issues with the project team: traffic flow, housekeeping, debris removal (how and when), etc.

_____

Appendix: Identify and communicate the responsibility for project monitoring that includes infection control concerns and risks. The ICRA may be modified throughout the project. Revisions must be communicated to the Project Manager.

Steps 1-3: Adapted with permission V Kennedy, B Barnard, St Luke Episcopal Hospital, Houston TX; C Fine, CA
Steps 4-14: Adapted with permission Fairview University Medical Center, Minneapolis MN
Forms modified and provided courtesy of Judene Bartley, ECSI Inc. Beverly Hills MI 2002

TABLE 31-4. INFECTION CONTROL CONSTRUCTION PERMIT

Location of Construction:
Project Coordinator:
Contractor Performing Work:
Supervisor:

Permit No:
Project Start Date:
Estimated Duration:
Permit Expiration Date:
Telephone:

Yes	No	Construction Activity	Yes	No	Infection Control Risk Group
		TYPE A: Inspection, noninvasive activity			GROUP 1: Low Risk
		TYPE B: Small scale, short duration, moderate to high levels			GROUP 2: Medium Risk
		TYPE C: Activity generates moderate to high levels of dust, requires greater 1 work shift for completion			GROUP 3: Medium/High Risk
		TYPE D: Extended duration and major construction activities requiring consecutive work shifts			GROUP 4: Highest Risk

	During Construction	Upon Completion of Construction
CLASS I	1. Use methods that minimize dust. 2. Immediately replace any ceiling tile displaced for visual inspection.	1. Clean work area when task is completed.
CLASS II	1. Prevent dust from dispersing into air. 2. Use mist (water) on work surfaces to control dust while cutting. 3. Seal unused doors with duct tape. 4. Block off and seal air vents. 5. Place dust mat at entrance and exit of work area. 6. Remove or isolate HVAC system in work areas. 7. Contain construction waste in tightly covered containers before transport.	1. Wipe work surfaces with disinfectant. 2. Wet mop and/or vacuum with HEPA-filtered vacuum before leaving work area. 3. Re-integrate HVAC system.
CLASS III Date Initial	1. Isolate HVAC system in area where work is being done to prevent contamination of the duct system. 2. Complete all critical barriers or implement control cube method before construction begins. 3. Maintain negative air pressure within work site; use HEPA-equipped air filtration units. 4. Contain construction waste in tightly covered containers before transport. Cover transport receptacles or carts.	1. Don't remove barriers until project is inspected and thoroughly cleaned. 2. Remove barrier materials carefully to minimize spreading dirt and debris created by construction. 3. Vacuum work area with HEPA-filtered vacuums. 4. Wet mop with disinfectant. Do not sweep. 5. Reintegrate HVAC system.

TABLE 31-4. INFECTION CONTROL CONSTRUCTION PERMIT (CONTINUED)

CLASS IV Date Initial	During Construction	Upon Completion of Construction
	1. Isolate HVAC system in area where work is being done to prevent contamination of duct system. 2. Complete all critical barriers or implement control cube method before construction begins. 3. Maintain negative air pressure within work site; use HEPA-equipped air filtration units. 4. Seal holes, pipes, conduits, and punctures appropriately. 5. Construct anteroom. All personnel must go through anteroom and be vacuumed with a HEPA vacuum cleaner before leaving work site or they can wear cloth or paper coveralls that are removed each time they leave the work site. 6. All personnel entering work site are required to wear shoe covers and change them each time they exit the work site. 7. Contain construction waste before transport in tightly covered containers. Cover transport receptacles or carts.	1. Do not remove barriers from work area until completed project is inspected and thoroughly cleaned. 2. Remove barrier materials carefully to minimize spreading dirt and debris created by construction. 3. Vacuum work area with HEPA-filtered vacuums. 4. Wet mop with disinfectant. 5. Re-integrate HVAC system.

Additional Requirements:

_____

Date_____Initials_____

Date_____Initials_____

Exceptions/Additions to this permit are noted by attached memoranda

Permit Request By:_____   Permit Authorized By:_____

Date:_____   Date:_____

Adapted with permission V Kennedy, B Barnard, St Luke Episcopal Hospital, Houston Tex. Forms modified and provided courtesy of Judene Bartley, ECSI Inc Beverly Hills MI 2002

---

precautions. Either the infection control team or the Project Manager should keep this permit on file and the contractor should post a copy at the job site (Table 31-4).

Construction Site Monitoring Tool

Someone (often an ICP) should inspect the worksite to make sure that the construction workers are following the guidelines. The Construction Site Monitoring Tool (Table 31-5) is useful for documenting the construction worker's compliance with the infection control policies and for identifying the contractors whose workers are most compliant with infection control practice. This information can be used when choosing contractors to do new projects.

Each facility should determine how often the site should be inspected and who will do the inspections. The hospital's size, the type of project, and the nature of sur-

---

TABLE 31-5. CONSTRUCTION SITE SURVEY TOOL

Date:_____   Time:_____   Time:_____

Barriers

Construction signs posted for the area	Yes	No	Yes	No
Doors properly closed and sealed	Yes	No	Yes	No
Floor area clean, no dust tracked	Yes	No	Yes	No

Air Handling

All windows closed behind barrier	Yes	No	Yes	No
Negative air at barrier entrance	Yes	No	Yes	No
Negative air machine running	Yes	No	Yes	No

Project Area

Debris removed in covered container daily	Yes	No	Yes	No
Designated route used for debris removal	Yes	No	Yes	No
Trash in appropriate container	Yes	No	Yes	No
Routine cleaning done on job site	Yes	No	Yes	No

Traffic Control

Restricted to construction workers and necessary staff only	Yes	No	Yes	No
All doors and exits free of debris	Yes	No	Yes	No

Dress Code

Appropriate for the area (OR, CSS, OB, BMTU)	Yes	No	Yes	No
Required to enter	Yes	No	Yes	No
Required to leave	Yes	No	Yes	No

OR = operating room; CSS = central sterile supply; OB = obstetrics; BMTU = bone marrow transplant unit

Comments:

Surveyor: _____

rounding patient care areas will affect this decision. In a small hospital, daily monitoring may be feasible. In a larger hospital, weekly monitoring may be more feasible. However, if the project is done in a highly sensitive area like a bone marrow transplant unit or an operating suite, daily inspections may be necessary. If infection control staff members teach the staff on the surrounding units what to look for, they can monitor the site almost continuously and save the infection control team considerable effort. If the unit staff members note breaches in infection control practice, they can contact the infection control personnel, who can address the issue.

Unit/Area Opening Worksheet

A checklist like the Unit/Area Opening Worksheet (Table 31-6) can help infection control personnel determine whether the unit is ready to open. For example, the tool directs the user to determine whether the unit has been cleaned thoroughly, the water system has been flushed, the ventilation system has been cleaned and balanced, and whether any deficits need to be corrected before the unit can open.

MAJOR INFECTION CONTROL ISSUES TO CONSIDER WHILE PLANNING MAINTENANCE, CONSTRUCTION, AND RENOVATION PROJECTS

Air Handling Systems

Generally, air-handling systems do not transmit nosocomial pathogens. However, at times, these systems can transmit pathogens such as *M. tuberculosis*, *Aspergillus* spp, *L. pneumophila*, and VZV. Air-handling systems can increase the risk of infection in other ways. For example, if the humidity level is high and the number of air exchanges is inadequate, walls, ceilings, and vents may drip water onto sterile supplies or clean surfaces. Thus, infection control personnel should make sure that the air-handling systems planned for new or renovated buildings will meet basic infection control requirements.

During the planning phase, infection control and engineering personnel should ensure that the air-handling systems will be adequate to provide the ventilation required for that area.[3] Patient rooms should have 6 air changes per hour (ACH), of which 2 ACH must be outside air. Operating rooms (ORs) and C-section delivery rooms require 15 ACH with 3 ACH of outside air. The relative humidity in ORs should be between 30% to 60% and the airflow should move from the OR to adjacent areas. AII

rooms require 12 ACH with 2 ACH of outside air and negative airflow with respect to adjacent areas. Air from these rooms should be exhausted to the outside away from air intakes or be recirculated after passing through HEPA filters. In addition, rooms in which high-risk procedures (such as bronchoscopy and aerosolized pentamidine treatments) are performed should have negative pressure or should have a flexible ventilation system that allows the pressure to be changed from neutral to negative. Bronchoscopy suites are required to have 12 ACH with outside air comprising 2 ACH. If a room that has special ventilation is renovated, the engineers should measure the ACH and the pressure relationships before and after the renovation to ensure that the renovation did not disrupt the air handling system within the room.[43]

When reviewing designs for a project, infection control personnel should ensure that exterior air intakes are placed at least 8 m from upwind (ie, the prevailing winds) of the exhaust outlets. The bottom of an intake should be at least 2 m above the ground or 1 m above the roof level. Intakes should be located away from cooling towers, trash compactors, loading docks, heliports, exhaust from biological safety hoods,[44] ethylene oxide sterilizers, aerators, and incinerators. Infection control and engineering personnel should evaluate the design and operation of ventilation systems carefully to ensure that potentially contaminated air is discharged safely to prevent airborne disease transmission.[45] Infection control personnel may need to tour the air intake and exhaust sites to make sure that they are placed properly.

Isolation Rooms

Given the resurgence of tuberculosis and the emergence of multiply-resistant bacterial pathogens and new viral pathogens, infection control personnel must ensure that the number, type, and placement of isolation rooms is adequate. The advent of new syndromes such as SARS suggests that HCFs may need more AII rooms than they did previously. In the past, some facilities have transferred patients with tuberculosis rather than create AII rooms. However, it may not be possible (or safe) to transport patients with SARS or smallpox from 1 facility to another and each facility may need AII rooms to accommodate such patients.

Infection control personnel should assess the patient population served by the facility to determine how many single rooms and how many AII rooms are necessary. Typically, a hospital should have one isolation bed for every 30 acute-care beds.[3] Pediatric areas require more single rooms, which can be used for isolation, per total beds than other areas of the hospital,[44] because respiratory or enteric infections that require isolation are more frequent in children than in adults.[46] The number of patients needing isolation on pediatric units will vary with patient age and the season.[46] In general, isolation rooms for non-

TABLE 31-6. INFECTION CONTROL UNIT/AREA OPENING WORKSHEET

Area Surveyed_____   Date_____

Surveyors are to check yes, no, or N/A for each criteria. A satisfactory review is required prior to reopening any unit/department.

Criteria	Yes	No	N/A	Comments
I. Contractor Final Cleanup				
a. Horizontal surfaces free of residual construction dust				
b. Installed equipment and cabinets properly cleaned				
c. Barriers cleaned and removed				
II. HVAC System				
a. HVAC system cleaned if not isolated				
b. New filters in place and operational				
c. HVAC system balanced as specified				
III. Plumbing System				
a. No visible leaks				
b. Plumbing system flushed within 24 hours prior to occupancy				
c. Sinks functional				
IV. Equipment				
a. Soap/towel dispensers/hand sanitizers installed and filled				
b. Refrigerators - checklist for temperature control				
c. Ice machine cleaned and flushed				
V. Final Cleaning				
a. Housekeeping final cleaning completed				
VI. Environmental Rounds				
a. Completion of Environmental Rounds				

Surveyors - Additional Comments:

Date_____
         Satisfactory Review
         Unsatisfactory Review

Unit Administrator_____
Infection Control_____
Facilities Management_____
Housekeeping_____

Developed by Jean Pottinger and Lori Goergen.

respiratory diseases do not require special features. If the isolation room has an anteroom, both the room and the anteroom should have handwashing sinks. Built-in nurse-server cabinets or isolation carts can be used to store necessary supplies such as gowns, masks, and gloves.

Patients who have infectious diseases, which are spread by respiratory droplets or droplet nuclei, often are seen first in emergency rooms and outpatient clinics. Thus, appropriate isolation rooms will be beneficial in these areas. In fact, the AIA Guideline states that emergency departments need at least 1 AII isolation room.

The requirements for air exchanges in AII rooms are discussed above in the section on air handling systems. Notably, some hospitals use flexible ventilation systems that allow some patient-care rooms to be either neutral or negative pressure. For such rooms care must be taken to ensure the airflow is appropriate for the patient in the room. Each AII room must have a handwashing station and storage area for clean and soiled material located directly outside or immediately inside the entry door. Each room must have a separate toilet room with a tub or shower and a handwashing station. The door must have a self-closing device and penetrations in walls, ceilings, and floors must be tightly sealed so that room is maintained at negative pressure to the surrounding environment.[45,47] A permanent monitor must assess the pressure status of the room continuously and a staff member must check the monitor daily. Anterooms are not required for AII except when imunosuppressed patients need AII. Infection control personnel must evaluate proposed AII isolation rooms during the design phase, because retrofitting regular patient rooms to meet the requirements of AII isolation rooms can be very costly.

Protective Environments

Protective environments include ORs and bone marrow transplant rooms. These areas must remain as free of airborne infectious agents as possible. The airflow within these areas must flow from a clean-to-less-clean.[43]

Handwashing Facilities

Each patient-care room, examination room, procedure room, and toilet room needs at least 1 handwashing sink that should be located as close to the room's exit as possible. Sinks should be large enough to prevent splashing. All sinks must have an associated soap dispenser (built-in stainless steel soap dispensers should not be used) and a paper-towel holder that are located at a level that is comfortable for the user. A trash receptacle should be placed near the sink, so paper towels can be discarded properly. Alcohol-based hand rubs should be located away from electrical outlets and switches[48] in places where HCWs are likely to use them.

A variety of mechanisms exist to control waterflow. Conventional hand controls are the least expensive, but may not be appropriate for all areas. Foot, knee, or electric eye controls allow staff members to wash their hands or scrub without touching the sink (no-touch method). Such sinks would be appropriate in operating suites, isolation rooms, and critical-care units. The electric-eye devices break frequently, and they are more expensive than the foot or knee controls. Infection control personnel should help unit staff and architects select the best equipment for the location and purpose.

Water Supply and Plumbing

Occasionally, the hospital's water supply will be disrupted intentionally or accidentally during construction projects. Hospitals should have emergency plans that are activated if the water supply to the hospital is disrupted or contaminated. Infection control personnel should help develop this plan, because water is crucial to many infection control practices and because contaminated water can spread pathogenic organisms.

During the summer of 1993, the University of Iowa Hospitals and Clinics, Iowa City, was faced with the possibility of losing its water supply because the Iowa River was flooding. Our contingency plan included water conservation measures such as shutting down drinking fountains and ice machines, replacing showers and full-tub or bed baths with partial baths, using alcohol-based hand cleaners rather than soap and water, and serving meals on disposable dishes. Our alternative water system was a well, which was tested for coliform organisms, nitrates, and iron. Our plant operations department was prepared to adjust the plumbing system in order to use the well water. The well water could be used if the water supply was shut down during hospital or road-construction projects. Hospitals that do not have wells must design alternative plans. If the water supply will be disrupted only for a short time, staff can fill large plastic containers with water to be used while the water system is turned off. If the water supply will be off for a longer period of time, the hospital may need to have a company deliver bottled water. During emergencies, agencies such as the National Guard may be able to provide water. If the water supply will be turned off for more than 4 hours, the contractor should do this work during times of nonpeak water use, such as evenings, nights, or weekends.

Space for Personal Protective Equipment

All patient care areas should store personal protective equipment, such as gloves, in areas where they are readily accessible. Sharps container must be accessible to workers who use, maintain, or dispose of sharps devices. The number of containers must be adequate, the size must be large enough for the sharps that will be disposed in that area, and HCWs must be able to safely access the opening when they need to discard sharps. Sharps containers should be 52 to 56 inches above the floor for use by HCWs who are standing or 38 to 42 inches above the floor for use by HCWs who are sitting.[49]

Waste

Infection control personnel should help clinical staff plan how urine and feces will be discarded in patient-care areas, clinics, and laboratories. A variety of bedpan flushing devices are available such as spray hoses, spray arms, or Vernacare units (Woodbridge, Ontario, Canada). Some of these options create splash hazards, clean poorly, or allow water to pool in hoses or nozzles. Waste disposal units such as Vernacare units are quite expensive. Soiled utility rooms should contain a clinical sink or a flushing-rim fixture and also a separate handwashing sink.[3]

FINISHES

General Considerations

During the design and development phase, infection control personnel should help the clinicians and architects choose the finishes-flooring, wall coverings, ceiling tiles, etc. Ideal finishes are those that are washable and easy to clean.[80] Porous or textured materials can be difficult to clean and thus may allow bacteria and fungi to grow. The finishes should be durable and able to withstand repeated cleaning. In addition, countertops, backsplashes, and floors should have as few joints as possible, so they are easy to clean.

Ceilings

Ceiling tiles should be appropriate for the areas in which they are being placed. Acoustical tiles may be used in hallways, waiting rooms, and standard patient rooms. Ceilings in semi-restricted areas, such as central sterile supply, radiology procedure rooms, minor surgical procedure rooms, and clean corridors in operating suites should not be perforated or have crevices where mold and bacteria could grow. The ceiling must be made of smooth, nonabsorptive material that can be washed and is capable of withstanding cleaning with chemicals. Perforated, serrated cut, or highly textured ceilings are not permitted. In restricted areas, such as ORs, all ceilings should be monolithic, washable, and capable of withstanding cleaning chemicals.[3] Cracks and perforations are not allowed. Ceilings in protective isolation rooms should be monolithic.

Floors

Floors should be easy to clean and should resist wear. Floors where food is prepared should be water-resistant

and floors that are walked on while wet should have a non-slip surface. The housekeeping department should use their cleaning procedures on samples of flooring to determine whether the materials can withstand cleaning and disinfection with germicidal cleaning solutions. Floors in ORs and delivery rooms used for C-sections should be monolithic and should not have joints. Floors in kitchens, soiled workrooms and other areas, which are frequently washed with water, should have tightly sealed joints.

Carpets decrease noise and have become popular in HCFs. There is no conclusive evidence that links carpet to illness but carpets can harbor microorganisms. Carpets should not be used in isolation rooms, protective environments, operating rooms, critical care units, kitchens, laboratories, autopsy rooms, or dialysis units. A good common sense rule is "do not use carpets in areas where liquids of any kind are likely to be spilled."

Walls

Walls should be washable and the finish should be smooth. Wall finishes in areas where blood or body fluids could splatter (eg, ORs and cardiac catheterization laboratories) should be fluid resistant (eg, vinyl) and easy to clean. Wall finishes around plumbing fixtures should be smooth and water resistant.[3] Wall bases and floors, especially around small pipes, should not have joints or should have joints that are sealed tightly.[3] In food preparation areas, walls should be free of spaces that harbor insects and rodents. In ORs, C-section rooms, and sterile processing rooms, walls should not have fissures, open joints, or crevices that permit dirt particles to enter the room.

Countertops

Countertops typically are composed of a nonporous solid material, such as Corian (duPont, Wilmington, Del), stainless steel, or laminate, with a protective sealant.

MINIMIZING THE RISK OF INFECTION DURING MAINTENANCE, CONSTRUCTION, AND RENOVATION

Air Handling Systems

Infection control personnel should collaborate with the facility's HVAC specialist to decide whether the HVAC system needs to be isolated during construction. During renovation or construction projects, selected air intakes (particularly those near excavation sites) and air ducts in the construction area need to be protected from dust by 1 of 3 methods: (1) shutting them down, (2) equipping them with additional filters, or (3) covering them with plastic. Engineering or maintenance personnel also should check air filters frequently and change them when necessary. Air-handling units in areas that care for immunocompromised patients should contain HEPA filters to decrease the amount of particulate matter and the number of microbes in the air.

For Class III or Class IV projects, the airflow should move from outside the construction sites into the site because air should flow from a clean area into a dirty area. Negative pressure or airflow into the construction site can be achieved by placing a HEPA-filtered negative airflow machine within the work zone. Ideally, the air from this machine would be exhausted directly to the outside. If this is not possible, the air can be exhausted into the air ducts and recirculated. A pressure monitor should be placed within the work zone to ensure that this area is maintained at negative pressure with respect to the adjacent areas. The contractor is responsible to monitor the airflow and to make sure the HEPA filters are clean and working properly.

A HEPA-filtered negative airflow machine may be required for other projects. For example, such machines would be necessary during work on the ceilings within patient care areas in Group 3 (ie, medium high risk) or Group 4 (highest risk) of the infection control construction matrix for Class I or Class II construction activities. Each contractor should own 1 or more of these machines and healthcare maintenance departments should have at least 1 machine that they can use during maintenance activities that generate dust.

The air quality must be maintained and monitored carefully in areas caring for immunocompromised patients, including patients receiving treatment for malignancies, patients with bone marrow or solid organ transplants, and premature neonates. We recommend that infection control personnel work with staff in the appropriate departments to develop policies that describe in detail what must be done when any modifications, renovations, demolition, or construction are done in their areas. Activities as seemingly minor as installing computer cables or conduits in the ceiling space could stir up *Aspergillus*-laden dust that would be hazardous for immunocompromised patients.

When working in areas housing immunocompromised patients, some precautions are needed in addition to those used on all patient-care areas (see section on Barriers). For example, existing air ducts and the space above the ceiling tiles must be cleaned with a HEPA-filtered vacuum before undertaking any project that involves opening these areas. The area inside the barrier must be cleaned and vacuumed (with a HEPA-filtered vacuum) before the barrier is removed and again after the barrier is removed. In addition to these precautions, portable HEPA filters could be placed in patients' rooms to ensure that the air is as clean as possible. Facilities that cannot implement appropriate precautions must move units to other areas of the hospital for the duration of the project.

Controlling Dust and Dirt

Construction and renovation projects create tremendous amounts of dust or debris that may carry microorganisms, such as *Aspergillus* spores.[57] Infection control personnel must collaborate with other staff to devise ways to prevent the dust and dirt from contaminating clean or sterile patient-care surfaces, supplies, and equipment.

Some general measures to limit dust and dirt and to minimize the risk of fungal infections in HCFs during maintenance, renovation, or construction include:
- Wet mop the area just outside the door to the construction site daily, or more often if necessary.
- Use a HEPA-filtered vacuum to clean adjacent carpeted areas daily, or more often if necessary.
- Shampoo carpets when the construction project is completed.
- Transport debris in containers with tight-fitting lids, or cover debris with a wet sheet.
- Remove debris as it is created; do not let it accumulate.
- Do not haul debris through patient-care areas, if possible.
- Remove debris through a window when construction occurs above the first floor, if possible.
- Remove debris after normal work hours, if possible, through an exit restricted to the construction crew.
- Designate an entrance, an elevator, and a hallway for use only by construction workers.
- If workers must traverse patient-care areas, they must remove dust from their bodies and clothes and then put on gowns, shoe covers, and head covers before walking through the unit. In particular areas of the hospital (eg, the operating suite), workers may need to wear protective clothing while working in the construction site.
- For small projects, the tool carts should be cleaned before entering the unit and left at the exit to the barrier. For larger projects, the carts and equipment should go into the area and stay behind the barrier until the project is done. Before removing carts and equipment from inside the barrier, the construction crew should clean the items and cover them with moist sheets. They should be moved off the unit by the designated route.

Barriers

Barriers are needed during maintenance, renovation, and construction projects to minimize the dispersion of dust. Commercially available portable drop-down cubicle barriers can be used for small, quick jobs, such as removing ceiling tiles to install computer cables. These units are equipped with either small HEPA-filtered negative airflow machines or connections for HEPA vacuums so that the space inside each cubicle is at negative pressure to the surrounding area. A closed door that is sealed with tape is an adequate barrier for enclosed short-term projects that make minimal dust. Plastic sheeting that is 3 to 8 mil thick or canvas barriers made specifically for dust control can be used for short-term projects that have minimal traffic and do not require fire rating. If plastic is used, contractors must inspect the integrity of the barrier several times during a work shift and they must repair holes, tears, or any defects in the plastic or canvass barrier immediately. A door can be created in the plastic barrier with a zipper or with a 2-foot overlap of the plastic. Anterooms, made of plastic, allow workers to don or remove protective attire or clean dust and debris off of their clothes and their carts before they leave the construction zone and enter a patient care area. Solid sheetrock barriers that are taped and finished are required for longer, more extensive projects. If the area is a high-risk area (eg, bone marrow transplant unit, operating suite), plastic barriers should be erected and the sheetrock barriers should be built behind the plastic barriers. Plastic barriers should be wiped down with a moist cloth before they are removed.

Facilities that are undergoing construction or renovation in particularly sensitive areas (eg, bone marrow transplant units if patients are on the unit) may want to document that the barriers are adequate. Particle counters that indicate the number of particles suspended in the air can be used for this purpose. The infection control personnel on the multidisciplinary team should determine during the ICRA whether particle counts are necessary. Particle counts should be obtained outdoors and compared with the indoor counts to ensure that the 90% filters are functioning properly. Thereafter, particle counts should be done in the areas adjacent to the work site before construction begins, during several days at the start of the project, and weekly until completion. Air cultures are not as useful for this task and should be reserved for special circumstances (eg, opening a bone marrow transplant unit) to document that the environment is not contaminated by fungi.

The work site should be kept as clean as possible to enhance the effectiveness of the barriers. HEPA-filtered vacuums should be used for cleaning the construction site and the workers' clothing before they leave the work site. If HEPA-filtered vacuums are not available, the site can be wet mopped but it should never be swept because sweeping disperses dust into the air. In addition, walk-off sticky mats should be placed just inside the entrance to the work site. A new mat should be used every day. Moist walk-off mats do not adequately remove dust from the wheels of carts as they exit a work site.

Traffic Patterns

To reduce the amount of dust and dirt in the hospital and the risk of exposure to infectious agents, patients, visitors, and staff may need to traverse the hospital by alternate routes. Infection control personnel should help identify the appropriate detours before construction begins. Staff should design these routes in a logical manner, so that they do not increase inadvertently the risk of nosocomial infections or of noninfectious hazards such as falls. They also should consider whether housekeeping personnel can maintain the new route, whether the new route interferes with the work done in the area, and whether the route meets minimum aesthetic requirements. If construction is necessary in or near operating suites, surgical personnel must be able to move from place to place without contaminating their surgical scrubs.

The routes by which inanimate items are transported throughout the hospital may need to be altered during construction. In general, all materials including food, linens, medical supplies and equipment, and janitorial supplies and equipment must be handled in a manner that minimizes the risk of contamination.[52] Before the construction project begins, infection control personnel should help the staff from the affected units plan the routes by which various supplies and equipment will be transported. Clean or sterile supplies and equipment must be transported to storage areas by a route that minimizes contamination from the construction site and prevents contact with soiled or contaminated trash and linen. To prevent unnecessary contamination with dirt and dust, used supplies and equipment should be moved in enclosed containers from the point of use to the point at which they will be processed.

Traffic patterns in critical areas, such as the operating suite, labor and delivery rooms, nurseries, laboratories, and pharmacies, may not be altered easily to meet these infection control requirements. In such cases, the construction crew may need to work during off hours and on weekends. If infection control requirements still cannot be met, some areas may need to relocated or closed temporarily.

Storage Areas

During construction, basic principles of infection control still apply. Thus, clinical areas must maintain appropriate storage areas, which may be difficult, because the allotted space may be small or may lack essential features. Before construction begins, infection control personnel should help the staff identify the locations in which they will store equipment and supplies. Temporary storage areas should allow staff to do the following:

➤ Easily monitor the supplies (eg, look at expiration dates)

➤ Store sterile supplies and equipment away from soiled items (ie, separate clean and dirty areas must be maintained)

➤ Store clean or sterile supplies at an appropriate distance from sinks to prevent the supplies from becoming wet

➤ Store contaminated wastes in a designated dirty area outside of direct patient-care areas

➤ Move items without placing them on the floor (ie, have adequate work space)

In addition, the temporary storage space should be clean, have adequate temperature and humidity control, and be free of rodents.

An outbreak of four surgical and burn wound infections that occurred when a large tertiary-care hospital renovated its central inventory control area illustrates the importance of storing supplies properly during construction.[22] The investigators identified several *Aspergillus* species on the outside packages of materials from the main floor of Inventory Control; on intravenous bags, the outsides of sterile paper wrappers, and storage bins in the pharmacy, which was adjacent to the area under construction; and from the outsides of packages containing burn dressings, elastic adhesive, Elastoplast (Beiersdorf AG, Hamburg, Germany), gloves, and disposable scissors, which were stored on the burn unit and in the intensive care unit. The investigators postulated that the supply boxes were contaminated during construction. The outside packages became contaminated when the boxes were opened, and the fungus was inoculated directly into the patients' wounds when the packages were torn open during dressing changes.[53]

One of the authors recently consulted with a hospital that was renovating several nursing stations during a time when the units were empty. The barriers were thin plastic that was not sealed and the areas being renovated were at positive pressure with respect to the surrounding areas. When the units closed, the staff left the supply carts in place and did not cover them. Consequently, the packages of clean and sterile supplies were covered with dust and grime. Supplies that could not be wiped with a disinfectant (eg, those that had paper wrappers) had to be discarded, costing the hospital thousands of dollars.

Final Check

After the project is completed, infection control personnel should inspect the area to make sure that all requirements have been met. Infection control personnel should verify the following steps have been done:

➤ Check the location of soap, alcohol-based hand hygiene products, and towel dispensers, the sharps container, and the wastebasket

➤ Check all areas to ensure that the appropriate flooring, ceiling tiles, and wall finishes have been installed

➤ Check all procedure rooms, kitchens, and utility rooms to ensure that they have the appropriate washable flooring and splash guards on sinks

➤ Inspect water faucets to ensure that they do not have aerators

➤ Check pressure and drainage in the water system

➤ Have personnel from maintenance or housekeeping run all faucets the day before patients occupy the unit to decrease the risk of infection from *Legionella* spp

➤ Evaluate the direction of air flow in negative-air-pressure rooms, and ensure that the air pressure monitors are placed and functioning properly

➤ Review the HVAC balance reports to ensure that system meets specification

In areas such as the bone marrow transplant unit or ORs, air sampling can be performed with an air sampling device such as the SAS compact air sampler (PBI International, Milan, Italy) to check for contaminated air. Alternatively, settle plates can be placed in various areas throughout the room for 30 min to 1 hour while ventilation is running and the room is vacant. The door should be closed and taped shut, so that persons do not enter the room while the settle plates are in place. If the ventilation system is running properly, the settle plates should be negative for pathogenic microbial growth.[44] A certified engineer can evaluate the effectiveness of laminar air flow.

THE COST OF INFECTION CONTROL MEASURES FOR MAINTENANCE, RENOVATION, AND CONSTRUCTION

There is no "rule of thumb" to determine the cost of the ICRA and the infection control measures. Douglas Erickson, a fellow of the American Society for Healthcare Engineering (ASHE), estimated that when the ICRA was first introduced, costs per contract increased by 25% but by last year this figure was down to 5%. He noted recently that some contractors were reporting that these measures actual reduced costs because they increased the pace of the project and prevented delays.[54]

The most accurate way to determine the cost of infection control measures is to add the cost of all the components (eg, the barriers, the HEPA-filtered negative-air machines, vacuums, walk-off mats, modifications to the

HVAC system, cleaning the work zone and surrounding areas, monitoring air pressure, and protective attire). Other costs to consider are special methods needed to minimize noise and vibration, and dust. For example, chipping by hand rather than with a rotohammer will take more time but will protect nearby patients from excessive noise and vibration. Generally, infection control precautions for large projects are best priced on a fixed set up cost (ie, the cost of barriers and ducting) plus the cost per day (eg, daily cost of renting negative air machines, maintaining barriers, cleaning work zones, and replacing walk-off mats). The longer the project takes the greater the cost.

Infection control precautions can make otherwise simple projects, such as carpet replacement and pulling wires more complicated and costly. For example, a project to replace 35,000 square feet of flooring at our hospital was bid at $147,000 without infection control measures and $180,000 once infection control precautions were included. The infection control measures added $33,000 to the cost of the project, which was about 1 extra dollar per square foot or an increase of 22% over the cost of conventional carpet replacement. However, 1 lawsuit resulting from *Aspergillus* spp infections would cost significantly more than this.

CONCLUSION

Construction and renovation projects pose special challenges for infection control personnel. In many hospitals, infection control personnel are the only clinical staff members who assist in all construction and renovation projects. Therefore, they may find themselves having to ensure that both infection control guidelines and general building codes are met. We would encourage infection control personnel to be involved in all phases of these projects to avert outbreaks and to ensure that newly constructed or renovated areas allow staff to follow good infection control practices. We would also encourage infection control personnel to maintain good relationships with the architects, contractors, facility maintenance personnel, and others involved in construction and renovation of HCFs so that together they can ensure that the area is safe and well designed

We think the role of infection control personnel in these projects will increase as the complexity and immunosuppression of hospitalized patients increase at a time when hospitals are required to decrease their budgets drastically and regulatory and accrediting agencies are increasing the number of infection control guidelines. Infection control aspects of construction and renovation projects require large amounts of time and hard work. We would argue that the time and energy invested before and during the project will save hours of time, huge sums of money, and the lives of patients and HCWs after the project is finished.

REFERENCES

1. Streifel AJ, Lauer JL, Vesley B, Juni B, Rhame FS. *Aspergillus fumigatus* and other thermotolerant fungi generated by hospital building demolition. *Am Soc Microbiol.* 1983;46:375-378.

2. Bartley, JM. APIC State-of-the-art report: the role of infection control during construction in health care facilities. *Am J Infect Control.* 2000;156-169.

3. American Institute of Architects, Guidelines for design and construction of hospital and health care facilities, 2001 edition, The American Institute of Architects, Washington, DC; 2001. American Institute of Architects (AIA) www.e-architects.com.

4. Mermel LA, Josephson S, Giorgio C, et al. Association of Legionnaires' disease with construction: contamination of potable water? *Infect Control Hosp Epidemiol.* 1995; 16:76-91.

5. Parry MF, Stampleman L, Hutchinson JH, et al. Waterborne *Legionella bozemanii* and nosocomial pneumonia in immunosuppressed patients. *Ann Intern Med.* 1985;103:205-210.

6. Thacker SB, Bennett JV, Tsai TF et al. An outbreak in 1965 of severe respiratory illness caused by Legionnaires' disease bacterium. *J Infect Dis.* 1978;138:512-519.

7. Haley CE, Cohen ML, Halter J et al. Nosocomial Legionnaire's disease: a continuing common-source epidemic at Wadsworth Medical Center. *Ann Intern Med.* 1979;90:583-586.

8. Kistemann T, Huneburg H, Exner M, Vacata V, Engelhart S. Role of increased environmental aspergillus exposure for patients with chronic obstructive pulmonary disease (COPD) treated with corticosteroids in an intensive care unit. *International Journal of Hygiene and Environmental Health.* 2002;204:347-351.

9. Oren I, Haddad N, Finkelstein R, Rowe JM. Invasive pulmonary aspergillosis in neutropenic patients during hospital construction: before and after chemoprophylaxis and institutions of HEPA filters. *Am J Hematology.* 2001;66:257-262.

10. Bryce EA, Walker M, Scharf S, Lim AT, Walsh A, Sharp N, et al. An outbreak of cutaneous aspergillosis in a tertiary-care hospital. *Infect Control Hosp Epidemiol.* 1996;17: 170-172.

11. Lueg EA, Ballagh RH, Forte V. Analysis of the recent cluster of invasive fungal sinusitis at the Toronto Hospital for Sick Children. *J Otolaryngol.* 1996;25:366-370.

12. Loo VG, Bertrand C, Dixon C, et al. Control of construction-associated nosocomial aspergillosis in an antiquated hematology unit. *Infect Control Hosp Epidemiol.* 1996; 17:360-364.

13. Sessa A, Meroni M, Battini G, et al. Nosocomial outbreak of *Aspergillus fumigatus* infection among patients in a renal unit? *Nephrol Dial Transplant*. 1996;11:1322-1324.

14. Alvarez M, Lopez Ponga B, Raon C, Garcia Gala J, Porto MC, Gonzales M, et al. Nosocomial outbreak caused by *Scedosporium prolificans* (*inflatum*): four fatal cases of leukemic patients. *J Clin Microbiol*. 1995;33:3290-3295.

15. Berg R. Nosocomial aspergillosis during hospital remodel. In: Soule BM, Larson EL, Preston GA, eds. *Infections and Nursing Practice: Prevention and Control*. St. Louis: Mosby, 1995:271-274.

16. American Health Consultants. Aspergillosis: a deadly dust may be in the wind during renovations. *Hosp Infect Control*. 1995;22:125-126.

17. American Health Consultants. Construction breaches tied to bone marrow infections. *Hosp Infect Control*. 1995; 22:130-131.

18. Iwen PC, Davis JC, Reed EC, et al. Airborne fungal spore monitoring in a protective environment during construction and correlation with an outbreak of invasive aspergillosis. *Infect Control Hosp Epidemiol*. 1994;15: 303-306.

19. Gerson SL, Parker P, Jacobs MR et al. Aspergillosis due to carpet contamination. *Infect Control Hosp Epidemiol*. 1994;15:221-223.

20. Flynn PM, Williams BG, Hethrington SV, Williams BF, Giannini MA, Pearson TA. *Aspergillus terreus* during hospital renovation [letter]. *Infect Control Hosp Epidemiol*. 1993;14:363-365.

21. Dewhurst AG, Cooper MJ, Khan SM, et al. Invasive aspergillosis in immunosuppressed patients: potential hazard of hospital building work. *BMJ*. 1990;301:802-804.

22. Jackson L, Klotz SA, Normand RE. A pseudoepidemic of Sporothrix cyanescens pneumonia occurring during renovation of a bronchoscopy suite. *J Med Vet Mycol*. 1990;28:455-459.

23. Hospital Infection Control. APIC coverage: dust from construction site carries pathogen into unit. *Hosp Infect Control*. 1990;17:73.

24. Humphreys H, Johnson EM, Warnock DW, Willats SM, Winter RJ, Speller DC. An outbreak of aspergillosis in a general intensive therapy unit. *J Hosp Infect*. 1991;18:167-168.

25. Barnes RA, Rogers TR. Control of an outbreak of nosocomial aspergillosis by laminar air-flow isolation. *J Hosp Infect*. 1989;14:89-94.

26. Weems JJ, David BJ, Tablan OC, et al. Construction activity: An independent risk factor for invasive aspergillosis and zygomycosis in patients with hematologic malignancy. *Infect Control*. 1987;8:71-75.

27. Perraud M, Piens MA, Nicoloyannis N, Girard P, Sepetjan M, Garin JP. Invasive nosocomial pulmonary aspergillosis: risk factors and hospital building works. *Epidemiol Infect*. 1987;99:407-412.

28. Opal SM, Asp AA, Cannady PB Jr, Morse PL, Burton LJ, Hammer PG II. Efficacy of infection control measures during a nosocomial outbreak of disseminated aspergillosis associated with hospital construction. *J Infect Dis*. 1986;153:634-637.

29. Krasinski K, Holzman RS, Hanna B, Greco MA, Graff M, Bhogal M. Nosocomial fungal infection during hospital renovation. *Infect Control Hosp Epidemiol*. 1985;6:278-282.

30. Grossman ME, Fithian EC, Behrens C, et al. Primary cutaneous aspergillosis in six leukemic children. *J Am Acad Dermatol*. 1985;12(2, part 1):313-318.

31. Sarubbi FA, Kopf HB, Wilson MB et al. Increased recovery of Aspergillus flavus from respiratory specimens during hospital construction. *Am Rev Respir Dis*. 1982;125:31-38.

32. Lentino JR, Rosenkranz MA, Michaels JA, Kurup VP, Rose HD, Rytel MW. Nosocomial aspergillosis: a retrospective review of air-borne disease secondary to road construction and contaminated air conditioners. *Am J Epidemiol*. 1982;116:430-7.

33. Arnow PM, Sadigh M, Costas C, et al. Endemic and epidemic aspergillosis associated with in-hospital replication of aspergillus organisms. *J Infect Dis*. 1991;164:998-1002.

34. Aisner J, Schimpff S, Bennett J, et al. Aspergillus infections in cancer patients. *JAMA*. 1976;235:411-412.

35. Centers for Disease Control and Prevention. Guidelines for preventing opportunistic infections among hematopoietic stem cell transplant recipients. *MMWR*. 2000;49(RR-10):1-125.

36. Miscellaneous gram-negative Bacilli. In: Murray PR, Rosenthal KS, Kobayashi GS, Pfaller MA. *Medical Microbiology*. 4th ed. St. Louis: Mosby; 2002:325-333.

37. American Society of Heating, Refrigerating and Air-Conditioning Engineers, Inc. Minimizing the Risk of Legionellosis Associated with Building Water Systems, ASHRE Guideline 12-2000.

38. Opportunistic mycoses. In: Murray PR, Rosenthal KS, Kobayashi GS, Pfaller MA. *Medical Microbiology*. 4th ed. St. Louis: Mosby; 2002:664-672.

39. Fox BC, Chamberlin L, Kulich P, et al. Heavy contamination of operating room air by penicillium species: Identification of the source and attempts at decontamination. *Am J Infect Control*. 1990;18:300-306.

40. D'Andrea C, New York City Department of Health and Mental Hygiene Bureau of Environmental and Occupational Disease and Epidemiology. *Guidelines on Assessment and Remediation of Fungi in Indoor Environments*. 2000:1-17.

41. Centers for Disease Control and Prevention. Healthcare Infection Control Practices Advisory Committee (HIC-PAC). Guidelines for environmental infection control in healthcare facilities. *MMWR*. 2003;52(RR-10):1-44.

42. Joint Commission on Accreditation of Healthcare Organizations. Comprehensive Accreditation Manual for Hospitals. The Official Handbook. Chicago, IL:JCAHO; 2003.

43. Streifel A. Health-Care IAQ Guidance for Infection Control. *HPAC Engineering*. 2000:28-36.

44. Soule BM, ed. The APIC Curriculum for Infection Control Practice, Volume II. Dubuque, Iowa: Kendall/Hunt Publishing Co;1983.

45. Neill HM. Isolation-room ventilation critical to control disease. *Health Facil Manage*. 1992;5:30-38.

46. Langley JM, Hanakowski M, Bortolussi R. Demand for isolation beds in a pediatric hospital. *Am J Infect Control*. 1994;22:207-211.

47. Centers for Disease Control and Prevention. Guidelines for preventing the transmission of *Mycobacterium tuberculosis* in health care facilities, 1994. *MMWR*. 1994;43:29.

48. Centers for Disease Control and Prevention. Guideline for hand hygiene in health-care settings. *MMWR*. 2002;51(No. RR-16):1-45.

49. US Department of Health and Human Services, National Institute for National Safety and Health (NIOSH). Selecting, evaluating and using sharps disposal containers. 1998;(No. 97-111):1-21, Cincinnati, Ohio.

50. Madden C. Environmental considerations in critical care interiors. *Crit Care Nurse Q*. 1991;14:43-49.

51. Opal SM, Asp AA, Cannady PB Jr, Morse PL, Burton LJ, Hammer PG II. Efficacy of infection control measures during a nosocomial outbreak of disseminated aspergillosis associated with hospital construction. *J Infect Dis*. 1986;153:634-637.

52. Fitch H. Hospital and industry can benefit by sharing contamination control knowledge. *Clean Rooms*. 1993;7:8-9.

53. Bryce EA, Walker M, Scharf S, et al. An outbreak of cutaneous aspergillosis in a tertiary-care hospital. *Infect Control Hosp Epidemiol*. 1996;17:170-172.

54. Downs P. Infection control expert hosted by local architecture, engineering firms. CNR News 2003. STL Construct NET. www.stlconstruction.com.

ABBREVIATIONS

AAMI: Association for the Advancement of Medical Instrumentation
ACH: air changes per hour
AFB: acid-fast bacilli
AHRQ: Agency for Healthcare Research and Quality
AII: airborne infection isolation
APIC: Association of Professionals in Infection Control
ASA: American Society of Anesthesiologists
ASM: American Society for Microbiology

BAL: bronchoalveolar lavage
BSE: bovine spongiform encephalopathy
BSI: bloodstream infection

CABG: coronary artery bypass graft
CAP: community-acquired pneumonia
CAPD: continuous ambulatory peritoneal dialysis
CDC: Centers for Disease Control and Prevention
CFU: colony-forming unit
CHF: congestive heart failure
CHICA-Canada: Community and Hospital Infection Control Association—Canada
CI: confidence interval
CJD: Creutzfeldt-Jakob disease
CMV: cytomegalovirus
COPD: chronic obstructive pulmonary disease
CPIS: clinical pulmonary infection score
CPU: central processing unit
CSHO: compliance safety and health officers
CVC: central venous catheter
CXR: chest radiograph

DICON: Duke Infection Control Outreach Network
DUE: drug utilization evaluation

ED: emergency department
EMS: emergency medical service
ESBL: extended-spectrum beta-lactamase

ETA: endotracheal aspirates
ETO: ethylene oxide

FEMA: Federal Emergency Management Agency
FMEA: failure modes and effects analysis

GI: gastrointestinal
GISA: glycopeptide-intermediate *Staphylococcus aureus*
GNB: gram-negative bacilli

HAV: hepatitis A virus
HBIG: hepatitis B immune globulin
HBeAg: hepatitis B "e" antigen
HBsAg: hepatitis B surface antigen
HBV: hepatitis B virus
HCF: healthcare facility
HCV: hepatitis C virus
HCW: healthcare worker
HDV: hepatitis D virus
HICPAC: Healthcare Infection Control Practices Advisory Committee
HIS: Hospital Infection Society
HIV: human immunodeficiency virus
HMOs: health maintenance organizations
HSV: Herpes simplex virus
HVAC: heating, ventilating, and air conditioning systems

ICP: infection control professional/practitioner
ICU: intensive care unit
ID: infectious disease
IDSA: Infectious Diseases Society of America
IM: intramuscularly
IOM: Institute of Medicine
ISG: immune serum globulin
IT: information technology
IV-CRIs: intravascular catheter-related infections
IVIG: intravenous immunoglobulin

JCAHO: Joint Commission on Accreditation of Healthcare Organizations

LOS: length of stay
LTBI: latent tuberculosis infection
LTCF: long-term care facility

MDR: multidrug-resistant
MDRE: multidrug-resistant Enterobacteriaceae
MDRO: multidrug-resistant organism
MICU: medical intensive care unit
MLEE: multilocus enzyme electrophoresis
MMR: measles, mumps, rubella
MMWR: *Morbidity and Mortality Weekly Report*
MPH: master in public health
MRSA: methicillin-resistant *Staphylococcus aureus*
MSCE: master of science in clinical epidemiology
MSSA: methicillin-susceptible *aureus*
MV: mechanical ventilation

NCCLS: National Committee for Clinical Laboratory Standards
NDMS: National Disaster Management System
NFID: National Foundation for Infectious Diseases
NIOSH: National Institute for Occupational Safety and Health
NIV: noninvasive ventilation
NNIS: National Nosocomial Infection Surveillance System
NP: nosocomial pneumonia
NRSA: National Institutes of Health's National Research Service Award

OPIM: other potentially infectious materials
OS: operating system
OSHA: Occupational Safety and Health Administration
OSHRC: Occupational Safety and Health Review Commission

PAPR: positive air pressure respirator
PCR: polymerase chain reaction
PCR-RFLP: polymerase chain reaction-restriction fragment length polymorphism
PEP: postexposure prophylaxis
PFGE: pulsed-field gel electrophoresis
PPD: purified protein derivative
PPE: personal protective equipment
PSB: protected specimen brush

RAM: Random Access Memory
RAPD: randomly amplified polymorphic DNA assay
RCA: root cause analysis
RCT: randomized controlled trial
REA: restriction endonuclease analysis
REP-PCR: polymerase chain reaction of repetitive chromosomal elements
RFLP: restriction fragment length polymorphism
R-PCR: realtime PCR
RSV: respiratory syncytial virus

SARS: severe acute respiratory syndrome
SDD: selective digestive decontamination
SENIC: Study on the Efficacy of Nosocomial Infection Control
SHEA: Society for Healthcare Epidemiology of America
SICU: surgical intensive care unit
SOJA: System of Objectified Judgment Analysis
SSI: surgical site infection

TST: tuberculin skin test

USB: Universal Serial Bus
UTI: urinary tract infection
UVGI: ultraviolet germicidal irradiation

VAP: ventilator-associated pneumonia
VISA: vancomycin-intermediate *Staphylococcus aureus*
VRE: vancomycin-resistant enterococci
VRSA: vancomycin-resistant *Staphylococcus aureus*
VSE: vancomycin-susceptible enterococci
VZIG: varicella-zoster immune globulin
VZV: varicella-zoster virus

WHO: World Health Organization

INDEX

AAMI (Association for the Advancement of Medical Instrumentation), 361
ACH (air changes per hour), 266, 361
Acinetobacter, 70, 72
acute-care settings, 184
adenovirus, 251
advanced model, infection control management, 19
adverse events, detecting and investigating, 299-300
AFB (acid-fast bacilli), 263, 268, 361
AHRQ (Agency for Healthcare Research and Quality), 361
AII (airborne infection isolation), 361
air handling systems, 351, 354-355
airborne infection isolation rooms, 268
airborne precautions, 145-147
ambulatory settings, 283-284
American Academy for Medical Microbiology, 155
American Board of Pathology, 155
American Institute of Architecture, *Guidelines for Design and Construction of Hospital and Healthcare Facilities*, 9
American National Standards Institute, 267
American Thoracic Society, 70
anthrax, 149, 229, 232
anti-rubella IgM, 252
antibacterial soap, 72-73
antibiotic resistance genotyping, 168
antibiotic-resistant gram-negative infections
antibiotic management, 195-196
   control measures, 192-195
   definition, 189
   mechanisms of resistance, 190-192
   microbiology and epidemiology, 189-190
   nonfermentative, 190
antibiotic use, 63
antibiotics, excessive use, 199
antimicrobial resistance, 169, 286-287
antimicrobial-resistant pathogens, 179, 280

antimicrobial stewardship
   antimicrobial cycling, 204
   antimicrobial optimization, 205
   antimicrobial order forms, 204
   computerized decision support, 204
   data collection, 200
   funding, 206
   goals, 199
   interventions, 200-203
   intravenous-to-oral conversion, 205
   management programs, 205-206
   organization and personnel, 199-200
   outcomes, 206
   restricting agents, 203-204
   success factors, 206-207
   surgical prophylaxis, 204
antimicrobial susceptibility testing, 166
APIC (Association of Professionals in Infection Control), 361
   AJIC (*The American Journal of Infection Control*), 11
   annual scientific meetings, 10
   APIC Text of Infection Control and Epidemiology, 9, 11
   certification in infection control, 155
   course in infection control and epidemiology, 9-10
   Infection Control Reference Service: The Experts' Guide to the Guidelines, 9, 11
   workshops, 9
arbitrarily primed PCR, 167-168
ASA (American Society of Anesthesiologists), 51, 361
ASM (American Society for Microbiology), 361
Aspergillus, 51, 339
Australian Group List of Biological Agents for Export Control, 223
automated claims data, 63

bacteremia, 100
bacterial diseases, 121-123, 157
BAL (bronchoalveolar lavage), 71, 361